THE ENCYCLOPEDIA OF

PARKINSON'S DISEASE

Anthony D. Mosley, M.D., M.S.
Medical Director
Booth Gardner Parkinson's Care Center
and Deborah S. Romaine

An Amaranth Book

☑®
Facts On File, Inc.

The Encyclopedia of Parkinson's Disease

Copyright © 2004 by Amaranth

All rights reserved. No part of this book may be reproduced or utilized in any form or by any means, electronic or mechanical, including photocopying, recording, or by any information storage or retrieval systems, without permission in writing from the publisher. For information contact:

Facts On File, Inc.
132 West 31st Street
New York NY 10001

Library of Congress Cataloging-in-Publication Data

Romaine, Deborah S., 1956
The encyclopedia of Parkinson's disease / Deborah S. Romaine ; Anthony D. Mosley.
p. cm.
"An Amaranth Book."
Includes bibliographical references and index.
ISBN 0-8160-5032-5 (alk. paper)
1. Parkinson's disease—Encyclopedias. I. Title.
RC382.R656 2004
616.8′33′003   dc21—2003052491

Facts On File books are available at special discounts when purchased in bulk quantities for businesses, associations, institutions, or sales promotions. Please call our Special Sales Department in New York at (212) 967-8800 or (800) 322-8755.

You can find Facts On File on the World Wide Web at http://www.factsonfile.com

Text and cover design by Cathy Rincon

Printed in the United States of America

VB FOF 10 9 8 7 6 5 4 3 2 1

This book is printed on acid-free paper.

For Gloria Shirley Chearneyi, with love;
may her journey through Parkinson's bring healing and hope.

CONTENTS

FOREWORD

Today is a very exciting time for clinicians in the field of Parkinson's disease. There has been a recent explosion of information about the disease from fields as diverse as genetics, epidemiology, and toxicology. There are about 1.2 million people with Parkinson's disease in the United States and Canada, roughly 3,500 people per million, with approximately 480 per million people newly diagnosed each year.

After decades of having only levodopa and anticholinergic agents available, a plethora of pharmacologic agents and the emergence of new surgical techniques have revolutionized treatment of the disease. In just the decade since I began my medical education surgery options have exploded with the development of deep brain stimulation therapy and investigations into dopaminergic cell replacement; dopamine agonist therapy has been revolutionized with the introduction of three new agonists (pergolide, pramipexole, and ropinerole) that have made the side-effect-prone bromocriptine obsolete in the treatment of Parkinson's disease; and researchers have elucidated much more information about the etiology and epidemiology of Parkinson's disease than was known before.

Some may ask, in this age of the World Wide Web and the rapid changes in the field, why one would undertake the task of publishing an encyclopedia on Parkinson's disease with so much factual and technical information. First, most of the people with Parkinson's disease are of a generation for whom the computer remains a foreboding and unfamiliar object; a book is more familiar and comfortable to such people. Also, the information available on the Web is diverse, with much of it of questionable validity as it has been posted by commercial interests seeking to make a sale, or individuals who may have their own motives other than providing balanced and timely information. I daily see patients who hunger for a comprehensive source of up-to-date information that is written for a lay audience and vetted by a movement-disorders physician as to clinical and scientific accuracy. I feel that this encyclopedia more than fulfills both of the above needs. It is among the most comprehensive treatises on Parkinson's disease for a lay audience that is currently available, and its encyclopedic format makes it perfect for use as a reference for those specific questions that patients and their family members often have. Entries are alphabetical, with relevant topics cross-referenced. My coauthor, Deb Romaine, and I have done our best to make this book indispensable for the investigation of questions related to Parkinson's disease by students from advanced elementary school science buffs to social work, nursing, and premedical students.

—Anthony D. Mosley, M.D., M.S.

ACKNOWLEDGMENTS

I wish to thank Deb Romaine, without whom this work would not have been conceivable. I also wish to thank my colleagues at the Evergreen Booth Gardner Parkinson's Care Center, my mentors during my neurology residency at UCLA, and especially Dr. Bill Marks and Dr. Phil Starr who honed my fledgling interest in movement disorders into expertise during my fellowship at UCSF. I also thank my wife and two daughters for enduring my absence from their lives during nights and weekends working on this book. Most of all, I thank my patients, from whom I continue to learn more and more about Parkinson's disease, and from whose insightful questions this work springs forth.

—Anthony D. Mosley, M.D., M.S.
Medical Director
Booth Gardner Parkinson's Care Center
Kirkland, Washington

AADC inhibitor medications   Drugs that block the action of AROMATIC AMINO ACID DECARBOXYLASE (AADC). This prevents the conversion of LEVODOPA to DOPAMINE in the bloodstream, thus avoiding side effects (for example nausea and lowering of standing blood pressure) and extending the length of time levodopa stays in the blood. This increases the amount of it that can cross the BLOOD-BRAIN BARRIER into the brain to be converted to dopamine. AADC inhibitors currently prescribed are CARBIDOPA (in the U.S.) and BENSERAZIDE (available in several other countries). Typically these are taken in combination with levodopa in products such as SINEMET (levodopa and carbidopa) and Madopar (levodopa and benserazide). Patients usually require roughly 75 mg–100 mg of carbidopa per day to avoid peripheral conversion of levodopa and the associated side effects, but some require more. Carbidopa is available by itself as Lodosyn.

See also ANTI-PARKINSON'S MEDICATIONS.

ablation   A surgical method that uses thermocoagulation (heat generated by electricity) or other means to destroy tissue. As a treatment for Parkinson's disease, ablation typically targets cells in the GLOBUS PALLIDUS that become overly active when DOPAMINE production declines. Destroying these cells results in a corresponding decrease in the abnormal movements that characterize Parkinson's disease. Modern technology allows surgeons to place the lesions with great precision and few complications. Because the depletion of dopamine-producing cells in the SUBSTANTIA NIGRA continues as Parkinson's disease progresses, ablation provides only temporary relief from symptoms.

In the usual open procedure, the patient remains awake, although sedated, during ablation to treat Parkinson's disease. The surgeon uses a local anesthetic to numb pain-sensing nerves in the skin of the scalp and the dura (the tissue that surrounds the brain); the brain itself contains no pain-sensing nerves, so it is not necessary to anesthetize brain tissue. The surgeon then guides a fine probe, or electrode, into the region believed to be the source of tremors and other movement abnormalities. The probe delivers electronic signals that the surgeon can listen to and display on a screen (oscilloscope) to help guide the probe's proper placement. Cells within the brain emit different and identifiable sound waves. When the probe is in the correct location, the surgeon releases small bursts of electricity or heat (or in some cases a destructive chemical like ethanol) that burn the area. The surgeon determines how much destruction is necessary by observing the changes in tremor activity. When the resulting scar heals, it permanently blocks the cells in the area and prevents them from sending signals to the muscles.

The primary risks associated with ablation are those that are possible risks with any surgery, such as reaction to the local anesthetic, bleeding, and infection. As well, there is the risk of damage to other brain tissue as the probe is inserted, which can cause problems with speech as well as localized paralysis. Often these complications lessen or go away when the damaged areas heal, although sometimes they are permanent. Because the size of the scar after healing determines the procedure's ultimate effectiveness, the precise outcome cannot be known for seven to 10 days or more after the surgery. Swelling at the site of the ablation often causes a more pronounced response during the healing phase. As Parkinson's disease progresses and dopamine depletion increases, tremors and other motor symptoms ultimately worsen.

An alternative to the "open" procedure is use of focused radiation (such as a gamma knife) in a "closed" procedure to cause a lesion. Though these procedures avoid any cutting of the scalp, skull, or dura, their targeting is completely based on imaging and lacks the precision of confirming the location by listening to the pattern of brain activity with a probe as is done in traditional "open" procedures. It also takes months before the exact extent of focused radiation induced lesions can be determined because irradiated neurons can take weeks to months to die.

Surgeons began using ablation to treat Parkinson's disease and other movement disorders in the 1940s, targeting the THALAMUS and other structures within the brain believed to be involved in the processes of movement, as well as the globus pallidus. However, technological limitations of the time made any surgery involving the brain risky and unpredictable. Some patients recovered from ablation to enjoy relatively symptom-free lives for a decade or longer, while others developed complications such as infection and unintended movement disturbances. When the medication LEVODOPA was introduced to the market in 1960, it replaced ablation as the treatment of choice for Parkinson's disease.

Recent refinements in medical technology allow surgeons to use DEEP BRAIN STIMULATION, which produces reversible and modifiable changes, instead of ablation. Ablation and other surgical procedures are usually options reserved for use to prolong best motor function in people who are not demented and can still walk, at least in their best medicated state, but in whom best attempts at medical therapy with ANTI-PARKINSON'S MEDICATIONS either lead to intolerable side effects or fail to resolve function-limiting motor fluctuations—fluctuating between "off" periods when medication is no longer effective and DYSKINESIAS. Today, ablative techniques are typically reserved for people who are poor candidates for open procedures due to underlying health conditions (for whom radiosurgical ablation is the only option), people who live in areas where they do not have access to specialists trained in the programming and management of deep brain stimulators, or possibly, people who are unlikely to comply with programming follow-up.

See also BRAIN TISSUE TRANSPLANT; DEEP BRAIN STIMULATION; PALLIDOTOMY; THALAMOTOMY.

accelerated aging   The theory that, for reasons unknown, certain parts of the brain deteriorate more quickly than others, resulting in diseases such as Parkinson's. With normal aging, the number of dopamine-producing cells in the SUBSTANTIA NIGRA declines at a slow rate. In a person with Parkinson's disease, this decline takes place rapidly and far ahead of the rate of decline of other brain cells. Researchers are exploring the connection between FREE RADICALS and ANTIOXIDANTS and accelerated aging. Some researchers believe that environmental factors, such as dietary habits and exposure to toxins, trigger accelerated aging. Other researchers believe hereditary factors are to blame.

See also AGING; APOPTOSIS; CHROMOSOMES LINKED TO PARKINSON'S DISEASE; ENVIRONMENTAL TRIGGERS; GENETIC PREDISPOSITION; PARKIN GENE.

aceruloplasminemia   A rare inherited (AUTOSOMAL RECESSIVE) disorder of iron metabolism, discovered in 1995, that causes Parkinson-like symptoms. A mutation of the ceruloplasmin gene on chromosome 3 prevents cells from making a protein called ceruloplasmin, which removes iron from cells. This defect allows iron to accumulate in the cells of the BASAL GANGLIA. The accumulated iron blocks the functions of these cells, causing damage similar to, and the gait disturbances and tremors characteristic of, Parkinson's disease. Aceruloplasminemia also results in accumulation of iron deposits in the pancreas (causing insulin-dependent diabetes), liver, and retina (causing vision problems and blindness). Although aceruloplasminemia is present from birth, it does not typically produce symptoms until early middle age (40 to 50 years). Treatment involves both trying to halt the iron accumulation with drugs called chelating agents, as well as treatment of motor symptoms with the same agents used for IDIOPATHIC Parkinson's disease.

The discovery of aceruloplasminemia marked the first time researchers could link the symptoms of Parkinson's disease to a genetic mutation and generated much excitement in the scientific community. Although this particular mutation is very rare and unlikely itself to be a cause of most cases of Parkinson's disease, it raises hope that further research will reveal other genetic connections and lead to new treatment approaches.

See also ALPHA-SYNUCLEIN GENE; CHELATION; GENE MAPPING; GENETIC PREDISPOSITION; PARKIN GENE.

acetylcholine   A MONOAMINE NEUROTRANSMITTER that plays a key role in the communication between nerve cells and muscle cells, between neurons in the brain, and in the autonomic NERVOUS SYSTEM. When the brain sends out a signal, for example, to make a voluntary muscle movement, the message travels along a network of nerves until it reaches the nerves that are in contact with the muscle group. When the neurons at the end of the line, the terminal neurons, receive the signal it triggers the release of acetylcholine into the synapse (the space between the nerve terminal and the muscle cells). The acetylcholine then serves as a chemical messenger, traveling across the synapse to activate receptors on the muscle cells, causing them to contract.

DOPAMINE, NOREPINEPHRINE, and serotonin are other monoamine neurotransmitters in the brain. In health, these neurotransmitters exist in balance. When disease causes one of them to exist either in excess or deficit, this balance shifts and alters the brain's function. Dopamine becomes increasingly deficient in Parkinson's disease, allowing excess levels of acetylcholine to accumulate. This, researchers believe, is what accounts for the TREMORS and DYSKINESIAS that are characteristic of Parkinson's disease..Medications called anticholinergics block the action of cholinergic neurons, thereby reducing the amount of acetylcholine they release. For a time, this reduction relieves many of the motor symptoms. As Parkinson's disease progresses, however, the imbalance increases and the symptoms return.

Acetylcholine plays a significant role in the processes of COGNITIVE FUNCTION, as well, and is deficient in DEMENTIAS such as Alzheimer's disease. Researchers are exploring whether anticholinergic medications used to treat the motor symptoms of Parkinson's disease might contribute to cognitive function losses and dementia that develop in some, but not all, people with Parkinson's disease. GLUTAMATE ANTAGONIST medications are sometimes successful in offsetting this effect. There does not seem to be a direct correlation between acetylcholine levels and Parkinson's disease.

The relative paucity of norepinephrine and dopamine, combined with the relative overabundance of cholinergic activity, also may account for the autonomic nervous system dysfunction commonly seen with Parkinson's disease. The sympathetic nervous system, which constricts vascular smooth muscle to raise blood pressure, depends on norepinephrine as its neurotransmitter, while the antagonist parasympathetic nervous system, which utilizes acetylcholine, relaxes blood vessels, lowering blood pressure. Hence the relative adrenergic deficit and cholinergic excess can lead to lowering of blood pressure, particularly with postural changes like standing.

acetylcholinesterase   An enzyme (substance that facilitates chemical reactions) CHOLINERGIC NEURONS produce that breaks down ACETYLCHOLINE into its two chemical components, choline and acetate. This process ends the acetylcholine cycle of activity. The faster acetylcholinesterase acts, the shorter the period of acetylcholine activity. When the activity period is too short, acetylcholine cannot function properly as a neurotransmitter and signals between neurons are "dropped." One theory as to the cause of ALZHEIMER'S DISEASE is that a dysfunction causes an accelerated release of acetylcholinesterase. The connection between acetylcholine and acetylcholinesterase and other dementias such as those that sometimes occur with Parkinson's disease is less clear and remains a matter of interest for researchers.

See also ANTI-PARKINSON'S MEDICATIONS.

acetylcholinesterase inhibitor   A medication that prevents the enzyme acetylcholinesterase from metabolizing acetylcholine. This extends the length of time acetylcholine is active in the brain. Acetyl-cholinesterase inhibitors are prescribed primarily to slow the decline in cognitive function that occurs with ALZHEIMER'S DISEASE. These medications seem to have a similar action in many people with Parkinson's disease. But as is typical with treatment approaches for Parkinson's disease, individual response varies widely. Not all people with Parkinson's-related dementia experience improvement with acetylcholinesterase inhibitors, and there seems to be no pattern to help identify who will and who will not. Although one medication in this class is not effective, another may, so use of these drugs is usually worthwhile to try to improve cognitive function if deterioration occurs. Acetyl-cholinesterase inhibitor medications available in the United States include DONEPEZIL (Aricept), GALANTAMINE (Reminyl), RIVASTIGMINE (Exelon), and TACRINE (Cognex).

See also ANTICHOLINERGIC MEDICATIONS; ANTI-PARKINSON'S MEDICATIONS; GLUTAMATE ANTAGONISTS.

activities of daily living (ADLs) The common functions of everyday life and tasks of daily routine. Clinicians use ADLs as a key measure of independence, treatment effectiveness (particularly as it relates to the fluctuating phenomenon), and, conversely, decline and care needs. Activities of daily living typically include such functions as bathing, toileting, dressing, cooking, eating, cleaning house, and performing other chores. ADLs, particularly those that require coordination and balance, become more difficult and eventually very limited as Parkinson's disease progresses. TREMORS and DYSKINESIAS interfere with the ability to manage tasks that require fine motor skills. Sometimes cognitive impairment becomes a factor as well. There are numerous scales that measure ADLs. The two most commonly used are the Unified Parkinson's Disease Rating Scale (UPDRS) and the Schwab and England Scale.

Unified Parkinson's Disease Rating Scale (UPDRS)

The Unified Parkinson's Disease Rating Scale (UPDRS) was developed to provide a consistent and objective measurement tool for assessing the progress of Parkinson's disease symptoms and the effectiveness of treatment approaches. It consists of a series of questions divided into six sections. Section II assesses ADLs and measures self-reported assessment, on a 0 through 4 point scale, of

- Speech
- Salivation
- Swallowing
- Handwriting
- Cutting of food/handling of utensils
- Dressing, hygiene
- Turning in bed/adjusting of bedclothes
- Falling unrelated to freezing
- Freezing when walking
- Walking
- Tremor
- Sensory complaints related to Parkinson's

The UPDRS integrates ADL scores with clinician assessment of motor function and other scales of measurement. Because of its comprehensiveness, UPDRS is a common tool for measuring and comparing the effectiveness of treatments and the results of clinical studies. Each of its six sections contains subsections with multiple questions or measures. The rating scale is the same as that used in the Common ADL Scale for Parkinson's Disease, 0 to 4, on which a smaller number indicates greater independence.

Schwab and England Scale of Capacity for Daily Living

The Schwab and England Scale of Capacity for Daily Living assesses functional capacity by percentage. Developed by R. S. Schwab and A. C. England Jr., this scale uses a percentage system to assign levels of independence and dependence, in which 100 percent represents complete independence and 0 percent complete dependence (bedridden). A presentation of the Schwab and England Scale would be similar to the following:

Level of Independence	ADL Capacity
100%	Able to do all chores without difficulty or impairment
90%	Able to do all chores but with some slowness (up to twice as long) or difficulty. Beginning to be aware of difficulty
80%	Able to do most chores but with some slowness (takes twice as long) and conscious of difficulty
70%	Difficulty and slowness doing chores, which take up to three or four times as long
60%	Can do most but not all chores, but with effort and very slowly; makes some mistakes
50%	Can do some chores but needs help with most; has difficulty with all and makes many mistakes
40%	Can help with a few chores but cannot do very many alone
30%	Can sometimes begin a few chores alone but cannot finish; needs much help
20%	Cannot do any chores alone (invalid)
10%	Helpless; total dependence
0%	Vegetative; bedridden; loss of swallowing, bladder or bowel functions

Source: Gillingham FJ, Donaldson MC, editors, Third Symposium of Parkinson's Disease, Edinburgh, Scotland, E&S Livingstone, 1969, pp. 152–157.

ADLs and Independent/Assisted Living Decisions

As a measure of a person's ability to live and function independently, ADLs factor into decisions regarding living arrangements. Most people with Parkinson's disease do not need to make significant changes in their living arrangements for years or decades after diagnosis. Awareness of changes in ADL measurements can help the person with Parkinson's disease and his or her caregivers to make minor adjustments as changes occur, helping to mitigate the effects of these changes. Adjustments range from simple accommodations such as removing throw rugs to prevent falls and arranging kitchen cabinets so that used items are within reach without the need to bend or stretch to exploring ADAPTIVE EQUIPMENT AND ASSIST DEVICES that can help maintain independence longer. Keeping pace with the changes as they occur helps reduce frustration with the progression of symptoms. Many people who have Parkinson's disease ultimately reach the point where it is necessary to consider assisted living arrangements. Consideration of ADLs helps make this decision process more objective and factors in the person's unique and specific needs.

See also AMBULATION; AMERICANS WITH DISABILITIES ACT; ASSISTED LIVING FACILITY; BATHING AND BATHROOM ORGANIZATION; BEDROOM COMFORT; CAREGIVING; CARE MANAGEMENT AND PLANNING; CLOTHING; DRESSING; DRIVING; FALLS, PREVENTING; FOOD PREPARATION; HOME SAFETY; INSTRUMENTAL ACTIVITIES OF DAILY LIVING; KITCHEN EFFICIENCY; LONG-TERM CARE; MEALS ON WHEELS; QUALITY OF LIFE; RESIDENTIAL CARE; RETIREMENT COMMUNITY; STAGING OF PARKINSON'S DISEASE; WORKPLACE ADAPTATIONS TO ACCOMMODATE PARKINSON'S.

acumassage See ALTERNATIVE THERAPIES.

acupressure See ALTERNATIVE THERAPIES.

acupuncture A centuries-old method of treatment in which a trained practitioner inserts very fine needles into specific points on the body. In the Eastern medicine perspective in which acupuncture originated, health is a state of balance and illness or disease a state of imbalance of the body's life energy, or chi. Chi flows along invisible energy channels in the body called meridians. These meridians roughly correspond to the body's physical nervous system. Acupuncture points along the meridians correlate to body organs, systems, and functions. These points often are in locations distant from their corresponding organs. For example, acupuncture points in the ear (auricular acupuncture) correlate to various body locations as well as certain areas within the brain related to addiction. Acupuncture is an integral element of traditional Chinese medicine (TCM) and other Eastern systems and is used for both diagnosis and treatment.

Western practitioners have adapted the concepts of acupuncture to Western principles of medicine. In the Western medicine perspective, acupuncture points correlate to locations along the nervous system. Needles inserted into these locations alter nerve impulses and stimulate the release of various chemicals that aid in pain relief and healing. It is likely, although not proven, that acupuncture causes cells to release chemicals called endorphins, the body's natural painkillers. Western practitioners often use mild electrical stimulation, heat, or cold applied to the inserted needles to intensify the acupuncture effect.

The National Institutes of Health (NIH) undertook a review of studies conducted to assess the effectiveness of acupuncture and in 1997 released a consensus statement:

> Acupuncture as a therapeutic intervention is widely practiced in the United States. While there have been many studies of its potential usefulness, many of these studies provide equivocal results because of design, sample size, and other factors. The issue is further complicated by inherent difficulties in the use of appropriate controls, such as placebos and sham acupuncture groups. However, promising results have emerged, for example, showing efficacy of acupuncture in adult postoperative and chemotherapy nausea and vomiting and in postoperative dental pain. There are other situations such as addiction, stroke rehabilitation, headache, menstrual cramps, tennis elbow, fibromyalgia, myofascial pain, osteoarthritis, low back pain, carpal tunnel syndrome, and asthma, in which acupuncture may be useful as an adjunct treatment or an acceptable alternative or be included in a comprehensive management program. Further research is likely to uncover additional areas where acupuncture interventions will be useful.
>
> —*Acupuncture. NIH Consensus Statement Online 1997 Nov 3–5; 15(5):1–34.*

Acupuncture and Parkinson's Disease

There are few structured studies of acupuncture and its effects on the symptoms of Parkinson's disease. However, surveys do suggest that more than half of people with Parkinson's disease use at least one alternative therapy in addition to conventional treatment, and acupuncture is among the most popular. People with Parkinson's disease who receive acupuncture treatments anecdotally report

a range of mild to moderate improvement in symptoms such as tremors, dyskinesias, gait difficulties, anxiety, stress, muscle rigidity, and pain. From a Western perspective the reasons for such effects are unclear. Acupuncture cannot cure Parkinson's disease, but as it does not interfere with conventional treatments, most doctors support its use as a complementary therapy.

Finding a Qualified Acupuncturist

As with any form of therapy or treatment, finding a qualified practitioner is essential. In the United States, most states require some form of training and licensing. In many states only those who are already licensed to practice as some form of health care provider—such as physician, chiropractor, dentist, registered nurse, naturopathic physician, TCM practitioner—can be licensed to practice acupuncture. In a few states, only a physician (medical doctor or doctor of osteopathy) can be so licensed. And in a few states, anyone who completes a minimal training program and passes the licensing test can become an acupuncturist.

Look for an acupuncturist who has both adequate training and experience; who always follows sterile techniques (uses sterile, disposable needles, new from the package for each treatment session) to prevent infection from needle-borne pathogens such as hepatitis; and, preferably who works frequently with people who have Parkinson's disease and other progressive, degenerative disorders. Doctors sometimes can recommend acupuncturists in the local community.

See also ALTERNATIVE THERAPIES; TAI CHI; YOGA.

adaptive equipment and assist devices   Items and modifications to help people with disabilities to perform common tasks and ACTIVITIES OF DAILY LIVING (ADLs). The TREMORS, RIGIDITY, BRADYKINESIA, and DYSKINESIA of Parkinson's disease can make everyday tasks, from holding and dialing a telephone to opening doorknobs and typing on a computer, difficult. There are many aids available to customize assistance to meet a person's specific needs. These include

• Mobility aids such as walking sticks, walkers, and wheelchairs

- Devices to hold books and papers in place to make reading and writing easier
- Replacement of buttons with hook-and-loop fasteners
- Shoehorns and zipper pulls
- Large button telephones
- Lever-style light switches, sound- or touch-activated lighting and appliances
- Lever-style door handles to replace conventional doorknobs
- Bed rails and trapeze
- Railings in bathrooms, wide-door showers with no sill
- Broad-handle eating and cooking utensils

Medicare and Medicaid provide limited coverage for certain adaptive equipment such as mobility aids, and private insurance might provide additional coverage. An OCCUPATIONAL THERAPIST can recommend appropriate aids and devices as well as evaluate the home environment and make suggestions for improving ease of access, preventing falls, and ensuring personal safety.

See also AMERICANS WITH DISABILITIES ACT; CHALLENGES OF DAILY LIVING; CLOTHING; COOKING; DEXTERITY, PHYSICAL; DRESSING; HOME SAFETY; KITCHEN EFFICIENCY; MOBILITY; READING; TASK SIMPLIFICATION; WALKING.

adaptive footwear   See SHOES.

adjunct therapies (adjunctive therapies)   Treatments given in conjunction with each other to provide benefits that one treatment alone cannot deliver, to supplement the primary treatment, or to offset undesired effects of the primary treatment. Typically adjunct therapies enter into the treatment picture when Parkinson's disease enters its middle and later stages as the effectiveness of LEVODOPA or dopamine agonist MONOTHERAPY wanes. DOPAMINE AGONIST MEDICATIONS, BROMOCRIPTINE, ROPINEROLE, PRAMIPEXOLE, and PERGOLIDE, for example, act on DOPAMINE RECEPTORS in the brain. Other medications usually used as adjunct therapies include ANTICHOLINERGIC MEDICATIONS, AMANTADINE MEDICATIONS, MONOAMINE OXIDASE INHIBITOR (MAOI) MEDICATIONS, and COMT inhibitor medications, though all of these except COMT inhibitors may potentially be used as monotherapy in early disease.

Adjunct therapies often involve various and changing combinations of medications. Although this ongoing variation can be frustrating for physicians and patients alike, it is partly the consequence of the wide variability of the course of Parkinson's disease and partly the consequence of reduced effectiveness of ANTI-PARKINSON MEDICATIONS and the development of motor fluctuations over time. Adjunct therapies also can include ABLATIVE SURGERY such as PALLIDOTOMY or THALAMOTOMY and DEEP BRAIN STIMULATION. Most doctors prefer to maintain monotherapy for as long as it adequately relieves symptoms before moving into adjunct therapies to reduce the risk of medication-induced side effects. The interval before adjunct therapies become part of the treatment package depends on multiple factors, however, and varies from individual to individual.

See also ALTERNATIVE THERAPIES; ANTI-PARKINSON'S MEDICATIONS; SUPPORTIVE THERAPIES; TREATMENT ALGORITHM.

adjusting to living with Parkinson's   Integrating the ongoing changes that become necessary as Parkinson's disease progresses. Living with Parkinson's disease is a process of continual adjustment for the person who has it as well as family members and caregivers. Many people are able to make relatively few accommodations for five to 10 years or more after diagnosis, provided that ANTI-PARKINSON'S MEDICATIONS control their symptoms with few side effects. During this time the disease continues to progress, however, and subtle changes are taking place whether or not they are readily apparent.

Physical Adjustments

As it is typically physical symptoms that cause a person to seek the medical attention that leads to a diagnosis of Parkinson's disease, it is the physical changes of the condition that become the focus of treatment and adjustment. A key question all people diagnosed with Parkinson's disease have is, What will happen to me? Unfortunately there is no clear answer to this question. There is neither predictability nor consistency to the progression of physical symptoms. Some days the body seems to work almost normally, while other days it behaves as though possessed. Simplifying the physical environment makes these variations easier to accommodate. Removing throw rugs, for example, eliminates potential obstacles when walking becomes difficult. Replacing round doorknobs with lever-type handles, adding railings in bathrooms, and rearranging kitchen cabinets to minimize reaching and stooping are other changes that are easy to make early on.

Conscious focus on physical functions seems to improve them for many people. Concentrating on moving one foot in front of the other, for example, as though lifting it through the effort of thought, sometimes overcomes problems such as FREEZING OF GAIT. Focusing on the tremor in a hand can sometimes temporarily calm it. Making every effort to continue using the body to the fullest extent possible helps to keep the body functioning as well as possible. Learning to compensate for changes, from brushing teeth with the less-affected hand to switching to slip-on shoes gives a sense of control.

Emotional Adjustments

Many emotions flood through a person who receives a diagnosis of Parkinson's disease. Fear and worry often lead the list as concerns about what the future holds more to the forefront, exacerbated by the unpredictable nature and many unknowns of the disease. There are fears and worries about what will happen to the person with Parkinson's as his or her body changes with the disease's progression. There can be disbelief or denial. Once a pattern of familiarity settles in regarding symptoms, frustration and anger might step in, as the person questions why this has happened to him or her. Depression and anxiety are common companions, as both elements of and responses to the symptoms of Parkinson's disease. Mood swings are also common.

As in any life-altering situation, it is important to have others to talk with and share these emotions. Friends and family need to know that it is all right that they do not have answers. What matters is that they are willing to listen, comfort, empathize, and support. Structured support groups, often sponsored by local Parkinson's disease organizations, senior centers, and health care centers, provide a safe environment for sharing reactions and feelings with others who are having similar experiences.

Social and Relationship Adjustments

The diagnosis of Parkinson's disease is a shock to family and friends as well. They are concerned for the person diagnosed, of course, and for themselves as well. What does this mean for their relationship with the person? The person who has Parkinson's disease also has these concerns. It is important to be open and honest in communicating about worries and fears. It is also important to recognize that relationships with spouses or significant others, children, siblings, and friends continue.

A person with Parkinson's disease sometimes is reluctant to socialize, especially when symptoms are less effectively controlled. GAIT and AMBULATION difficulties might make a brief trip to the grocery store take three or four times longer and appear awkward enough to draw attention. Changes in bladder function alter the context of nearly any social outing. Yet with compassion, planning, and a sense of humor, adaptations not only are possible but also help to maintain joy and pleasure in living.

Planning and Preparation for Future Needs

It is challenging to plan for the unknown yet essential to prepare for the future. There are many facets of planning to consider, from medical care and insurance needs to the possibility of assisted or residential living arrangements. Who will be the primary caregiver? Who will make care and other decisions for the person with Parkinson's disease when that becomes necessary? Making these determinations before the needs arise averts much anguish among family and friends, allowing the person's wishes to be fulfilled to the extent possible. Financial and estate planning makes management of assets more efficient and effective.

See also COMPASSION; COPING WITH DIAGNOSIS OF PARKINSON'S; COPING WITH ONGOING CARE OF PARKINSON'S; DENIAL AND ACCEPTANCE; EARLY-ONSET PARKINSON'S; FAMILY RELATIONSHIPS; GOING PUBLIC;

JOY; LEGAL CONCERNS; MARRIAGE RELATIONSHIP; OPTIMISM; PARENT/CHILD RELATIONSHIPS; PRECLINICAL PARKINSON'S DISEASE; QUALITY OF LIFE; RETIREMENT; SHOPPING.

adrenal glands   A pair of glands located one above each kidney in the central abdomen. They are sometimes called the suprarenal (above the kidneys) glands. The adrenal glands are part of the body's endocrine system, a network of structures that produce hormones (chemicals secreted directly into the bloodstream). Each adrenal gland is actually two distinct structures, the adrenal cortex and the adrenal medulla.

Adrenal Cortex

The adrenal cortex is the outer portion of the adrenal gland's structure and wraps around the adrenal medulla. The adrenal cortex is key to the body's metabolic functions. The hormones it produces, called corticosteroids, include

- Aldosterone, which regulates blood pressure and blood volume by controlling the amount of sodium that the kidneys filter from the blood.
- Cortisol, which regulates the way the body metabolizes energy (uses fats, carbohydrates, and proteins) and suppresses inflammation. Cortisol plays a key role in immune functions and also is known as the body's stress hormone; the adrenal cortex releases more cortisol when the body experiences stress.
- Small amounts of androgen, the male sex hormone (in men and women alike).

Adrenal Medulla

The adrenal medulla, which lies within the adrenal cortex, is actually made of nerve tissue. It produces EPINEPHRINE and NOREPINEPHRINE. These hormones have numerous functions within the body, particularly in the cardiovascular system. They affect the constriction and relaxation of smooth muscle tissue in the arteries and veins, the force and rate of the heartbeat, and blood pressure. Because other tissues in the body produce these hormones, the adrenal medulla is considered nonessential for life: That is, it is possible to live without the functions it

fulfills and experience no life-threatening complications as a result.

Adrenal Medulla and Parkinson's Disease

The adrenal medulla has no direct correlation to Parkinson's disease. However, because the brain produces epinephrine and norepinephrine, it has drawn the attention of researchers as a potential source for replacing these substances in the brain through ALLOGRAFT. The adrenal medulla produces and releases epinephrine and norepinephrine into the blood. This makes them hormones. When the neurons in the brain produce and release epinephrine and norepinephrine during synapses, these substances are considered NEUROTRANSMITTERS. They are CATECHOLAMINES, the same chemical family to which dopamine belongs. Chemically, these substances are identical wherever in the body they are produced. In the body, some norepinephrine converts to dopamine that body systems other than the brain, such as the cardiovascular system, use. This dopamine cannot cross the BLOOD-BRAIN BARRIER, however, so it cannot affect the brain. But what if there was a way to circumvent the blood-brain barrier? The prospect intrigued researchers studying Parkinson's disease, arousing speculation that adrenal medulla cells, if transplanted into the brain of a person with Parkinson's disease, might be able to replace dying substantia nigra cells and continue to provide the brain with an adequate supply of dopamine. Although this is a solution that seems sound on its surface, so far ADRENAL MEDULLARY TRANSPLANT has not succeeded as a treatment for Parkinson's disease.

See also BRAIN TISSUE TRANSPLANT.

adrenal medullary transplant   An AUTOGRAFT in which surgeons remove the medulla portion of one ADRENAL GLAND and transplant it into the brain's caudate nucleus. The procedure is also called adrenal-to-brain transplant. Adrenal medullary transplant is an effort to sidestep the BLOOD-BRAIN BARRIER by "planting" adrenal medulla cells in the caudate in the hope that they will continue to function and produce the components that the brain can convert to dopamine. The premise for this approach came about in the 1980s, when researchers were able to remove adrenal medullary cells from the body and cultivate them in the laboratory, leading to speculation that the cells could also grow in other parts of the body.

The paired adrenal glands cap the top of each kidney in the central abdomen. Transplanting adrenal medullary tissue to the caudate requires two simultaneous surgeries with separate surgical teams, one to remove one adrenal medulla and the other to implant the adrenal medullary tissue in the caudate. Only one adrenal medulla is removed. Because the surgery is lengthy, complex, and involves multiple body systems, complications are common and often serious, sometimes fatal. At present, the American Academy of Neurology classifies adrenal medullary transplant as "unacceptable" as a treatment option because it entails these complications, because there is little objective evidence that the procedure produces long-term benefits, and because other surgical treatments produce results that are at least as effective without such high risk.

Only about 60 adrenal medullary transplants have been performed in the United States and Canada since the 1980s, with mixed results. Among people who recovered from the surgery without major complications, Parkinson's symptoms such as TREMORS, BRADYKINESIA, and DYSKINESIA seemed to improve. All remained on medication therapy, although some were able to reduce the amount of LEVODOPA they were taking. It does not appear that the transplanted adrenal medulla cells survive very long after transplant; one study that followed patients who died within two years of surgery found at autopsy that there were no remaining adrenal medulla cells in the caudate. Other surgical interventions such as PALLIDOTOMY, THALAMOTOMY, DEEP BRAIN STIMULATION (DBS), retinal pigmented epithelial cell transplant, and STEM CELL IMPLANT produce similar results with significantly less risk.

See also FETAL DOPAMINERGIC CELL TRANSPLANT; FETAL PORCINE BRAIN CELL TRANSPLANT.

adult stem cells See STEM CELL.

advance directives Documents providing written instructions regarding treatment decisions should a person become incapacitated and unable to express such desires when care is needed. Advance directives are particularly important with regard to end-of-life care for people with progressive conditions such as Parkinson's disease. Each state has procedures and processes for creating and implementing advance directives. In most states, two documents comprise advance directives, a living will and a durable power of attorney for health care (DPHC). Local Parkinson's disease support groups, senior centers and programs, hospitals, medical clinics, physician offices, and extended care facilities such as assisted living centers, skilled nursing facilities, and long-term care centers typically have information about advance directives specific to relevant laws, regulations, and procedures to follow to make certain advance directives are valid and followed if needed.

It is important for family members or close friends to know about advance directives and the desires these documents specify. The person who is most responsible for assisting with care, or who would be most likely to make health care decisions on the incapacitated person's behalf, should receive copies of advance directive documents. Copies also should go to the physician responsible for care for inclusion in the medical record. The earlier in the course of a progressive condition such as Parkinson's disease that advance directives are prepared, the better. A person may always modify or withdraw advance directives.

Living Will

A living will stipulates a person's preferences for medical treatment at the end of life, including whether to initiate or continue cardiopulmonary resuscitation (CPR), lifesaving measures such as mechanical ventilation, and other considerations. The easiest way to prepare a living will is to fill out and sign standardized forms available through many health care providers, bookstores, and stationery stores. It is important to use forms of documents that follow relevant state laws and procedures. Some states require the signatures of witnesses to make a living will valid, while others require only the signature of the person completing the living will. The person who signs a living will can change or revoke it at any time, even during a medical crisis when death seems imminent if the person is capable of communicating his or her wishes.

Durable Power of Attorney for Health Care (DPHC)

Durable power of attorney for health care (DPHC), called health care proxy in some states, is a legal document that gives one person the right to make medical treatment decisions on behalf of another person. This can be a trusted family member or friend. In most states, it cannot be a doctor, nurse, or other health care professional unless there is a relationship by blood, adoption, or marriage.

Because DPHC is a legal document, it is more formal than a living will and requires the signatures of two witnesses (in most states). Typically the person to whom the DPHC is assigned (sometimes called the health care agent) cannot be one of the witnesses, although health care professionals and employees can. It is a good idea to designate a primary and an alternate health care agent; some DPHC forms require this. A DPHC can be changed simply by replacing it with a revised document. Make sure all copies, including those provided for inclusion with health care records at the doctor's office and at the hospital, are replaced.

A DPHC assignee, or health care agent, is authorized to make decisions regarding the person's medical treatment including end of life decisions. It is important that this assignee understand the person's desires and be willing to make sure they are honored. These desires might include those expressed in a living will as well as other preferences related to matters such as surgery and emergency medical care. A DPHC covers any circumstance in which the person becomes unable to make his or her own health care decisions, not only the end of life. Because it is not possible to anticipate when or how such an inability might occur, it is a good idea to have a DPHC prepared.

See also END OF LIFE CARE; ESTATE PLANNING; FINANCIAL PLANNING; HOSPITALIZATION; HOSPICE; MEDICAID; MEDICAL MANAGEMENT; PALLIATIVE CARE; PLANNING FOR THE FUTURE.

age-related dementia   See DEMENTIA.

aging   The natural process of cell growth, decline, and death. Although aging is an inevitable and familiar process, there is much about it that scientists can observe and even measure but do not fully understand. At what point does the body cease to replace cells that die? Is this a biological or chronological point? Why does it—and aging—occur at seemingly different rates in different people? Can an individual influence his or her rate of aging through lifestyle choices? Why and how? Why do apparently identical choices have different outcomes from one person to another? These and myriad other questions intrigue researchers and guide numerous research studies, yet the answers remain elusive.

Age-Related Health Changes

As the body ages, it becomes less resilient in its ability to resist and recover from the ailments common to everyday life. What were mild aches and discomforts in youth and middle age can become obstacles that interfere with favorite activities as well as the ACTIVITIES OF DAILY LIVING (ADLs). Many of these changes, as the best scientists understand them, are biological in nature. The body, as it grows older, changes in terms of the way it functions. Certain processes become slower, and others (such as menstruation) stop altogether. The likelihood of developing many common health problems—arthritis, cancer, diabetes, and heart disease, to name just a few—likewise increases with age. The reasons are likely a blend of genetics and environment (including lifestyle). Modern medicine has become more successful in treating these conditions, often delaying them for years and even decades. These interventions do not delay the aging process, however. Eventually the body's tissues and organ systems wear out whether or not diseases develop.

Age-Related Changes in the Brain

As a function of aging, cells die throughout the body. This is true in the brain just as it is elsewhere in the body. With increasing age, parts of the brain such as the hippocampus shrink. As well, neurotransmitters in the brain and throughout the body become less active; it takes more stimulation to initiate their actions. One result might be that cognitive functions such as deductive reasoning and memory recall take a little longer. Experience allows most people to function without much noticeable change, however. An older person might occasionally forget where he or she put the car keys, for example, but knows where the keys are likely to be and easily finds them. Age-related changes in the brain can be difficult to distinguish from health conditions (such as Alzheimer's disease) involving brain functions or can compound the effects of disease or injury (such as with stroke).

Age-Related Parkinson's Disease

Changes related to aging in the brain also take place in the SUBSTANTIA NIGRA, where the brain's dopamine-producing neurons reside. Some scientists speculate that everyone who lives long enough will eventually experience enough depletion of these neurons to result in symptoms such as those that occur with Parkinson's disease. But does this mean everyone who lives long enough (a significant variable in itself) will develop actual Parkinson's disease? Or is Parkinson's disease just a name given to what is really a natural and normal process of aging? Most researchers believe neither idea is entirely accurate, although there are components of evidence for both. One estimate is that every decade after age 40, the substantia nigra loses 10 percent of its dopamine-producing cells through the normal processes of aging. Yet the brain can function remarkably well with limited resources; scientists estimate that the substantia nigra can adequately compensate for dopamine depletion until it has as little as 20 percent of the dopamine-producing neurons of a healthy brain. Even though there is a correlation between aging and Parkinson's disease, aging is not the only reason Parkinson's disease occurs.

About a third of people older than age 75 have at least some of the symptoms of Parkinson's disease, although often the symptoms are mild enough that the person does not seek treatment for them or they are discovered incidentally in relation to other health concerns. Most people diagnosed with Parkinson's disease are older than age 60, and the progression of the disease for them is usually gradual. Most will die of causes other than Parkinson's disease. One theory as to the cause of Parkinson's disease is that it is the consequence of accelerated aging, in which the neurons of the substantia nigra age more rapidly than cells elsewhere in the body to leave the brain "older" than the rest of the body. What triggers such an acceleration, if this is in fact what happens, remains a mystery. As well, it fails to explain EARLY-ONSET PARKINSON'S disease and the vast variations among individuals in the course of the disease. Many of these same questions apply as well to other degenerative diseases that are more prevalent in old age.

See also ACCELERATED AGING; APOPTOSIS; DEMENTIA.

agitation   Intense feelings and behaviors that often appear as excitement or extreme restlessness. In general, agitation can be a sign of many conditions including psychosis and age-related dementia. Agitation in Parkinson's disease can occur as a consequence of the disease's progression (as a function of DEMENTIA and COGNITIVE IMPAIRMENT), a reaction to frustration and lack of understanding about changes taking place, or an adverse effect of medication. More often than not, the cause is a combination of these factors.

Cognitive function serves as a gatekeeper of sorts between thoughts or feelings and behavior. Structure and routine in everyday activities help a person with diminishing cognition to maintain familiarity. Responding calmly and with soothing words and actions can help restore a sense of order when there are disruptions of routine.

Many ANTI-PARKINSON'S MEDICATIONS can cause agitation; they are more likely to do so as the disease becomes more advanced and doses must be increased to maintain symptom control. ANTICHOLINERGIC MEDICATIONS are often responsible. Often adjusting the dose or switching to different ADJUNCT THERAPIES can mitigate agitation and other side effects of medications. Sometimes persistent agitation is a signal that the diagnosis of Parkinson's disease is incorrect. This is something to suspect if the person's response to LEVODOPA has been less than expected or if stopping levodopa ends agitation.

See also ANXIETY; BEHAVIOR, EMOTIONAL; CONFUSION; DELUSIONS; DEPRESSION; HALLUCINATION; MEMORY IMPAIRMENT; MENTAL STATUS; SUNDOWNING.

agonist   A drug or substance that acts as a NEUROTRANSMITTER. Such a substance sometimes is called a receptor agonist. A DOPAMINE AGONIST taken to treat the symptoms of Parkinson's disease, for example, activates DOPAMINE RECEPTORS in the brain, binding with them in the same manner as does dopamine. The binding is not as strong or as comprehensive as that of the natural neurotransmitter, however, so that effect is more limited. This can be an advantage in a therapeutic context, because an agonist can be used to target a specific receptor to minimize adverse effects that would result if all receptors sensitive to the natural neurotransmitter were activated.

See also ANTAGONIST.

akathisia   An inability to sit still, typically as an aspect of AGITATION or ANXIETY. In people with Parkinson's disease, akathisia is relatively rare and when it does occur is often an adverse reaction to a medication used to treat the disease. Drugs commonly responsible include ANTIPSYCHOTICS and ANTIDEPRESSANTS. The person feels and acts so excited and so "wound up" that he or she moves continually, crossing and uncrossing the legs or moving the feet as if walking in place. Sometimes the person repeatedly jumps up and then sits back down. When akathisia is drug-induced, the best treatment is to reduce the medication dosage until this symptom goes away. If reducing the dose is not the best therapeutic choice, sometimes adding a benzodiazepine medication lessens agitation enough to calm the akathisia.

See also RESTLESS LEG SYNDROME; ROCKING.

akinesia   The absence or lack of movement. Akinesia typically manifests in Parkinson's disease as temporary episodes of "freezing" during movement or difficulty in starting movement such as walking. Although akinesia is one of the classic symptoms of moderate to advanced Parkinson's disease, not all people with Parkinson's develop it. As Parkinson's progresses, those who have akinesia find that episodes become more frequent and last longer. The prevailing perception of akinesia is that it is a consequence of dopamine depletion. However, some recent studies suggest that serotonin and norepinephrine are also depleted in people with akinesia due to Parkinson's disease and are exploring the possible need to add therapies that raise the levels of these NEUROTRANSMITTERS as well. Akinesia also can be an adverse effect of medication therapies to treat other Parkinson's symptoms, such as antipsychotics and other medications with dopamine antagonist actions. When this is the case, akinesia typically goes away when the drug is stopped.

See also AMBULATION; BRADYKINESIA; BRADYPHRENIA; GAIT; MOTOR FLUCTUATION; POSTURAL INSTABILITY.

alcohol and Parkinson's disease   Recent studies show that people who regularly drink light to moderate amounts of alcohol have a lower incidence of Parkinson's disease than people who drink no alcohol at all. The reasons for these findings remain unclear, however. No clinicians are recommending alcohol consumption as a means to reduce the risk of, or prevent, Parkinson's disease. Excessive alcohol consumption carries its own set of risks irrespective of Parkinson's disease and may contribute to accelerated or worsened dementia and other symptoms in people who already have Parkinson's disease.

Ale, beer, wine, sherry, liqueurs, and most hard liquors contain an enzyme called tyramine that can interact with MONOAMINE OXIDASE INHIBITOR (MAOI) MEDICATIONS sometimes used to treat Parkinson's symptoms. Because of this, people who are taking MAOIs should avoid drinking alcohol. As well, alcohol is a central nervous system depressant and can cause many symptoms that mimic, exacerbate, or mask symptoms of Parkinson's disease, including lethargy, drowsiness, and movement and coordination difficulties. As well, other anti-Parkinson's medications are contraindicated in alcoholism because alcohol consumption causes changes in the brain and the body, because the drugs and the alcohol interact, or because the combination of the drugs and the alcohol overwhelms the liver's ability to metabolize these substances.

Ali, Muhammad The three-time world heavyweight boxing champion who developed Parkinson's disease after his 21-year boxing career ended in 1981. A year later Ali was diagnosed with Parkinson's disease. Although Ali exhibits classic Parkinson's symptoms, it is likely that Ali's form of the disease was brought on by the repeated blows to the head he sustained in his career as a boxer. Ali retreated to a fairly private life until 1996, when he emerged again as a public figure, this time to champion the cause of research to find a cure for Parkinson's disease.

Ali became a spokesperson for the National Parkinson's Disease Foundation. And as the final torchbearer who lit the Olympic flame at the 1996 Summer Olympic Games, Ali became the face of Parkinson's disease. His walk up the steps to the Olympic cauldron was painstakingly slow. When Ali reached out to touch his torch to the cauldron, 3.5 billion people around the world watched on television as the hands of the man once known as "The Greatest" shook with the characteristic TREMORS of Parkinson's. The moment was one of the most moving in American sports, and it catapulted Parkinson's disease into the public spotlight.

Although Parkinson's has robbed Ali of his voice, he remains an outspoken advocate for Parkinson's research. In 2002 he joined actor MICHAEL J. FOX and others to testify before the U.S. Congress about the urgent need for additional funding and support, with his wife, Lonnie, speaking on his behalf. Ali founded and continues to support the Muhammad Ali Parkinson Research Center at Barrow Neurological Institute in Phoenix, Arizona. For more information about the center and its activities, contact:

Muhammad Ali Parkinson Research Center
Barrow Neurological Institute
500 W. Thomas Road
Suite 720
Phoenix, AZ 85013
(602) 406-4931 or (800) 273-8182
http://www.thebni.com

See also RENO, JANET; WHITE, MAURICE.

allograft Transplanted tissues or organs from a donor other than the recipient; also called nonself transplant. Allografts sometimes used as treatment for Parkinson's disease include NEURAL GRAFTS and STEM CELL IMPLANTS. Most such procedures are still considered experimental and are not consistently successful. Donor tissues and organs are carefully screened for pathogens and other contaminants before use. A slight risk of infection or other problems remains, however. As well, there is the possibility that the recipient's body will reject the transplanted tissue, negating the effects of the transplant and potentially causing additional health problems.

See also AUTOGRAFT; INVESTIGATIONAL TREATMENTS; XENOGRAFT.

alpha-adenosine receptor A substance or drug that blocks the action of alpha-adenosine, a neurochemical in the brain that plays a role in electrical conductivity among neurons. At present, such substances are experimental, and their effectiveness as viable treatment options for Parkinson's disease remains unclear.

See also ANTI-PARKINSON'S MEDICATIONS; CLINICAL PHARMACOLOGY TRIALS; INVESTIGATIONAL NEW DRUG.

alpha-adrenergic agonist Drug or substance that acts as a NEUROTRANSMITTER to activate certain EPINEPHRINE (also called adrenaline) receptors in smooth muscle tissue, increasing the amounts of epinephrine that can bind to these receptors. Epinephrine, like DOPAMINE, belongs to the catecholamine chemical family. Among its effects, it raises blood pressure, opens the airways, and increases blood flow to the muscles to allow them to increase activity such as is necessary during exercise. Alpha-adrenergic agonists are sometimes used to treat erectile dysfunction and orthostatic hypotension.

See also BETA-ADRENERGIC AGONIST.

alpha-adrenergic blocker (antagonist) Drug or substance that blocks the action of certain epinephrine receptors in the brain and other parts of the body, decreasing the effect of epinephrine. These medications, often simply called alpha-blockers, typically are prescribed to lower blood pressure. They are also sometimes prescribed to treat bladder spasms that occur with Parkinson's disease.

See also BETA-ADRENERGIC BLOCKER; URINARY RETENTION.

alpha-synuclein gene The first gene identified as having a role in familial predisposition to Parkinson's disease. Discovered in 1997 by researchers at the National Human Genome Research Institute (NHGRI) at the National Institute of Health (NIH), the alpha-synuclein gene is one of a cluster of similar genes located on chromosome 4; it regulates how the body makes and uses alpha-synuclein protein. This protein has a role in the function of neurons in the brain.

Only a handful of families have been found to have mutations of the alpha-synuclein gene, and in these families the mutations cause autosomal dominantly inherited Parkinson's disease: The disease is passed from generation to generation with each child of an affected parent having a 50-50 chance of inheriting it. Notably, the proportion of those people with the genetic mutation who develop the disease is much less than 100 percent, suggesting that additional nongenetic factors may be important in developing the disease even in people with the mutation.

The LEWY BODY deposits that characteristically develop in the brain of people with Parkinson's disease contain accumulations of alpha-synuclein protein; healthy brains do not have these deposits. The alpha-synuclein gene group already had been identified by scientists as having a key role in neuron activity in the brain. Researchers isolated a mutation, an error, in one pair of the 400 sets of genetic codes that the gene structure comprises. This tiny defect has significant implications for understanding of diseases such as Alzheimer's and Parkinson's that researchers hope will lead to more effective treatments as well as a possible cure or prevention.

Researchers are fairly certain that the alpha-synuclein gene mutation and other gene mutations since discovered do not themselves cause Parkinson's disease, nor are they likely to be the sole focus of new treatment approaches. Most scientists still think that even with a genetic predisposition for Parkinson's disease, there are additional factors that cause the mutation to result in development of the disease. These factors are likely environmental as well as perhaps other genetic triggers.

See also ENVIRONMENTAL TRIGGERS; GENE MAPPING; GENETIC PREDISPOSITION; PARKIN GENE; UBIQUITIN.

alpha-tocopherol The primary active ingredient of vitamin E. Vitamin E is a potent ANTIOXIDANT. Some studies have shown that people who take antioxidants regularly and long term are less likely to develop many health problems typically related to AGING and deterioration, from heart disease and cancer to conditions such as Parkinson's disease. This has led to speculation that high doses of antioxidants such as vitamin E could also play a role in treatment for such conditions. Clinical studies have failed to support this speculation. One of the most extensive was the 10-year multicenter DATATOP (Deprenyl and Tocopherol Antioxidative Therapy for Parkinson's Disease) study. In this and other studies, alpha-tocopherol had no effect on the course of Parkinson's disease.

It is possible that alpha-tocopherol and other antioxidants have a preventive effect for conditions such as Parkinson's disease, as some studies suggest. Yet once the disease develops, these substances have no effect in terms of slowing the disease's progress. They do not appear to do any harm, however, and many people take antioxidants along with conventional ANTI-PARKINSON'S MEDICATIONS.

See also ALTERNATIVE THERAPIES; FREE RADICAL; METABOLIC NEEDS; NUTRITION AND DIET; PROOXIDANT.

alprazolam A drug in the benzodiazepine family that is taken as a muscle relaxant, sleeping aid, or ANTIANXIETY MEDICATION. There is some evidence that alprazolam also has antidepressant effects, a helpful secondary benefit when mild DEPRESSION also is present. Alprazolam, like other benzodiazepines, acts to reduce communication among nerve cells in the brain, slowing brain activity. This effect reduces ANXIETY and often causes drowsiness, although alprazolam seems to cause less drowsiness than some of the other benzodiazepines. Alprazolam, along with other benzodiazepine medications, also slows nerve responses throughout the body, thus helping to relieve muscle spasms. It is sometimes useful for RESTLESS LEG SYNDROME (RLS) and muscle rigidity. The trade name for alprazolam is Xanax.

See also ANTI-PARKINSON'S MEDICATIONS; ANXIETY; BETA-ADRENERGIC BLOCKERS.

alternative therapies Treatments and remedies that are outside the realm of conventional medicine. These therapies are supportive and complementary, not primary treatments for Parkinson's disease. Those commonly used include:

- Acumassage and acupressure—rubbing or applying pressure to common acupuncture points
- Aromatherapy—the use of essential oils and fragrances
- Aquatic therapy—treatment that takes advantage of the buoyancy of the body in water, which reduces resistance, allowing freer range of motion and expression of movement
- Herbal remedies—natural botanical substances used or taken to promote healing and health. Herbalists recommend EVENING PRIMROSE OIL, milk thistle, and passion flower for Parkinson's disease, and there is some evidence that these might have therapeutic or protective health effects.
- Homeopathy—a system of treatment popular in Europe that uses diluted amounts of natural substances to stimulate the body's own healing responses
- Massage therapy—treatment that helps to relax muscles and relieve spasms and rigidity
- Music therapy—method that helps to relieve stress and anxiety
- Nutritional and vitamin supplements, including ANTIOXIDANT THERAPY
- Reiki—an energy healing method

None of these and no other alternative therapy can take the place of conventional treatment for people with anything but possibly very mild symptoms. It is important to continue with conventional medical care and to make sure the physician overseeing this care is aware of any and all alternative therapies being used. Sometimes people are reluctant to tell their doctor that they are using alternative therapies, but most physicians are supportive of methods that help relieve symptoms without creating further problems. Herbal remedies, vitamin supplements, and nutritional supplements are drugs and as such can interfere with the actions of medications so it is particularly important to talk with the doctor about these substances before starting them. It is a good idea for people who are using alternative therapies to keep a written journal of what they do or take, both to monitor the effectiveness of these therapies and to record them in case there are interactions with other treatments.

The National Institutes of Health (NIH) has established the National Center for Complementary and Alternative Medicine (NCCAM) to study, monitor, and report on alternative and complementary therapies. To contact NCCAM, write to them or visit their website:

NCCAM, National Institutes of Health
Bethesda, MD 20892
http://www.nccam.nih.gov

This is an excellent objective resource that lists sources, clinical studies that it supports, and warnings and advisories about fraudulent or hazardous practices.

See also ACUPUNCTURE; NUTRITION AND DIET; STRESS REDUCTION TECHNIQUES; TAI CHI; VITAMINS; YOGA.

Alzheimer's disease A progressive, degenerative brain disease that affects cognition, memory, and physical functioning. A German physician named Alois Alzheimer was the first to observe and document the progression of symptoms in 1907; as a result the disease bears his name. Although doctors had long been familiar with what was then called senility (a gradual mental decline that takes place in old age, as a result of aging), Alzheimer's disease occurred in younger people and the decline was more rapid as well as more severe. Through the decades, doctors and researchers observed a clear pattern and sequence to the changes of Alzheimer's disease and recognized that the symptoms of mental confusion and memory loss reflected specific and extensive damage to the parts of the brain responsible for these functions. About 4 million Americans have Alzheimer's disease.

As with Parkinson's disease, definitive diagnosis of Alzheimer's disease is not possible until autopsy after death. Instead, doctors focus on ruling out other potential causes that might produce the same symptoms. Some such potential causes, such as hypothyroidism (underactive thyroid), vitamin B_{12} deficiency (which can be a consequence of simple nutritional deficiency or long-term alcoholism), and certain brain tumors, are treatable. Also as with Parkinson's disease, however, the symptoms of Alzheimer's disease become progressively worse over time and the likely diagnosis becomes more clear.

The Pathology of Alzheimer's Disease

In Alzheimer's disease, the brain becomes clogged with protein deposits called amyloid plaques, which occur outside of neurons. These deposits interrupt neuronal communication and functions. As well, neurons become entangled and intertwined, rendering them unable to function. A second critical element of the pathology of Alzheimer's disease is the occurrence of tangled deposits of a protein named tau. These so-called neurofibrillary tangles (NFTs), resemble clumps of thread. NFTs disrupt neuronal function and are thought to play a key role in causing neuronal cell death.

In Alzheimer's disease, a drastic decline in ACETYLCHOLINE, seems to be a predilection for the death of certain key cholinergic neurons which causes a neurotransmitter essential for cognitive functions including reasoning and memory. Drugs new to the market in recent years, called ACETYL-CHOLINESTERASE INHIBITORS, appear able to delay this decline and corresponding progression of symptoms in some but not all people with Alzheimer's disease. Acetylcholinesterase inhibitor medications currently available in the United States include DONEPEZIL (Aricept), GALANTAMINE (Reminyl), RIVASTIGMINE (Exelon), and TACRINE (Cognex).

Alzheimer's disease was one of the first degenerative disorders for which researchers were able to identify genetic mutations. The first of these was the discovery that people with Down syndrome, a chromosomal disorder also known as trisomy 21, almost always develop early-onset Alzheimer's disease when they live past their 40s. Researchers also observed that Alzheimer's disease appeared to run in families or have a familial predisposition. This led to the discovery, over the past decade, of nearly a dozen genes that often are mutated in people with Alzheimer's disease, particularly early-onset (before age 60) disease.

Why Alzheimer's Disease Interests Parkinson's Disease Researchers

Although the symptoms and mechanisms of Alzheimer's disease and Parkinson's disease are distinct from one another, there are similarities that intrigue researchers. Both are progressive, degenerative conditions that affect brain function, and there are overlaps in the kinds of damage they produce. Cognitive decline and dementia are the primary consequences of Alzheimer's disease, although physical functions become affected in later stages of the disease in some people. Physical dysfunction (motor movement) is the hallmark of Parkinson's disease, although cognition and dementia affect some people in later stages of the disease.

- Each has a form that begins as an aspect of aging, in which case the symptoms tend to progress gradually over years and even decades.
- Both also can occur prematurely, that is, in people who are not in old age (early onset). When this is the case, the symptoms tend to begin dramatically and progress rapidly.
- Both have genetic components that are most likely activated by environmental (including personal health) factors.
- Each involves the depletion of an essential neurotransmitter in the brain (acetylcholine in Alzheimer's disease and dopamine in Parkinson's disease).

Researchers are hopeful that these similarities mean that findings relative to one condition have application to the other as well as to many of the progressive, degenerative diseases that currently are little understood and for which there are few treatment options such as AMYOTROPHIC LATERAL SCLEROSIS (ALS) and MULTIPLE SCLEROSIS.

See also GENE MAPPING; HUMAN GENOME PROJECT.

amantadine   An antiviral drug, brand name Symmetrel, that also stimulates DOPAMINE release. Approved for use in the United States in the 1960s, amantadine's primary use is to prevent or shorten the course of infection with influenza A. Recent research shows promising results in treating hepatitis C as well. Doctors identified amantadine's ability to mitigate mild motor symptoms in Parkinson's disease when people who had the disease took the drug to treat influenza and noticed improvement in their Parkinson's symptoms. Doctors now often prescribe amantadine as a MONOTHERAPY in the early stages of Parkinson's disease; it usually remains effective for 18 to 24 months. In later stages of Parkinson's, amantadine is sometimes effective as an ADJUNCT THERAPY to LEVODOPA and other ANTI-CHOLINERGIC MEDICATIONS to help offset ON-STATE and OFF-STATE fluctuations.

Researchers do not fully understand how amantadine works to neutralize the symptoms of Parkinson's disease. It appears to stimulate dopamine production or release, although the precise mechanisms by which it does so remain a mystery. Many researchers think that amantadine's blocking (antagonism) of NMDA-type glutamate receptors is the key to explaining its anti-dyskinetic effect. Amantadine's side effects are similar to those of anticholinergics, and they can include visual hallucinations, swelling of the ankles and feet, and discolored skin (LIVIDO RETICULARIS). When amantadine ceases to be effective, it must be discontinued gradually and under a doctor's supervision rather than suddenly stopped. Sudden withdrawal of the drug can result in rapid and severe worsening of Parkinson symptoms.

See also ANTI-PARKINSON'S MEDICATIONS.

ambulation   The ability to move from place to place by walking. Ambulation becomes more diffi-cult as Parkinson's disease advances. Changes in gait are marked by shortened stride, shuffling, and freezing of gait. Balance also becomes affected, contributing to the stooped posture characteristic of Parkinson's disease.

See also COORDINATION; GAIT; MOBILITY; PATTERNED MOVEMENT; POSTURAL INSTABILITY; POSTURAL RIGHTING REFLEX; RANGE OF MOTION.

American Parkinson Disease Association, Inc.   A not-for-profit organization that funds and supports research and education. The American Parkinson Disease Association (APDA) provides resources and information for people with Parkinson's disease, caregivers, and health care professionals. The main contact for the APDA is

The American Parkinson Disease Association, Inc.
1250 Hylan Boulevard
Suite 4B
Staten Island, NY 10305-4399
(718) 981-8001 or (800) 223-2732
http://www.adaparkinsons.org

The ADPA's website lists the contact information for state chapters and local support groups. Founded in 1960, the ADPA today sponsors 55 information and referral centers, 65 chapters, and more than 800 support groups throughout the United States. The ADPA is also a cofounder of the World Parkinson's Disease Association (WPDA), whose 20-some member organizations are national Parkinson's disease associations around the world.

Americans with Disabilities Act (ADA)   Federal legislation passed in the United States in 1990 to give persons with disabilities equitable access to employment, housing, transportation, and other opportunities. In brief, the ADA requires businesses (except the federal government and its agencies) to make reasonable accommodations for qualified individuals with disabilities. There are many interpretations of this law, and many variations in its implementation. In general, the ADA has the broadest implications in the workplace and prohibits employers from firing individuals solely on the basis of disability.

The majority of people diagnosed with Parkinson's disease are older than age 65 and have already retired or are near enough to retirement that it becomes a feasible option and employment rights are less of a concern. Those who are younger than age 65 often want to maintain the most normal life possible for as long as possible, and for them that means remaining employed. At what point is it necessary to let an employer know that a disabling condition exists? Technically, there are no laws or regulations that establish this responsibility, although conditions of employment might stipulate otherwise. Many people are reluctant to let others, particularly employers, know of potentially disabling health conditions; this is a personal decision that needs to take into account the nature of the job. The ADA does not provide guidance in this area. The U.S. Department of Justice oversees enforcement of the ADA and can provide additional information about the act and its requirements. For further information contact

U.S. Department of Justice
950 Pennsylvania Avenue, NW
Civil Rights Division
Disability Rights Section—NYAV
Washington, DC 20530
(800) 514-0301 (voice)
(800) 514-0383 (TTY)
http://www.ada.gov

See also GOING PUBLIC; LIFESTYLE FACTORS; RETIREMENT; WORKPLACE ADAPTATIONS TO ACCOMMODATE PARKINSON'S; WORKPLACE RELATIONSHIPS.

amino acid Chemical substance that composes the basic structure of proteins. Proteins are key to numerous functions that take place within cells, including the synthesis (manufacture) of many substances essential for life. Although there are only about 20 amino acids, they can form into nearly countless structures through the ways in which they align and configure themselves. The body can manufacture 12 amino acids from compounds that exist within it. These are called the nonessential amino acids. The body must acquire the remaining eight amino acids through the diet. Dietary proteins from animal sources, such as meats and dairy products, supply all eight of these amino acids. Dietary proteins from nonanimal sources—vegetables, fruits, grains, nuts, legumes, and beans—supply some of them. Combining different plant-based foods can provide the full range of essential amino acids. Nearly all body processes require amino acids, so it is important to meet the body's dietary needs for them.

Amino acids are digested and absorbed into the bloodstream through the small intestine. The mechanics of this process limit the amounts of amino acids that the body can absorb in the normal length of time it takes for food to move through the digestive system. All amino acids that enter the body, regardless of source, compete for digestion and absorption. LEVODOPA, the cornerstone of ANTIPARKINSON'S MEDICATION therapy, is an amino acid that, once within the body, becomes metabolized into dopamine.

Because levodopa is taken orally and absorbed into the bloodstream through the intestines, it too competes for absorption. When levodopa doses are relatively small, typically the case early in the course of the disease, this is not so much a problem. When doses increase as symptoms intensify, however, dietary amino acids can crowd out levodopa, with the result that less of it enters the bloodstream than the dose would suggest. This of course affects levodopa's effectiveness. Typically this results in raising the dose as an attempt to get more levodopa into the body. If dietary protein consumption is high, however, this strategy becomes counterproductive. It is more effective to separate levodopa doses from eating protein to limit the competition for absorption.

See also EATING; FOODS TO AVOID; FOODS TO EAT; METABOLIC NEEDS; NUTRITION AND DIET; PROTEIN; PROTEIN RESTRICTIONS, DIETARY.

amino acid decarboxylase See AROMATIC AMINO ACID DECARBOXYLASE.

amitriptyline A tricyclic ANTIDEPRESSANT MEDICATION. Common brand names include Elavil and Endep. Amitriptyline causes significant drowsiness in many people and might be prescribed if both depression and difficulty in sleeping are problems.

Alcohol compounds the drowsiness, so people taking amitriptyline should not drink alcoholic beverages. Amitriptyline also has many potential anticholinergic side effects, including dry mouth, difficulty urinating, and even CONFUSION and HALLUCINATIONS in some people. Amitriptyline cannot be taken with MONOAMINE OXIDASE INHIBITOR (MAOI) MEDICATIONS, which are sometimes prescribed for people with Parkinson's disease to inhibit APOPTOSIS. Triavil is a brand-name product that contains a combination of perphenazine, an ANTIPSYCHOTIC MEDICATION, and amitriptyline that sometimes is prescribed to treat hallucinations. Perphenazine can cause Parkinson's-like symptoms, however, so it is usually not an appropriate medication for a person with Parkinson's disease because it can worsen symptoms such as DYSKINESIAS and TREMORS.

See also ANTI-PARKINSON'S MEDICATIONS; DEPRESSION; SELECTIVE SEROTONIN REUPTAKE INHIBITOR (SSRI) MEDICATIONS.

amyotrophic lateral sclerosis (ALS)   A progressive, degenerative disease in which the NEURONS in the BRAIN and spinal cord that control muscles die off, resulting in inability to use the muscles. ALS is also called Lou Gehrig's disease, so named after the famous baseball player whose diagnosis with and death of the disease gave it public prominence. In its early stages, ALS begins with mild muscle twitching, fatigue, and weakness and can be difficult to distinguish from other neuro degenerative disorders such as Parkinson's disease without a careful neurologic exam. These conditions sometimes are mistaken for one another until symptoms progress. Diagnosis of ALS commonly hinges on electromyographic testing.

ALS progresses relatively rapidly once symptoms become apparent, however, making diagnosis fairly certain. In most people ALS progresses from initial symptoms to dependence on mechanical ventilation and death inside five years, although some people have survived as long as 20 years. There are no effective treatments for ALS, although a drug called riluzole provides some NEUROPROTECTIVE EFFECTS that appear to extend the length of time a person with ALS can breathe without mechanical assistance for a few months if started early in the disease.

ALS interests researchers studying Parkinson's disease because ALS, as do Parkinson's and Alzheimer's diseases, destroys motor neurons, depletes neurotransmitters, and has both familial (genetic) and IDIOPATHIC forms. ALS and Parkinson's also can occur together, and ALS, an Alzheimer's type of dementia, and parkinsonism frequently occur together in the native Chamorro population of Guam. Studies have identified a defective gene present in a small percentage of those diagnosed with ALS, although for most people the cause is unknown. Unlike Parkinson's and Alzheimer's, ALS does not have among its symptoms cognitive impairment or dementia. About 5,000 Americans are diagnosed with ALS each year.

See also GUAM AMYOTROPHIC LATERAL SCLEROSIS PARKINSONISM DEMENTIA COMPLEX (GUAMALS-PDC); MOTOR SYSTEM DISORDERS; MOVEMENT DISORDERS; MULTIPLE SCLEROSIS; MUSCULAR DYSTROPHY.

antagonist   A drug or substance that blocks the effects of a biochemical action in the body, also called a blocker.

antianxiety medication   A drug that relieves the symptoms of anxiety. Commonly prescribed among these drugs are the benzodiazepines such as ALPRAZOLAM (trade name Xanax) and DIAZEPAM (trade name Valium). The main side effects of these medications are drowsiness and dependence. Many of the antidepressants (especially the SSRIs) and buspirone are better choices for daily medication of chronic anxiety.

anticholinergic medication   A drug that counters the effects of ACETYLCHOLINE, a NEUROTRANSMITTER that stimulates muscle activity. These medications are used in Parkinson's disease to reduce tremors and were the first drugs used to treat Parkinson's. Anticholinergics commonly prescribed for Parkinson's include TRIHEXYPHENIDYL, BENZTROPINE, procyclidine, and biperiden, all of which act mainly at the muscarinic type of acetylcholine receptor. Side effects, which increase with long-term use, can include vision problems, excessive dryness of mucous membranes, CONSTIPATION, URINARY RETENTION, and drowsiness. A recent report raises the possibility that long-term use of these anti-muscarinic agents might promote the later development of dementia.

antidepressant medication A drug that relieves depression. There are three major kinds of antidepressants: TRICYCLIC ANTIDEPRESSANT MEDICATIONS, SELECTIVE SEROTONIN REUPTAKE INHIBITOR (SSRI) MEDICATIONS, and MONOAMINE OXIDASE INHIBITOR (MAOI) MEDICATION. Antidepressant medications affect DOPAMINE mechanisms in the brain, sometimes worsening symptoms such as TREMORS and DYSKINESIAS. The MAOI SELEGILINE, one of the ANTI-PARKINSON'S MEDICATIONS, is sometimes used because of its neuroprotective qualities. Other antidepressant medications cannot be taken at the same time as nonselective MAOIs, and special attention should be paid to starting them slowly and monitoring closely for side effects if they are given with selective MAOIs.

antihistamine medication A drug that blocks histamine response, typically used to treat or prevent allergic reactions. These drugs have mild anticholinergic effects and are often effective in relieving mild to moderate tremors in people with Parkinson's disease. DIPHENHYDRAMINE (Benadryl), available without a prescription, is the antihistamine usually used. The primary side effect is drowsiness.

antioxidant A substance such as certain vitamins that counters oxidation. Oxidation is a by-product of metabolism that many health experts believe causes damage to cells and tissues. Scientists have demonstrated that oxidation damages the genetic structure, or deoxyribonucleic acid (DNA), of cells, and that this is how many disease processes such as cancer begin. Although the concept of using antioxidants to -prevent oxidation damage and thus the disease process that results is intriguing, so far studies have failed to demonstrate that this method is effective.

antioxidative therapy Consumption of high levels of antioxidant vitamins C, E, and beta-carotene (which converts to vitamin A in the body), as well as COENZYME Q-10. Health experts disagree about whether these antioxidants must be ingested from natural sources (foods such as fruits and vegeta-

bles) or can be equally effective when taken as supplements.

See also METABOLIC NEEDS; NUTRITION AND DIET; VITAMINS.

anti-Parkinson's medications The general classification for drugs that counteract or mitigate the symptoms of Parkinson's disease. Medications remain the primary treatment approach for Parkinson's disease. There is no established regimen of medication therapy that works consistently for all people who have Parkinson's; finding an effective regimen is a matter of trial and error. It also requires ongoing adjustment as the symptoms develop resistance to certain drugs or become more advanced. DOPAMINERGIC MEDICATIONS are the cornerstone of medication treatment for Parkinson's disease. These drugs, which mimic the actions of dopamine in the brain, include LEVODOPA (which is converted to dopamine in the brain) and the DOPAMINE AGONISTS, which mimic the actions of dopamine by activating DOPAMINE RECEPTORS in the BRAIN. CATECHOL-O-METHYLTRANSFERASE (COMT) INHIBITOR medications extend the time levodopa remains active in the bloodstream, increasing the amount of it that crosses the BLOOD-BRAIN BARRIER and is available for conversion to dopamine.

Although levodopa is often referred to as the "gold standard" of medication therapy for Parkinson's, experts in treating Parkinson's disease disagree on when is the optimal time to begin it because motor fluctuations tend to occur only after a person has been on levodopa for a few years. Most clinicians prefer to use DOPAMINE AGONISTS as MONOTHERAPY to control symptoms in the early stages of Parkinson's, at least in younger people. Eventually nearly everyone with Parkinson's disease moves from monotherapy to ADJUNCT THERAPIES as the disease progresses and symptoms worsen. Other medications used in treating Parkinson's disease target specific symptoms such as TREMORS (ANTICHOLINERGIC MEDICATIONS and ANTIHISTAMINE MEDICATIONS) or attempt to slow the progress of the disease (NEUROPROTECTIVE THERAPIES).

Ongoing research into new drugs and drug treatments shows considerable promise, particularly in the area of neuroprotective therapies.

SUMMARY OF ANTI-PARKINSON'S MEDICATIONS

Drug or Drug Group	Common Drugs in Group	Use
Amantadine	Amantadine	stimulates dopamine release
Anticholinergics	trihexyphenidyl, benztropine, procyclidine, biperiden	reduce tremors
Antihistamines	diphenhydramine	anticholinergic effect
COMT inhibitors	tolcapone, entacapone	increase the duration and effectiveness of levodopa
Dopamine agonists	pergolide, bromocriptine, ropinirole, pramipexole	mimic the action of dopamine
Levodopa/carbidopa	Sinemet, Atamet	converted to dopamine in the brain
MAOI-B inhibitors	Selegiline, rasagiline	improve dopamine metabolism in the brain; neuroprotection

Gene research also is providing new understanding of how cells function in health and in disease, with the hope that this direction too will lead to new treatments and perhaps cure and prevention as well.

antipsychotic medication   Drug taken to mitigate the symptoms of psychotic conditions such as schizophrenia and personality disorders. Antipsychotic medications are not often used by people with Parkinson's disease because they block DOPAMINE RECEPTORS in the brain. ANTIPSYCHOTIC MEDICATIONS are commonly divided into two classes: typical and atypical antipsychotics. Typical antipsychotics have a higher risk of side effects expressed as movement problems in general, particularly the tardive disorders of abnormal movement that occur after being on the drug for some time. Atypical antipsychotics have an overall lower risk of tardive disorders of movement, but many of them are not much safer than typical antipsychotics when it comes to the risk of causing or worsening parkinsonian motor symptoms. QUETIAPINE and clozapine are typically the safest choices to avoid worsening Parkinson's symptoms.

anxiety   Intense feelings of fear and worry. In people with Parkinson's disease, anxiety is both a symptom and a reaction. Palpitations (rapid, pounding heartbeat), sweating, and shortness of breath often accompany anxiety. Anxiety often accompanies, or becomes more intense during, WEARING-OFF STATE and OFF-STATE episodes, when physical symptoms such as RIGIDITY, TREMORS, and AKINESIA worsen. Anxiety is also a component of DEPRESSION. As long as cognition is unimpaired, talking through worries and fears can help to dispel them and the anxiety that accompanies them. Antianxiety medications often are necessary to provide long-term relief, however.

See also ANTI-PARKINSON'S MEDICATIONS.

apathy   A lack of motivation, interest, and energy. Apathy is an early and progressive symptom of DEMENTIA in Parkinson's disease. As well, apathy is a symptom of DEPRESSION, which also occurs as a symptom of Parkinson's as well as a response to the diagnosis and progression of Parkinson's disease. Taking an ANTIDEPRESSANT MEDICATION can relieve both depression and apathy. Apathy also can become an expression of COGNITIVE IMPAIRMENT in later stages of Parkinson's disease. When this occurs, sometimes taking medications used to treat ALZHEIMER'S DISEASE such as RIVASTIGMINE (Exelon) improves cognition and counteracts apathy. Increased social interaction also sometimes counteracts apathy by increasing exposure to stimulating environments and events.

LONELINESS and isolation can be problems for people with Parkinson's disease, especially those who have symptoms that are not well controlled by medication or who are particularly self-conscious about their symptoms. Even limited contact with other people, such as walking or sitting in a park or other public location, can be beneficial. Watching and being around others are often uplifting and provide a different perspective. As Parkinson's disease progresses, once-favorite activities that require fine motor skills and coordination become difficult or impossible to continue. This can cause an increased sense of frustration and loss of interest in life. Getting out and about helps pique interest in new activities. If the person with Parkinson's is reluctant or becomes unable to leave home, visits from family members and friends also help stimulate interest.

People with Parkinson's disease sometimes give the impression of apathy because of altered facial expressions and lack of control over facial muscles, the so-called masked face appearance that characterizes later stages of Parkinson's. This impression can be false, as apathy is a function of behavior, not of appearance.

See also EMBARRASSMENT; PSYCHOSOCIAL FACTORS; QUALITY OF LIFE; SHOPPING; SOCIAL INTERACTION.

apomorphine   A DOPAMINE AGONIST medication that extends the effectiveness of LEVODOPA by stimulating DOPAMINE RECEPTORS in the BRAIN. Although apomorphine is, as its name implies, chemically related to the narcotic morphine, apomorphine stimulates the central NERVOUS SYSTEM (CNS), whereas morphine is a CNS depressant. When given by subcutaneous injection, apomorphine is a potent RESCUE DRUG that provides immediate and dramatic relief (usually within 15 minutes) of severe Parkinson's symptoms that are no longer responding to levodopa. Apomorphine specifically targets D1 dopamine receptors, unlike ergot-based dopamine agonists such as PERGOLIDE, which target D2 dopamine receptors. D1 dopamine receptors have the broadest distribution within the brain, so stimulating them produces a rapid and intense response. A major drawback to apomorphine is that when given in doses high enough for the drug to function as a dopamine agonist, it causes vomiting. Apomorphine's predictability in causing vomiting is so consistent, in fact, that veterinarians use the drug to induce vomiting in animals. To counter this emetic effect when giving apomorphine as a dopamine agonist, doctors administer it in tandem with an antiemetic medication, usually DOMPERIDONE.

Its potency and serious side effects make apomorphine appropriate only for severe symptoms, and it is in widespread clinical use of in Europe but still awaiting FDA approval for use in the U.S. Apomorphine cannot be absorbed through the intestine well enough to reach the blood levels necessary for it to act as a dopamine agonist in the brain, so injection is currently the typical route of administration. Preparations administered through a patch placed on the skin or a nasal spray are alternatives that so far have not proved as effective for treating symptoms of Parkinson's disease. They have, however, led to the discovery that in weaker doses apomorphine has the effect of stimulating sexual desire. D1 dopamine receptors in the brain play a role in perceptions of pleasure, including sexual arousal. A sublingual (tablet that dissolves under the tongue) form of apomorphine, marketed under the brand name Uprima, received approval in Europe in 2001 as a treatment for male erectile dysfunction but is not approved for use in the United States because of its potential side effects.

See also ANTI-PARKINSON'S MEDICATIONS; FLUCTUATING PHENOMENON; LEVODOPA; OFF-STATE; SEXUAL DYSFUNCTION; SEXUALITY; WEARING-OFF STATE.

apoptosis   The point in the life cycle of a cell at which a stimulus or trigger sets in motion a sequence of events that cause the cell to die, often referred to as programmed cell death. This process keeps cell growth and death in check and protects the body from harm that damaged or defective cells might cause. Various factors, internal and external, activate the sequence of events that initiates apoptosis. Some researchers believe interference with apoptosis causes many diseases such as cancer, in which cells grow without control, and degenerative conditions such as Parkinson's disease, in which cells die prematurely.

Parkinson's disease results when too many DOPAMINERGIC NEURONS (dopamine-producing cells) in the SUBSTANTIA NIGRA of the brain die, creating a shortage of the vital neurotransmitter DOPAMINE. Although findings are incomplete, some research suggests that a combination of genetic factors and damage from free radicals inappropriately activates apoptosis, causing these cells to die rapidly and in great numbers. One direction of potential treatment focuses on therapies, including medications and genetic interventions, that delay or halt apoptosis to keep cells alive. Although research in this area is promising, it has yet to yield conclusive results.

apoptosis inhibitor A drug or substance such as a genetic intervention (gene therapy) that delays or stops APOPTOSIS, or programmed cell death. Such a delay could slow the progression of diseases that result from apoptosis dysfunction. One approach is for such substances to attack one or more of the several proteins and enzymes known to have key roles in the apoptosis sequence of events, interrupting the process. Genetic therapies look at introducing genetically engineered cells into tissues, such as the SUBSTANTIA NIGRA, or creating other forms of genetic interference where apoptosis has gone awry in an attempt to halt the sequence. Many of these approaches are still in the research or experimental stages.

A group of drugs that doctors have prescribed for decades to treat depression, MONOAMINE OXIDASE INHIBITOR (MAOI) MEDICATIONS seem also to function as apoptosis inhibitors in some people with Parkinson's disease. These medications work by altering the way the brain metabolizes a MONOAMINE NEURO-TRANSMITTER such as DOPAMINE. This alteration prolongs the activity of these neurotransmitters. MAOIs are particularly effective during the early stage of Parkinson's disease, at which time they often are able to stabilize the brain's dopamine levels enough to prevent the symptoms that later characterize Parkinson's, such as TREMORS and DYSKINESIAS.

See also NEUROPROTECTIVE EFFECT; NEUROPROTEC-TIVE THERAPIES.

Archimedes spiral A simple drawing exercise in which a person traces or copies a spiral. The test reveals the effects of tremor and aids in determining whether the person has Parkinson's disease or another movement disorder. The spiral is named after the famed ancient mathematician Archimedes, who developed it according to a precise mathematical formula.

See also DIAGNOSING PARKINSON'S; MICROGRAPHIA.

arm swing The movement of the arm with each stride during walking. A diminished arm swing, particularly one that is asymmetrical (existing only on, or more pronounced on, one side), is an early sign of Parkinson's disease. Arm movement helps with balance when walking. In normal AMBULA-TION, the arms and legs move in opposition to each other with equal momentum. The right arm swings back when the left leg steps forward, then swings forward as the left leg pulls back. The BASAL GAN-GLIA control this arm movement. As the DOPAMINE depletion of Parkinson's disease affects the basal ganglia, arm swing shortens comparably to stride. Typically, when walking is reduced to a shuffle, arm swing is nonexistent. The degree to which arm swing is reduced is one of the measures of the progression of Parkinson's disease and of the effectiveness of treatment. Arm swing is nearly normal during the ON-STATE and can become minimal or nonexistent during the OFF-STATE. Consciously moving or swinging the arms helps to improve balance and stability during walking.

aromatherapy See ALTERNATIVE THERAPIES.

aromatic amino acid decarboxylase (AADC) An enzyme that metabolizes, or breaks down, LEV-ODOPA in the blood before it can cross the BLOOD-BRAIN BARRIER and enter the BRAIN. AADC's very rapid action necessitates dosages of levodopa that are much higher than would otherwise constitute an adequate supply for the brain to convert to DOPAMINE. AADC INHIBITOR MEDICATIONS can slow AADC's action. AADC is sometimes called amino acid decarboxylase.

See also ANTI-PARKINSON'S MEDICATIONS.

Artane See TRIHEXYPHENIDYL.

assisted living facility A residential center that provides limited care for people who need help with some aspects of the activities of daily living but who otherwise are fairly independent. Most use an ACTIVITIES OF DAILY LIVING (ADL) scale such as the Schwab and England Scale of Capacity for Daily Living or the UNIFIED PARKINSON'S DISEASE RATING SCALE (UPDRS) to determine an individual's level of independence. Residents typically live individually in small apartments. Assisted living facilities have staff who can help with bathing, toileting, dressing, eating, and housekeeping activities. They also offer physical and occupational therapy, group activities and outings, and social programs to reduce isolation and encourage social interaction. An assisted living facility can arrange for nursing and other health care services but does not itself provide them. Most assisted living facilities allow a person to reside in them as long as he or she is not bedridden.

State agencies accredit or license assisted living facilities according to state laws and regulations and federal MEDICARE regulations. Some facilities offer a continuum of care at the same location, from retirement communities (fully independent living) to assisted living (partially independent) and long-term care centers (fully dependent living). It is a good idea to explore all of these options to learn what is available, how much it costs, and what the application procedures are. Always visit facilities of interest for tours and for talks with staff and other residents, preferably more than once and at different times of the day. Most facilities charge a set rate, usually monthly, that includes a range of services including meals, housekeeping services, basic utilities, and laundry. Ask for an itemized list of included services and the procedures for obtaining billed services. It is important to know whether services such as transportation to and from doctor's appointments, to community events and activities, and for shopping are available, and whether there is an additional charge for them.

See also LONG-TERM CARE FACILITY; MEDICAID; MEDICARE; RESIDENTIAL CARE; RETIREMENT COMMUNITY; SKILLED NURSING FACILITY.

asymmetrical symptoms Symptoms that occur on only or primarily one side of the body, the right or the left, sometimes called unilateral symptoms. The side of the body on which symptoms appear is opposite the side of the brain that is affected. Asymmetrical symptoms are typical of Parkinson's disease and are among the factors that distinguish it from other movement disorders, aiding in its diagnosis. When symptoms similar to those to Parkinson's disease are present but are symmetrical or bilateral (present equally on both sides of the body), the condition responsible is not likely to be Parkinson's disease. As Parkinson's disease progresses and more of the brain becomes affected, symptoms begin to affect both sides of the body. Even when this happens, however, symptoms typically remain more dominant on one side than the other.

See also AUTONOMIC DYSFUNCTION; NERVOUS SYSTEM; DIAGNOSING PARKINSON'S; TREMOR-PREDOMINANT PARKINSON'S.

Atamet See SINEMET.

ataxia Lack of coordination involving muscles in the fingers, hands, arms, legs, and sometimes neck and head. Ataxia results from damage to the cerebellum (the section of the brain responsible for functions of muscle coordination), the BASAL GANGLIA, the spinal cord, or the peripheral nerve pathways that are related to motor movement. Ataxia can affect balance and speech and can also occur as an independent condition or as a symptom related to other conditions such as stroke, exposure to toxins, infection, and head trauma. Some forms of ataxia are hereditary, correlating to specific gene mutations. Ataxia also is common in various movement disorders such as MULTIPLE SYSTEM ATROPHY (MSA), Freidreich's ataxia (a recessively inherited genetic disorder), or the spinocerebellar ataxias (SCA 1-8 and 10-12, which are familial disorders with an autosomal dominant inheritance). The finding of ataxia with parkinsonism strongly argues against Parkinson's disease and in favor of MSA, SCA-2, or SCA-3 (Machado-Joseph disease). The movements of ataxia often are such that they give the appearance of intoxication, which can be embarrassing for the person who has them.

SYMPTOMS COMPARISON

	Parkinson's Disease	Ataxia
Standing	Feet close together	Feet wide apart
Walking	Narrow gait with small steps	Broad gait with long steps
Muscle tone	Increased (rigid)	Decreased (flaccid)
Tremor	With muscle relaxation	With muscle contraction

Some medications taken to relieve the symptoms of Parkinson's disease also can cause ataxia. Those most likely to produce this effect are BENZODI-AZEPINES (taken for anxiety and muscle relaxation). In most cases, reducing the dosage or switching to another drug improves the ataxia.

See also AKINESIA; BALANCE; BRADYKINESIA; BRADYPHRENIA; CONDITIONS SIMILAR TO PARKINSON'S; DYSKINESIA; DYSPHAGIA; POSTURAL INSTABILITY.

athetosis Involuntary movements that are slow, writhing, flowing or rhythmic, and repeating. These movements can involve any part, or all, of the body and sometimes are called athetoid movements. Athetosis signals damage to the BASAL GAN-GLIA. In Parkinson's disease, athetosis is a secondary symptom that is a side effect of prolonged treatment with LEVODOPA and most commonly involves the fingers, hands, and arms. It develops as Parkinson's disease progresses and the SUBSTANTIA NIGRA'S capacity to produce dopamine dwindles. This decrease in dopamine production causes a higher level of more dopamine to circulate in the brain than the brain's dopamine receptors are able to receive, causing an imbalance that generates abnormal movement. Athetosis is a side effect as well of other medication therapies that interfere with dopamine functions, such as antipsychotics, for similar reasons. In other movement disorders such as cerebral palsy and HUNTINGTON'S DISEASE, athetosis is a primary symptom that often accompanies other DYSKINESIAS and results from damage caused by the disease itself rather than by its treatment.

Treatment for athetosis in Parkinson's focuses on moderating the dopaminergic effects of drugs such as levodopa. Generally therapy employs a combination of implementing ADJUNCT THERAPIES

and reducing the levodopa dosage. The time frame during which athetosis develops in Parkinson's varies among individuals, although most who take levodopa long term (as is currently the conventional treatment approach) eventually experience problems. Some people can have decades of levodopa treatment with few adverse effects, other people begin to experience adverse effects within a few years.

See also ANTI-PARKINSON'S MEDICATIONS.

Ativan See LORAZEPAM.

atrophy The wasting away of body tissue such as organs or muscle. In Parkinson's disease, atrophy of the SUBSTANTIA NIGRA occurs as the loss of dopamine-producing cells progresses. When physical activity diminishes in later stages of Parkinson's disease, muscles also begin to atrophy. Regular exercise, physical therapy, and occupational therapy can help preserve muscle tone and strength because muscle tissue is not actually affected by the disease process as it is in movement disorders such as AMYOTROPHIC LATERAL SCLEROSIS (ALS). Atrophy can be an important distinguishing trait in early diagnosis of movement disorders because it is not a key factor in Parkinson's disease.

atropine, sublingual An ANTICHOLINERGIC MED-ICATION placed under the tongue. Some studies report that placing a drop or two of liquid atropine solution (ophthalmic) under the tongue helps to reduce the excessive DROOLING (SIALORRHEA) that often becomes a problem with Parkinson's disease. Atropine has strong anticholinergic effects: That is, it acts on the mucous membranes to reduce their secretions. When used directly in the mouth, atropine acts only on the salivary glands, minimizing the side effects of taking ANTICHOLINERGIC MED-ICATIONS systemically.

See also ANTI-PARKINSON'S MEDICATIONS.

augmentation An increase in symptoms, often as a consequence of treatment with ANTI-PARKINSON'S MEDICATIONS.

autograft   Transplant of cells or tissue from one's own body to another location in the body. The experimental procedure ADRENAL MEDULLARY TRANSPLANT is an example of an autograft as potential treatment for Parkinson's disease. The primary advantage of an autograft is that because the tissue or organ is the person's there is no risk of rejection.

See also ALLOGRAFT; STEM CELL IMPLANT.

automatic reflexes   Spontaneous actions the body takes without conscious awareness or intervention, such as swallowing and blinking. In Parkinson's disease automatic reflexes, which are regulated by the autonomic nervous system, gradually diminish and eventually disappear. This is the result of disruption to the BASAL GANGLIA that occurs when dopamine depletion affects the balance of DOPAMINE and ACETYLCHOLINE in the brain. Reduced swallowing and blinking are early symptoms of Parkinson's disease.

autonomic dysfunction   Changes to body functions regulated by the autonomic NERVOUS SYSTEM that are the result of injury or disease. As Parkinson's disease progresses, the NEUROTRANSMITTER imbalances affect other organ systems in addition to the SUBSTANTIA NIGRA and affect motor movement processes. These include changes in how the body adjusts blood pressure and heart rate. ANTI-PARKINSON'S MEDICATIONS further affect these autonomic functions. Orthostatic hypotension (blood pressure that drops with change of position, usually from lying down or sitting to standing), for example, is a common side effect of drugs such as levodopa, dopamine agonists, and selegiline. Distinguishing the autonomic dysfunctions that result from Parkinson's disease and those that result from the medications used to treat it becomes difficult.

See also HYPOTENSION; SECONDARY SYMPTOMS.

autonomic nervous system   See NERVOUS SYSTEM.

autosomal dominant inheritance   Pattern of genetic transmittal in which a mutated gene in one parent can carry through to the offspring regardless of whether the same mutated gene is present in the other parent. Only one mutated copy is needed, and the disease passes from generation to generation: each child has a 50-50 chance of receiving the mutant gene from the parent with the mutation. This means only that the mutated gene, if transmitted, becomes part of the genetic structure of the offspring, not necessarily that the mutation will cause a defect or disease. Environmental factors (conditions inside as well as outside the body) appear responsible for initiating the events that interact with the mutated gene to permit a disease to develop. The ALPHA-SYNUCLEIN GENE mutation for Parkinson's disease is autosomal dominant.

autosomal recessive inheritance   Pattern of genetic transmittal in which the same mutated gene must be present in both parents to carry through to the offspring. Though genetic, there typically is no history of the disorder in prior generations because carriers of the mutation are unaffected. These disorders may appear sporadic unless one comes from a family where other siblings are affected—a rarity in these days of smaller families because each child of two carrier parents only has a 25 percent chance of getting both mutated genes. As with AUTOSOMAL DOMINANT INHERITANCE, the presence of the mutated gene does not necessarily mean the defect or disease will be present; environmental factors appear to trigger disease development. The PARKIN GENE mutation for Parkinson's disease is autosomal recessive.

axon   The long, taillike segment that extends from the bottom of a NEURON to conduct signals to other neurons or muscle cells. An axon ends in a synapse, or corridor, between the cells. Although axons come very close to one another, they do not actually make contact. Instead, the receptor cell releases an appropriate NEUROTRANSMITTER, a chemical, that conducts or transports the signal from the axon of one neuron to the DENDRITE (receiving structure) of the other neuron. The neurotransmitter must be present in the correct amount and for the correct length of time for the communication to be complete. In Parkinson's disease there is not enough DOPAMINE, the neurotransmitter that carries movement signals between neurons in the basal ganglia, a structure that regulates movement. This disrupts the signal transmission, producing the dyskinesias and other motor movement dysfunctions characteristic of Parkinson's disease.

Axons typically are covered in a sheath that helps to contain and insulate the nerve signal as it passes through. In certain diseases such as MULTIPLE SCLEROSIS this sheath is destroyed, and as a result, the signal becomes diffuse or dissipates before it reaches the synapse. In other diseases such as Alzheimer's disease the axons become entangled and coated in protein plaques, which prevent signals from traveling through them.

See also DENDRITE; NEUROCHEMISTRY; NEURONS; NEUROTROPHIC FACTORS (NEUROTROPHIC PROTEINS).

baclofen A drug taken to relax muscles and to relieve muscle spasms (antispasmodic). Baclofen works in part by intercepting nerve signals as they leave the spinal cord, reducing the frequency and intensity of messages that reach muscle cells. It also has an AGONIST effect on the pain receptors in the BRAIN, stimulating the release of GAMMA-AMINOBUTYRIC ACID (GABA). GABA acts to slow the release of ACETYLCHOLINE, helping to restore balance between acetylcholine and DOPAMINE in the brain and to reduce the number of nerve signals to muscles in the body. Baclofen's first approved use in the United States was as a treatment to relieve the muscle spasms of MULTIPLE SCLEROSIS. Its use has since expanded to relieve similar symptoms in other neuromuscular conditions including spinal cord injury and cerebral palsy. In people with Parkinson's disease, baclofen sometimes is effective in relieving DYSTONIA and particularly stiffness and spasms in the feet but does not help rigidity, tremor, bradykinesia, or other symptoms of parkinsonism.

Baclofen is available in oral and injectable forms as the brand-name product Lioresal and also as a generic. Because it is a CENTRAL NERVOUS SYSTEM (CNS) DEPRESSANT, baclofen often causes drowsiness, slowed reactions, confusion, weakness, and dizziness, all of which make it very unlikely that the vast majority of people with Parkinson's will be able to tolerate significant amounts of oral or intravenous baclofen. Continuous infusion of baclofen directly into the fluid space around the brain lessens these side effects, is useful for patients with spasticity, and does seem useful for dystonia, but it still does not treat the cardinal symptoms of Parkinson's disease. Baclofen in any form is rarely used by movement disorders experts for people with Parkinson's disease. Baclofen can interact with other drugs to intensify the side effects of either or both. Such interactions are a particular risk with TRICYCLIC ANTIDEPRESSANT MEDICATIONS and MONOAMINE OXIDASE INHIBITOR (MAOI) MEDICATION. Typically the dose is gradually increased until it achieves the expected results in relieving muscle spasms and cramps. This approach minimizes undesired side effects, particularly drowsiness.

See also INTRATHECAL BACLOFEN THERAPY.

balance A state of equilibrium. Parkinson's disease causes a progressive loss of the ability to maintain the body in balance, particularly during movement. MOVEMENT and balance are intricate functions that require the close integration of multiple events. The BASAL GANGLIA play a key role in this integration. Sensory signals enter the brain from all parts of the body; the cortex then integrates this information and prepares instructions for a motor response, which is modified via feedback of information from the basal ganglia and cerebellum before being sent out to the muscles. The basal ganglia help to fine-tune movements to keep the body stable whether walking, standing, or sitting. The depletion of DOPAMINE level and corresponding increase of ACETYLCHOLINE level in the brain as Parkinson's progresses set the stage for this integration to deteriorate. Inadequate amounts of dopamine cause the nerve signals that regulate movement and coordination to be incomplete, yet the excess of acetylcholine increases the number of these signals. The messages the basal ganglia sends become erratic and distorted, generating muscle response that is dysfunctional. The resulting loss of balance has unique characteristics which include

- Stooped posture when walking, standing, or sitting
- Small, shuffling steps that sometimes become more rapid when balance becomes jeopardized when walking (festination)
- Taking many small steps, rather than pivoting on the ball of the foot, to change direction or turn
- Unawareness that balance is threatened or has already been lost
- Tendency to lean forward or backward when starting to walk (POSTURAL INSTABILITY)
- Tendency to tip or fall forward or backward if bumped during walking, with an inability to self-correct
- Start hesitation and freezing of gait (FOG)

The primary hazard of these balance disturbances as they develop is falling, with the potential for injury; in the later stage of Parkinson's disease they can combine with other symptoms such as RIGIDITY and DYSKINESIA to make movement virtually impossible. Remaining as physically active as possible for as long as possible helps to maintain movement and balance. Structured, flowing movements such as those of TAI CHI can improve balance and flexibility. Techniques to improve balance include

- Focusing conscious effort on the actions of movement, such as thinking about and watching the foot lift, move forward, and move back to the floor
- Hand rails in hallways, stairways, bathrooms, and other locations where changes of position are essential
- Chairs with firm cushions and sturdy arms
- Use of WALKING AIDS such as a walker for stability during movement
- Patience in allowing for the extra time movement requires

See also BODY SCHEME; COORDINATION; DEXTERITY, PHYSICAL; FALLS; HOME SAFETY; ROCKING; SUBSTANTIA NIGRA.

basal ganglia   The collective term for the clusters of nerve cells that control voluntary muscle movement. The basal ganglia are part of the EXTRAPYRAMIDAL SYSTEM within the autonomic NERVOUS SYSTEM. Not all of their functions and interactions are clearly understood. Located in the brain at the base of the cerebrum adjacent to the cerebellum and above the BRAINSTEM, the basal ganglia consist of five distinct and identifiable bilateral structures:

- *Caudate* (also called the caudate nucleus), which means "having a tail," in reference to this structure's commalike shape
- *Putamen*, which means "shell" and wraps around the outside of the globus pallidus
- *Globus pallidus,* which are round pale structures (sometimes called the pallidum) with two distinct parts that have different functions, the globus pallidus interna (GPi) and globus pallidus externa (GPe)
- *Substantia nigra,* a structure which includes dark pigmented cells whose primary function is to produce dopamine
- *Subthalamic nucleus* (STN), a small structure located beneath the THALAMUS

Sometimes the motor portion of the thalamus, an oval paired structure on either side of the central fluid space (third ventricle) of the brain that is mostly devoted to serving as a relay station between sensory organs and the sensory cortex, is included as being part of the basal ganglia.

The caudate and the putamen form the STRIATUM, the collective functions of which control the smoothness and continuity of muscle activity during movement. Parkinson's disease starts with the death of dopamine-producing cells in the substantia nigra, which reduces the amount of DOPAMINE present in the striatum and other structures of the basal ganglia (and other structures in the brain as well). This reduction results in an imbalance between dopamine and ACETYLCHOLINE, allowing acetylcholine to overwhelm the striatum with signals to the body's muscles. The striatum's dysfunction produces the TREMORS, DYSKINESIAS, RIGIDITY, and other muscle-related symptoms of Parkinson's disease. The function of the subthalamic nucleus closely tied to the function of the striatum, providing vital feedback to help regulate the output of the striatum.

Treatment with levodopa, the current therapeutic standard in Parkinson's disease, targets the basal ganglia, increasing the amount of dopamine present and stimulating the dopamine receptors of these structures, temporarily improving their ability to carry out functions related to movement. This effect is most pronounced in the caudate and putamen. Functional imaging technologies such as SINGLE PHOTON EMISSION TOMOGRAPHY (SPECT) and POSITRON EMISSION TOMOGRAPHY (PET) make it possible to observe the changes and functions of the basal ganglia, providing objective information that may correspond to treatment effectiveness and disease progression. DEEP BRAIN STIMULATION (DBS) of the subthalamic nucleus (STN) and globus pallidus interna (GPi) have both been shown to be effective treatments for all the cardinal symptoms of Parkinson's disease, though only STN DBS is associated with being able to significantly reduce anti-Parkinson's medications.

In the 1990s researchers began experimenting with FETAL DOPAMINERGIC CELL TRANSPLANT, a procedure in which dopamine-producing cells from fetal brain tissue are injected into the caudate or the putamen, where they "take root" and replace the cells damaged by Parkinson's disease to restore the supply of dopamine and the striatum's ability to function. The results have been fairly promising, but a bit mixed overall in light of a recent large randomized controlled trial. These mixed results as well as the controversy surrounding use of fetal cells have caused a virtual moratorium on human studies of the procedure in the United States for the time being. Other potentially successful interventions directly into the basal ganglia include retinal pigment epithelium cell transplants and direct infusion of glial derived neurotrophic factor (GDNF) into the striatum.

See also ABLATION; ADRENAL MEDULLARY TRANSPLANT; HOPE FOR A PARKINSON'S CURE; NERVOUS SYSTEM; PALLIDOTOMY; THALAMOTOMY.

bathing and bathroom organization   Techniques to accommodate the restrictions and limitations Parkinson's disease imposes on the mobility and coordination necessary to maintain good personal hygiene. Bathing personal hygiene, particularly independently, become increasingly challenging as Parkinson's disease progresses. Organizing the bathroom to accommodate changing needs improves both efficiency and safety.

General

- As much as is practical, arrange items in the bathroom to be within easy reach of the person's stronger side. This may or may not be the side that was dominant before Parkinson's.
- Place commonly used items on shelves, open if possible, that do not require reaching or bending.
- Replace area rugs with nonslip bath mats.
- If cognitive impairment is a problem, print signs with instructions in large, dark letters for steps to follow to perform tasks such as using the toilet, washing hands, or shampooing hair.

Toilet

- Install a raised toilet seat and grab rails. Lowering the body to sit and raising it to stand are actions that require coordination and balance.
- Relocate the toilet tissue dispenser to be within easy reach, if necessary. Make sure the roll is full or place a replacement roll (unpackaged) within easy reach, such as on a small shelf near the dispenser.

Sink

- Install lever-type water controls.
- Use a pump soap dispenser with a broad head.
- Use broad-handled combs and brushes.
- Use an electric toothbrush that has a broad handle and toothpaste in an easy-to-dispense container (ask the dentist or check in the children's products section).

Shower and Tub

- Adjust the temperature of the hot water heater to no higher than 120 degrees to prevent scalding injuries.
- Install grab rails for tubs and showers.

- Install nonslip mats, in a contrasting color, on the floor of the shower or tub.
- Install lever-type water controls.
- Use soap-on-a-rope, and always provide a full bar, which is easy to grip.

See also BODY CARE.

Beck Depression Inventory (BDI) A series of questions that help to identify and quantify the presence and extent of clinical DEPRESSION using criteria consistent with the *Diagnostic and Statistical Manual of Mental Health Disorders—Fourth Edition (DSM-IV)*. The original BDI was published in 1961 by the psychiatrist Aaron T. Beck, M.D. Currently in use is the Beck Depression Inventory II (BDI-II), issued in 1996. The full BDI-II features 21 areas with four statements that the person completing the inventory chooses among for the one that best identifies his or her response. The BDI is designed to be quick to take (less than 10 minutes) and self-administered, although an interviewer can ask the questions and record the responses.

Depression is one of the earliest symptoms in about 20 percent of those diagnosed with Parkinson's disease and becomes a significant symptom in about 40 percent as Parkinson's disease progresses. Because it is easy to administer and to take, the BDI is a popular tool for helping to assess whether depression is present in a person with Parkinson's disease. Depression can be difficult to diagnose in Parkinson's as symptoms tend to fluctuate, decreasing during an ON-STATE and increasing during an OFF-STATE. The BDI is most effective when it is one element of a comprehensive evaluation for depression; by itself, it does not provide a conclusive diagnosis, although its results are considered highly reliable.

The Psychological Corporation owns the copyright to all versions of the BDI issued after 1977 and produces the BDI in written, computerized, and short-form formats. For more information about the BDI, including purchase and scoring information, contact

The Psychological Corporation
19500 Bulverde
San Antonio, TX 78259

(800) 872-1726
(800) 232-1223 (fax)
http://www.psychcorp.com

See also HAMILTON DEPRESSION RATING SCALE.

bedroom comfort Techniques to accommodate the restrictions and limitations Parkinson's disease imposes on the mobility, flexibility, and coordination needed to adjust bedclothes, turn in bed, and manage other actions to make restful sleep possible. People with Parkinson's have trouble with these tasks.

- Use sheets that have a slick surface, such as satin, to make moving and turning easier.
- Wear pajamas that are comfortable but not baggy and are made of a fabric that moves easily over the sheets. Nightgowns tend to gather and bunch.
- Install an overhead trapeze and bedrails so the person has something to grip for support when getting in and out of bed and turning in bed.
- Have a minimum of furniture in the room so it is easy to get into and out of bed.
- Place a bedside table or stand within easy reach, which might mean moving it to about shoulder level after the person is in bed.
- If excessive drooling is a problem, use an absorbent pillowcase.
- Use touch-activated lamps and install lever-type light switches.

See also ADAPTIVE EQUIPMENT AND ASSIST DEVICES; HOME SAFETY; SLEEP DISTURBANCES.

bedsores Ulcers on the skin that result from extended pressure, also called decubitus ulcers. Bedsores are so-called because they tend to develop in people who are bedridden and infrequently change position. However, any condition that limits movement, such as Parkinson's disease, places a person at risk for developing these wounds. Continued pressure compresses blood vessels near the skin's surface, preventing oxygen exchange with the tissues in the area. The cells die and the skin deteriorates, exposing the underlying tissues. Nearly all bedsores are preventable through frequent changes in position (every two hours for someone who is totally bedridden) and good BODY CARE to maintain the health of the skin. Once they develop, bedsores can become easily infected and require medical intervention.

For anyone who has significant difficulty turning in bed or is completely confined to bed, the caregiver should check closely for early signs of bedsores every day. Such signs include redness or other discoloration, irritation, or breaks in the skin. Treatment consists of keeping the area of the sore clean, dry, and free of pressure. Sometimes antibiotics are necessary, either applied topically or taken orally, to fight or prevent infection. Untreated bedsores are painful and increase debilitation. The skin and tissue over bony areas such as the hips, knees, shoulders, and elbows are most vulnerable to bedsores. Placing a sheepskin beneath the person helps to cushion the skin. Air or water mattress pads also can help.

See also HOME HEALTH CARE.

behavior, emotional The actions that result from the changes in the brain with Parkinson's disease. Although Parkinson's disease is thought of primarily as a degenerative condition affecting movement, the changes that take place in the brain also affect emotions and emotional response. This effect is believed to be the result of shifts in the balance of NEUROTRANSMITTERS in the brain. ANXIETY and DEPRESSION are the most common emotional symptoms of Parkinson's disease. The drugs that treat these symptoms act on the brain to affect the production or action of neurotransmitters. MOOD SWINGS are also common in people with Parkinson's, and sometimes outbursts of anger and aggressive behavior accompany the DEMENTIA of late stage disease. With cognitive decline deterioration of inhibitions regarding inappropriate emotional expression occurs, leading to outbursts that are inappropriate. This is most likely a consequence of physical damage to the brain.

Treatment for emotional symptoms is generally pharmacological and targets the conditions as if they exist independently of the Parkinson's,

although many people with Parkinson's disease find it helpful to talk about their fears and concerns in SUPPORT GROUPS or with a therapist. Because dopamine depletion is already present, doctors try to use ANTIANXIETY MEDICATIONS and ANTIDEPRESSANT MEDICATIONS that have minimal effect on this neurotransmitter. ANTI-PARKINSON'S MEDICATIONS such as ANTICHOLINERGIC MEDICATIONS, which suppress ACETYLCHOLINE, further alter the brain's biochemical balances and sometimes cause disturbances in emotion (typically depression or anxiety).

For some people with Parkinson's disease, the volatility of emotions is more distressing than the physical symptoms. It is possible to swing from euphoria to deep, almost suicidal depression within hours or to feel and respond with inappropriately intense emotion such as anger. The prevailing belief is that these emotional swings result from fluctuating dopamine levels, although few studies have focused on this possibility. Dopamine is known to have a role in perceptions of pleasure and euphoria, and in addiction.

Another factor of emotional behavior in Parkinson's disease is its expression. Parkinson's affects the muscles of the face—the characteristic masked face—to leave no outward expression of emotion. This effect makes the person appear emotionless, which is seldom the case. People, of course, do not respond to the person's emotions because the visual cues that are critical to understanding them are not clear or are not present. This can feed frustration and depression in the person with Parkinson's.

See also MEDICATION SIDE EFFECTS; PSYCHOSOCIAL FACTORS; PSYCHOTHERAPY; SOCIAL INTERACTION.

belladonna A chemical compound that has ANTICHOLINERGIC qualities. One of the oldest medicinal extracts known, belladonna derives from the deadly nightshade plant. Belladonna is an alkaloid that is chemically related to drugs such as atropine, scopolamine, and strychnine. Its strongest action is to relax smooth (involuntary) muscle. The name means "pretty lady" in reference to the practice in ancient times of touching the juice of the plant to a woman's eye to cause the pupil to dilate, then considered a sign of beauty. The evolution of this practice has medical applications today. Doctors use topical drops containing belladonna alkaloids, usually atropine or scopolamine, to dilate the pupils to examine and perform surgery on the eye. Anesthesiologists also use these drugs for their effects in relaxing smooth muscle, especially in the intestines. When they are taken systemically, however, the margin between therapeutic and lethal doses among these drugs is particularly narrow, and poisoning is a significant risk. There are numerous synthetic (laboratory-manufactured) drugs that are much safer to use.

As an anticholinergic, belladonna blocks the release of ACETYLCHOLINE in the brain. This slows the reactions of muscles throughout the body. Before the discovery of drugs such as LEVODOPA, belladonna was the main pharmacological treatment for Parkinson's disease. It was effective in controlling the tremors of early Parkinson's, but its dangerous toxicity level made it less than ideal and overdoses were common. Doctors today rarely prescribe low doses of belladonna or a derivative drug to help relieve the sialorrhea (excessive saliva production and drooling) that develops in later stages of Parkinson's disease; again there are numerous synthetic drugs that are just as effective and safer to use.

Benadryl   See DIPHENHYDRAMINE.

benserazide   A DOPA DECARBOXYLASE (DDC) INHIBITOR DRUG taken in combination with levodopa to increase the amount of LEVODOPA that crosses the BLOOD-BRAIN BARRIER to become converted into DOPAMINE. DDC acts quickly to metabolize levodopa as it enters the bloodstream from the intestines. As well as limiting the amount of levodopa that reaches the brain, this action puts into circulation a level of dopamine that causes numerous undesired side effects including nausea, low blood pressure (HYPOTENSION), and irregular heart rate. Combining levodopa with a DDC inhibitor such as benserazide mitigates this process. Levodopa/benserazide is sold under the brand name Madopar in the United States and Prolopa in Canada, in varying strengths that com-

bine the two drugs in a four-to-one ratio. It is available in a regular release form taken three or four times a day and an extended release form (Madopar CR) taken once daily. Treatment generally starts with small doses increased gradually over six to eight weeks until symptoms (TREMORS and DYSKINESIA) are controlled.

See also ANTI-PARKINSON'S MEDICATIONS; ENTACAPONE; FAVA BEANS; SINEMET.

benztropine   One of the ANTICHOLINERGIC MEDICATIONS taken as an adjunct therapy to relieve the TREMORS and RIGIDITY of Parkinson's disease. Benztropine is sold in the United States as the brand name product Cogentin, which is available as an injection or a tablet. It also has some ANTIHISTAMINE effect. As other anticholinergics can, benztropine can cause dryness of mucous tissues such as the mouth, for that reason it is sometimes prescribed for people with Parkinson's disease. It also restricts perspiration (sweating); that property is a benefit when excessive sweating is a symptom but can result in symptoms of heat exhaustion. An undesired side effect of benztropine is that it can cause or worsen symptoms of DEMENTIA such as confusion and disorientation. A recent study of postmortem brain pathology samples has even suggested that the long-term use of benztropine or other anticholinergics in people with Parkinson's raises the risk of developing Alzheimer's disease.

See also ANTI-PARKINSON'S MEDICATIONS.

bereavement   See GRIEF.

beta-adrenergic agonist   A drug that acts as a NEUROTRANSMITTER to activate certain epinephrine (also called adrenaline) receptors in smooth muscle tissue, increasing the level of epinephrine that can bind to these receptors. Epinephrine, like DOPAMINE, belongs to the CATECHOLAMINE family of biochemicals. Among its effects it raises blood pressure and opens the airways. Beta-adrenergic agonists are used to treat HYPOTENSION (low blood pressure) and asthma. These drugs also increase blood flow to the muscles and therefore can exacerbate symptoms such as DYSKINESIAS and TREMORS. People with Parkinson's should use caution in taking them, but they are very useful in avoiding the risk of passing out and falling in people who have significant orthostatic hypotension.

See also ALPHA-ADRENERGIC AGONIST.

beta-adrenergic blocker (antagonist) A drug that inhibits, or blocks, the action of receptors in certain cells in the body, particularly smooth muscle such as the heart and arteries, that respond to epinephrine (also called adrenaline). These drugs are often simply called beta-blockers and typically are prescribed to treat high blood pressure (hypertension). Beta-blockers are sometimes effective in treating migraine headaches, calming anxiety, and relieving tremors, although they are more commonly used to treat ESSENTIAL TREMOR than the tremors of Parkinson's disease. When anxiety and tremors are both present, as sometimes occurs in Parkinson's a beta-blocker can be an effective therapeutic choice for treating both conditions with minimal side effects. Commonly prescribed beta-blockers include propanolol (such as the brand name product Inderal), nadolol (such as the brand name product Corgard), and metoprolol (such as the brand name Lopressor). ORTHOSTATIC HYPOTENSION and erectile dysfunction are among the undesired side effects of beta-blockers.

See also ALPHA-ADRENERGIC BLOCKER.

bioavailability The amount of a drug or substance that enters the bloodstream and has an effect. There is usually an inverse relationship between a drug's dosage and its bioavailability: That is, the lower the bioavailability, the higher the dosage that is needed to deliver a therapeutic effect. For example, 95 percent of an oral levodopa dose is converted to dopamine before it can reach the blood-brain barrier, leaving just 5 percent of the dose therapeutically available. This means it is necessary to take a dose of 500 mg for 25 mg to reach the brain.

Bioavailability is an important factor in calculating appropriate dosages, particularly with drugs such as levodopa that have significant side effects when they are present in the body in large amounts. High levels of peripheral dopamine circulating in the body, for example, can cause rapid or irregular heart rate, nausea, lightheadedness, and other unpleasant symptoms. With levodopa, it is possible to reduce the dosage by taking the levodopa in combination with CARBIDOPA (SINEMET) or BENSERAZIDE (Madopar), drugs that delay the enzyme response that breaks down the levodopa to dopamine in the body. Delaying this conversion extends levodopa's bioavailability to 10 to 30 percent, thereby significantly lowering the needed dosage and reducing the side effects.

Factors that can influence bioavailability include whether the drug is taken before, during, or after a meal and what foods or drinks the meal contains. These factors affect the level of the drug that is absorbed from the intestines into the bloodstream. Foods that delay movement through the intestines can increase the amount, while foods that speed movement through the intestines (such as those high in fiber) can reduce it. Some foods interact chemically with certain drugs, interactions that the drug's patient information sheet or package label identifies. Levodopa, an AMINO ACID, competes for absorption with other amino acids, including dietary proteins, that are being digested and metabolized as the body can only accept so much amino acid at one time.

bioethics The study of, and guidelines for, moral and ethical issues in medicine and medical research. Bioethics has far-reaching implications in areas of research and treatment and is often at the core of disagreement and debate around matters such as using animals for research and experimentation, using people in research studies, calculating the benefit-to-risk ratio of treatment options, and making treatment decisions including end of life choices and care. Current bioethical flash points in Parkinson's research are fetal STEM CELL research and fetal stem cell therapy.

All research facilities are required to have bioethics guidelines that include elements such as informed consent and full disclosure of risks and benefits. This is particularly important when studies involve the use of placebos (inert substances), so human volunteers know whether they are forgoing medical care by participating in the study and what the possible consequences are. For conditions such as Parkinson's disease that at present have no cure and treatment options that are less than ideal, people often are willing to try experimental drugs and procedures in the hope that the outcome will be better than what conventional approaches can provide. It is essential for researchers to present realistic expectations for both benefit and risk.

See also CLINICAL RESEARCH STUDIES; INFORMED CONSENT; INVESTIGATIONAL NEW DRUG.

biofeedback A method of learning to identify body signals to control body responses. Learning biofeedback techniques requires training and guidance from a therapist who specializes in this area, but once learned the techniques can be used anywhere at any time. There are different approaches and forms of biofeedback. The most common uses sensors attached to the fingertips. These sensors measure the tiniest changes in perspiration, which electrodes convey to a machine that converts them into visible (lights) or audible (tones) signals. Increased perspiration is one of the body's earliest responses to various stressful stimuli, ranging from physical pain to emotional stress and anxiety.

Biofeedback integrates the identification of such stimuli with methods to reduce their stress. In response to the lights or tones from the biofeedback machine, the person focuses on the method he or she prefers, which can be visualization, guided imagery, meditation, breath control or breathing exercises, or another STRESS REDUCTION TECHNIQUE. As the method begins to calm the person, the intensity of biofeedback signals decreases. When the level of perspiration that the fingertip sensors detect falls below the stress threshold, the signals stop.

With practice, the person learns to identify his or her stress responses without signals from the sensors and machine and implements the appropriate method to stop the response. It generally takes six to 15 sessions to reach this point, when the machine is no longer necessary. The person can practice biofeedback anywhere at any time. Biofeedback is also an effective treatment for migraine headaches and some kinds of chronic pain.

See also ALTERNATIVE THERAPIES; LIFESTYLE FACTORS; MEDITATION; YOGA.

biomarker A common factor that is always present in a particular disease or medical condition. Biomarkers can be gene mutations such as those that identify HUNTINGTON'S DISEASE cellular changes such as those that identify cancer, or an abnormal level of a chemical such as glucose in the blood that identifies diabetes. The presence of a biomarker makes it possible to diagnose conclusively, and sometimes even screen for, the condition. At present, there are no biomarkers for Parkinson's disease. As a result, as many as 20 percent of those diagnosed with Parkinson's disease are found later to have a different medical condition. It is likely that even more people, who do have the disease, are not diagnosed accurately, although this percentage is more difficult to determine. Such diagnostic uncertainty means that some people receive unnecessary treatment and others may fail to receive treatment that could delay a condition's progress (although unfortunately there is no such treatment to date for Parkinson's disease).

Research to identify biomarkers for Parkinson's is ongoing; some of the most promising results have been gained from increased understanding of the brain's biochemical functions. Sophisticated imaging techniques such as Functional Magnetic Resonance Imaging (FMRI), SINGLE PHOTON EMISSION TOMOGRAPHY (SPECT), and POSITRON EMISSION TOMOGRAPHY (PET) make it possible for researchers to "see" the inner workings of the brain, gaining new insights and information.

See also CLINICAL RESEARCH STUDIES; CONDITIONS SIMILAR TO PARKINSON'S; DIAGNOSING PARKINSON'S; HOPE FOR A PARKINSON'S CURE; NEUROTROPHIC FACTORS.

blepharospasm Involuntary contraction involving the muscles of the eyelid that causes the eyelid to close. The closure can be brief or prolonged, may be partial or complete, and may involve one or both eyes. When blepharospasm involves both eyes simultaneously, it can cause complete inability to see (temporary blindness). Blepharospasm can occur as an independent, IDIOPATHIC condition; as a symptom of brain or nerve damage; or in neuro-logic conditions such as Parkinson's disease. In Parkinson's disease, blepharospasm can be the result of rigidity that affects the muscles of the eyelids and other facial features or a consequence of long-term LEVODOPA treatment. Bright lights and exposure to environmental irritants such as wind and dust can cause or worsen blepharospasm episodes regardless of their cause.

Most people receive long-term and nearly complete relief from BOTULINUM TOXIN THERAPY (BTX) injections into the eyelids, which paralyze small segments of the muscles. Muscle relaxants such as CLONAZEPAM or baclofen and ANTICHOLINERGIC MEDICATIONS such as TRIHEXYPHENIDYL also provide relief, although they have systemic effects that are sometimes undesired (drowsiness with muscle relaxants and drowsiness or excessive drying of mucous tissues with anticholinergics). If blepharospasm is a likely side effect of a levodopa dosage, usually reduction of the dosage is necessary to relieve the blepharospasm fully. Generally when the levodopa dosage is to blame, there are other symptoms (such as nausea and DYSKINESIA) as well.

See also BLURRY VISION; EYE MOVEMENTS; MEDICATION SIDE EFFECTS; MYOCLONUS; VISION PROBLEMS.

blink rate The number of times in a minute that the eyelids close spontaneously. In a healthy person, the blink rate ranges from 10 closures per minute during activities such as reading or watching television to 30 closures per minute during conversation. In a person with Parkinson's disease, the blink rate can be as slow as zero to five closures in a minute regardless of activity. This is a manifestation of dopamine depletion in the STRIATUM, the brain structure responsible for muscle movement and coordination, that results in rigidity of the muscles of the eyelids. This rigidity causes the lids to stay open.

One function of blinking is to bathe the eye in tears to help flush away irritants and debris. When spontaneous blinking is reduced, the eye can become dry and painful. Usually the person with Parkinson's can consciously blink; making the effort to do so on a regular basis during waking hours can help offset decreased spontaneous

blinking. Using artificial tear eye drops to keep the eye lubricated and clear of debris helps reduce irritation.

Sometimes rigidity can affect the lower eyelid to the extent that it pulls somewhat away from the surface of the eye. This allows tears to spill over the lid and run down the face, giving the impression that the person is crying. Blink rate returns to normal or near-normal when treatment, such as administration of DOPAMINE AGONIST MEDICATIONS, early in the disease or LEVODOPA as Parkinson's progresses, restores other muscle function. As treatment effectiveness declines in later stages of the disease, blink rate again slows as other symptoms also worsen.

See also BLEPHAROSPASM; BLURRY VISION; EYE MOVEMENTS; VISION PROBLEMS.

blood-brain barrier A dense layer of endothelial cells that line the interior of blood vessels in the brain to form a semipermeable membrane that significantly limits the molecules that can pass from the blood into the brain. The blood-brain barrier is a protective mechanism that prevents potentially harmful substances from affecting the brain. Glucose and oxygen, the main fuel sources for cells, easily cross the blood-brain barrier. Other molecules are able to cross the blood-brain barrier after binding with endothelial transport proteins. Among them are choline, essential for making acetycholine, and amino acids. As LEVODOPA is an amino acid, it is among the molecules that can make the passage. DOPAMINE, along with other NEUROTRANSMITTERS, cannot. These restrictions help the brain to maintain the intricate and delicate biochemical balance that makes its functions possible.

Although scientists have known of the blood-brain barrier's existence since the early 1900s, there is little understanding of the exact way it works. In capillaries throughout the rest of the body the endothelial cells are less tightly aligned than those in the capillaries in the brain, a structure that allows broad passage of molecules between the blood and body tissues. What causes this layer to "tighten" in the brain remains a mystery that scientists are only now beginning to unravel. In 2000, researchers at the University of

Maryland School of Medicine isolated two proteins that appear to activate the transport proteins that bind with the molecules that are permitted to make the passage. The binding excludes far more molecules than it permits, and the selection process appears to accommodate factors in addition to the molecule's size. The molecules of certain diseases, for example, are able to cross the blood-brain barrier while antibiotics and other therapeutic drugs cannot.

The blood-brain barrier presents a key challenge in treating a diverse range of neurological disorders including ALZHEIMER'S DISEASE, MULTIPLE SCLEROSIS, AMYOTROPHIC LATERAL SCLEROSIS (ALS), MUSCULAR DYSTROPHY, and of course Parkinson's disease. Were it possible to manipulate access across the blood-brain barrier, it would be possible to target therapies to act directly on the involved portions of the brain. Because the potential of such an approach is both tantalizing and promising, there is much ongoing research in this area.

See also HOPE FOR A PARKINSON'S CURE; MEDICATION MANAGEMENT.

blurry vision   Difficulty in seeing clearly. Many people with Parkinson's disease experience VISION PROBLEMS. Blurry vision is one of the most common and likely results from a combination of factors, include

- Inadequate tears, either as a side effect of treatment with ANTICHOLINERGIC MEDICATIONS or as a result of eyelid rigidity and reduced BLINK RATE that allow tears to escape instead of lubricating the eye. TRICYCLIC ANTIDEPRESSANT MEDICATIONS and ANTIHISTAMINE MEDICATIONS also can cause dry eyes.

- Excessive tearing as a consequence of irritants that have entered the eye because of reduced spontaneous BLINK RATE.

- Parkinson's-related BRADYKINESIA affecting the muscles that control the eyes, causing slowed eye movements. This condition can make focusing difficult.

- Other Parkinson's-related disturbances of muscle activity affecting the muscles that control the eyes that can influence focus by preventing the eyes from properly aligning when looking at close objects.

- Cataracts, cloudy growths within the lens of the eye, that appear to form a film over it. Cataracts are common with increasing age and are not related to Parkinson's disease.

- Anticholinergic medications may cause the pupil to enlarge such that light does not focus on the retina as it should. A common parlor trick, in which a person who requires glasses can clearly see through a pinhole held up to their eye without wearing glasses, illustrates this principle.

- People with the rare form of glaucoma known as angle-closure glaucoma might have an acute worsening of their vision with starting levodopa. This would be an indication that the pressure inside the eye is going up and that levodopa should be immediately discontinued.

It is not appropriate to assume blurry vision is just another symptom of Parkinson's. There are many treatable reasons for vision problems, and it is important to have a comprehensive eye examination by an ophthalmologist to make sure that one or more of them is not responsible.

body care   Maintaining of good personal hygiene. Many people with Parkinson's disease experience excess sweating and changes in the skin and hair. The skin may become very oily, especially on the face. The scalp, too, may become oily or develop dandruff. More frequent washing and shampooing can relieve these symptoms. Skin astringents can help dry the oiliness of the skin, and dandruff-control shampoos can improve the appearance of the hair. Some people with Parkinson's find that they have the opposite problem, however: dry skin and hair.

Excess sweating can be either a consequence of damage to the structures of the brain and autonomic nervous system that occur with Parkinson's disease or the side effect of the wearing off of ANTI-PARKINSON'S MEDICATIONS, especially LEVODOPA. DOPAMINE plays a role in the brain's temperature response mechanisms. As Parkinson's progresses, some people experience profuse, drenching sweating with OFF-STATE episodes. BETA-ADRENERGIC

BLOCKER medications or adjustment of the dosing of anti-Parkinson's medications can sometimes mitigate this symptom.

The movement dysfunctions of Parkinson's make body care and personal hygiene difficult to handle independently. TREMORS and RIGIDITY can prevent a person from holding a bar of soap or applying it to the body. Balance problems present falling hazards in the shower or bath. Applying skin care products such as lotions and taking care of needs such as shaving may require assistance. It is also important to protect the body from bruises, scrapes, and cuts and to take care of these injuries when they occur. As movement becomes more restricted the possibility of pressure sores or BEDSORES increases. Frequent changes of position, whether sitting or lying down, can help prevent this.

See also BATHING AND BATHROOM ORGANIZATION; BEDROOM COMFORT; DENTAL CARE AND HYGIENE.

body image The perception a person has about his or her physical appearance. The physical changes that take place as Parkinson's disease progresses can be distressing for the person with Parkinson's as well as for friends and family members. RIGIDITY, TREMORS, and DYSKINESIAS alter the way the body looks and feels. It is often especially difficult to lose the ability to make facial expressions, as much human communication takes place in this way. Self-consciousness is common and can cause the person to limit social interactions such as going shopping, out to dinner, or to the movies—activities that he or she once enjoyed. It is important, albeit difficult, to remember that the changes that Parkinson's disease causes are beyond control. Concern about body image can lead to DEPRESSION, and depression (which affects about 40 percent of those who have Parkinson's disease) can feed worries about body image.

See also SELF-ESTEEM.

body scheme An internalized sense of body parts and where they are in relation to each other. The body scheme represents a learned model that the brain stores to help it maintain a constant, although not conscious, awareness of the body's position. This model becomes the backdrop or foundation for the feedback loop that provides brain structures involved in movement—such as the BASAL GANGLIA and the cerebellum—the information they need to send nerve signals to the muscles. The body scheme streamlines the neural communication process by allowing the BRAIN to send what amount to preprogrammed messages for common movements. Signals back from the muscles, as well as other body structures such as the balance organs of the inner ear, then allow for fine-tuning. All of this takes place at incredible speed so that movement appears smooth and continuous.

The body scheme tends to remain as originally learned even when the physical structure or function of the body changes until those changes have been present for some time. An adolescent who experiences a rapid and dramatic growth spurt seems not to have any sense that he is suddenly six inches taller and constantly hits his head until his body scheme finally readjusts. Someone who gains a substantial amount of weight might continually misjudge the amount of space his or her body requires—not because he or she is unaware that the body's size has increased but because the body scheme still perceives the body as small. A person who loses a limb tends to act as though the limb is still present, and often perceives that it is, although obviously it is not. Movement messages might still attempt to signal for an amputated arm to reach out to hold open a door, for example, because that is what the body scheme is programmed to do. The body scheme also accommodates physical responses to the environment. A person who is unusually tall continually ducks when going through doorways because the body scheme has become programmed to do so even when there is adequate head clearance. Over time, however, the body scheme readjusts and adapts to the new set of circumstances.

People with Parkinson's disease tend not to have an awareness of where their bodies are or what their bodies are doing. The brain fails to recognize that the body scheme and the body are no longer synchronized, even to the extent of responding as though signals sent have achieved the intended results. The brain may not perceive, for example, that the feet are not moving and continue to send movement messages to them as though they are still engaged in the activity of walking. Similarly the brain fails to respond to loss of balance with signals for corrective movements, allowing the person to fall without making any apparent effort to regain balance or stop the fall. Any responses that do take place happen too slowly to be effective. For the person with Parkinson's disease, paying constant, conscious attention to movement, location of body parts, and the surroundings helps to overcome disorientation to body scheme.

See also BALANCE; EQUILIBRIUM; FALLS; GAIT; GAIT DISTURBANCE.

botulinum toxin therapy Treatment for SPASTIC-ITY and DYSTONIA that consists of injecting small amounts of botulinum toxin into the affected muscles to paralyze them. Botulinum toxin is a protein that blocks ACETYLCHOLINE release. If botulinum toxin enters the body systemically, as in botulism poisoning, it acts on all muscles, creating a dangerous and potentially fatal paralysis. When injected into a specific muscle group, it affects only those muscles. The amount of botulinum toxin used in muscle injections is also very small, further limiting the severity of any inadvertent transfer of it in the systemic circulation. In people with Parkinson's, botulinum toxin therapy is often effective in relieving BLEPHAROSPASMS and severe foot or other dystonias. A treatment typically relieves symptoms for three to six months. This treatment is one of the ADJUNCT THERAPIES; it does not eliminate the need for ANTI-PARKINSON'S MEDICATIONS. Two types of botulinum toxin currently are available on the market, and their actions are roughly the same though their dosing is different. Therapeutic botulinum toxin type A is marketed under the brand name product Botox and botulinum toxin type B is marketed as Myobloc.

bradykinesia Slowness of movement. Bradykinesia is one of the CARDINAL SYMPTOMS, and earliest symptoms, of Parkinson's disease. Typically, it begins with the kinds of slowness that are easy to attribute to the normal changes of aging. There might be some hesitation or difficulty in rising from a chair, in getting out of bed, or in starting to walk.

Reactions, such as to unexpected obstacles or the appearance of other people when walking, are also slow. The person might trip over the obstacle or bump into someone else, even though to an observer it appears that there was plenty of time to react and avoid. As Parkinson's disease emerges more completely, bradykinesia begins to affect other aspects of movement. It can become difficult to hold cooking and eating utensils, for example, or to brush the teeth, comb the hair, button the shirt, and participate in the myriad ACTIVITIES OF DAILY LIVING. It also becomes difficult to do more than one thing at once and to engage in repetitive movements.

Because this slowness appears to be intentional, family members and friends often become impatient. However, the person with Parkinson's might not even recognize that his or her movements have slowed, or realize the extent to which they have slowed, in this early stage of the disease's development unless someone else points it out. Later in the course of the disease bradykinesia becomes frustrating for the person with Parkinson's as well because the slowness extends to additional symptoms such as start hesitation and freezing of gait, as the person wants to move but the muscles will not. Bradykinesia also affects muscles involved with swallowing, speech, facial expressions, and handwriting, slowing these functions as well.

Bradykinesia remains a hallmark symptom of Parkinson's, worsening as the disease progresses. It is the result of the growing imbalance in the brain, particularly in the BASAL GANGLIA, between DOPAMINE and ACETYLCHOLINE levels. As dopamine-producing cells in the SUBSTANTIA NIGRA die off, the level of dopamine diminishes. Without dopamine to facilitate the intricate intercommunications among neurons that make smooth, consistent, coordinated movement possible, acetylcholine-transmitted signals to the muscles become erratic and jumbled. Muscles respond inappropriately and dysfunctionally, and TREMORS, RIGIDITY, and other DYSKINESIAS also emerge. Bradykinesia accounts for much of the difficulty with BALANCE and WALKING that plagues people with Parkinson's disease. Movement requires smooth and continuous interaction between the body's muscles and the brain. A disruption anywhere in the process spawns further disruptions, as when the wheel of a train falls off the track.

Treatment with LEVODOPA, DOPAMINE AGONIST MEDICATIONS such as PRAMIPEXOLE or ROPINEROLE and other ANTI-PARKINSON'S MEDICATIONS can restore relatively normal muscle function and movement for years and even decades in the majority of people diagnosed with Parkinson's disease. PHYSICAL THERAPY including RANGE OF MOTION exercises and OCCUPATIONAL THERAPY for training in using ADAPTIVE EQUIPMENT AND ASSIST DEVICES can mitigate the disruption bradykinesia and other Parkinson's symptoms cause in daily living. Staying as active as possible, maintaining a sense of humor, and enlisting the assistance and support of friends and family are also helpful. For the person with Parkinson's, it is especially important to cultivate conscious awareness of the body's movements and to plan them. Walking from the bedroom to the kitchen, for example, might require maneuvering narrow spaces (hallways), corners, and stairs. Knowing that these challenges are going to occur, and where they are, allows additional time to respond.

See also ADJUSTING TO LIVING WITH PARKINSON'S; AKINESIA; COGWHEELING; DAILY LIVING CHALLENGES; DIAGNOSING PARKINSON'S; GAIT; GAIT DISTURBANCES; PATTERNED MOVEMENTS.

bradyphrenia   Slowness of thinking and COGNITIVE FUNCTIONS. A person with bradyphrenia might hesitate in responding to a question or stop talking in midsentence, forget how to perform formerly familiar activities such as prepare a sandwich or unlock a door, or find once-common functions such as balancing a checkbook or counting out money to pay for a purchase at the store incomprehensible mysteries. Typically these problems appear in the later stages of Parkinson's disease and fluctuate, as do motor impairment symptoms. That is, they worsen during OFF-STATE times and improve, with ANTI-PARKINSON'S MEDICATIONS, during ON-STATE times.

There is some debate about whether, and to what extent, bradyphrenia is a manifestation of Parkinson's disease. Almost everyone who has Parkinson's to some degree during the course of the disease shows the four characteristic neuromuscular CARDINAL SYMPTOMS: resting TREMOR, BRADYKINESIA, RIGIDITY, and POSTURAL INSTABILITY. Only about half of those with Parkinson's disease experience problems with cognitive functions such as concentration, memory, and thought processes. Some neurologists believe that bradyphrenia and cognitive impairment are the result of other deteriorations that are concurrently taking place in the brain such as those caused by ALZHEIMER'S DISEASE.

This is an intriguing concept because there is such a high cross-incidence of Alzheimer's and Parkinson's. This assessment draws from observations that some but not all people with Parkinson's disease develop cognitive impairments and some but not all people with Alzheimer's disease develop motor impairments. Still other neurologists believe that cognition impairments in elderly people with Parkinson's occur as part of the normal aging process or reflect an ACCELERATED AGING process, drawing attention because the other symptoms of Parkinson's make all impairments more obvious.

Bradyphrenia frequently responds to ANTI-PARKINSON'S MEDICATIONS taken to relieve motor impairments. However, in some people these drugs, particularly ANTICHOLINERGIC DRUGS, cause or exacerbate cognitive impairment. Although anticholinergic drugs can improve movement and motor function by establishing a better balance between acetylcholine and dopamine levels in the brain, the suppression of acetylcholine production can reduce thinking capability and memory, as acetylcholine is essential for cognitive function. Finding a therapeutic balance is often a matter of trial and error, and sometimes of making choices about which emphasis is more important for the person with Parkinson's disease. New ACETYLCHOLINESTERASE INHIBITOR drugs being used to treat cognitive decline and dementia in people with Alzheimer's disease, such as DONEPEZIL (sold as the brand name product Aricept) and RIVASTIGMINE (sold as the brand name product Exelon), sometimes improve cognitive function in people with Parkinson's disease.

Some people find that memory and thinking abilities improve with vitamin B_6 and vitamin B_{12} supplementation. *Ginkgo biloba* is helpful for some people, but those taking aspirin or other "blood-thinning" agents must use caution. Because the potential for thyroid deficiency (hypothyroidism) increases with age and because that deficiency can cause problems with concentration and memory, anyone showing signs of cognitive impairment should be tested for it. Cognitive symptoms cease when thyroid hormone replacement therapy restores blood thyroid levels to normal. Activities that require thinking, concentration, and memory help maintain cognitive functions. Because these activities also require fine motor coordination—such as writing for crossword puzzles, holding books and turning pages for READING, moving game pieces for board games like chess—being creative in finding ways to overcome limitations or finding alternative activities often becomes necessary. There are assist devices to hold books open, and art supply stores carry "fat" pencils and gripping devices that attach to any pen or pencil to make it easier to hold. A friend or family member might enjoy helping with a board game. Listening to books on tape or to music is another alternative that activates the brain; a large-button tape player, such as those marketed for young children, makes this activity easier.

See also ADAPTIVE EQUIPMENT AND ASSIST DEVICES; ADJUSTING TO LIVING WITH PARKINSON'S; APOPTOSIS; CONFUSION; DAILY LIVING CHALLENGES; DEXTERITY, MENTAL.

brain The primary organ of the NERVOUS SYSTEM, responsible for all conscious thought and voluntary actions as well as the unconscious, automatic functions that sustain life such as breathing and heart rate. The brain, which weighs two and a half to three pounds in a healthy adult, consists of three major parts: the cerebrum, cerebellum, and brainstem. The cerebrum is sometimes called the "conscious" brain because it handles the functions of consciousness and voluntary actions, and the cerebellum and brainstem the "unconscious" brain because they handle involuntary actions that do not require or respond to conscious intervention.

Coordinating their functions requires close interaction among neurons that comprise these structures, which send a multitude of signals, in the form of electrical impulses, throughout the brain. Visualization through an electron microscope shows that a single neuron in the brain can connect with a thousand other neurons in nearly countless combinations. In this way, millions of transmissions take place every second. NEUROTRANSMITTERS such as DOPAMINE, epinephrine, NOREPINEPHRINE, serotonin, and ACETYLCHOLINE facilitate specific kinds of transmissions.

Cerebrum

The cerebrum is the largest and most sophisticated structure of the brain. Its pair of lobes, the right and left hemispheres, fill most of the skull. The cerebrum's hemispheres are contralateral: That is, functions of the right hemisphere relate to the left side of the body and functions of the left hemisphere relate to the right side of the body. Each hemisphere has functionally distinct (but not physically apparent) areas that manage specialized functions, generally divided into four lobes that bear the names of the bones of the skull above them. The lobes have comparable but not identical functions in each hemisphere. Because the lobes are not physically distinct from one another, their functions overlap and also are closely integrated.

The cerebrum's billions of nerve cells, or NEURONS, conduct all cognitive functions such as

Cerebral Lobe	Location	General Functions	Effect of Parkinson's Disease
Frontal	Front (forehead)	Thought, speech, and voluntary muscle actions	Bradyphrenia; voice modulation and speech problems; dyskinesia, tremors, rigidity that interferes with or prevents intended muscle actions
Temporal	Side	Auditory information; language, and word meanings	Cognitive and memory disturbances
Parietal	Top	Sensory information such as touch, taste, pressure, pain, temperature	Occasional disturbances in taste and smell
Occipital	Back	Visual information	Inability to control eye muscles that can distort visual information that travels from the eyes to the brain

thought, language, and memory and also handle sensory and voluntary movement functions. The outer layer of cells are called the cerebral cortex; these densely packed neuron bodies have a grayish appearance. The cerebral cortex is the region of the cerebrum where most cognitive functions take place. The inner layer of the cerebrum is called white matter; it contains mostly AXONS enclosed in protective MYELIN SHEATHS, which give them their whitish appearance. The white matter is the region of the cerebrum that carries sensory and motor information to and from the brain. The motor areas of the cerebral cortex direct the voluntary muscle movements such as walking, climbing, running, dancing, and other activities, although it is the cerebellum and BASAL GANGLIA that give feedback which affects the specific instructions the muscles that carry out these movements receive.

Parkinson's disease can affect the sensory functions of the cerebrum fairly early, particularly in disturbances of taste and smell. Although the association between DOPAMINE depletion and Parkinson's disease focuses on motor impairment, there is evidence that it also has a direct effect on the functioning of the frontal lobe. Cognitive impairments typically occur later in the disease, and not in all people with Parkinson's. BRADYPHRENIA, MEMORY PROBLEMS, and thought disturbances that effect reasoning and activities such as math calculations are among the cognitive impairments that are common. Speech difficulties and slowness to respond due to rigidity of the muscles of the face and mouth can give an incorrect impression that there is cognitive impairment. Cognitive impairment also can be the result of ALZHEIMER'S DISEASE, which affects many people who have Parkinson's disease.

Although Parkinson's disease does not directly affect the cerebral cortex's control over voluntary muscle actions (as do other neurologic disorders such as CEREBRAL PALSY), motor impairment symptoms that result when dopamine depletion occurs alter the normal muscle response. When there is a decision to engage in voluntary movement—such as to rise from a seated position and walk across the room—the cerebral cortex sends a barrage of signals to the cerebellum and to the basal ganglia. This transmittal route seems to remain undisturbed in Parkinson's disease. Rather, problems arise after

the signals enter the cerebellum and the basal ganglia, where there is insufficient dopamine to continue the communication. The cerebellum and the basal ganglia are unable to send out the correct and appropriate feedback signals back to the cerebral cortex and muscles resulting in erratic signals to the muscles, causing motor impairment symptoms such as TREMORS, freezing and BRADYKINESIA. ANTI-PARKINSON'S MEDICATIONS can also cause motor impairment symptoms such as dyskinesias, but these are not related to cerebral functions.

Cerebellum

The cerebellum regulates balance, posture, and coordination. Located below the cerebrum and behind the brainstem, the cerebellum is connected to both of these structures. Like the cerebrum, the cerebellum has two hemispheres, each with an outer layer of cortex and an inner layer of white matter. The cerebellum's cortex has no cognitive function. Instead, as does the white matter, it participates in the functions of voluntary movement. Between the cortex and the white matter is a layer called Purkinje's cells, which have extraordinarily long DENDRITES. Purkinje's cells form an extensive network that rapidly sends and receives nerve impulses related to movement. The cerebellum continually responds to these impulses by sending back other impulses, which adjust muscle response and balance to keep movement smooth and continuous. Unlike the cerebrum, the hemispheres of the cerebellum are ipsilateral: They correlate to the same side of the body. The left cerebellar hemisphere acts on the left side of the body and the right cerebellar hemisphere acts on the right side of the body.

Brainstem

The brainstem, located within the protective base of the skull, is the most primitive structure of the nervous system and controls the body's basic and involuntary functions. Approximately three inches in length, the brainstem bridges the cerebrum and the spinal cord, connecting these two structures and functioning as the conduit for communication between the brain and the body. The cerebellum attaches to the back of the brainstem. Ten of the 12 pairs of cranial nerves, the body's primary nerve "highways" for transmitting nerve signals between the brain and the body including those responsible for movement and motor functions, pass through the brain stem. Changes take place in the brainstem as Parkinson's disease progresses; scientists do not fully understand whether they are in response to or part of the disease process.

Reticular formation A network of nerves that forms the core of the brainstem, the reticular formation traverses and integrates with the brainstem's other functional structures. Although the reticular formation's primary function is to regulate breathing and heart rate, certain locations also participate in posture, movement, and level of consciousness.

Midbrain The midbrain joins directly to the cerebrum; the basal ganglia extend from beneath the cerebrum into the midbrain. The midbrain contains the SUBSTANTIA NIGRA. The pigmented dopamine-producing cells of the substantia nigra cells die as Parkinson's disease progresses, causing the decline of dopamine available in the brain. Tumors of the midbrain (not related to Parkinson's disease) can cause DYSTONIA (muscle rigidity and spasms).

Pons Bearing the Latin name for its function, the pons is a tissue "bridge" between the midbrain and the medulla oblongata, containing a mix of cells common to each structure. It also extends thick fibers of nerves, resembling cables, into the cerebellum. The pons also contains the paramedian pontine reticular formation (PPRF), a cluster of nerves responsible for horizontal eye movements. These movements are sometimes impaired in people with Parkinson's disease. An area of the pons called the locus ceruleus contains cells that make and store NOREPINEPHRINE, a NEUROTRANSMITTER essential for cognitive functions. Recent research shows that these cells die as Parkinson's disease advances, presenting a possible explanation for DEMENTIA, MEMORY IMPAIRMENT, and COGNITIVE DYSFUNCTION.

Medulla oblongata *Medulla* means "marrow," a reference to the thick nerve bundles that this structure contains; *oblongata* refers to its cylindrical appearance. The medulla oblongata merges into the top of the spinal cord, although its functions are separate, and is similar in appearance to the spinal cord. It contains the nerve centers that regulate breathing, heart rate, blood pressure, and digestion. Most of the nerve bundles, including the ninth through the 12th cranial nerves, that pass through the medulla oblongata cross at the point of exit from the medulla so those nuclei on the left serve nerves going to the right side of the body and those nuclei on the right serve nerves going to the left side of the body.

See also NERVOUS SYSTEM.

brain-derived neurotrophic factors (BDNFs) Natural substances, usually proteins, that stimulate the growth of new nerve cells (neurons) in the brain. BDNFs, which were discovered in the 1980s, are found primarily in the cells of the developing fetal brain. They are the critical substances in FETAL DOPAMINERGIC CELL TRANSPLANT and FETAL PORCINE BRAIN CELL TRANSPLANT, both of which are experimental treatments in the early stages of research. When BDNFs from dopamine-producing cells are experimentally injected into the STRIATUM of an animal with an experimental model of Parkinson's disease, they cause new dopamine-producing cells to start growing. This represents exciting potential in treatment for not only Parkinson's disease but other conditions and injuries caused by damage to brain or nerve cells such as stroke and spinal cord injuries.

The body produces a number of different NEUROTROPHIC FACTORS, or nerve-generating substances; ongoing research is exploring their potential as well. Other research is focusing on developing sources of BDNFs such as genetically engineering them in the laboratory, because using donor sources (human or animal) is controversial as well as limiting. The molecules of BDNFs and other neurotrophic factors are too large to pass through the blood-brain barrier; therefore, at present any therapeutic use of these substances involves injecting them directly into the brain.

See also BASAL GANGLIA.

brain tissue transplant Experimental treatment in which dopaminergic cells are injected into the brain of a person with Parkinson's disease. Sources of these cells have included human fetal dopaminergic cells, porcine fetal dopaminergic cells, human retinal pigment epithelial cells, and autograft using adrenal medullary tissue (which has limited dopamine-producing capabilities). The risk-to-benefit ratio of brain tissue transplant still remains unacceptably high. Results are inconsistent and complications can be significant. However, research continues in this area and there is much hope that future treatment for Parkinson's disease (as well as other neurodegenerative conditions) will incorporate the kind of long-lasting or even permanent effects that such transplants could make possible.

See also ADRENAL MEDULLARY TRANSPLANT; FETAL DOPAMINERGIC CELL TRANSPLANT; FETAL PORCINE BRAIN CELL TRANSPLANT; HOPE FOR A PARKINSON'S CURE; RETINAL CELL IMPLANT.

breath control The ability to adjust one's breathing. The RIGIDITY of Parkinson's disease often affects the muscles of the throat, neck, and trunk of the body. This has a twofold effect. One is that it creates a slumping posture that restricts the movement of the lungs, limiting the amount of air that each breath draws in. As well, the muscles do not respond as they should, often producing shallow breathing. The other effect is that speech becomes difficult. Poor breath control creates problems in modulating the tone of the voice, as it restricts the force with which the person can push air through the vocal cords.

People with Parkinson's disease can improve breath control through YOGA breathing and other methods such as repeating a one-syllable word as many times as possible on the same breath, singing, and blowing into a musical instrument or even a bottle in such a way as to generate sound. Consciously working on projecting the voice and singing are exercises that many speech pathologists employ. Physical activities such as stretching and RANGE OF MOTION EXERCISES to improve posture and the chest's ability to expand are also helpful. Regular physical activity such as swimming helps to keep muscles more flexible and improve lung capacity.

breathing exercises See YOGA.

bromocriptine A DOPAMINE RECEPTOR AGONIST DRUG that mimics the action of DOPAMINE, stimulating DOPAMINE RECEPTORS in the brain. Bromacriptine (Parlodel) is an ergot alkaloid that primarily binds with the D2 receptors in the STRIATUM, although it also has an effect on D1 receptors. It has been in use to treat Parkinson's disease since 1975 and until recently has been primarily an adjunct therapy to enhance the effectiveness of LEVODOPA and relieve fluctuating response. New research suggests that bromocriptine and other dopamine agonists are as effective as levodopa as MONOTHERAPY in relieving symptoms in people newly diagnosed with Parkinson's disease. This treatment approach extends the period that ANTI-PARKINSON'S MEDICATIONS are useful. Levodopa-induced motor complications, such as dyskinesias and on-off phenomenon, can be avoided.

Bromocriptine can take three or four months to reach full effectiveness or to be found to be ineffective. Common side effects include drowsiness, ORTHOSTATIC HYPOTENSION, nausea, headache, and tingling in the hands and feet called ergotism. These side effects, if they occur, usually go away by the time the drug reaches full effectiveness. Some people develop hallucinations and even psychosis while taking bromocriptine; when this happens, trying a different dopamine agonist is the often best response. Fibrosis of a number of organs is also a risk that accompanies the use of bromocriptine and other ergot-derived dopamine agonists. Bromocriptine interacts with the antibiotic erythromycin, so these two drugs should not be taken at the same time. Bromocriptine also acts to lower blood levels of the hormone prolactin, with the potential to increase sexual desire. Bromocriptine is available in generic form and as the brand name product Parlodel. In the opinion of most experts, the newer nonergotamine agonists ropinerole and pramipexole are the dopamine agonists of first choice, followed by pergolide and other ergotamine agonists such as cabergoline and bromocriptine.

bruxism Involuntarily grinding the teeth together. The RIGIDITY and SPASMS of Parkinson's disease can affect the muscles of the jaw, causing the jaw to clamp shut. This puts tremendous force on the teeth and can cause them to wear down over time or even break. It also can interfere with eating, drinking, and speaking when it prevents the mouth from opening.

Bruxism, as do many Parkinson's symptoms, tends to lessen or disappear during an ON-STATE and worsen or return during an OFF-STATE. Treatment for bruxism, then, is the same as for other motor symptoms of Parkinson's disease. Muscle relaxants (antispasmodic drugs) such as CLONAZEPAM or ANTI-CHOLINERGIC MEDICATIONS such as TRIHEXYPHENIDYL sometimes provide relief, although they can have undesired systemic effects such as drowsiness and, with anticholinergics, DRY MOUTH. When bruxism is so severe that it prevents opening the mouth and chewing, BOTULINUM TOXIN THERAPY is often effective for immediate and long-term relief. These injections paralyze small segments of the muscles, causing them to relax.

See also DYSTONIA; SWALLOWING.

burnout   The sense of being physically, mentally, and emotionally exhausted. Burnout is a significant risk for family members who are the primary caregivers for loved ones who have Parkinson's disease. In the early stages of Parkinson's disease, the person generally has a high level of independent function and can adequately manage most if not all the ACTIVITIES OF DAILY LIVING (ADLs) and the tasks that he or she performed before the onset of symptoms. As the disease progresses, however, independence declines. The person becomes more reliant on others for assistance with everyday functions from bathing and dressing to eating and moving. Caregivers often feel frustrated and guilty because their best efforts cannot change the course of the disease. By the late stages of Parkinson's, the person becomes totally dependent and requires constant attention even at night. Difficulty managing bedclothes and turning in bed makes sleeping difficult as well,

leaving the caregiver sleep-deprived and physically exhausted.

The emotional challenges of caring for a loved one who has Parkinson's disease also can become overwhelming, particularly as the disease progresses. MOOD SWINGS, ANXIETY or DEPRESSION (or both), COGNITIVE IMPAIRMENT, and DEMENTIA are difficult symptoms for caregivers to accommodate and may result in erratic or inappropriate behavior. Caregivers often feel that they are watching their loved one slip away or turn into a stranger yet are helpless to intervene; emotional distress and depression can result.

Common signs of burnout include:

- Feeling hopeless and helpless
- Feeling that there is no life beyond caring for the person with Parkinson's
- Absence of interests and activities that do not involve caring for the person with Parkinson's
- Weight loss or weight gain
- Changes in sleep habits (sleeping too much, insomnia, or waking up too early)
- Lack of energy
- Frequent illnesses
- Continual complaining, irritability, and negative attitude

RESPITE CARE, in which someone else stays with the person who has Parkinson's disease so the caregiver can get away for a few hours, and SUPPORT GROUPS in which caregivers can share their experiences, frustrations, and fears are among the means that can help caregivers prevent burnout. It helps, too, if other family members, friends, or even neighbors can step in for a few hours here and there to give the primary caregiver a break and can listen to and be supportive of the caregiver.

See also CAREGIVER WELL-BEING; COPING WITH ONGOING CARE OF PARKINSON'S; GRIEF.

cabergoline A long-acting DOPAMINE AGONIST MEDICATION taken to counter the adverse effects of LEVODOPA. Cabergoline is a synthetic ergot alkaloid that targets D2 DOPAMINE RECEPTOR. As other dopamine agonists are, cabergoline is effective as MONOTHERAPY in DE NOVO PARKINSON'S DISEASE (newly diagnosed disease for which no treatment has yet started) and EARLY-ONSET PARKINSON'S DISEASE; it is also effective as one of the ADJUNCT THERAPIES prescribed in late-stage Parkinson's disease to minimize OFF-STATE episodes. Its key advantage is its very long half-life of 65 hours, which permits once-a-day dosage. This dosage has the advantage of maintaining stable levels of the drug in the body, greatly reducing fluctuations and allowing lower dosages of levodopa when cabergoline is taken as an adjunct therapy. Other dopamine agonists have half-lives of eight to 12 hours and require two, three, or four doses daily. Though a pergolide dose has a half-life of 12–27 hours, it typically requires three-times-a-day dosing to obtain a steady clinical effect.

Overall, there is little published experience with the use of Cabergoline in the treatment of Parkinson's disease, but randomized controlled studies support its use as monotherapy in early disease to avoid the onset of dyskinesias and as adjunct therapy with levodopa in people with advanced Parkinson's disease and motor fluctuations (off-on fluctuating phenomenon and dyskinesias).

Cabergoline may cause fewer problems with COGNITIVE IMPAIRMENT, DEMENTIA, and PSYCHOSIS than do other dopamine agonists, perhaps because it is taken less frequently. Other adverse side effects, which are the same as for all ergot-derived dopamine agonists, include drowsiness, ORTHOSTATIC HYPOTENSION, nausea, headache, and tingling in the hands and feet called ergotism. These side effects, if they occur, usually end by the time the drug reaches full effectiveness. It also carries some risk of causing fibrotic changes in a few organs, similar to other ergot-derived medications. As for other dopamine agonists cabergoline dosage is titrated, or gradually increased, until it reaches the level that provides maximal effectiveness, a process that can take three or four months. It also must be tapered off when stopping the drug to prevent sudden and severe Parkinson's symptoms. Cabergoline is available in the United States as the brand name product Dostinex.

See also ANTI-PARKINSON'S MEDICATIONS; BROMOCRIPTINE; MEDICATION MANAGEMENT; PERGOLIDE; PRAMIPEXOLE; ROPINIROLE.

caffeine A stimulant drug common in drinks such as coffee, tea, and cola, and in foods including chocolate. Caffeine is an ingredient of hundreds of medications because of its ability to potentiate, or enhance, the effectiveness of pain drugs and because of its diuretic ("water pill") action. Recent studies suggest a connection between caffeine consumption and a reduced likelihood of development of Parkinson's disease, although the connection is not clear. This is in part because the actions of caffeine are not entirely understood and in part because the cause of Parkinson's disease remains a mystery.

Some scientists believe caffeine blocks ALPHA-ADENOSINE RECEPTOR activation in the brain. Alpha-adenosine is a NEUROTRANSMITTER that facilitates signals among neurons, particularly to depress messages related to pleasure. Blocking alpha-adenosine from binding with alpha-adenosine receptors allows these messages to get through. Researchers hypothesize that blocking the release of alpha-adenosine also extends the effectiveness of the neurotransmitter DOPAMINE. In the context of Parkinson's disease the focus is on dopamine's role in the processes of movement, as it is a shortage of dopamine that causes the symptoms of Parkinson's disease. But dopamine also acts on dopamine receptors in other parts of the brain that are part of emotional response as well as addiction to drugs such as NICOTINE and cocaine. If researchers can gain more complete understanding of the connections among caffeine, alpha-adenosine, and dopamine, it is possible they also will gain understanding of how Parkinson's disease develops and progresses.

Other scientists think caffeine has a protective effect on various neurotransmitter receptors. There is some evidence that as dopamine levels drop with advancing Parkinson's disease, levels of the neurotransmitter GLUTAMATE rise. Glutamate overstimulates certain receptors, causing premature death of the neurons that contain them. Caffeine appears to function as a GLUTAMATE ANTAGONIST to block the glutamate from binding with sensitive receptors, preventing if from activating the receptors.

Caffeine affects cells elsewhere in the body as well. It increases muscle contractions, including of the heart. It causes the kidneys to extract more fluid from the blood, increasing urine output. And caffeine acts on the ADRENAL GLANDS to increase their production of peripheral epinephrine and NOREPINEPHRINE, neurotransmitters that affect neuron communication outside the brain. Researchers do not believe any of these actions has an effect on Parkinson's disease. Excessive caffeine intake can overstimulate muscles to the extent of causing them to twitch and can overstimulate the heart to the point of palpitations (extra but usually harmless beats) and increased blood pressure. It also can cause or exacerbate SLEEP DISTURBANCES.

It is possible that other factors account for the finding that people in whom Parkinson's disease is developing stop drinking coffee and other caffeinated beverages long before symptoms become apparent. Among the early, and at that time inconclusive, symptoms of Parkinson's disease are changes in perceptions of taste and smell. These changes could result in a distaste for caffeinated beverages years and even decades before Parkinson's disease manifests, giving the false impression that there is a link between caffeine and Parkinson's. And many people find that they become increasingly intolerant of caffeinated beverages as they grow older, as a result of problems such as gastroesophageal reflux disorder (GERD), or of the stimulant effect of caffeine itself. As the risk for Parkinson's disease also increases with age, what appears to be a correlation could be nothing more than a coincidence.

At present, there is no conclusive evidence that caffeine prevents development of Parkinson's disease. Nor is there any evidence that consuming caffeine after Parkinson's has been diagnosed has any effect, positive or negative, on the course of the disease. Research continues to explore the connections between caffeine and Parkinson's disease.

CAFFEINE IN COMMON DRINKS AND FOODS		
Product	Approximate Amount	Caffeine Content
Drip-brewed coffee	12 ounces (typical mug)	280 mg
Percolator-brewed coffee	12 ounces (typical mug)	250 mg
Instant coffee	12 ounces (typical mug)	160 mg
Espresso	1 shot (2 ounces)	100 mg
Brewed tea	6 ounces (typical cup)	50 mg
Iced tea	12 ounces (typical glass)	75 mg
Colas	12 ounces	40 mg
Energy drinks	8 ounces	130 mg
Milk chocolate candy	1 ounce	8 mg
Dark chocolate candy	1 ounce	20 mg

See also NEUROPROTECTIVE EFFECT; NEUROPROTECTIVE THERAPIES; NICOTINE.

calcium   A mineral essential for the strength and health of bones and teeth and for the conduction of nerve signals that cause muscle contractions. Calcium is ingested from dietary sources or supplement, and requires vitamin D for proper absorption into the bloodstream. With advancing age, the body becomes less efficient at extracting calcium from dietary sources, making it necessary to consume greater amounts to meet the body's needs. The typical adult requires 1,000 mg of calcium daily before age 65 and 1,500 mg of calcium daily after age 65. Women past menopause who are not taking ESTROGEN or hormone replacement therapy need 1,500 mg of calcium after age 50.

Calcium, along with magnesium and potassium, is essential for conducting nerve impulses, particularly nerve signals to muscles. An imbalance of calcium in the bloodstream interferes with this conductivity. Too low a calcium level can result in slowed muscle response; too high a level can cause abnormal muscle contractions. Abnormalities in blood calcium levels also affect the heart and can cause irregularities in heart contractions.

When calcium blood levels drop below what is necessary to supply the body's needs, the body begins to dissolve calcium from the bones. This process weakens and thins bone structure, increasing vulnerability to fractures. Bone loss of 20 percent or more constitutes the clinical condition osteoporosis, which is a risk to health that can result in deformity and spontaneous fracture (bones that break without a precipitating injury). As Parkinson's progresses BALANCE and stability become increasingly fragile, putting the person at great risk for FALLS and for fractures if the bones are weakened by calcium depletion.

The most efficient way to get calcium is through diet, for as long as this is practical. Because swallowing becomes a problem for many people with Parkinson's and because taste preferences change as the disease advances, diet may not remain an adequate means of meeting the body's needs for long. Common dietary sources of calcium include milk and milk products (cheese, yogurt, sour cream, cottage cheese, ice cream), fortified soy milk, tofu, bok choy (Chinese cabbage), almonds, mustard greens, turnip greens, kale, broccoli, calcium-fortified orange juice, and fortified grain products such as breads and cereals. Product labels tell how much calcium a serving of the food contains.

For the person with Parkinson's disease, assuring adequate calcium intake is especially important yet challenging. Because Parkinson's typically affects the muscles of swallowing, eating many of the foods that are high in calcium becomes difficult. As well, changes in perceptions of taste and

smell affect the person's dietary likes and dislikes. And with advancing disease, appetite diminishes. The person loses interest in eating or may eat only small amounts of favorite foods.

When the person can no longer meet his or her calcium needs through diet, a supplement becomes necessary. Many calcium tablets are large and hard to swallow even for people without impaired swallowing ability. Chewable forms that can be crushed and mixed with soft food such as applesauce or pudding are often easier to take. Most calcium products sold as supplements also contain vitamin D, as the body cannot absorb calcium without it. Chewable antacid tablets that contain calcium carbonate are a good source of calcium but must be taken with a vitamin supplement that includes vitamin D.

See also NUTRITION AND DIET; VITAMINS.

cancer and Parkinson's   Some scientists believe there are connections between the cell dysfunctions that cause cancer and those that result in degenerative diseases such as Parkinson's disease, ALZHEIMER'S DISEASE, and MULTIPLE SCLEROSIS. These diseases develop as a result of uncontrolled cell activity—unrestrained growth in cancer and uninhibited death in degenerative conditions. One theory holds that these are opposite ends of the same spectrum and reflect a dysfunction of APOPTOSIS, the process of programmed cell death. Other theories point to external environmental factors such as exposure to toxins or to internal changes that take place under the misdirection of faulty genes. There are certain commonalities that exist in such diseases including changes in the functioning of GLIAL CELLS (cells in the brain that facilitate communication among NEURONS) and lowered levels of GLUTATHIONE, an ANTIOXIDANT found in the brain. Research in either area—cancer or degenerative diseases—often leads to findings that provide new understandings and treatments in both.

See also COENZYME Q-10; FREE RADICALS; GENE THERAPY; NEUROTROPHIC FACTORS.

carbidopa   A DOPA DECARBOXYLASE (DDC) INHIBITOR drug taken in combination with LEVODOPA to treat the neuromuscular symptoms of

Parkinson's disease. DDC is an enzyme the body releases that acts quickly to metabolize levodopa, which is an AMINO ACID, into dopamine as levodopa enters the bloodstream from the intestines. Because of the fast action of DDC levodopa dosages must be much higher than the amount needed to reach the brain to accommodate this level of loss. Without a DDC inhibitor, dopamine levels in the body's peripheral circulation become high enough to cause numerous undesired side effects including nausea, low blood pressure (HYPOTENSION), and irregular heart rate. Taking a DDC inhibitor such as carbidopa in combination with oral levodopa slows the metabolism of levodopa into peripheral dopamine.

As a DDC inhibitor, carbidopa suppresses the activity of DDC. This decreases the amount of levodopa that is metabolized in the intestine, allowing higher levels to reach the brain, where the levodopa can then cross the blood-brain barrier and be metabolized into dopamine in the brain. This action permits use of lower dosages of levodopa and therefore reduces undesired side effects. Carbidopa became available in combination with levodopa as the product Sinemet in 1967 and almost always is taken as a combination product, as its only therapeutic value is to delay levodopa's metabolism. The combination of both drugs is available in generic forms as well as the brand name products Sinemet, SINEMET CR (a CONTROLLED RELEASE form of the drug) and Atamet. A person usually requires about 75 mg. per day of carbidopa to effectively suppress DDC, though some require more. It usually is combined with levodopa in a ratio of one to four, although doctors can prescribe additional carbidopa alone (brand name Lodosyn) in those people on very low doses of levodopa (such that they aren't getting a full 75 milligrams of carbidopa per day) or for those who require more than the usual amount of carbidopa to block the peripheral conversion of dopamine. The one-to-ten ratio found in the 10/100 formulations of carbidopa/levodopa is only appropriate for people who are taking greater than eight tablets per day. These 10/100 preparations of carbidopa/levodopa are shunned by most experts since many physicians less familiar with Parkinson's disease mistakenly use these tablets to start de novo patients, due to erroneously believing that they're avoiding side effects by giving less medicine. Dosing frequency ranges from two or three times a day at the start of treatment to multiple doses each day in the later stages. Any side effects that occur are caused by the levodopa component.

See also ANTI-PARKINSON'S MEDICATIONS; BENSERAZIDE; ENTACAPONE; FAVA BEANS.

cardinal symptoms The four core, or classic, symptoms that identify Parkinson's disease; the word *cardinal* means "prime" or "fundamental." They are

- Resting TREMORS
- Bradykinesia
- Rigidity
- Postural instability

Because there is no definitive diagnostic test for Parkinson's disease, doctors must base diagnosis on an evaluation of the symptoms. This can be a challenge, particularly early in the disease, as a number of degenerative neuromuscular disorders start with one of these symptoms, especially tremors. When only one of the cardinal symptoms is present and others do not develop, there is a good likelihood that the condition is something other than Parkinson's disease. The presence of so-called red flags—dementia within the first two years of symptoms, postural instability with falls within the first two years of symptoms, certain eye movement abnormalities, or signs of cerebellar or pyramidal motor system dysfunction—also argues for a diagnosis other than Parkinson's disease. When two or more of the cardinal symptoms are present without any red flags, they point to a diagnosis of Parkinson's disease; when three or all four are present and they improve with LEVODOPA, the diagnosis is considered conclusive. Nearly everyone with Parkinson's has all of the cardinal symptoms at some point in the disease's progress.

See also COGWHEELING; CONDITIONS SIMILAR TO PARKINSON'S; DIAGNOSING PARKINSON'S; SECONDARY SYMPTOMS.

caregiver well-being The health and other needs of those who are caring for the person with Parkinson's disease. When the needs of the person with Parkinson's increase as the disease advances, the caregiver finds it more difficult to pay attention to his or her own needs. This is more likely to occur when there is a single person functioning as caregiver, especially when there are no other family members or other family members are unwilling to share in caregiving responsibilities. The caregiver might feel overwhelmed by the tasks and responsibilities of caring for the person and feel frustrated, angry, and helpless about his or her inability to make conditions better. As a result, the caregiver becomes vulnerable to physical illness and emotional distress.

SUPPORT GROUPS offer a safe and caring environment for caregivers to share their feelings and concerns. Drawing other family members and friends into caregiving, even in small ways such as reading to the person with Parkinson's or just being present so the caregiver can get away for an hour or two, can provide much needed relief for the caregiver. RESPITE CARE, in which a trained individual (such as a nursing assistant) goes to the home to take care of the person with Parkinson's so the caregiver can take a break, is sometimes a covered service of LONG-TERM CARE INSURANCE. Some retirement communities, assisted living centers, and long-term care facilities offer SHORT STAY SERVICES in which the person with Parkinson's stays for several days or a week in the facility to allow the caregiver longer breaks.

Most caregivers are also dealing with their own emotions about their changing relationships with the person with Parkinson's disease. They have been husbands, wives, daughters, sons, sisters, brothers, significant others in some fashion, who have had established roles and hopes for the future that suddenly change with the diagnosis of Parkinson's. All attention focuses on the person with Parkinson's; as a result, caregivers may feel that their emotions and experiences are not important. Some caregivers describe their situation as living in limbo—nothing is the same, yet nothing changes.

It is essential for caregivers to recognize and accept that their feelings and needs are valid and not feel guilty about desiring to take breaks from their caregiving responsibilities or about feeling sad and frustrated about the changes that are taking place in their loved ones and with their relationships. As much as possible, such breaks should incorporate activities that are unrelated to caregiving and are done solely for the caregiver's enjoyment, such as seeing a movie.

See also ADJUSTING TO LIVING WITH PARKINSON'S; CHANGING ROLES; DAILY LIVING CHALLENGES; FAMILY RELATIONSHIPS.

caregiving The functions of meeting the physical, emotional, and social needs of the person with Parkinson's disease. Caregiving encompasses the full spectrum of potential needs and affects the caregiver as well as the person with Parkinson's disease. In the early stages of the disease and for as long as ANTI-PARKINSON'S MEDICATIONS adequately control symptoms, the person with Parkinson's often needs very little assistance. ADAPTIVE EQUIPMENT AND ASSIST DEVICES extend independence as the disease progresses. As the disease advances and symptoms are more severe and less controlled by medications, however, caregiving needs increase. For those whose Parkinson's reaches the end stage in which there is complete inability to function, full-time caregiving becomes necessary.

See also ADJUSTING TO LIVING WITH PARKINSON'S; CAREGIVER WELL-BEING; COPING WITH ONGOING CARE OF PARKINSON'S; RESPITE CARE.

care management and planning The process of establishing long-term procedures for taking care of the medical and supportive needs of the person with Parkinson's disease. As Parkinson's can extend over several decades of the person's life and for most who have the condition is not the cause of death, care management and planning are essential.

One of the most pressing concerns for the person with Parkinson's disease is appropriate medical care. The person will have more extensive health care needs than if he or she did not have the condition. Parkinson's itself requires treatment, of course, and also sets the stage for a variety of secondary symptoms or complications of primary treatment that themselves require medical intervention. It becomes important to have access to a network of health care services that can meet the full spectrum of medical and supportive needs. This includes doctors, medical centers and hospitals, pharmacies, physical and occupational therapists, HOME HEALTH CARE, and extended care services such as ASSISTED LIVING CENTERS, SKILLED NURSING FACILITIES, or a LONG-TERM CARE FACILITY.

Specialized Medical Needs

For most people, the journey to a diagnosis of Parkinson's disease begins with a visit to a PRIMARY CARE PHYSICIAN who is a family practitioner or an internist. The physician suspects a neurological problem and refers the person to a NEUROLOGIST, a physician who specializes in diagnosis and treatment of conditions involving the BRAIN and NERVOUS SYSTEM. For many people with Parkinson's disease, this specialist is the doctor who takes over care of the Parkinson's disease. A neurologist has in-depth knowledge about conditions such as Parkinson's disease, understands the ways in which ANTI-PARKINSON'S MEDICATIONS are most effective, and is up-to-date on the latest treatments. Some neurologists subspecialize in movement disorders such as Parkinson's disease.

For people who live in or near metropolitan areas, where such specialists and the health care systems that support them are easily accessible, shifting care to a specialist presents little problem. For those who live in rural areas, however, a doctor appointment can be an all-day event, although with the sophistication of today's technology this is becoming less of a challenge. It is becoming possible for doctors in rural areas to be in regular communication with specialists in cities hundreds of miles away or even across the country, helping to limit travel for such consultation. Interactive video is being investigated as a way for a distant specialist to "examine" a person remotely, through teleconsultations that are nearly as useful as in-person office visits. Unfortunately some elements of the neurologic examination important in people with Parkinson's disease (such as testing for rigidity) do require the specialist to actually lay hands on the person. Many barriers currently exist to the adoption of teleconferences, including the expense of having (or accessing) suitable equipment for both the primary care physician and the specialist, reim-

bursement issues (most insurers, including Medicare, do not have clear policies regarding payment for such services), and physician licensing issues if teleconsultations are done across state lines.

For the person with Parkinson's, consulting a doctor often requires additional planning beyond scheduling appointments. Health insurance coverage through managed care plans or health maintenance organizations (HMOs) typically specify the health care providers (including doctors and hospitals) patients must use and require and preauthorization of many diagnostic tests and treatment procedures (particularly surgery). Transportation to and from health care visits also might be a concern, if the doctor is some distance away or if the person's independence has slipped to the point at which safe driving is no longer possible. Generally the primary caregiver should accompany the person with Parkinson's to health care appointments so he or she has a clear picture of the person's health status. This becomes increasingly important as Parkinson's progresses and symptoms intensify, particularly if COGNITIVE IMPAIRMENT develops.

Maintaining Overall Health Care Needs

When Parkinson's disease develops, all emphasis shifts to getting the symptoms under control. This shift tends to guide medical care decisions, as well it should for optimal management of the Parkinson's. But this focus should not preclude attention to overall health care needs, as it sometimes does. It remains important for the person with Parkinson's disease to continue seeing a primary care doctor to manage other health conditions and tend to other routine health matters such as physical exams and screenings for high blood pressure, high blood cholesterol level, heart disease, diabetes, and breast, colon, and prostate cancer, as well as other conditions that become more common with aging. Parkinson's does not usually cause medical states that require hospitalization. Generally, having Parkinson's disease has little or no effect on other health conditions except for potential drug interactions.

Medications and Drug Interactions

ANTI-PARKINSON'S MEDICATIONS remain the cornerstone of treatment and can restore near-normal function for years or decades. Their effectiveness requires regular monitoring and adjustment, particularly in the months following diagnosis and later as Parkinson's disease progresses. Anti-Parkinson's medications can have serious interactions with a wide range of other drugs. The person with Parkinson's should carry a list of the medications he or she is taking and take no additional drugs until a pharmacist or the patient's physician confirms that they will not cause interactions. It is always a good idea to compare this list with the records in the medical chart at office visits, to make sure both are accurate and current.

Health Care Expenses

The costs of receiving treatment for Parkinson's disease can be significant. Medications alone can cost several thousand dollars a year. Private health insurance and MEDICAID (government-funded assistance) typically cover drug costs, whereas MEDICARE does not. Anyone who has health insurance should understand the plan's limitations and exclusions. Insurers are required to have a process for answering specific questions and addressing concerns and complaints. Every state's insurance commissioner can answer general health insurance questions and address concerns and complaints about insurers.

People who are younger and working when diagnosed are likely to have employer-sponsored group health insurance. Although insurance regulations vary among states, in most states an insurer must continue coverage for a person enrolled in a group health insurance plan to the full extent of the plan's coverage limitations. Insurance coverage through individual plans generally falls under different regulations. People who are retired but not yet eligible for Medicare sometimes have health insurance benefits through their pension packages. Generally the same regulations and procedures apply to these group plans as to any other group plan, and the plan covers medical expenses related to Parkinson's disease as it covers any other eligible health care service. Whatever the health insurance status of the person with Parkinson's, it is essential to know payment or reimbursement levels and procedures.

Those who are past age 67 when diagnosed with Parkinson's generally are eligible for Medicare coverage. Health insurance plans—group, individual, or Medicare—do not pay for most long-term care services. Most plans have some level of benefit for short-term skilled nursing facility or home health care while recovering from a hospitalization for a serious illness or surgery. Medicaid, which operates under different names from state to state, is state-funded public assistance for health care services that is available to people who meet certain income-related criteria. Many of these programs have strict guidelines for the kinds of treatment and medications they cover. Medicaid does pay for long-term care, once the person qualifies.

Assisted Living and Long-Term Care Considerations

Although Parkinson's disease can strike at any age, it remains a condition primarily associated with aging and afflicts those beyond age 65 more frequently than those who are younger. Living arrangements become a consideration with increasing age, and having a chronic, progressive disease such as Parkinson's can narrow the field of options. Although it is difficult to acknowledge that it might become necessary for the person with Parkinson's to enter an assisted living environment of some sort, plans to do so make the decision process easier for all involved. Family members and caregivers often feel more comfortable knowing their loved one has been involved in the decision and knowing they can honor his or her wishes. Many assisted living and long-term care facilities have waiting lists that can be months to years long, so making early decisions helps assure that the desired arrangements will be available when they are needed.

See also ADJUSTING TO LIVING WITH PARKINSON'S; DENIAL AND ACCEPTANCE; DENTAL CARE AND HYGIENE; ESTATE PLANNING; FINANCIAL PLANNING; GOING PUBLIC; HOME HEALTH CARE; MEDICAL MANAGEMENT; MEDICATION SIDE EFFECTS; SELF-CARE TECHNIQUES.

carotid body cell graft   A surgical procedure in which DOPAMINERGIC CELLS are removed from the carotid body and transplanted into the SUBSTANTIA NIGRA, putamen, or STRIATUM of a person with Parkinson's disease. This is typically an AUTOGRAFT, transplanting the person's own carotid body cells to reduce the likelihood of rejection and other complications.

The carotid body is a small structure located within each of the two carotid arteries that carry blood through the neck to the head. Its cells sense changes in the oxygen content and the pressure of blood flowing through the carotid artery. When oxygen levels or blood pressure drop below the needs of the BRAIN, the carotid body produces large quantities of dopamine. Peripheral dopamine (elsewhere in the body than the brain) causes breathing and heart rate to quicken, increasing both oxygenation and blood pressure.

The dopaminergic activity of the carotid body, as does that of the adrenal medulla, presents an enticing possibility that a person's own tissues could correct the imbalance of dopamine in the brain that causes the movement symptoms of Parkinson's disease. However, research studies have been very small and their results inconsistent. Although carotid body cells produce dopamine, they do not function in the same way as the dopaminergic cells in the brain. The transplanted carotid body cells seem to mitigate symptoms (TREMORS and DYSKINESIAS) for a time after transplant but then die off; the effect is similar to that of ADRENAL MEDULLARY TRANSPLANT, with surgery on the carotid body carrying significantly more risk. Carotid body cell graft remains an experimental procedure of very little promise.

See also ABLATION.

catecholamine   The chemical family whose major members are DOPAMINE, epinephrine, and NOREPINEPHRINE. Structurally, a catecholamine contains molecules of catechol, an organic compound, and of amine, a nitrogen compound. The amino acid tyrosine is a key source of both compounds. Dopamine is exclusively a NEUROTRANSMITTER; epinephrine and norepinephrine function as neurotransmitters as well as hormones. The three major catecholamines have key roles in brain and peripheral activities related to the functions of movement. As hormones, epinephrine and norepinephrine act on specific receptor targets in precise locations to help to regulate heartbeat, blood pressure, and the body's stress response. As neurotransmitters, they act on any adregenergic or noradregenergic neuron in any location within the body.

There is no chemical difference between catecholamines produced in the brain and those produced in the body. The BLOOD-BRAIN BARRIER prevents peripherally produced catecholamines, among many substances, from having direct contact with the brain as a protective measure. In the body, the catecholamines can be metabolized from one to another—dopamine to norepinephrine, norepinephrine to epinephrine—to meet the body's peripheral needs. These conversions do not take place in the brain.

Current thinking is that there are intricate and complex connections among the body's catecholamines, such that when one is affected, all are affected. Research in the late 1990s revealed that in addition to the depletion of dopaminergic neurons in the brain that is the characteristic trait of Parkinson's, people with Parkinson's also have fewer noradrenergic neurons in the heart. This finding provides a possible explanation for the symptom of ORTHOSTATIC HYPOTENSION (a sudden drop in blood pressure when rising from a lying or sitting position to standing) that many people with Parkinson's disease experience. Such a connection renews hope that future treatments for Parkinson's might include methods to convert one catecholamine into another to restore appropriate levels of the one in deficit—dopamine, in the case of Parkinson's disease.

Because the catecholamines are closely related and because the body metabolizes dopamine into norepinephrine and norepinephrine into epinephrine, one line of research has explored the possibility that these metabolisms could be manipulated to reverse the process to use epinephrine or norepinephrine to produce dopamine. Some of this research has used autografts to implant adrenergic and noradrenergic cells into the STRIATUM and SUBSTANTIA NIGRA. This research has not been very fruitful, however. As well, catecholamine metabolism in the brain seems limited to the process of synthesizing, or manufacturing, dopamine from its source ingredients, namely, TYROSINE and dihydrophenylalanine (DOPA).

See also ADRENAL MEDULLARY TRANSPLANT; CAROTID BODY CELL GRAFT; MONOAMINE NEUROTRANSMITTER; MONOAMINE OXIDASE.

Catecholamine	Where Produced	Functions in the Brain	Functions in the Body
Dopamine	**Brain:** substantia nigra, striatum, midbrain, cerebellum, thalamus, hypothalamus **Body:** carotid body	Neurotransmitter that facilitates nerve cell communication for smooth, coordinated movement	Metabolized into epinephrine, in which form it stimulates cell activity to increase heartbeat, blood pressure, and breathing
Epinephrine	**Brain:** adrenergic neurons throughout the cerebrum **Body:** adrenal medulla	Neurotransmitter that facilitates nerve cell communication for the sympathetic nervous system	Hormone that stimulates the the body's stress response: constricts blood vessels, increases the strength and rate of the heart's pumping action, and dilates the airways
Norepinephrine	**Brain:** noradrenergic neurons throughout **Body:** adrenal medulla	Neurotransmitter that facilitates nerve cell communication for the sympathetic nervous system	Constricts blood vessels to maintain sufficient blood pressure

catechol-*o*-methyltransferase (COMT) One of the two key enzymes, the other of which is DOPA DECARBOXYLASE (DDC), that metabolize DOPAMINE in the BRAIN and peripheral body and LEVODOPA as it enters the bloodstream. COMT metabolizes levodopa to 3-*O*-METHYLDOPA (3-OMD). Whereas levodopa can cross the blood-brain barrier, 3-OMD cannot. Such rapid metabolic responses are the body's way of protecting the brain from excessive amounts of dopamine, which would be very damaging. When dopamine is depleted, as occurs in Parkinson's disease, and the brain can benefit from additional dopamine, this protective mechanism becomes counterproductive. Both COMT and DDC act peripherally and are also present in the brain.

Research efforts focusing on ways to extend levodopa and dopamine availability have resulted in the development of drugs to inhibit levodopa and dopamine metabolism. The first of such drugs was the DDC INHIBITOR carbidopa, which became available in 1967 and now is routinely taken in combination with levodopa (in products such as in SINEMET). This slows the DDC arm of the metabolism process. However, when this happens, COMT action intensifies to compensate. In 1993 the first of the COMT INHIBITOR medications, TOLCAPONE, was introduced to shut down COMT's role in levodopa metabolism. Added in combination with the drug regimen as adjunct therapies, DDC inhibitors and COMT inhibitors are highly effective in many

(although not all) people with moderate to severe Parkinson's disease for whom on–off state fluctuations have become severe or unpredictable.

See also MONOAMINE OXIDASE.

catechol-*o*-methyltransferase (COMT) inhibitor A drug that prevents the actions of the enzyme CATECHOL-*O*-methyltransferase (COMT), which metabolizes LEVODOPA and DOPAMINE. COMT's action limits the amount of levodopa that crosses the BLOOD-BRAIN BARRIER for metabolism to dopamine and limits the length of time dopamine remains active. Inhibiting this action extends the amount of levodopa that is available to cross the blood-brain barrier and appears to extend the time dopamine remains active in the SUBSTANTIA NIGRA and STRIATUM. COMT inhibitors have no effect on the rate at which levodopa enters the bloodstream from the intestines.

COMT inhibitors were first used as one of the ADJUNCT THERAPIES in the 1990s. The first introduced was TOLCAPONE, which can be highly effective but has a high risk of side effects including diarrhea and a risk of worsening levodopa induced side effects such as DYSKINESIA. Adjusting the levodopa dose can improve or eliminate the dyskinesias. The diarrhea usually ends in time (up to several months) but can be serious enough that the person prefers to stop taking the tolcapone. Rarely, tolcapone also causes liver damage, which can be severe if not caught very early. Frequent, regular liver function tests are necessary for people taking tolcapone. ENTACAPONE, the other COMT inhibitor currently available in the United States, does not cause any liver problems, and is generally the drug of choice for initial COMT inhibitor treatment though most experts feel that it has somewhat less potency than tolcapone in extending the therapeutic effects of levodopa.

When a person with Parkinson's starts taking a COMT inhibitor, there is often an increase in dyskinesias and other side effects (such as nausea) that signal high levels of dopamine in the bloodstream. This happens because the COMT inhibitor extends the effectiveness of levodopa, allowing more of it to be metabolized to dopamine. This is a great benefit in the brain, but the higher amounts circulating peripherally (elsewhere in the body than the brain) cause side effects. Lowering the levodopa dosage typically relieves these side effects. Because COMT inhibitors are new treatments, as yet there are no findings about their long-term effectiveness.

See also ANTI-PARKINSON'S MEDICATIONS; MEDICATION MANAGEMENT; MONOAMINE OXIDASE INHIBITOR (MAOI) MEDICATION; TREATMENT ALGORITHM.

caudate See BASAL GANGLIA.

causes of Parkinson's See PARKINSON'S DISEASE, CAUSES OF.

central nervous system See NERVOUS SYSTEM.

central nervous system (CNS) depressant A drug that slows the actions of the brain and nerve structures, affecting consciousness and voluntary and involuntary actions and movement. These can include functions such as breathing, heart rate, and blood pressure. Side effects such as sleepiness indicate that a drug is a CNS depressant. muscle relaxant drugs (antispasmodics), particularly benzodiazepines such as CLONAZEPAM and DIAZEPAM; ANTIHISTAMINE DRUGS; and ANTIPSYCHOTIC DRUGS have pronounced CNS depressant effects. Other ANTI-PARKINSON'S MEDICATIONS such

as ANTICHOLINERGIC DRUGS are more subtle CNS depressants. The body can adjust to many of these drugs so the CNS symptoms are not apparent, generally over a period of two weeks to two months.

See also DAYTIME SLEEPINESS; MEDICATION SIDE EFFECTS; NERVOUS SYSTEM.

cerebellum See BRAIN.

cerebral cortex See BRAIN.

cerebrum See BRAIN.

changing roles The shifts in responsibilities and relationships that take place between the person with Parkinson's and others as Parkinson's disease progresses. In particular they affect FAMILY RELATIONSHIPS involving spouses or significant others, children, and siblings. The person who has been the family leader many now be the one who needs assistance and support. FRIENDSHIPS based on common interests might founder when the interests can no longer be shared. Colleagues or coworkers may be uncertain about the person's capabilities. These are not easy transitions for the person with Parkinson's or for others. Family and friends should be compassionate yet honest with each other and with the person who has Parkinson's.

See also ADJUSTING TO LIVING WITH PARKINSON'S; SELF-ESTEEM; MARRIAGE RELATIONSHIP; PARENT/CHILD RELATIONSHIPS; SOCIAL INTERACTION; WORKPLACE RELATIONSHIPS.

chelation Treatment of diseases involving the abnormal handling and accumulation in the body of metals such as copper with an agent that binds to the metal and promotes its excretion.

See also ACERULOPLASMINEMIA; WILSON'S DISEASE.

chemical toxins Poisons that can cause illness, injury, and disease. A number of chemical toxins have been considered or implicated as CAUSES OF PARKINSON'S DISEASE. Contact can be environmental, as with pesticides and herbicides, or ingested, as with drugs or metals such as mercury. Chemical toxins that scientists suspect might increase the risk of, or contribute to causing, Parkinson's disease include the following:

- Pesticides and herbicides: A number of studies have shown that people who have a higher than usual exposure to chemicals used to control insects and weeds have Parkinson's disease more often than people without such exposure. Researchers have been able to create a Parkinson's model (an induced disease state that produces the dopamine depletion and corresponding symptoms of Parkinson's) in laboratory animals by giving them repeated injections of the commonly used pesticide rotenone. One action of rotenone is inhibition of COMPLEX I, which allows toxins to accumulate within cells.

- Polychlorinated biphenyls (PCBs): There are thousands of these chemicals, most of which were in common use in thousands of products and applications until their use was banned in the United States in the 1970s. Some scientists believe PCBs contribute to accelerated aging with a corresponding decline in the number of dopaminergic cells in the SUBSTANTIA NIGRA and in this way contribute to an increased risk for Parkinson's disease. PCBs are linked to many health problems including birth defects, cancer, and chronic conditions other than Parkinson's. Despite being banned for more than 30 years, PCBs remain a significant and pervasive environmental contaminant that causes exposure through such unlikely sources as eating foods such as contaminated fish, dairy products, and meat products.

- Drugs and medications: Some drugs, most notably powerful antipsychotics such as haloperidol (used to treat schizophrenia), affect dopamine levels in the brain, creating Parkinson's-like symptoms. These symptoms are not always reversible and sometimes persist after the person stops taking the drug. When they do, the condition is considered DRUG-INDUCED PARKINSON'S and ANTI-PARKINSON'S MEDICATIONS often provide relief. The inadvertent contaminant of attempts to synthesize an illegal drug 1-METHYL-4-PHENYL-1,2,3,6-TETRAHYDROPYRIDINE

(MPTP), a synthetic hormone, produces rapid, severe, and irreversible Parkinson's disease that does not respond to anti-Parkinson's medications, leading to rapid decline and usually death within a short time.

- Mercury and other metals: There is some evidence connecting prolonged exposure to high levels of mercury and Parkinson's disease, although the link is not clearly understood. Mercury, as are other metals, is a neurotoxin. It accumulates in nerve cells, interfering with their ability to function. ACERULOPLASMINEMIA, for example, is a form of Parkinson's disease caused by the accumulation of iron in the cells of the brain that results from a genetic defect that prevents the body from metabolizing iron. Mercury, lead, and other metals can similarly accumulate to cause a range of neurological damage.

Chemical toxins cause cell death and affect other organ systems as well as the brain and NERVOUS SYSTEM. Whereas most other tissues in the body can replace the destroyed cells, the brain cannot. Limiting or preventing exposure to chemical toxins is the most effective means of reducing the risks associated with them.

chiropractic A system of healing that emphasizes proper alignment, or realignment through physical manipulation, of the spine. The DYSTONIA (muscle rigidity) that develops as a consequence of long-term LEVODOPA therapy often causes discomfort and pain. The stooped, tight posture that is characteristic of Parkinson's disease also can result in aching and stiffness as muscles are held in distorted positions.

Gentle chiropractic manipulations can help relax muscles and relieve stiffness and tension in the neck and back. Manual manipulation (use of only the hands) is the most appropriate method for people with Parkinson's disease, as muscles with impaired function do not respond in the same ways to these therapies as do unimpaired muscles. Chiropractic manipulation is a SUPPORTIVE THERAPY that can provide short-term relief of the discomfort that Parkinson's symptoms can cause. Chiropractic manipulation can temporarily improve BALANCE,

POSTURAL STABILITY, and MOBILITY by increasing flexibility and range of motion. It does not treat the symptoms or the dopamine depletion that causes the symptoms of Parkinson's disease, and it cannot cure or alter the progression of Parkinson's. Special care should be taken to avoid potential injury during neck manipulations, particularly in people who also have histories of vascular disease or the risk factors (smoking, hypertension, high cholesterol, elderly age) for vascular disease.

Today's chiropractors receive extensive education and training in body structure and function, with an emphasis on the back and spine, and must pass certification tests and be licensed before they can practice. When choosing a chiropractor, look for one who has experience treating people with neuromuscular conditions. Health care providers and Parkinson's support groups often can make recommendations within their local communities.

See also ALTERNATIVE THERAPIES; EXERCISE AND ACTIVITY; PHYSICAL THERAPY.

choline acetyltransferase An enzyme that catalyzes, or facilitates, the bonding between choline and acetate to produce ACETYLCHOLINE, a key NEUROTRANSMITTER in the processes of movement. In a sense, choline acetyltransferase functions as a "factory" that produces acetylcholine. A CHOLINERGIC NEURON takes in molecules of choline and acetate separately by active transport. A waiting choline acetyltransferase molecule accepts the choline and acetate molecules and holds them until the chemical reactions necessary to allow them to bond into acetylcholine take place. The choline acetyltransferase molecule then releases the newly formed acetylcholine molecule and is ready to start the cycle again. Acetylcholine molecules are stored in vesicles within the cholinergic neuron AXON and are released into the SYNAPSE when the cholinergic neuron "fires" (depolarizes). Once in the synapse, acetylcholine activates receptors on other neurons (or muscle cells) and is metabolized by acetylcholinesterase back into choline and acetate.

People with ALZHEIMER'S DISEASE have decreased levels of choline acetyltransferase, which is a key factor in the depletion of acetylcholine that is the hallmark of this degenerative

disease. Acetylcholine is critical for COGNITIVE FUNCTION, and its depletion results in COGNITIVE IMPAIRMENT including MEMORY LOSS and DEMENTIA. The role of choline acetyltransferase in Alzheimer's disease interests researchers studying Parkinson's disease for two reasons. First, about 20 percent of people who have either Alzheimer's or Parkinson's have the other disease as well. This raises the strong possibility that there are connections between the two conditions.

Second, there are commonalities in the GENE MUTATIONS found in some people who have Alzheimer's, Parkinson's, or both. Gaining more complete understanding of the role of choline acetyltransferase might shed light on causes of and lead to potential new treatments for both Alzheimer's and Parkinson's. Although acetylcholine levels do not directly affect Parkinson's disease, suppressing acetylcholine production with ANTICHOLINERGIC DRUGS lowers the level of acetylcholine circulating in the brain and improves its balance with the level of dopamine circulating in the brain. This process helps to control DYSKINESIAS in the early and middle stages of Parkinson's. A recent report implicates that the long-term use of anticholinergic medications in people with Parkinson's disease may increase the risk of developing Alzheimer's disease even further.

See also ACETYLCHOLINESTERASE; ACETYLCHOLINESTERASE INHIBITOR; ANTI-PARKINSON'S MEDICATIONS; GENE THERAPY; NEUROTROPHIC FACTORS.

cholinergic neuron A nerve cell that produces ACETYLCHOLINE, a NEUROTRANSMITTER that has a key role in movement. Cholinergic and DOPAMINERGIC NEURONS comprise much of the structure of the BASAL GANGLIA, the part of the brain that regulates muscle movement and that Parkinson's disease affects. The hallmarks of Parkinson's are the death of dopaminergic neurons, particularly in the SUBSTANTIA NIGRA, and the resulting depletion of DOPAMINE in the brain.

Smooth, coordinated movement relies on an intricate, complex choreography of nerve and muscle communication. This process requires an appropriate balance of neurotransmitters. As dopaminergic neurons diminish, the actions of cholinergic neurons become more pronounced. Although cholinergic neurons in the brain continue to produce normal amounts of acetylcholine, the depletion of dopamine results in an imbalance of these two neurotransmitters. The excess acetylcholine overwhelms nerve signals to the muscles, sending confusing and sometimes conflicting messages that result in the rigidity and tremors of Parkinson's disease.

ANTICHOLINERGIC DRUGS block the action of cholinergic neurons to reduce the amount of acetylcholine circulating in the brain. This process reduces tremor and rigidity in the early and middle stages. As dopaminergic neurons continue to die as the Parkinson's progresses, the imbalance of neurotransmitters increases to the extent that suppression of the action of cholinergic neurons can no longer compensate. Cholinergic neurons also are present in peripheral muscle tissue, where they release acetylcholine in response to nerve impulses transmitted from the brain to direct movement. As well cholinergic neurons and acetylcholine are crucial to COGNITIVE FUNCTION. A recent report implicates that the long-term use of anticholinergic medications in people with Parkinson's disease may further increase their already elevated risk of developing Alzheimer's disease.

cholinesterase   See ACETYLCHOLINESTERASE.

cholinesterase inhibitor   See ACETYLCHOLINESTERASE INHIBITOR.

chorea   Involuntary, unpredictable, and rapid movements that can affect nearly any voluntary muscle group in the body. These abnormal motions have the appearance of dancing; the word *chorea* comes from the Greek word for "dance." Chorea can be a symptom of injury or illness involving the brain or a side effect of medications that affect brain function. In people with Parkinson's disease, chorea appears as a secondary symptom that is a side effect of ANTI-PARKINSON'S MEDICATIONS. Chorea can occur alone or in combination with ATHETOSIS, a slower form of involuntary move-

ments that typically have a writhing character. The latter is called CHOREOATHETOSIS.

Reducing chorea is a matter of trying to adjust the doses and timing of anti-Parkinson's medications to provide maximal relief of primary Parkinson's symptoms (such as TREMOR, RIGIDITY, BRADYKINESIA, AND AKINESIA) with a minimum of undesired side effects. Sometimes dividing the daily dosages of these medications into smaller, more frequent doses mitigates chorea and other involuntary, dysfunctional movements. It is often useful to add adjunctive therapies to reduce levodopa induced CHOREIFORM DYSKINESIA; AMANTADINE is a particularly effective addition in reducing choreiform dyskinesia. In Parkinson's later stages, it is often not possible to establish a balance between primary symptom relief and creation of secondary symptoms. This remains one of the most significant challenges in treatments for Parkinson's disease.

Chorea may also occur as a side effect of the long-term use of antipsychotic medications, which is called tardive dyskinesia. Classically tardive dyskinesia predominantly involves the tongue and mouth, though all areas of the body can become involved.

When it appears without other DYSKINESIAS, chorea is a primary symptom of HUNTINGTON'S DISEASE, a hereditary condition in which there is a progressive degeneration of the BASAL GANGLIA. Nonmedication induced chorea may also be a sign of brain lesions or tumors involving the midbrain or cerebellum, and brain injury resulting from trauma or stroke.

See also ABLATION; ACETYLCHOLINE; DEEP BRAIN STIMULATION; DYSTONIA; MEDICATION MANAGEMENT; MEDICATION SIDE EFFECTS; MOTOR SYSTEM DISORDERS; MOVEMENT; PALLIDOTOMY; THALAMOTOMY.

choreiform dyskinesia   A term used to describe CHOREA that is drug-induced rather than caused by illness or injury. In the context of Parkinson's disease, choreiform dyskinesia is a side effect of LEVODOPA therapy and usually appears when blood levels of levodopa are high though some people with Parkinson's experience biphasic dyskinesias: experiencing chorea both when levodopa is peaking and later when it falls. By contrast, DYSTONIA (muscle rigidity and stiffness) usually appears when blood levels of levodopa are low. These two secondary symptoms typify on/off fluctuations. Relieving choreiform dyskinesia requires adjusting the dosages and timing of ANTI-PARKINSON'S MEDICATIONS to reduce blood levels of levodopa. AMANTADINE is of particular value in decreasing choreiform dyskinesia when it is added as an ADJUNCTIVE THERAPY. DOPAMINE AGONIST MEDICATIONS (such as PERGOLIDE and BROMOCRIPTINE), COMT INHIBITOR MEDICATIONS (TOLCAPONE and ENTACAPONE), and MAOI-B inhibitors (such as SELEGILINE) also often are effective ADJUNCT THERAPIES that can improve the effectiveness of levodopa at lower blood levels.

chromosomes linked to Parkinson's disease In recent years researchers have identified a number of chromosomes that appear to have an involvement in the development of Parkinson's disease. A chromosome is a cellular structure that contains hundreds or thousands of genes, which are the base units of inherited information that determine many of the characteristics of an individual's existence. A normal cell contains 23 pairs of chromosomes; in health, the pairs have identical structure, except for the unmatched X-Y sex chromosomes in men (women have matched X-X sex chromosomes). Each cell repeats this pairing and structure (except ova, or eggs, and sperm, which each contain half the chromosomes and blend to create a full chromosomal complement at conception).

Genes line each chromosome in a particular and identical order for every appearance of that chromosome in every cell. All of the genes on chromosome 4, for example, are in exactly the same location on every chromosome 4 in every cell. It is this consistent presence that allows the characteristics of their genetic coding to manifest, somewhat in the way that aligning tumblers in a lock allows the lock to open. If just one tumbler is out of alignment, the lock does not open. Such is the case with genes and chromosomes, although of course in a much more intricate and complex manner; all must be precisely aligned to display their characteristics.

There can be mutations (changes or "errors" in the gene's content) of a particular gene that appear in that gene in every cell or minor aberrations in a single presence of the gene. Generally single aberrations do not interfere with health although mutations create differences that can be either benign or harmful.

Locating the chromosome in which the genes responsible for certain traits reside is the first step in identifying and possibly correcting GENE MUTATIONS that cause diseases. The extent to which gene mutations cause Parkinson's disease remains unknown. Most researchers believe it is a combination of genetic and environmental factors that converge to permit Parkinson's to develop. Recent research suggests that genetic factors might be more prevalent and significant than long assumed, however. Scientists can now link mutations in defined areas on chromosomes 1, 2, 4, 5, 6, 8, 9, and 17 to Parkinson's disease, although the role that these mutations play and the specific genes that are involved remain unclear.

Researchers discovered the PARKIN GENE, located on chromosome 6, in the 1990s and subsequently have discovered a number of other genes that seem specific to Parkinson's disease, particularly EARLY-ONSET PARKINSON'S, in some way. Some of these genes relate only to Parkinson's, and others have broader effects on health and disease throughout the body. As technology is rapidly evolving to allow more precise examination of chromosomal and genetic structures, there is a continuous stream of new discoveries about the extent to which genetic factors influence Parkinson's disease regardless of the age of onset. These are spawning a number of experimental GENE THERAPIES that show great promise for changing the course of Parkinson's disease and strengthen HOPE FOR A CURE FOR PARKINSON'S.

See also ALPHA-SYNUCLEIN GENE; AUTOSOMAL DOMINANT INHERITANCE; AUTOSOMAL RECESSIVE INHERITANCE; ENVIRONMENTAL TRIGGERS; GENE MAPPING; HUMAN GENOME PROJECT; RISK FACTORS FOR PARKINSON'S.

cigarette smoking See NICOTINE.

cisapride   A prokinetic drug that increases the motility of the gastrointestinal tract. As Parkinson's disease progresses, it affects the muscle activity of smooth (involuntary) muscle tissue such as that of the digestive system. Many people with moderate to advanced Parkinson's have DYSPHAGIA (difficulty in swallowing) and chronic CONSTIPATION, reflecting the slowed activity of the muscles responsible for moving food down the esophagus and through the intestines and colon. Cisapride works by increasing the release of ACETYLCHOLINE in the muscles of the gastrointestinal tract, which stimulates them to contract more frequently and intensely. This action moves food through the digestive system more quickly, helping to relieve symptoms of dysphagia and constipation.

Cisapride's action also seems to have a slight effect on reducing on/off fluctuations, which researchers believe occur in part because LEVODOPA digestion becomes delayed. Later in the course of Parkinson's disease gastric emptying (the length of time food remains in the stomach before moving into the small intestine to begin the digestive process) can become significantly extended. This in turn delays the levodopa's absorption, allowing levels of DOPAMINE in the brain to drop precipitously low. It becomes necessary to compensate by taking larger levodopa doses more frequently. By moving the stomach's contents more quickly into the intestines, cisapride moves levodopa into the bloodstream faster (although it does not increase the amount of levodopa that is absorbed).

Cisapride is rarely prescribed in the United States since access to it is very restricted due to its association with a number of serious side effects including very dangerous alterations in heart rhythm, liver toxicity, and bone marrow suppression (production of all the major types of blood cells can precipitously fall). Its formal indication is to treat gastroesophageal reflux disorder (GERD) in people who do not have Parkinson's disease and is sold as the brand name product Propulsid in the United States. Grapefruit and grapefruit juice increase the amount of cisapride that is absorbed and should not be consumed while taking cisapride. Cisapride can cause adverse interactions with many of the drugs taken to treat Parkinson's disease (especially ANTICHOLINERGICS, ANTIHISTAMINES, AMANTADINE, and ANTI-PARKINSON'S MEDICATIONS that target DYSKINESIAS). Before one considers adding cisapride, it is important to evaluate the overall medication regimen as well as the potential serious side effects of cisapride. It may be necessary to monitor drug blood levels and effectiveness, and to adjust dosages and their timing, when adding cisapride. Most experts do not believe that cisapride has much of a role in the management of Parkinson's disease.

See also DOPA DECARBOXYLASE; DOPA DECARBOXYLASE INHIBITOR; GASTRIC MOTILITY; PERISTALSIS.

clinical pharmacology trials   Controlled research studies that test the effectiveness of new drugs. These are also called clinical pharmacology studies, clinical trials, or clinical studies. The process of taking a new drug from concept to prescription is lengthy and costly and involves many levels of research and testing. Most of these processes take place in the laboratory, making sure the new drug is as safe as possible before expanding its testing to humans. Laboratory testing is called preclinical testing. In the United States, the Food and Drug Administration (FDA) oversees drug testing and determines whether a drug is approved for clinical use (treatment of people).

Until a drug receives FDA approval, it is classified as an INVESTIGATIONAL NEW DRUG (IND). This designation imposes strict limitations on the drug's availability and use. Drugs in the later phases of clinical testing are sometimes made available for treatment purposes under specific and limited circumstances in what is known as an expanded access protocol, as when a person who has Parkinson's would clearly benefit from the drug but cannot qualify to participate in clinical trials.

Researchers recruit volunteers to participate in clinical pharmacology trials, which typically take place in four phases.

Phase I is the first and preliminary test of the investigational new drug in humans. These studies are generally small and intended to determine whether laboratory findings—benefits and risks—are the same in people as in test animals. Researchers look in particular for unexpected side effects that affect the drug's safety. Nearly always, the volunteers for phase I studies are healthy individuals who have no signs or symptoms of the condition the drug is intended to treat, to provide a base of information about how an undiseased human body responds to the drug. Phase I clinical trials tend to have a short duration, often just weeks.

Phase II trials are randomized, controlled studies that involve larger groups of volunteers, who, for investigational ANTI-PARKINSON'S MEDICATIONS, have Parkinson's disease. The goal in this phase is to demonstrate effectiveness in a small group and to confirm safety. The stage of disease might be narrowly defined or open, depending on the drug's intended use. Researchers might want to test an investigational new drug's effectiveness in EARLY-ONSET PARKINSON'S, for example, and so limit study enrollment to people with Parkinson's who are younger than age 40. Phase II clinical trials can last months to years, depending on the study's design and the parameters researchers want to measure. Typically there are at least two groups of study participants, those who receive the investigational new drug and those who receive a standard treatment (or occasionally a PLACEBO, an inert substance designed to look or taste like the investigational new drug). For the most objective results, studies are double-blinded—neither the researchers nor the participants know which participants are receiving the new drug and which are receiving standard treatment to prove the drug's effectiveness for people with Parkinson's as a whole.

Phase III trials expand the new drug's use to a broad base of people with Parkinson's disease, typically chosen from medical centers in different locations across the country to get a diverse selection of participants. Like phase II trials, phase III trials are randomized and controlled, often are double-blinded, and last for several years. This is the final level of testing before the investigational new drug enters therapeutic use (if approved by the FDA), so researchers aim to account for as many variables as possible.

Phase IV studies continue to collect data after an investigational new drug receives FDA approval for marketing and use for the approved purposes. This data collection phase continues for as long as the drug is on the market.

All CLINICAL RESEARCH STUDIES, pharmacological and nonpharmacological, follow strict guidelines and procedures to make them as safe as possible for participants. The FDA must approve and closely oversee all clinical pharmacology studies. Researchers must fully disclose all potential risks of participating in the study, and participants must sign a statement of INFORMED CONSENT verifying that they understand these risks and agreeing to comply with any conditions of the study. Generally research studies provide any necessary medical care related to the study during participation. Some studies, especially phase I trials, pay volunteers for participation.

Because treatment options for Parkinson's disease are less than ideal, many people with Parkinson's are eager to participate in research studies that could result in more effective treatments. The advantage to participating in clinical pharmacology studies is that the drug being tested might provide greater relief from symptoms than do currently approved treatments. When the study ends, study participants have the knowledge to discuss with their doctors the value of continuing with the new drug. New anti-Parkinson's medications that have caused significant improvements for many people with Parkinson's include COMT INHIBITOR MEDICATIONS and the nonergot DOPAMINE AGONIST MEDICATIONS, drugs that received FDA approval in the 1990s.

Sometimes a clinical pharmacology trial examines a new use for a drug approved for other purposes, such as AMANTADINE, which was originally approved as an antiviral agent. After amantadine had been in use for several years, doctors noticed that people with Parkinson's who took the drug to prevent or shorten the course of an influenza infection also noticed significant improvement in their Parkinson's symptoms while they were taking the amantadine. This observation opened a new avenue of research, and amantadine subsequently received formal approval for use as an anti-Parkinson's medication. It is important to note that many drugs that have been approved for one use are commonly used off-label by physicians for other conditions; many drug firms are loathe to seek formal approval for off-label uses due to the time and expense it takes to gain formal FDA approval; doctors can already prescribe the medication off-label; and additional indications often don't extend a firm's exclusive rights to manufacture a drug.

See also HOPE FOR A PARKINSON'S CURE; PHARMACOTHERAPY; TREATMENT ALGORITHM.

clinical research studies Controlled tests to determine the effectiveness of new treatment approaches, also called clinical research trials. Clinical research studies can involve new devices such as DEEP BRAIN STIMULATION (DBS), new surgeries, or other new procedures for treating medical conditions such as Parkinson's disease. A CLINICAL PHARMACOLOGY TRIAL is a type of clinical research study that evaluates the effectiveness of new drugs and is under the oversight of the U.S. Food and Drug Administration (FDA). Clinical research trials follow medical, legal, and ethical guidelines established by federal regulations. Although there is inherent risk in participating in a clinical research study, these guidelines strive to establish an environment in which participant safety and well-being are the defining parameters.

At any given time, there are thousands of clinical research trials taking place at government agencies, research facilities, medical centers and hospitals, and health care practice groups throughout the country. The website www.clinicaltrials.gov, produced and maintained by the National Institutes of Health (NIH), provides extensive information about clinical research trials for people who might be interested in participating in them. The website also lists the trials that are currently seeking participants.

The NIH identifies four primary classifications of clinical research trials:

- Treatment trials—studies that are exploring new treatment options, such as new drugs and stem cell therapy, for people who already have a disease such as Parkinson's.
- Prevention trials—studies that seek ways to prevent people from acquiring or developing

diseases such as Parkinson's, such as COENZYME Q-10 supplementation and NEUROPROTECTIVE THERAPIES.

- Screening trials—studies that attempt to find practical ways to identify the presence of a disease such as Parkinson's in its earliest stages, particularly before symptoms signal that the disease has already caused damage.
- Quality of life trials—studies looking for ways to improve and sustain the well-being, aside from health status, of people who have chronic or degenerative diseases such as Parkinson's.

Regardless of type, clinical research trials all include certain key elements. A clinical research trial starts with a protocol, which is the researchers' statement of what they expect to find through the study, what benefits and risks are possible for participants, and how the trial will be conducted in details. All participants must receive and sign a statement INFORMED CONSENT, which explains the protocol and the participant's rights and responsibilities.

Clinical research trials have both benefits and risks, and it is important to understand both fully as well as to have realistic expectations when beginning the trial. Most of the time, the research team provides whatever medical care is necessary as a result of participation in the trial although participants typically continue to receive care through their regular health care providers. People with Parkinson's who enroll in clinical research trials should notify their doctors and make sure that they do not make any changes in their care without first talking with the researchers.

See also CLINICAL PHARMACOLOGY TRIALS; FETAL DOPAMINERGIC CELL TRANSPLANT; FETAL PORCINE BRAIN CELL TRANSPLANT; HOPE FOR A PARKINSON'S CURE; INVESTIGATIONAL NEW DRUG; INVESTIGATIONAL TREATMENTS.

clonazepam A muscle relaxant and antispasmodic drug in the benzodiazepine family. It is also used to treat seizures, anxiety, insomnia and pain related to chronic conditions such as fibromyalgia. In Parkinson's disease clonazepam helps to relieve RESTLESS LEG SYNDROME, and DYSTONIA (muscle rigidity). It also is useful in treating the movement disorder MYOCLONUS. As other benzodiazepines are, clonazepam is a CENTRAL NERVOUS SYSTEM (CNS) DEPRESSANT that works by inhibiting the actions of certain neurotransmitters in the brain, most notably GAMMA-AMINOBUTYRIC ACID (GABA).

There are many potential drug interactions with clonazepam, including with many of the commonly used ANTI-PARKINSON'S MEDICATIONS. Clonazepam may slightly decrease the amount of levodopa that is absorbed into the bloodstream, making it necessary to adjust the levodopa dosage to compensate. The most common undesired side effect is drowsiness, which gradually recedes in most people after two to six weeks of taking the medication as the body adjusts to the drug. This same adjustment process sometimes continues, however, making clonazepam less effective over time. Clonazepam is available in the United States in generic forms and as the brand name product Klonopin. Due to clonazepam's long duration, this drowsiness, as well as other hangover effects such as dizziness, imbalance, confusion, and slowing of thinking, may be big issues in people with Parkinson's who already have fatigue, balance problems, or cognitive difficulty.

See also ALPRAZOLAM; DIAZEPAM; LORAZEPAM; TEMAZEPAM.

clothing As Parkinson's disease progresses, the inability to control voluntary movement, especially fine movement, makes common activities exceedingly difficult. Before Parkinson's disease begins a person's primary concerns regarding clothing may be fit and fashion; clothing choices after Parkinson's begins are selections based on ease of wear. Buttons, zippers, and belts can be impossible to manage, pantyhose and neckties a nightmare. Elastic waists, pullover shirts and tops, and hook-and-loop fasteners (such as Velcro) are far less frustrating, as are slip-on shoes instead of shoes with laces. Men might find it easier to wear boxers instead of briefs, and women to opt for camisoles or T-shirts instead of bras. Fabrics can make a difference, too, in ease of putting on, comfort while wearing, and ease of laundering. Lighter jersey cotton knits slip on more easily than heavier sweat-shirt kinds of fabrics and are convenient to layer for warmth as well as quick removal if desired.

The easier items of clothing are for the person with Parkinson's to put on and take off, the more independent the person can remain. Laying out clothing in the order in which the person will put it on eases the frustration of moving around to find items. It also encourages the person to sit on the edge of a bed or on a chair to get dressed. As BALANCE and POSTURAL INSTABILITY are problems for nearly everyone with Parkinson's, sitting to dress reduces the risk of FALLS. For some people, this means learning new methods after years of other habits. Until impairment forces the matter, most people do not even think about the processes of everyday activities such as getting dressed and often do not realize how much they rely on steadiness and balance to step into a pair of pants or align the buttons of a blouse. It is helpful to maintain creativity and a sense of humor about clothing options and the process of DRESSING and undressing.

Selections of adaptive clothing are improving as the demand for them increases and generally offer the same range of styles and fashions as regular clothing. There are retailers that specialize in adaptive clothing or provide clothes for people who have special needs. Many of these offer mail order and online shopping. Some styles of clothing are designed for easy on/easy off dressing, such as athletic warm-up pants with snap-away sides and loose-fitting tops. As styles have become more casual and people wear athletic clothing just about everywhere, manufacturers have broadened the color and variety of clothing items that are available. Western-style shirts for men and women typically have snaps, which are easier to manage than buttons.

Other options are to replace buttons on existing clothing with snaps or to sew hook-and-loop fasteners under buttons so the buttons are still there for appearance but the hook-and-loop fasteners do the job of holding the garment closed. For women, elastic-waist skirts are easier to manage than dresses. Elastic-waist pants for women are available in a broad range of styles from jeans to fashionable dress slacks and are a good option when replacing pantyhose with knee-high stockings or socks.

See also ADAPTIVE EQUIPMENT AND ASSIST DEVICES; ADJUSTING TO LIVING WITH PARKINSON'S.

coenzyme Q-10   A naturally occurring substance that facilitates mitochondrial energy production within the cell. It is also available in the form of a dietary supplement, marketed as an ANTIOXIDANT. Coenzyme Q-10's name refers to its function as a coenzyme and its chemical structure; it is also called ubiquinone. A coenzyme is a chemical compound that supplements the functions of enzymes, which are proteins that facilitate chemical reactions within the body. Coenzyme Q-10 molecules are vital components of the mitochondrial electron transport chain, serving to transfer electrons to maintain a steady supply of oxygen to meet cellular energy needs.

Recent research shows that people with Parkinson's have lower levels of coenzyme Q-10 than people without the disease. In several animal studies, administration of coenzyme Q-10 supplements to raise the body's levels of this substance seems to slow the loss of dopaminergic cells in the SUBSTANTIA NIGRA and other parts of the brain. The increased levels of coenzyme Q-10 also raise the levels of COMPLEX I, another substance critical to mitochondrial metabolism that is present at a lower than normal level in people with Parkinson's.

As an antioxidant, coenzyme Q-10 prevents some FREE RADICALS from forming and inactivates those that do form. Coenzyme Q-10 is popular as a dietary supplement for this purpose. Many people with Parkinson's disease, particularly those in the early stages, take coenzyme Q-10 for its antioxidant effects even though its effectiveness in slowing the progress of Parkinson's has not yet been proved through controlled research studies. Preliminary studies suggest that high doses of the supplement are safe and may slow the progression of motor disability early in the course of Parkinson's disease. There is currently debate as to whether this indicates a possible protective effect. Such high doses of Q-10 are expensive, the 1200 milligrams per day dose used in the recent clinical study typically costs around $200 per month, and insurance usually won't pay for supplements such as Q-10. Experts agree that more studies are necessary before it can become a recommended treatment.

See also CHEMICAL TOXINS; LIPOPOLYSACCHARIDES; MITOCHONDRIAL DYSFUNCTION; PARKINSON'S DISEASE, CAUSES OF.

coffee consumption   See CAFFEINE.

cognitive function   The collective abilities to think, reason, analyze, and remember. From the Latin word meaning "to come to know," cognition encompasses awareness and judgment. This term reflects the significance not only of receiving information, but of processing it and of being able to act (or not act, as the case might be) appropriately. The functions of cognition are complex and take place primarily in the frontal and temporal lobes of the brain's cerebrum. The NEUROTRANSMITTER ACETYLCHOLINE is essential for cognitive function, and DOPAMINE plays a role as well.

In the early stages of Parkinson's disease, cognitive functions typically remain normal though it is not unusual for there to be mild problems finding words or mild slowing of cognitive processing speed. Some people with Parkinson's experience severe and fluctuating COGNITIVE IMPAIRMENT as the disease progresses; this is widely variable. Brain functions other than those directly involved in cognition sometimes become factors in cognitive function. Parkinson's disease often affects the muscles that control movement of the eyes; as a result distorted visual images are sent to the BRAIN. This process alters spatial judgment, causing the person with Parkinson's to make errors that appear to be impairments of cognitive function when in fact the misjudgments are responses to incorrect information that has reached the brain. Parkinson's disease also often affects the muscles that control the vocal cords and mouth structures necessary for speech, causing impairments that again appear to be problems of cognition but are not. As the disease progresses some degree of cognitive impairment becomes common.

See also ALZHEIMER'S DISEASE; COMMUNICATION SKILLS.

cognitive impairment   A reduced ability or an inability to think, reason, analyze, or remember. Diminished awareness and inappropriate judgment are key signs of cognitive impairment. Some degree of cognitive deterioration occurs with the natural process of aging, generally noticeable as forgetfulness. When this deterioration interferes with everyday activities, it becomes a clinical concern. Cognitive impairment is the primary symptom of ALZHEIMER'S DISEASE and can be a symptom of many neurological disorders including MULTIPLE SCLEROSIS, HUNTINGTON'S DISEASE, and PARKINSON'S DISEASE. Injury to the BRAIN, as through trauma or stroke, also can cause impaired cognition.

In Parkinson's disease, the presence and degree of cognitive impairment are highly variable. Many researchers believe that the NEUROTRANSMITTER imbalance in the brain, particularly between ACETYLCHOLINE and DOPAMINE, that develops as Parkinson's progresses inevitably interferes with cognition even if there are no obvious problems. Both of these neurotransmitters facilitate neuron communication related to thought processes and MEMORY, and as dopamine levels drop, the concentration of acetylcholine rises. Other researchers believe that cognitive impairment results from factors other than Parkinson's disease, such as the coexistence of Alzheimer's disease (which commonly develops in people with Parkinson's, with some estimates as high as 25 percent) the development of cortical Lewy bodies (making the diagnosis Lewy body dementia rather than Parkinson's), or deterioration that would have taken place without Parkinson's.

For most people with late stage Parkinson's, cognitive impairment is significant. Also for most people with Parkinson's cognitive impairment typically develops slowly and does not become significant until the disease's late stages. This makes it possible to compensate for impairments for quite a long time. The person with Parkinson's can develop methods to aid memory, such as posting notes and carrying a small notebook with directions to commonly visited locations. Family members and caregivers can help by reminding the person of scheduled events using conversational prompts to make sure the person knows where he or she is going. It is common for cognitive impairment to ebb and flow with on/off fluctuations, and helpful to notice whether such a pattern is present. The person with Parkinson's usually does not recognize that his or her cognitive functions are impaired.

Drugs called ACETYLCHOLINESTERASE INHIBITORS that enhance cognitive function are now available. They include DONEPEZIL (Aricept), GALANTAMINE (Reminyl), RIVASTIGMINE (Exelon), and TACRINE (Cognex). They work by extending the period of activity of acetylcholine in the brain. Although these drugs are intended to treat Alzheimer's disease, in which acetylcholine depletion is a key factor, many doctors are prescribing them for people with cognitive impairment related to Parkinson's. Rivastigmine has particularly strong published evidence of its usefulness and safety in Parkinson's disease with dementia. As is the case in Alzheimer's, some people with Parkinson's have improved COGNITIVE FUNCTION with these drugs and others experience no effect.

Bradyphrenia

BRADYPHRENIA is a slowness of the thought process. The person with Parkinson's might take a long time to answer a question or provide information, sometimes stopping in midsentence as if the thought has been lost. Patience gives the person a chance to regain his or her thoughts, and gentle prompting can sometimes help close a gap that persists.

Memory

Changes in memory begin with forgetfulness about common events and tasks. The person with Parkinson's might forget an appointment or a meeting or not remember how to get to the produce section of the grocery store. He or she may forget the names of familiar people or how to run water for a bath or cook scrambled eggs as though he or she has never done these things. The person may be able to follow written directions that outline the steps of the task or may need supervision and assistance.

Concentration and Focus

It is common for the person with Parkinson's to lose focus when engaged in daily activities. He or she may walk away in the middle of a conversation or appear to be listening but then start talking about something entirely unrelated. Establishing and maintaining eye contact help to determine whether the person with Parkinson's is focused on the conversation at hand, and frequent "check back" inquiries can help to confirm that the person has heard what was being said. Problems with concentration and focus also make it difficult for the person with Parkinson's to engage in any one task for very long, for example, watching a movie, reading a book, or even cooking a meal. Inobtrusive observation and redirection can help avert disasters. Many ANTI-PARKINSON'S MEDICATIONS, especially levodopa and the dopamine agonists, can adversely affect the ability to concentrate.

Logic and Planning

Cognitive impairment often interferes with the person's ability to organize thoughts in a logical fashion, creating the sense of a haphazard approach to activities and tasks. The person may attempt to lay out the day's clothing, for example, and place garments all around the bedroom or even in other rooms in apparently random fashion. It is difficult for the person to figure out what to do first, what to do next, and what to do last. Notes that present simple, step-by-step lists can sometimes help.

See also ADJUSTING TO LIVING WITH PARKINSON'S; DEMENTIA; FLUCTUATING PHENOMENON; LEWY BODY; LEWY BODY DISEASE; MEMORY IMPAIRMENT; READING; TASK SIMPLIFICATION.

cogwheeling The form of muscle RIGIDITY characteristic of tremor in which muscles move with slight hesitations, in a pattern of ratcheting movement that resembles that of a cogwheel. The symptom is also called cogwheel rigidity. It often is an early sign of Parkinson's especially if there is also the constant, nonspeed dependent "lead pipe" rigidity that is characteristic of PARKINSONISM. The rigidity results from delays and confusion in the nerve signals being sent to the muscles, which cause changes in muscle tone. These changes are usually not noticeable during intentful movement but obvious with passive movement (when the limb is held relaxed and is manipulated by someone else).

Most people with Parkinson's do not notice cogwheeling as a symptom, although they may perceive that their muscles ache and feel stiff. Cogwheeling is apparent to a doctor during examination and often easiest to detect at the wrist or ankle. To test for cogwheeling, the doctor holds the arm or leg and instructs the person to relax the muscles and let the doctor manipulate the hand or foot. When cogwheeling is present, the manipulations reveal the characteristic pattern of movement of initial resistance, relaxation, and resistance again. This pattern gives the impression of start-and-stop movement, although it can be quite subtle in the early stages of Parkinson's. Cogwheeling is most apparent during movement at joints and can appear at any movable joint in the body.

Treatment with ANTI-PARKINSON'S MEDICATIONS, especially LEVODOPA, generally relieves cogwheeling completely in the early stages. Cogwheeling can be a symptom of a condition other than Parkinson's such as essential tremor, lesions of the basal ganglia, or lesions of the cerebellum or its tracts (cerebellar tremor), the brainstem (rubral tremor), or of other parts of the brain involved in movement. Diagnostic imaging such as MAGNETIC RESONANCE IMAGING (MRI) or COMPUTED TOMOGRAPHY (CT) SCANNING can help distinguish these other causes from Parkinson's. Parkinson's disease is likely when cogwheeling appears with other CARDINAL SYMPTOMS such as tremor and BRADYKINESIA. As do other symptoms of Parkinson's, cogwheeling typically affects one side of the body or affects one side more prominently than the other.

See also BALANCE; DIAGNOSING PARKINSON'S DISEASE; GAIT DISTURBANCES; LEAD PIPE RESISTANCE; MYOCLONUS.

color perception The ability of the brain to interpret signals from the eye that present color properly. People with Parkinson's disease often have distorted color perception. The reasons for this are not clearly understood but probably reflect depletion of DOPAMINERGIC NEURONS in the retina, the structure within the eye that collects visual information and transmits it to the brain. Limited research has been done in this area. Although doctors know that the retina is one of the structures in the body that have dopamine-producing cells, they do not know the extent to which those cells are affected by the processes that cause depletion of the dopaminergic neurons in the SUBSTANTIA NIGRA. Such a depletion in the retina could cause faulty signals to be sent to the brain.

People with Parkinson's disease also tend to have other visual disturbances, including BLURRY VISION and difficulty in perceiving contrast. These are problems that can affect color perception. The specialized cells in the retina that perceive color, called rods, require bright light and good contrast to properly perceive colors. This is why colors appear washed out in dim light, even to people who have no visual disturbances. Coexisting problems in perceiving contrast may also have an effect on color perception, interfering with the ability of the rods to detect enough of colors to present their signals properly to the brain.

Color perception disturbances can involve colors at any point along the color spectrum, although blues and yellows seem to be affected more often than other colors in people with Parkinson's. Disturbances in color perception are annoying but do not usually affect the person's ability to function unless the person is still driving, in which case confusion with red/green interpretation presents a hazard. The person with Parkinson's should have a complete eye examination, including testing for color perception, at least once a year.

See also BLEPHAROSPASM; EYE MOVEMENTS; VISION PROBLEMS.

communication skills   The cognitive abilities necessary to speak, listen, write, think, and otherwise exchange information. The changes that take place in various structures within the BRAIN as a consequence of Parkinson's disease have a significant effect on communication skills. Parkinson's disease typically affects the muscles that control the face, swallowing, and the structures of the mouth, causing the masked face appearance that is a characteristic trait of Parkinson's and also alters the tone, volume, clarity, and inflection of the voice. People with Parkinson's often have difficulty in forming words and pushing sounds through the vocal cords as a result of RIGIDITY and BRADYKINESIA involving the muscles of the mouth and throat, a symptom called DYSARTHRIA. These symptoms also can affect breathing, further restricting SPEECH.

Speech therapy is an important element of SUPPORTIVE THERAPIES for people with Parkinson's. A speech therapist can teach the person specific exercises to improve speech quality. Breathing exercises improve lung capacity and BREATH CONTROL, both of which help to increase the volume of speech. The muscles that control the vocal cords also become affected, causing changes in the pitch, tone, and modulation of the voice. When the vocal cords do not close completely, air can move around them, causing the voice to become soft and sometimes raspy, depending on the extent to which the cords remain open. As a consequence of these involvements, people with Parkinson's often speak in a monotone, lacking tonal expression, so that the voice sounds flat and uninterested. Changes in speech can make the person with Parkinson's difficult to understand, although the person often does not recognize that these changes have taken place and so becomes frustrated when others have trouble hearing or understanding.

Communication skills extend beyond the capacity of speech. Facial expressions are crucial for expressing emotion. Laughing, frowning, and even crying are all actions that involve extensive use of the facial muscles to convey messages of feeling and emotion. When these actions are lacking, as they characteristically are in Parkinson's, there is the perception that the person is uninterested and uninvolved. One of the most frustrating aspects of Parkinson's for people who have the disease as well as for their loved ones is the loss of facial expression that limits their ability to share nonverbal communication, particularly JOY and happiness. ANTI-PARKINSON'S MEDICATIONS sometimes relieve speech-related symptoms.

See also COORDINATION; DYSPHAGIA; DYSPHASIA; YOGA.

compassion   The ability to feel and express kindness, sympathy, and patience. Parkinson's is a chronic, degenerative disease that requires ongoing medical and supportive care, but most of those who have it are able to lead relatively normal lives for quite some time, years and even decades, with ANTI-PARKINSON'S MEDICATIONS and other treatments. Compassion is an important aspect of coping with Parkinson's, as it is important to recognize and remember that this is not just a disease but a life-changing experience for all whose lives touch the person with Parkinson's. Inherent in compassion is the element of hope—hope for effective treatment, hope for minimal debilitation, hope for loved ones' capacity to cope, and hope for a cure.

The many technical aspects of treating Parkinson's often overshadow compassion. In the rush to establish appropriate clinical treatments to relieve symptoms and restore function, doctors and health care providers tend to focus on the clinical aspects of the disease; that focus can make their approach seem harsh and cold. People with Parkinson's often feel that their doctors are treating the disease without regard for the person who has it. It is important for people with Parkinson's and their loved ones to establish and maintain a human connection with their doctors, to ensure that the clinical dimensions of Parkinson's do not overshadow the person who has it. The lack of human connection is one of the primary complaints people with chronic conditions that require constant care express about health care providers.

Compassion becomes a greater challenge when Parkinson's enters its later stages and the person with Parkinson's requires extensive or even complete care. It is draining, emotionally and physically, for caregivers to meet the demands such care exerts. Compassion toward the person with Parkinson's helps to put these demands in a context that has meaning greater than the actions of the care, and to restore a sense of the caring that was present before Parkinson's. This is especially important when there are COGNITIVE IMPAIRMENTS that cause the person who has the disease to display uncharacteristic EMOTIONS and behavior. Compassion is the element of caring that helps people remember that these are the manifestations of the disease, not the choices of the person.

See also ADJUSTING TO LIVING WITH PARKINSON'S; BEHAVIOR, EMOTIONAL; CAREGIVER WELL-BEING; EMPATHY; FAMILY RELATIONSHIPS; LONELINESS; MARRIAGE RELATIONSHIP; MOOD SWINGS; OPTIMISM.

complex I An enzyme within cell mitochondria that scientists believe helps cells to resist damage from FREE RADICALS, the natural molecular by-products of energy generation within the cell. Some studies have shown that cells in the brain and throughout the body of people with Parkinson's disease have low levels of complex I, leading to speculation that free radical damage plays a role in the development of Parkinson's and other neurodegenerative diseases such as ALZHEIMER'S DISEASE and AMYOTROPHIC LATERAL SCLEROSIS (ALS). Extended or repeated environmental stress, which can range from internal factors such as disease and injury to external factors such as exposure to CHEMICAL TOXINS, increases the body's energy demands.

Mitochondria are structures within cells that generate energy. As cells generate higher levels of energy, they also produce higher levels of waste, including free radicals. In health, complex I is the counterbalance in this process, rendering free radicals harmless. In the body's normal chemical reactions molecules combine and bind with each other to form substances that the body needs, from the cell fuel adenosine triphosphate (ATP) to NEUROTRANSMITTERS such as dopamine. Free radicals are unstable molecules that bind with any other molecules that are "open" to create chemical structures that cannot meet the body's needs and can interrupt normal body processes.

When this occurs in excess and over time, as with continued or repeated exposure to ENDOTOXINS or EXOTOXINS (internal or external environmental stress), the result is cell and tissue damage that scientists believe opens an entry for many diseases ranging from cancer to DEGENERATIVE CONDITIONS such as Parkinson's disease. Whether and which diseases develop then becomes a matter of interactions among various factors including GENETIC PREDISPOSITION or GENE MUTATION, other health conditions and overall health status, and the nature of exposure to environmental stresses.

Complex I interferes with the binding process of free radicals, preventing them from joining with other molecules. The body's natural defenses are then able to dismantle the free radicals into harmless molecular structures and bind them in ways that allow them to be removed from the body as waste. When complex I is in short supply, it cannot keep up with the production of free radicals. What is not clear is whether the disease process initiates the decline in complex I or whether reduced complex I level allows disease to develop; research continues to explore these connections. COENZYME Q-10, a naturally occurring substance in the body, seems to perform functions similar to those of complex I in neutralizing free radicals.

See also APOPTOSIS; LIPOPOLYSACCHARIDES; MITO-CHONDRIAL DYSFUNCTION; MITOCHONDRIAL ELECTRON TRANSPORT CHAIN; PARKINSON'S DISEASE, CAUSES OF.

computed tomography (CT) scan   A sophisticated, noninvasive imaging technology that combines X rays with computer images to create longitudinal "slices" of an organ, part of the body, or the entire body. CT scan is sometimes used to look for structural damage to the basal ganglia in ruling out other causes for what may appear to be Parkinson's disease, though magnetic resonance imaging (MRI) is a more sensitive technique for this purpose. CT scan also is sometimes used to determine appropriate probe placement during ablative surgeries such as THALAMOTOMY and PALLI-DOTOMY or during insertion of electrodes for DEEP BRAIN STIMULATION (DBS), although MRI is more commonly used for this procedure as well.

There is no special preparation necessary for a CT scan, and there is no discomfort during the procedure. A CT scan of the brain takes about 15 minutes, though a complete second scan is required if a scan with intravenously injected contrast is desired. For a CT scan, the person lies on a table that moves into the doughnut-shaped scanner. The scanner contains a moving camera that takes numerous pictures as a narrow X-ray beam through the part of the body that is being scanned. The table moves forward in small increments to repeat the process until the imaging is completed. A computer then assembles the collected pictures to create multidimensional views of the body part.

The exposure to radiation is well within safe limits although significantly higher than that of a single-image X ray such as of an arm or a leg. It is high enough that doctors use CT scanning only when the procedure is likely to provide clinically

useful information: that is, information that aids in diagnosis or treatment selections. Iodinated contrast agents add more risk as iodine allergies are not uncommon and because the contrast agent can damage the kidneys in people who have even mild pre-existing kidney problems. For someone with early symptoms of Parkinson's disease, it could be used to rule out other potential causes of the symptoms such as stroke or tumor. For most people with Parkinson's disease, CT scans do not provide clinically useful information. As yet there are no definitive diagnostic tests for Parkinson's, and symptom response determines treatment options.

See also POSITRON EMISSION TOMOGRAPHY; SINGLE PHOTON EMISSION COMPUTED TOMOGRAPHY.

computer, personal   A technology gift for the person with Parkinson's disease. The personal computer allows people with disabilities of all kinds to communicate and explore without regard for mobility and other limitations. With telephone line and an Internet service provider (ISP) account, the computer becomes a gateway to the world, giving unprecedented access to information, communication, and recreation. There are numerous adaptive aids available for computers that make them easy to use for the person with Parkinson's disease. The Microsoft website www.microsoft.com/enable/ provides an up-to-date listing of available accessibility products (hardware and software) and suggestions for improving accessibility.

Dvorak Keyboard Layouts
TREMORS and BRADYKINESIA involving the hands are common symptoms of Parkinson's, and they can make any task that requires dexterity and coordination, such as typing, quite difficult. The traditional QWERTY keyboard configuration that is standard on personal computers is a carryover from the typewriter, in which its primary purpose was to prevent the keys from jamming. QWERTY refers to the first six letters of the top row of letters and as a keyboard configuration requires significant cross-reaching to strike commonly used keys. Designed by August Dvorak in the 1930s, Dvorak keyboard layouts break with tradition by putting the com-

monly used keys in the keyboard's home row, significantly reducing the amount of cross-reaching that is necessary to use the keyboard. This arrangement makes typing much easier for people who have limited dexterity in their fingers, type with just one hand, type with just one finger, or type with an assist device called a wand. Dvorak keyboard layouts have two-hand, left hand, and right hand versions and are sold at most retail stores that sell computers.

Optical Sensor Pointing Devices and Touch-Activated Screens

The mouse makes software commands easy for people without physical impairments, but for the person with Parkinson's who has tremors and limited dexterity, this pointing device can be difficult to use. Unlike the typical mouse or trackball, the optical sensor pointing device does not require contact with a surface. Instead, it uses digital images to send signals to the computer. Touch-activated screens can be pricey but are worth the investment for people who use the computer often but have serious dexterity challenges. The person touches a point on the screen to signal a command that otherwise would be sent by using the keyboard or pointing device. Touching with a finger or a wand activates the screen.

Accessibility Software

Computer operating systems (such as Microsoft's Windows) incorporate accessibility options into this software. Through menu options, the computer's user can customize the operating system to help overcome the limitations of disabilities. Options typically include using extra large screen images, preprogrammed or customized keyboard shortcut commands, commands to ignore input such as repeated key strokes, and adding sounds to common functions so they are audible as well as visible.

Voice Recognition Software

Voice, or speech, recognition software allows the computer's user to speak into a microphone to activate certain commands, rather than typing them on a keyboard or using a pointing device. Voice recognition software must be "trained" to recog-

nize and respond to the person's voice in a potentially time-consuming process. All voice recognition software is equally effective; it is best to discuss particular needs with a knowledgeable computer representative who can recommend an appropriate product. A voice that is very soft or devoid of tone and inflection can be difficult for the software to recognize consistently.

COMT   See CATECHOL-*O*-METHYLTRANSFERASE.

COMT inhibitor   See CATECHOL-*O*-METHYLTRANSFERASE (COMT) INHIBITOR.

conditions similar to Parkinson's   There are numerous neuromuscular conditions that have symptoms similar to those of PARKINSON'S DISEASE. Some estimates place misdiagnosis at 20 to 30 percent for either a diagnosis of Parkinson's that is instead another condition or a diagnosis of another condition that is instead Parkinson's disease. Misdiagnosis is more likely in the early stages when symptoms are less obvious and less clearly defined and has greater clinical significance when it delays therapy for a treatable condition such as a tumor that could be surgically removed. Related conditions known collectively as PARKINSONISM have symptoms that are similar to those of classic Parkinson's disease but have specific, identifiable causes and lack some of the characteristic changes in the brain that accompany depletion of DOPAMINERGIC NEURONS such as the presence of LEWY BODIES.

When Parkinson's disease seems the most likely diagnosis based on the symptoms that are present, many doctors prescribe a test regimen of LEVODOPA therapy. When the diagnosis is Parkinson's, levodopa causes the symptoms to improve or go away entirely. If there is no improvement after two or three months of levodopa therapy, the diagnosis is not likely to be Parkinson's disease. When doubt remains, imaging technologies such as COMPUTED TOMOGRAPHY (CT) SCAN and MAGNETIC RESONANCE IMAGING (MRI) can sometimes identify causes that are not Parkinson's, such as tumors or brain injury due to stroke or trauma. Conditions sometimes or often confused with Parkinson's disease, particularly in their early stages, include:

- LESIONS and tumors of the BASAL GANGLIA (especially the SUBSTANTIA NIGRA), thalamus, or cerebellum
- Medication induced parkinsonism
- Multiple system atrophy (MSA)
- Progressive supranuclear palsy (PSP)
- Corticobasal degeneration (CBGD)
- Normal pressure hydrocephalus
- Spinocerebellar ataxia-3 (Machado Joseph Disease)
- AMYOTROPHIC LATERAL SCLEROSIS (ALS)
- GUAM AMYOTROPHIC LATERAL SCLEROSIS–PARKINSONISM DEMENTIA COMPLEX (GUAM ALS-PDC)
- BENIGN ESSENTIAL TREMOR

As either Parkinson's disease or the other condition progresses or fails to respond as expected to the attempted treatment, the true diagnosis typically emerges.

See also PARKINSON'S DISEASE, CAUSES OF; DIAGNOSING PARKINSON'S.

confusion A state of disorganized COGNITIVE FUNCTION that affects memory, analytical thinking, and judgment. Confusion can be temporary, transient, or progressive. A number of factors can cause temporary confusion in the person with Parkinson's disease, including adverse drug reactions and factors unrelated to Parkinson's disease, as temporary confusion becomes more common with aging. Transient confusion, which comes and goes, often accompanies OFF-STATE episodes as Parkinson's enters the later stages. Confusion that becomes persistent and progressively worse with additional COGNITIVE IMPAIRMENT can be the result of factors not related to Parkinson's disease, such as ALZHEIMER'S DISEASE or non-Alzheimer's DEMENTIA that accompanies the mental deterioration of aging.

Caregivers and family members can help redirect the person's confusion with gentle reminders about tasks and locations. Patience is often the most effective approach, particularly when confusion is temporary or transient. Confusion that results from an adverse drug reaction generally ends after the drug's effect wears off and typically does not return unless the drug is taken again. Medications to improve cognitive function are sometimes helpful with progressive confusion.

See also DEMENTIA; MEDICATION MANAGEMENT; MEDICATION SIDE EFFECTS; MEMORY IMPAIRMENT.

constipation Difficulty and delay in bowel movements. Constipation is an early but inconclusive symptom of Parkinson's that tends to become more severe as the disease progresses. This is because the muscles of the intestinal tract are affected by the changes in muscle activity that Parkinson's causes, and their function becomes slow. Constipation also is a common side effect of many ANTI-PARKINSON'S MEDICATIONS.

The best treatment for constipation is prevention, to the extent that this is possible. A diet high in fiber (fruits, vegetables, whole grains, and whole grain products), drinking of plenty of water and nonalcoholic liquids, and walking are the most effective lifestyle preventive measures. Because Parkinson's affects SWALLOWING, BALANCE, and POSTURAL STABILITY, these methods are not always practical or possible for the person with Parkinson's. Stool softeners are often useful and fiber supplements also can help. Conventional laxatives are helpful, but chronic daily use can lead to dependency on them to avoid severe constipation. The realization that most people are perfectly fine if they go without a bowel movement for a couple of days per week, and implementing other measures, usually results in a fairly rare need for laxatives.

See also EXERCISE AND ACTIVITY; NUTRITION AND DIET.

controlled release medication A drug that contains coatings or binders that delay its dissolving and absorption into the body; also called a sustained release medication. Controlled release medications deliver a stable stream of the active drug into the bloodstream, preventing the peaks and troughs common with intermittent doses. Many oral medications begin dissolving in the stomach and enter the bloodstream rapidly. Most controlled release medications are designed to dissolve slowly and further into the digestive process, parceling out the drug's entry into the bloodstream. Digestive disturbances such as constipation or diarrhea, and even the foods eaten during the course of a day, can affect the effectiveness of controlled release medications. Controlled release forms of levodopa have a less predictable response as Parkinson's disease progresses, with its effects frequently being delayed and reduced due to digestive disturbances and its increased time in the gut making it more susceptible to competition from dietary protein. When ON–OFF state fluctuations become severe, sometimes it becomes necessary to augment controlled release LEVODOPA such as SINEMET CR with doses of regular release levodopa or just to convert over completely to regular release formulations.

See also ANTI-PARKINSON'S MEDICATIONS; DOPAMINE DEGRADATION; MEDICATION MANAGEMENT.

cooking The process of preparing foods for meals. In the early and middle stages of Parkinson's, moderate adaptations can allow the person with Parkinson's to function relatively independently in the kitchen. These include using wide-handled measuring implements and cooking utensils, rearranging cupboards to put commonly used items within reach without stretching or bending, and storing spices and seasonings in containers with flip-tops or other easy-open configurations. Other adaptations that are helpful include replacing knob-style with lever-style kitchen faucets, cabinet handles, and drawer pulls and removing throw rugs that can be tripping hazards. Kitchen equipment such as a food processor (with large, easy to push buttons), microwave oven, crockpot, and bread-making machine provide ways to simplify preparation and cooking tasks that require physical dexterity or strength.

Cooking often becomes a significant challenge for the person with Parkinson's as the disease advances, and safety becomes a critical concern. Physical symptoms such as TREMORS, BRADYKINESIA and other DYSKINESIAS make holding measuring and cooking utensils difficult, raising the risk of spills that can become slipping hazards. Symptoms that affect the person's mobility and balance also present safety risks. COGNITIVE IMPAIRMENT creates another set of hazards, as the person with Parkinson's may forget about a stove burner that is on or a food item that is in the oven. The caregiver or other family member might prepare meals and store them in containers that the person with Parkinson's can take from the freezer or refrigerator and heat in the microwave. It is generally safer for the person whose Parkinson's disease is in later stages to cook only with supervision and assistance.

See also KITCHEN EFFICIENCY.

coordination The ability of muscle groups to function in a harmonized, productive manner. In health, movement is an intricate and complex choreography of brain and body, muscles and nerves, action and reaction, cells and chemicals. These elements integrate to generate smooth, uninterrupted muscle activity. When injury or disease interrupts any of these elements, movement becomes impaired. In Parkinson's disease, the depletion of DOPAMINERGIC NEURONS and DOPAMINE in the regions of the brain that control movement sets in motion a cascade of mistiming and imbalance of muscle response that results in the disease's characteristic TREMORS, BRADYKINESIA, and RIGIDITY. These symptoms inhibit coordination and MOBILITY as well as fine motor movements that tasks such as fastening buttons require.

In the early and into the middle stages of Parkinson's disease, ANTI-PARKINSON'S MEDICATIONS typically restore muscle functions to near-normal. The person with Parkinson's can reinforce this effect with concentrated effort and regular activity to improve coordination. Physical therapy can teach the person specific techniques. TAI CHI, a form of martial arts that emphasizes flowing, fluid movement, improves coordination and BALANCE. Activities such as playing table tennis and other games that require focus and repetition of movement can help to maintain both physical coordination and HAND-TO-EYE COORDINATION.

See also AMBULATION; HOME SAFETY; OCCUPATIONAL THERAPY; POSTURAL INSTABILITY.

coping with diagnosis of Parkinson's   The diagnosis of Parkinson's disease is life-changing. People react in many different ways to receiving the news that the cause of their symptoms is Parkinson's, ranging from acceptance to denial, from relief to anger. Those who clearly have the cardinal symptoms might feel a sense of relief at finally having an explanation, and younger people or those whose disease is in the very early stages might feel disbelief. Because there is no definitive test for Parkinson's disease, some people wish to exhaust every possible alternative before accepting a diagnosis of Parkinson's. Doctors, too, desire to rule out other causes of symptoms that might be treated in other ways. Their willingness to perform additional tests and procedures, even when they are certain of the diagnosis, sometimes raises expectations that the diagnosis is wrong. Most people experience the spectrum of emotions in response to being diagnosed with Parkinson's and may vacillate among responses before accepting the diagnosis. It is not uncommon for a person to accept diagnosis before treatment and then deny diagnosis after ANTI-PARKINSON'S MEDICATIONS relieve the symptoms and his or her functioning returns to apparent normal status.

The diagnosis of Parkinson's most significantly affects the person who has it, of course, but it also affects others in the person's circle of family, friends, and coworkers if the person is employed. All know the diagnosis means changes in their relationships, but no one knows exactly what they will entail. Friends and family members often are unsure what to say to the recently diagnosed person or how to behave toward him or her. Straightforward expressions of concern and compassion are usually the best approach. It is also important and beneficial to maintain friendships and relationships, although this can become challenging if common interests are based on activities that become difficult for the person with Parkinson's.

Most people are concerned about what the future holds for them. Will they remain independent, or will they need continuous care? At what point in the disease, in their lives, will they no longer be able to function as they desire? These are issues that relate to everyone regardless of health status, of course, but being diagnosed with a chronic, progressive disease puts them at the forefront. Because the course of Parkinson's disease is so individual, it is nearly impossible for doctors or anyone to predict how long a person will enjoy relatively symptom-free living with ANTI-PARKINSON'S MEDICATIONS or what direction the disease will take. Younger people may feel a sense of hopelessness because they see their future as cut short, although they may be in a position to benefit from new discoveries and treatment approaches. People of any age who are diagnosed with Parkinson's disease in the next five or ten years may never experience the full range of symptoms, given the dramatic findings of ongoing research.

At the same time, there is the reality that Parkinson's is a neurodegenerative disease. It is important to begin planning for future medical and supportive care needs sooner rather than later, so the person with Parkinson's can fully participate in decisions.

See also CAREGIVER WELL-BEING; CHANGING ROLES; COPING WITH ONGOING CARE OF PARKINSON'S; FAMILY RELATIONSHIPS; HOPE FOR A PARKINSON'S CURE; PSYCHOTHERAPY.

coping with ongoing care of Parkinson's   Regardless of symptom severity at diagnosis, Parkinson's disease requires ongoing care and attention to the physical, emotional, and financial needs such care encompasses.

Physical Needs

In the early stages of Parkinson's disease symptoms do not usually create unusual physical needs, particularly when ANTI-PARKINSON'S MEDICATIONS suppress them. Mild TREMORS and occasional BRADYKINESIA are annoying but do not interfere with the ACTIVITIES OF DAILY LIVING (ADLs). In the middle and late stages of Parkinson's disease, anti-Parkinson's medications can no longer suppress symptoms and often begin to cause symptoms of their own, particularly DYSKINESIA. As RIGIDITY, tremors, and POSTURAL INSTABILITY intensify, the person with Parkinson's needs increasingly higher levels of assistance with physical needs in all facets of daily activity from personal hygiene to mobility. Cognitive impairment sometimes becomes a factor as well, inhibiting the person's ability to remember how to perform what were once ordinary tasks and functions.

It is more comfortable for both the person with Parkinson's and others in the household to transition to anticipated needs before there is a crisis that makes the need obvious. Planning to accommodate changes in physical abilities and needs may include:

- Removing throw rugs and furnishings that might present tripping hazards, to reduce the risk of falls

- Anticipating the need for additional support when walking, such as a walker or a wheelchair

- Installing hand railings and grip bars in locations such as hallways, stairways, and bathrooms

- Replacing round doorknobs with lever-type designs or removing interior doors that are not necessary

- When purchasing clothing and shoes, looking for hook-and-loop closures instead of buttons, snaps, and zippers, or items that pull on

- Begin acquiring cooking and eating utensils with broad handles for easier gripping

Physical needs vary widely along the course of Parkinson's and from person to person among those who have Parkinson's.

Emotional and Social Needs

Living with a chronic, degenerative disease can be an emotional roller coaster for the person who has Parkinson's as well as family and friends. The unpredictable course of the disease, including the uncertainties of how the person will respond to treatment, combined with the physical changes that are taking place in the brain, can result in MOOD SWINGS and emotional behavior that seem out of character for the person. It is important for those who are close to the person with Parkinson's to be supportive and compassionate.

Expenses and Financial Resources

When most people set up their retirement funds and pension plans, they do so with the vision of living comfortably and in reasonable health as they enter old age. Not many people consider the possibility that they may have special needs that zap their plans in record time or expect that there will be other resources to cover the unexpected. Health insurance and Medicare will help with medical expenses; other costs can quickly become overwhelming. Accommodating such needs often means readjusting plans and expectations.

See also ADJUSTING TO LIVING WITH PARKINSON'S; DENIAL AND ACCEPTANCE; ESTATE PLANNING; FINANCIAL PLANNING; GOING PUBLIC; LONG-TERM CARE INSURANCE; MEDICAL MANAGEMENT.

corpus striatum   See STRIATUM.

corticobasal degeneration (CBD)   A rare and serious degenerative brain disease that, in its early stages, mimics Parkinson's disease. CBD may begin with mild TREMOR and BRADYKINESIA in one limb, often an arm, but stiffness seems to be more pronounced than is typical for nonyoung onset Parkinson's disease. It then rapidly progresses to involve other parts of the body, but tends to remain asymmetric with the originally involved side being much worse than the other side. One of the key distinguishing factors in differentiating CBD from Parkinson's is that CBD symptoms do not improve with LEVODOPA whereas Parkinson's symptoms do. CBD also advances quickly to affect speech and swallowing. CBD nearly always develops in people after age 60 and affects large portions of the brain including the CEREBRUM, often causing significant COGNITIVE IMPAIRMENT as well as DYSTONIA. A peculiar phenomenon of "alien limb syndrome" in which a clumsy limb may seemingly undertake movements on its own, sometimes with the feeling that the limb itself seems to not be one's own, commonly occurs in CBD. CBD's cause is unknown and its course progressive, resulting in nearly complete immobility within five to 10 years. At present, there are no known treatments that relieve the symptoms. Although CBD itself is not usually a cause of death, its end-stage immobility typically leads to fatal bacterial infections such as pneumonia.

See also CONDITIONS SIMILAR TO PARKINSON'S.

Creutzfeldt-Jakob disease   (CJD)   A rare, pro-gressive, and fatal condition that causes brain tis-sue to waste away, resulting in a characteristic spongelike appearance of the brain that is appar-ent at autopsy. Most cases of traditional CJD are random, although the condition seems to have a hereditary connection in some families. Tradi-tional CJD can also be acquired through receipt of tissue such as corneal transplants from an affected individual and has been reported after consump-tion of infected animals. The early symptoms are often vague and are mistaken for the symptoms of other conditions such as Parkinson's disease, depending on the parts of the brain that are first affected. Early signs of CJD can include motor dysfunctions such as TREMORS as well as DEPRES-SION, ANXIETY, and COGNITIVE IMPAIRMENT. CJD progresses rapidly within a few months to dementia, delirium, and myoclonus, such that there is little chance for confusing it for Parkin-son's disease. Death commonly occurs in less than one year with CJD. There is no conclusive method to diagnose CJD until autopsy after death, though late CJD has a fairly characteristic ELECTROENCEPHALOGRAM (EEG) and has been reported to have some characteristic findings on certain MAGNETIC RESONANCE IMAGING (MRI) sequences. Nor are there any treatments to relieve symptoms or delay progression. In this regard, it distinguishes itself from Parkinson's dis-ease quite quickly, as symptoms of Parkinson's disease respond to LEVODOPA therapy.

Random and hereditary forms of CJD tend to appear after age 60, although researchers believe the disease is present for years before symptoms appear. From the time symptoms become apparent, deterioration is rapid, and the disease is generally fatal within a year. The person may become inca-pacitated within weeks or months of the onset of symptoms, however. Researchers are uncertain about what causes CJD, although most believe the culprit is a mutated prion—a portion of a protein structure that goes awry. Although this line of study is promising, scientists do not yet know what causes the mutation or how it results in disease as prions contain neither DNA nor RNA, the genetic machinery viruses require to take over the bodies cells to replicate themselves.

CJD has attracted much public attention in recent years as a result of "mad cow disease" in Europe and other parts of the world. This infectious disease affects cattle, and eating contaminated meat spreads the infection to people in the form of variant Creutzfeldt-Jakob disease (vCJD). Doctors believe, but are not certain, that the infectious agent is a mutated prion; research continues to explore this possibility. The symptoms and progres-sion of vCJD are very similar to those of classic CJD; symptoms can follow infection by as long as 20 years. Classic CJD differs from vCJD in a num-ber of ways, including means of contracting the dis-ease, length of time until symptoms are apparent, and interval between the onset of symptoms and death. Although classic CJD can be passed from one person to another, such as through trans-planted tissue when the presence of CJD in the donor was unknown and in several instances through incompletely sterilized surgical instru-ments used in neurological surgery, doctors do not consider it infectious.

As with other progressive, degenerative dis-eases, there is speculation that CJD develops through an interaction between GENETIC PREDISPO-SITION and environmental factors. Although doc-tors have known of CJD for many decades and it affects populations around the world, there is little understanding of this disease and how it develops. It does not appear to be related to Parkinson's dis-ease in any way and resembles Parkinson's only in its very early stages.

cytokines   Chemicals the body produces that cause inflammation and other damage in certain cells as a result of immune activity. The most com-mon cytokines are the interleukins and tumor necrosis factor (TNF), which have been implicated as causative factors in the development of many health conditions including heart disease and can-cer. Researchers have found that brain cells in people with Parkinson's disease contain elevated levels of cytokines, along with a corresponding decrease in NEUROTROPHIC FACTORS that help to protect nerve cells from attack and damage. Actions that increase neurotrophic factors seem to cause cytokine levels to drop. Some researchers speculate that the increase in cytokines alters APOPTOSIS, the normal process of programmed cell death. It is not clear whether the increase in cytokine levels causes a decline in neurotrophic factors, or whether the decline in neurotrophic factors permits an increase in cytokine levels. Nor do scientists know precisely what roles cytokines play in health or in disease.

daily living challenges The variable nature and progressive course of Parkinson's disease alter the ways in which the person with Parkinson's confronts and accommodates everyday activities and tasks. Parkinson's disease presents an inconsistent spectrum of experience among those who have it; although the disease is progressive, its course follows no precise pattern. As well, each person's abilities along the arc of illness are both unique and erratic. By the middle stages of Parkinson's, most people experience unpredictable spirals and plateaus in their abilities to manage the ACTIVITIES OF DAILY LIVING (ADLs).

ANTI-PARKINSON'S MEDICATIONS control symptoms fairly completely for most people in the early stages of Parkinson's. Adjustments are minor; the person may take a little more time to button a shirt or engage a jacket zipper, but not so much more that it becomes a disruption in daily routine. As the disease progresses and the medications become less effective, however, symptoms interfere with many aspects of everyday life from getting out of bed to bathing, dressing, and eating. One of the most frustrating dimensions of Parkinson's disease is that there is no consistency or predictability to the extent of this interference for most people. A person may feel in a nearly normal and function normally one morning and be almost incapacitated the next or experience extreme fluctuations from one hour to the next and then have few symptoms for days.

It is important for the person with Parkinson's to remain as active as possible, and to engage as fully as possible in everyday activities. Research and anecdotal evidence support the "Use it or lose it" premise: If the person stops performing a particular activity, such as walking, regaining it becomes difficult. Physical therapy and occupational therapy can help the person find alternative ways to accomplish specific tasks. ADAPTIVE EQUIPMENT AND ASSIST DEVICES are also useful. Most people who are still employed at the time they are diagnosed prefer to continue working as long as that is feasible. They may find it necessary to explore workplace adaptations and accommodations.

Mental activities are as important as physical activities. Sometimes they create a greater challenge than physical activities do, particularly when the person can no longer do what he or she used to enjoy such as read or perform functions related to work or hobbies. Some people are able to continue variations on former favorite activities by making creative adaptations such as listening to books on tape. The COMPUTER also provides a means of staying in touch with interests and events.

Personality and attitude have much to do with how a person adjusts and adapts to the ever-changing circumstances that Parkinson's disease presents. DEPRESSION often becomes more of a factor as abilities decline and even fundamental functions become nearly impossible. Support groups give people the opportunity to share their feelings and experiences with others. They provide a good venue for discussing alternative solutions for common problems as well as talking about worries and FEARS.

See also ADJUSTING TO LIVING WITH PARKINSON'S; AMERICANS WITH DISABILITIES ACT; COPING WITH DIAGNOSIS OF PARKINSON'S; COPING WITH ONGOING CARE OF PARKINSON'S; QUALITY OF LIFE; WORKPLACE ADAPTATIONS TO ACCOMMODATE PARKINSON'S.

Dalmane See TRAZODONE.

dandruff   A common condition in which the skin of the scalp sheds an unusually high number of dead cells. The clinical term for dandruff is *pityriasis capitis*. The most common cause is SEBACEOUS DERMATITIS, in which the sebaceous glands of the skin secrete excessive amounts of sebum, an oily substance. This irritates and inflames the skin, causing yellowish red scaly patches that itch. The excess sebum gives hair a "greasy" appearance that makes it look and feel unclean. Because a sebaceous gland surrounds each hair root, sebaceous dermatitis is more pronounced in areas where there are concentrations of hair, such as on the head as well as in the beard area and on the chest in men.

The most effective treatment is shampooing once or twice daily with a dandruff shampoo that contains one or more of the ingredients salicylic acid, coal tar, selenium, zinc, and piroctone. These substances help to reduce sebum secretion and accumulation. Generally shampoos that are available without prescription do the job. Prescription medicated shampoos include ketaconazole or hydrocortisone to reduce inflammation and itching. For stubborn dandruff the doctor might prescribe ketaconazole cream or recommend over-the-counter hydrocortisone cream massaged into the scaly patches.

An extension hose and sprayer attached to a sink faucet make shampooing easier and reduce the risk of falls in the shower or tub. In later stages of the disease, the person with Parkinson's will need help with body hygiene tasks such as shampooing. Dandruff that does not seem to improve with medicated shampoo may indicate a bacterial or yeast infection of the skin or hair follicles and should be evaluated by a physician. Such infections require appropriate medication. Scratching increases the likelihood of infection.

In people with Parkinson's and other neurological conditions, dandruff and other problems such as OILY SKIN and excessive SWEATING develop as a consequence of the disease's effects on the autonomic NERVOUS SYSTEM. However, dandruff becomes increasingly common with age and is in itself not a symptom of Parkinson's disease.

See also BODY CARE; HYGIENE; LIVIDO RETICULARIS.

day-night reversal   A pattern of staying awake all night and sleeping during the day. This was a key symptom in diagnosing post-encephalitic PARKINSONISM from Von Economo's encephalitis, though some degree of this problem is not uncommon in idiopathic Parkinson's disease as one of numerous SLEEP DISTURBANCES. Sometimes there are factors that make it difficult for the person to sleep at night such as NIGHTMARES, RESTLESS LEG SYNDROME, WEARING-OFF EFFECT that causes a surge in Parkinson's symptoms, URINARY FREQUENCY, and mobility problems that impede becoming comfortable. In other situations, the person just feels awake and alert at night.

In day–night reversal, the person's sense of day and night is completely reversed with full wakefulness at night and extended sleep during the day. This is a different phenomenon from DAYTIME SLEEPINESS, in which the person feels sleepy or falls asleep in short episodes. Adjusting the ANTI-PARKINSON MEDICATION regimen sometimes helps restore a normal pattern of sleeping at night and being awake during the day, if the drugs are responsible for the periods of wakefulness and sleepiness.

See also BEDROOM COMFORT.

daytime sleepiness   (daytime somnolence)   The overwhelming and uncontrollable desire to sleep, or sudden falling asleep, during the day that many people with Parkinson's disease experience. Sometimes called excessive daytime sleepiness (EDS), daytime sleepiness can occur for one or a combination of several reasons:

• As a side effect of ANTI-PARKINSON'S MEDICATIONS, particularly DOPAMINE AGONIST MEDICATIONS such as PRAMIPEXOLE and ROPINIROLE. LEVODOPA may also cause episodes of sleepiness.

• Progression of Parkinson's that interferes with brain function. Daytime sleepiness increases in frequency and intensity as Parkinson's progresses.

• Disturbed nighttime sleep. Many people with Parkinson's have trouble sleeping at night, leaving them tired and unrested during the day. This condition can be the result of medications, symptoms such as RESTLESS LEG SYNDROME or DYSKINESIA, or an increased need to sleep that is common with aging.

Daytime sleepiness can strike at any time and during any activity. It is particularly hazardous when one is DRIVING or engaged in other functions that are potentially harmful to the person with Parkinson's or to others. Suddenly falling asleep without first feeling drowsiness is uncommon but does happen. Feeling drowsy and then dozing off into sleep is most likely to occur during periods of little activity such as reading and watching television. For some people daytime sleepiness has an element of predictability in being more likely to happen at certain times of the day or in relation to certain events (such as medication doses), although for most people it is seemingly random.

Treatment for daytime sleepiness targets identifying and mitigating the source. For some people, adjusting the regimen of anti-Parkinson's medications, particularly ADJUNCT THERAPIES with levodopa and dopamine agonist combinations, reduces or eliminates daytime sleepiness. This might involve changing to different drugs or altering the dosage and timing of current medications and can take time and patience. It is also important to do what is possible to assure restful sleep at night. Sometimes changes in the medication regimen improve nighttime sleep. Relaxation techniques, MEDITATION, and certain YOGA postures are often helpful, and sleep medications are an option when other methods are less than successful. The stimulant drug MODAFINIL (name brand Provigil), which typically is prescribed to treat narcolepsy, provides relief for some people.

See also BEDROOM COMFORT; EPWORTH SLEEPINESS SCALE; FATIGUE; PARKINSON'S DISEASE SLEEP SCALE; SLEEP DISTURBANCES.

decarboxylase   See DOPA DECARBOXYLASE.

decarboxylase inhibitor   See DOPA DECARBOXYLASE INHIBITOR.

deep brain stimulation (DBS)   A procedure for treating TREMORS in which implanted electrodes deliver electrical stimulation to structures of the brain that are responsible for movement. The most common placement for DBS electrodes is within the THALAMUS, the globus pallidus, or the subthalamic nucleus (STN). Thalamic stimulation was the first target approved by the U.S. FDA, but it is only effective in reducing tremor, hence it is rarely done in people with Parkinson's today and is largely reserved for other tremor disorders such as ESSENTIAL TREMOR.

As rigidity, slowness, incoordination, and even balance can be improved (as well as tremor) by pallidal (GPi) or subthalamic nucleus (STN) DBS, these are the procedures of choice for people with Parkinson's. Though there have not been any head-to-head studies to date, most movement disorders experts agree that STN DBS reliably allows a reduction in medications and does seem to be associated with slightly better reported motor improvements to date.

GPi and STN DBS are almost always done bilaterally, though many centers like to do a staged approach where only one side is placed at a time, typically a month or two apart. There are some theoretical reasons for avoiding unilateral (one sided) STN stimulation in the long run. Thalamic DBS is typically bilateral as well, since the condition it is usually used to treat, essential tremor, is so symmetric, though it is done unilaterally in many patients.

Deep brain stimulation is done as a stereotactic surgical procedure in which a circular frame holds the head in a precise position. A small hole drilled into the bone of the skull (with local anesthesia to numb the nerves of the skin and bone) gives access to the brain. Using MAGNETIC RESONANCE IMAGING (MRI) for guidance, the neurosurgeon slowly and carefully inserts the micro electrode (a very tiny electrode) into the brain. The person is sedated but awake during the surgery so he or she can respond to the neurosurgeon's instructions and questions. The normal awake firing patterns (neurophysiology) of neurons is also critical so that the surgeon can verify the location of the tip of the microelectrode as he or she maps their way to the target. Typically a handful of mapping passes are required to find the ideal location for each stimulating electrode. This technique helps to assure that the electrode is in the appropriate location. The neurosurgeon tests the adequacy of the stimulating electrode's placement by hooking it up to a handheld device to determine the thresholds at which stimulation causes side effects, as well as noting how the test stimulation effects motor signs such as tremor or rigidity.

Once the electrode is in place, the surgeon implants a battery-controlled modulator, similar to a pacemaker, under the skin in the chest and runs a thin connecting wire under the skin from the electrode's base in the scalp, behind the ear, down the neck, and to the modulator. The modulator then delivers a programmed impulse of electricity at preset intervals to alter the abnormal pattern of activity at the target and thereby reduce symptoms.

Unlike those of ablative surgery, the effects of DBS are temporary and adjustable. This feature allows DBS to be continually altered to optimally control symptoms with minimal adverse effects; the vast majority of patients have demonstrated clear benefit from DBS at four or more years after implantation. DBS is expensive but, as a U.S. FDA approved therapy for Parkinson's, it is covered by most health insurances, including Medicare. There is a risk of stroke (currently estimated as 1 to 2 percent), a risk of worsened cognitive abilities (almost exclusively in those with some pre-existing cognitive impairment), and a risk of adverse consequences from damage to surrounding brain structures from implantation, and there is a continued risk of infection as well as equipment malfunction because there is a device left in the body. Many side effects that develop post implantation (such as voice changes, swallowing changes, and stimulation induced dyskinesias) can be solved with proper reprogramming and management of medications. STN DBS also is associated with a weight gain of about seventeen pounds on average.

Studies indicate that GPi and STN DBS only prolong the on-time: It is rare that they achieve a better response than the person's best on-medications function. DBS is not appropriate for patients who do not at least have brief periods of demonstrable good response to anti-Parkinson's medications. Given the fact that either DBS procedure just prolongs on-time, and the clear risks of DBS surgery described above, most experts reserve these procedures for those patients who (1) have severe motor fluctuations; (2) are able to walk and have reasonable function in their best on-medications state; or (3) have failed attempts at optimal medical management with a number of medications, including frequent dosing of levodopa.

See also ABLATION; SURGERY.

degenerative condition   A disease that becomes progressively worse, resulting from deterioration or impairment of a body process or system. Typically, treatment can delay but not halt the progression of a degenerative condition. The most common degenerative condition is arthritis. Many degenerative conditions cause decreasing functional abilities that may progress to a state of disability or debilitation, but few are themselves fatal. Degenerative conditions are more common with age. As a degenerative condition of the NERVOUS SYSTEM, Parkinson's disease belongs to the subclassification of NEURODEGENERATIVE disorders.

Some degenerative conditions such as rheumatoid arthritis and MULTIPLE SCLEROSIS are autoimmune disorders in which the body's immune system "attacks" a particular structure or organ system. Most degenerative conditions, including Parkinson's disease, appear to emerge as the convergence of various genetic and environmental factors with symptoms that typically surge and recede as the condition progresses. Generally, treatment requires ongoing adjustment, in part because the body seems to develop a resistance to the actions of particular therapies (especially drugs) and in part because deterioration continues. DOPAMINE AGONISTS, for example, LEVODOPA, only work as MONOTHERAPY for a few years before the most potent treatment for Parkinson's disease is required. In turn, levodopa typically works very well only for a few years before its potency in controlling the symptoms of Parkinson's begins to wane and motor fluctuations develop.

See also ADJUNCT THERAPIES; PARKINSON'S DISEASE, CAUSES OF.

delirium   An episode of an alteration in the level of consciousness characterized by marked mental confusion, fluctuations between decreased arousal (stupor) and agitation, and DISORIENTATION. In Parkinson's disease, delirium tends to be more common in those who are elderly and who also have DEMENTIA. It often is generated by ANTI-PARKINSON'S MEDICATIONS, particularly anticholinergic medications and dopamine agonist medications, although LEVODOPA, selegiline, amantadine, and many other medications can be causes. Delirium also is a symptom of cognitive impairment that may or may not be a consequence of the Parkinson's. It is more likely if ALZHEIMER'S DISEASE is also present or if there is a history of alcoholism or drug abuse. Even fairly minor infections or mild problems with the body's steady state, like dehydration, may cause delirium in individuals with dementia, but delirium should always be evaluated. Potentially life-threatening situations such as bleeding or infection in the brain, which are particular risks if there has been any surgical treatment of Parkinson's, and stroke also cause delirium. It is essential to identify the cause of delirium promptly; diagnostic imaging such as COMPUTED TOMOGRAPHY (CT) SCAN or MAGNETIC RESONANCE IMAGING (MRI), and in some cases spinal tap to examine the fluid around the brain, can usually diagnose or rule out the critical causes.

During an episode of delirium, confusion and disorientation can be severe; the person does not recognize people, places, and events that should be familiar. Episodes may last hours or days. Delirium can cause a person to behave unpredictably, with wide and sudden swings in mood and actions. Sometimes behavior is angry and violent, without apparent provocation. Delirium and psychosis often appear in tandem, and determining whether they are related to the Parkinson's or are symptoms of other conditions such as Alzheimer's disease, other age-related DEMENTIA, or psychiatric illness such as schizophrenia can be a clinical challenge.

Because anti-Parkinson's medications are often the culprit when delirium is manifested in a person with Parkinson's, the first treatment approach is adjustment of their dosages. Levodopa tends to be a safer choice than dopamine agonists and anticholinergics, and has a much higher potential symptomatic benefit though similar delirium risk to amantadine and selegiline, hence demented patients are typically taken off of the other agents

and maintained on the maximum dose of levodopa they can tolerate without developing delirium or psychosis. Sometimes taking smaller doses more frequently is enough of an adjustment to end the delirium, or manipulations across the spectrum of anti-Parkinson's medications may be required to find the adjustments that relieve the Parkinson's symptoms without causing delirium. Generally, if changes in the drug regimen end the delirium, the doctor can reasonably conclude that the anti-Parkinson's drugs induced the delirium and any related symptoms such as HALLUCINATIONS, DELUSIONS, or psychosis.

Other drugs known to cause delirium and related psychotic symptoms in people with Parkinson's disease are muscle relaxants and antispasmotic drugs, TRICYCLIC ANTIDEPRESSANT MEDICATIONS, narcotic pain reliever drugs, benzodiazepines, and over-the-counter cold and flu products.

Delirium that continues despite efforts to adjust the anti-Parkinson's medication regimen requires evaluation and treatment. Doctors often prescribe the atypical antipsychotic drug QUETIAPINE, commonly available in the United States as the brand name product Seroquel, for this purpose. Quetiapine affects the brain's dopamine receptors differently than do conventional antipsychotic medications and seems to calm psychotic symptoms without interfering with the actions of anti-Parkinson's medications. Clozapine is another good choice for treating psychosis and delirium in people with Parkinson's, but it requires close monitoring of white blood cell counts as it can adversely affect them.

See also AGITATION; ANXIETY; DIAGNOSING PARKINSON'S; NEUROCHEMISTRY; NEUROPSYCHIATRY; SUNDOWNING.

delusion   A false belief that something is real although in fact it is untrue or imagined. The person having a delusion is unable to understand that his or her belief is unreal, no matter how rational and reasonable the efforts to explain it. Often delusions are harmless and family members tend to humor the individual. Occasionally delusions are paranoid, and the person believes and fears that others intend to harm him or her in some way. This idea can cause the person to refuse to participate in necessary activities such as eating or taking medication.

Delusions, HALLUCINATIONS and illusions are often thought to be the same phenomenon. A delusion involves false beliefs. Whereas a hallucination is a false sensory perception manufactured within the brain. Illusions are incorrectly interpreted messages related to sight, sound, hearing, touch, or taste and are not considered a definite sign of psychosis. Delusions, hallucinations, and +illusions are common in Parkinson's disease and may be caused by the disease itself or arise as a side effect of the ANTI-PARKINSON'S MEDICATIONS used to treat it. Delusions also tend to accompany DEMENTIA, are more common with advancing age, and can be a symptom of DEPRESSION. Delusions are usually more distressing for family members and friends than for the person who is having them.

Treatment for delusions in the person with Parkinson's should start with an evaluation of the anti-Parkinson's drug regimen. Because anti-Parkinson's medications alter the brain's NEUROCHEMISTRY, they often cause other disturbances in brain function. Delusions tend to surface in the later stages of Parkinson's when the two forces of the disease's progression and the need for increasingly higher amounts of medications to control its motor symptoms collaborate to produce an unstable neurochemical environment in the brain. Sometimes it is not possible to eliminate delusions and related symptoms completely without increasing motor symptoms. Atypical ANTIPSYCHOTIC MEDICATIONS, especially quetiapine may be helpful in treating delusions in people with Parkinson's, but any atypical antipsychotic should be used with caution as these drugs act on the brain's DOPAMINE RECEPTOR, and may create additional disturbances in movement. Typical antipsychotics should be avoided for the same reason. Some drugs used to treat HYPERTENSION can also cause delusions and hallucinations, particularly in people with Parkinson's.

See also AGITATION; ANXIETY; DELIRIUM; MEDICATION SIDE EFFECTS; MENTAL STATUS; NEUROPSYCHIATRY; PARANOIA.

dementia COGNITIVE IMPAIRMENT severe enough to interfere with everyday activities and functions. Dementia includes dysfunctions of memory, logic, reasoning, and analytical thinking. AGITATION, ANXIETY, and problems with memory and language (such as difficulty in finding the right words) are often the earliest signs of dementia. DELIRIUM, DELUSIONS, HALLUCINATIONS, PARANOIA, and SLEEP DISTURBANCES often are present later in dementia. The degree to which dementia is apparent fluctuates, particularly early on, when the person might have extended periods of normal COGNITIVE FUNCTION with infrequent and minor interruptions of cognitive impairment. Because these inconsistencies are unpredictable, managing them is more difficult than managing symptoms of dementia that is constant. However, dementia represents progressive degeneration of brain function and gradually worsens with time.

The older the person with Parkinson's, the more likely that dementia will develop or already is present. This is likely an interaction of the progression of the Parkinson's and the deteriorations that occur with aging. In a person who already has dementia at the time Parkinson's disease is diagnosed, treatment with DOPAMINERGIC MEDICATIONS such as AMANTADINE and SELEGILINE or with DOPAMINE AGONIST MEDICATIONS such as PERGOLIDE and BROMOCRIPTINE is likely to worsen the dementia. ANTICHOLINERGIC MEDICATIONS such as BENZTROPINE, TRIHEXYPHENIDYL, and biperiden, prescribed to relieve TREMORS, can worsen cognitive impairment overall, further contributing to dementia.

Those who are closest to the person, such as family members, friends, and caregivers, typically notice the signs of dementia although the person with Parkinson's does not. A health care provider can gather some idea as to the presence and extent of dementia by using a tool called the MINI-MENTAL STATUS EXAMINATION (MMSE), a short series of questions that gauge the person's orientation to time and place as well as ability to use language, follow multistep directions, and perform analytical tasks such as sequentially subtracting or adding numbers.

There are several forms of dementia that can accompany Parkinson's disease. There is some debate as to how dementia and Parkinson's are related.

Some researchers believe that dementia exists independently but concurrently with Parkinson's. Others believe that there is an overall connection between dementia and various NEURODEGENERATIVE conditions including Parkinson's disease as well as ALZHEIMER'S DISEASE.

Lewy Body Dementia

The LEWY BODY is a deposit of proteins, particularly ALPHA-SYNUCLEIN, within a NEURON that has a characteristic shape and structure. These deposits, which so far can only be detected at autopsy, are not present in the brain of people without neurodegenerative conditions but are typically found in the brain of people with Parkinson's disease. They are virtually restricted to the SUBSTANTIA NIGRA and other structures of the MIDBRAIN and BASAL GANGLIA in people with Parkinson's. In people with Parkinson's who develop dementia later, Lewy bodies are usually present in other parts of the brain as well. Some people who have dementia long before the onset of parkinsonian motor features also have Lewy bodies present in regions of the brain responsible for cognitive function but not in those related to movement. These people are said to have Lewy body dementia.

A number of researchers believe that Parkinson's disease and dementia are both Lewy body disorders and that the symptoms reflect the areas of the brain where Lewy bodies exist. When both motor and cognitive symptoms are present, these researchers refer to the condition as DIFFUSE LEWY BODY DISEASE. However, a person with Parkinson's disease can have Lewy body dementia or non–Lewy body dementia. Because there is no way as yet to determine the presence or absence of Lewy bodies in a living person, these distinctions remain incompletely understood.

People who have Lewy body dementia tend not to tolerate the conventional medications, such as ANTIPSYCHOTIC and ANTIANXIETY MEDICATIONS, that are sometimes effective in other forms of dementia. These drugs act to inhibit the brain's dopamine receptors, thereby increasing motor symptoms such as TREMOR and BRADYKINESIA. Two of the ACETYLCHOLINESTERASE INHIBITOR drugs currently available to treat cognitive impairment in Alzheimer's disease that sometimes help are RIVASTIGMINE and DONEPEZIL. Rivastigmine has been proven effective in Lewy body dementia in several studies, including a randomized controlled trial, and does not worsen the motor symptoms of Parkinson's. Donepezil's usefulness in Lewy body dementia is supported by at least one open label trial, though there are some reports of it worsening parkinsonian motor symptoms. Galantamine has been reported to help in a number of cases. Tacrine has been reported to help in few cases, but it has been more frequently reported to harm motor function. Two atypical antipsychotic drugs, so called because they have different mechanisms of action from conventional antipsychotic drugs, that sometimes reduce dementia symptoms in Lewy body dementia and dementia in Parkinson's are QUETIAPINE (Seroquel) and CLOZAPINE (Clozaril).

Alzheimer's Dementia

Deterioration of cognitive function is a recognized natural dimension of aging. Estimates project that beyond age 85, most people have some level of dementia. So-called age related dementia is usually Alzheimer's disease. The dementia of Alzheimer's disease has different characteristics from those of Parkinson's disease but often coexists with Parkinson's. Experts estimate that as many as a third of those who have one of these diseases also have the other. Rather than Lewy bodies, protein deposits called amyloid plaques accumulate and interfere with neuron communication in Alzheimer's disease. The dementia of Alzheimer's is less variable and more obviously progressive than the dementia of Parkinson's and has predictable patterns of ebb and flow such as SUNDOWNING, or the worsening of dementia symptoms toward the end of the day.

Anticholinergic medications used as adjunct therapies for Parkinson's disease can worsen the dementia of Alzheimer's disease as they further inhibit the actions of acetylcholine, which is already in short supply in Alzheimer's. A recent report even hints at links between the use of these anticholinergic medications in people with Parkinson's and an increase in the risk of developing Alzheimer's. Acetylcholinesterase inhibitors often diminish the symptoms of dementia in Alzheimer's disease.

Multiinfarct Dementia

Multiinfarct dementia is cognitive impairment that is the result of damage from strokes or small vessel ischemic changes. It typically progresses in a stepwise fashion as more infarcts (strokes) occur. These infarcts are the result of either progressive narrowing of vessels from atherosclerosis such that they eventually plug up (occlude), or from small clots having broken loose from other parts of the body making their way to the brain, where they lodged inside the arteries, disrupting the flow of blood to a portion of the brain. The location of the infarct, or clot and blockage, determines the nature and extent of the damage, which generally is small but becomes cumulative. Sometimes this form of dementia shows up on a COMPUTED TOMOGRAPHY (CT) SCAN or MAGNETIC RESONANCE IMAGING (MRI) of the head. The only value in knowing that the dementia is the result of multiple infarctions is that treating the underlying cause, which is commonly hypertension, may be possible. Drugs such as those taken for the dementia of Alzheimer's disease are not effective in multiinfarct dementia. Anti-Parkinson's medications have no effect on multiinfarct dementia; however, it is not always easy to determine that multiinfarct dementia is the form of dementia present.

See also ALPHA-SYNUCLEIN GENE; APATHY; DEPRESSION; MEDICATION SIDE EFFECTS; NEUROPSYCHIATRY.

dendrite The branchlike structure that extends from the top of a neuron to receive signals. Like AXONS (the taillike structures that extend from the bottom of a neuron to send signals), dendrites reach into the synapse, or corridor, between nerve cells. Although dendrites and axons come very close to one another, they do not actually touch. Instead, they rely on NEUROTRANSMITTERS to convey impulses between them. When the neurotransmitter is in short supply the signals become scrambled or are incomplete. DOPAMINE, the neurotransmitter necessary for transmitting nerve impulses related to movement, is diminished in Parkinson's disease. This low level prevents nerve signals from properly moving among neurons, interfering with smooth and coordinated movement.

See also AXON; NEUROCHEMISTRY; NEUROPROTECTIVE EFFECT; NEUROPROTECTIVE THERAPIES; NEUROTROPHIC FACTORS.

denial and acceptance Denial, or refusal to accept the truth, of a difficult situation is a normal human coping mechanism. It allows a person to process the information in the background of consciousness while continuing in the usual activities of living. For most people, a diagnosis of Parkinson's disease is a shock even if it might have been anticipated or the person is relieved to learn that there is an explanation for the symptoms. Denial is the mind's way of dealing with this shock. Acceptance is the necessary next step for returning to a healthy perception of the situation. It might begin gradually or in pieces, depending on the person's typical methods for processing challenge and difficulty. Acceptance acknowledges the truth and reality of the Parkinson's diagnosis and initiates realistic expectations about its treatment and prognosis.

The Cycle of Denial and Acceptance

The denial segment of the cycle often begins before diagnosis with the first symptoms that come and go, making them easy to ignore, such as a mild and occasional TREMOR in a single finger or an arm that ever so lightly trembles when it is doing nothing. This is the most effective and efficient response for the mind at this point because it permits everyday functioning to continue and is not the result of conscious thought and decision. Rather, it is a series of subconscious adjustments in perception and behavior. By the time there are a pattern and progression to these symptoms the mind is conditioned to ignore them, as it continues to do until the symptoms begin to defy control or to interfere with regular activities.

After diagnosis, the focus on treatment and the physical challenges of Parkinson's disease often overlooks the emotional components. This emphasis can leave the person with Parkinson's, or family members, feeling confused and alone in coming to grips with what the diagnosis means in terms of health as well as the bigger picture of life plans. Denial helps to protect the person from the emotional stress of these feelings. Typically, when the diagnosis is Parkinson's, the confirming evidence is whether the symptoms respond to ANTI-PARKINSON'S MEDICATIONS. Although there is no conclusive diagnostic test for Parkinson's, CONDITIONS SIMILAR TO PARKINSON'S do not respond to treatment with DOPAMINE AGONISTS or LEVODOPA. For many people this is the point at which the reality of the diagnosis begins to sink in and the transition to acceptance begins. For others, however, the remission of symptoms with treatment instead feeds the denial. A person might continue seeking opinions from different medical specialists, who often feel obliged to repeat tests or run additional tests because misdiagnosis is a possibility.

When Denial Becomes Dysfunctional

There is no defined length of time in which it is "normal" for a person to move from denial to acceptance. However, denial becomes dysfunctional and unhealthy when it persists despite incontrovertible evidence, such as when the person refuses to acknowledge that symptoms improve with levodopa and recur when the levodopa dosage reaches the end of its effectiveness or refuses treatment altogether even though symptoms are becoming more profound. Denial that continues in this manner prevents the person, and sometimes family members, from initiating adaptations that can help control motor symptoms, such as increasing the level of exercise, and from exploring treatment options that are most successful in the early stages of Parkinson's. If denial prevents the person from participating in treatment, symptoms worsen and become more difficult to control later in the course of the disease.

There is a line of thinking that persistent denial could allow a person to enjoy a higher quality of life during the earlier stages of Parkinson's because he or she will continue with everyday activities as though nothing is wrong. This logic is controversial, as most experts agree that treatment provides the best opportunity to preserve daily function, and there is now some evidence that some treatments may have the potential to slow the disease. Acceptance allows the person with Parkinson's to make reasonable and realistic plans for the future and allows family members to make appropriate adjustments.

Denial and Acceptance Issues for Family Members

Sometimes family members struggle with denial and acceptance issues, for the same reasons as the person with Parkinson's. Their attitudes can increase emotional stress for the person with Parkinson's, particularly when he or she has moved from denial to acceptance but the family member has not. Many people with Parkinson's experience numerous cycles of denial and acceptance throughout the course of the disease, often in response to the ebb and flow of symptoms. These cycles can help the person to cope with the challenges of changing and unpredictable circumstances.

Dealing with Denial

The course of Parkinson's disease is such that when denial persists, confrontations with reality become increasingly frequent. It becomes challenging and eventually impossible for the person to mask or hide symptoms such as TREMORS, BRADYKINESIA, START HESITATION, GAIT DISTURBANCES, and BALANCE problems. A single significant event, such as a fall or an automobile accident, may force the person to recognize that he or she has a serious medical problem, although more often a gradual shifting of perspective occurs.

Denial, even when it becomes dysfunctional or when it appears to be deliberate and intentful, remains a primarily subconscious coping mechanism. Family and friends can help by being compassionate and understanding of the difficulty the person with Parkinson's is having with accepting the diagnosis. An attitude that is calm, compassionate, and matter-of-fact about the situation can help the person to feel less threatened. A mental health professional may be able to help the person who persists in denial despite clear and obvious evidence move toward acceptance, although the person is likely to believe that there is no need for such help.

Sometimes because of concerns about what effects acknowledging the Parkinson's might have on career or job situations, a person presents an outward image that his or her health is fine. This is not an extension of denial but rather a conscious and deliberate structure of privacy and protection the person creates as a safeguard in certain circumstances or situations. Many people are able to accept their Parkinson's fully but choose to be selective in how and with whom they share the information.

See also EMBARRASSMENT; GOING PUBLIC; GRIEF; SOCIAL INTERACTIONS; PROGNOSIS; STRESS; WORK-PLACE RELATIONSHIPS.

de novo Parkinson's disease   Newly diagnosed Parkinson's disease for which the person has not yet received treatment. Currently, experts believe that the therapeutic goal with most de novo Parkinson's disease should be to delay treatment with LEVODOPA for as long as possible. This is because on-off fluctuations and dyskinesias typically do not develop until after a person has been on levodopa for at least a few years.

Some scientists believe that although levodopa ultimately becomes the only effective course of treatment for Parkinson's disease, in the process of relieving motor symptoms it also may contribute to the depletion of DOPAMINERGIC NEURONS in the BRAIN, though all human studies, almost all animal studies, and many cell culture studies all do not support any finding that levodopa is toxic. Beginning treatment with DOPAMINE AGONISTS that mimic the action of dopamine and with NEUROPROTECTIVE THERAPIES delays the need for levodopa and may help to preserve dopaminergic neurons, according to recent functional imaging studies of people with Parkinson's on ropinerole and pramipexole. After a few years of monotherapy on dopamine agonists (or if a patient either can't or is very unlikely to tolerate a dopamine agonist) addition to levodopa to the anti-Parkinson's medication regimen is usually required.

See also DIAGNOSING PARKINSON'S; CABERGOLINE; SECOND OPINION; THERAPEUTIC WINDOW; TREATMENT ALGORITHM.

dental care and hygiene   Regular care and cleaning of the mouth and teeth. Brushing and flossing are essential for good oral health but require good DEXTERITY and COORDINATION, abilities that become more difficult as Parkinson's disease progresses. A wide-handled toothbrush is easier to grip and manipulate early in the disease than an ordinary

one. An electric toothbrush can help accommodate coordination and strength problems that develop. A person in the later stages of Parkinson's often needs help with oral hygiene.

ANTICHOLINERGIC MEDICATIONS taken to control the neuromuscular symptoms of Parkinson's disease cause the salivary glands to produce less saliva. These drugs sometimes are taken specifically for this effect as excessive saliva production is often a problem for people with Parkinson's disease. Lowered saliva production also occurs as a natural function of aging and can be a side effect of numerous other drugs including ANTI-PARKINSON'S MEDICATIONS and over-the-counter cold medications. Saliva helps to rinse food debris and bacteria from the mouth, so when the mouth becomes dry it creates an ideal environment in which infection can flourish. Infection can take the form of dental cavities, periodontal disease (inflamed and infected gums), and sores in the mouth.

The following methods can reduce the risk for infection and related problems:

- Brushing the teeth on awakening, before going to bed, and after eating.

- Rinsing the mouth frequently with water. Mouthwashes contain ingredients that can be irritating and drying, so they are not a good choice unless a dentist specifically recommends them.

- Avoiding sticky or chewy foods.

- Receiving prophylactic dental care (cleanings by a dentist or dental hygienist) every six months or more frequently if needed.

- Giving prompt attention to dental problems while they are minor, including toothache and bleeding gums (which can be signs of infection).

See also BATHING AND BATHROOM ORGANIZATION; BODY CARE; COPING WITH ONGOING CARE OF PARKINSON'S; DROOLING; HYGIENE.

Deprenyl   See SELEGILINE.

depression   A prolonged or intense state in which a person feels deep sadness, hopelessness, helplessness, worthlessness, or guilt. Most people experience brief periods of these feelings, often related to events or circumstances in their life such as the loss of a loved one. This response is normal and is not usually considered depression. Such a period constitutes depression when it interferes with everyday activities and enjoyment of life. Often the person with depression does not recognize that there is anything wrong. Common symptoms of depression include

- Loss of interest in everyday activities and in the joy of life in general (called anhedonia)
- Changes in sleep patterns, especially excessive sleeping without a feeling of being rested
- Inability to concentrate or make decisions
- Changes in eating habits (overeating or loss of appetite)
- Withdrawal from social activities and other people, increasing amounts of time spent alone
- Wide and frequent MOOD SWINGS
- Lack of facial expression or response to external events (diminished affect)
- In severe depression, thoughts of suicide

Clinicians generally use depression inventories such as the BECK DEPRESSION INVENTORY (BDI) or the HAMILTON DEPRESSION RATING SCALE (HDRS) to quantify the symptoms of depression and the extent to which they affect the person's daily living experience, emotional well-being, and perceptions about prognosis. These tools consist of a series of questions that the person (or caregiver) answers. The score is a general assessment of whether a clinical depression exists but care must be taken in interpreting the scores of many depression instruments in people with Parkinson's as many symptoms of Parkinson's can be confused for symptoms of depression. The PARKINSON'S DISEASE QUALITY OF LIFE QUESTIONNAIRE (PDQL), the HOEHN AND YAHR STAGE SCALE, and the UNIFIED PARKINSON'S DISEASE RATING SCALE (UPDRS) also have sections that evaluate and rate depression.

Depression can be a response to external situations or events, such as the diagnosis or symptoms of Parkinson's disease, or exist without apparent cause, in which case it is called an exogenous depression. Depression also can be an integral element of the overall presentation of symptoms in Parkinson's disease, in which case it is called an endogenous depression. Depression is more common with increasing age. Some of the symptoms of depression overlap with those of Parkinson's disease, making distinguishing the two conditions difficult, particularly in older people when a diagnosis of Parkinson's has not yet been made. Researchers believe that about 40 percent of people who have Parkinson's disease also experience depression; one in five had depression before being diagnosed with Parkinson's.

The Role of Monoamine Neurotransmitters

DOPAMINE and SEROTONIN are MONOAMINE NEURO-TRANSMITTERS in the brain that facilitate brain activity related to mood and emotion. In the brain, dopamine also has functions related to movement. EPINEPHRINE, NOREPINEPHRINE, and ACETYLCHOLINE are also monoamine neurotransmitters. In health, these biochemicals exist in balance. When disease affects one of them, the balance is altered. Scientists know that interrelationships exist among these neurotransmitters but do not yet fully understand what they are and how they affect brain activity and function.

In Parkinson's, the affected monoamine neurotransmitter is dopamine. Although the primary disruption is in the SUBSTANTIA NIGRA and other structures of the BASAL GANGLIA related to movement, scientists speculate that the depletion of dopamine affects other brain activities as well even though these functions depend on activation of different DOPAMINE RECEPTORS than do the functions of movement. ANTIPSYCHOTIC MEDICATIONS used to treat conditions such as dementia target these other dopamine receptors but also affect the receptors for movement.

Antidepressant medications work by increasing the levels of norepinephrine and serotonin, although they do so through different mechanisms. MONOAMINE OXIDASE INHIBITOR (MAOI) MEDICATIONS, the earliest group of antidepressant drugs used, work by preventing metabolism of monoamine neurotransmitters. This effect extends the length of time these neurotransmitters are available in the brain. Certain MAOIs such as selegilene and rasalagine, called selective because they target and affect just one or two dopamine receptors are theorized to have potential as NEURO-PROTECTIVE THERAPY as treatment for early stage Parkinson's disease or as one of the ADJUNCT THER-APIES later in the disease by apparently protecting DOPAMINERGIC NEURONS from damage caused by the by-products of metabolism, but they have only been proven to have a symptomatic effect on relieving Parkinson's symptoms to date. However, because of their action on dopamine receptors, general MAOIs typically are not prescribed to treat depression in people with Parkinson's disease.

Antidepressant drugs called SELECTIVE SEROTONIN REUPTAKE INHIBITOR (SSRI) MEDICATIONS function in a different way to produce the same result that MAOIs produce. SSRIs slow the biochemical processes that allow serotonin to be reabsorbed into the brain's neurochemical system after being metabolized. This effect extends serotonin's presence in the brain, keeping its levels higher and elevating mood.

Anti-Parkinson's Medications and Depression

The drugs taken to treat the symptoms of Parkinson's disease do not themselves contribute to depression, but most of them interact in some way with antidepressant drugs. Those most likely to cause problems are the MAOIs, for which there is a broad range of possible and potentially severe interactions. MAOIs also cannot be taken at the same time as any other antidepressant medication, or within two weeks of administration of another MAOI. This category includes the selective MAOI-B drugs SELEGILINE and rasalagine, sometimes taken as monotherapy in early disease or as an adjunct therapy in mild to advanced disease. Tricyclic antidepressants also have anticholinergic effects, as do many ANTI-PARKINSON'S MEDICATIONS. The SSRIs, trazadone, and venlafaxine are the least likely to interact with most anti-Parkinson's medications.

Treating Depression in the Person with Parkinson's Disease

Depression requires treatment when it continues to interfere with a person's enjoyment of and partici-

pation in the activities of life. The available options are as follows:

- PSYCHOTHERAPY without medication: Many people benefit from talking through their worries and fears with a professional who can help them put their concerns in perspective.

- Psychotherapy with medication: Antidepressants address the biochemical aspect of depression, and therapy helps the person to address any emotional issues that are contributing to the depression.

- Antidepressant medications: When the depression is endogenous (arising from the biochemical imbalances in the brain), antidepressants are often the most effective treatment. It is essential to evaluate the anti-Parkinson's medication regimen to select drugs that are least likely to have drug interactions.

- ELECTROCONVULSIVE THERAPY (ECT): For very severe depression, electroconvulsive therapy, in which an electrical impulse "shocks" the brain. This procedure realigns the brain's electrical activity, producing significant improvement of depression in some people. ECT also seems to relieve the DYSKINESIAS of Parkinson's; researchers do not entirely understand why this occurs.

The choice of treatment depends on the person's symptoms, stage of Parkinson's disease, and anti-Parkinson's medication regimen. The potential for drug interactions makes consideration of all dimensions of the person's condition before choosing an antidepressant medication important.

Depression As a Risk Factor for Development of Parkinson's

People who have depression are three times more likely to have Parkinson's disease than people who do not have depression. Scientists are uncertain whether this correlation suggests that depression is one of the earliest symptoms of Parkinson's or that the neurochemical disturbance in the brain with depression creates a cascading effect that can progress to involve the dopamine system as it affects movement. This remains an area of interest in research.

Depression in Caregivers and Other Family Members

Parkinson's also changes the lives of loved ones. Although depression is common among those who are close to the person with Parkinson's, it often is not recognized because the focus is on the person with Parkinson's. Such depression usually is generated by the stress of caring for the person with Parkinson's and the distress of seeing a loved one experience the changes and symptoms of Parkinson's. Support groups can provide safe environments and opportunities to share worries, concerns, and frustrations with others who understand them firsthand. Psychotherapy and antidepressant medications are treatment options when depression persists.

See also CAREGIVER WELL-BEING; MEDICATION SIDE EFFECTS; MENTAL STATUS; PARANOIA; PRECLINICAL PARKINSON'S DISEASE; PSYCHOSIS; PSYCHOSOCIAL FACTORS; QUALITY OF LIFE.

dermatitis, sebaceous   An inflammation of the skin caused by obstruction of the sebaceous glands; also called seborrheic dermatitis. In people with Parkinson's the most commonly affected areas are the face, particularly around the eyebrows, and the scalp, where the inflammation often causes DANDRUFF. Sebaceous dermatitis makes the skin appear and feel oily and unclean, even when it has just been washed. It is thought that the disruptions of the autonomic NERVOUS SYSTEM that Parkinson's disease causes are responsible for these changes in the skin. ANTI-PARKINSON'S MEDICATIONS usually relieve dermatitis and oily skin, although in some people these drugs instead cause these problems to worsen.

Keeping the skin clean and dry helps to improve the appearance of sebaceous dermatitis. Cleanliness often necessitates frequent washing with astringent, or drying, skin care solutions. It is important first to rule out other kinds of skin problems that have other treatments, such as acne or rosacea. In some people sebaceous dermatitis is an early symptom of Parkinson's; this association is generally recognized in retrospect,

after other symptoms have made the diagnosis obvious.

See also BODY CARE; HYGIENE; LIVIDO RETICULARIS; SWEATING.

desipramine   A TRICYCLIC ANTIDEPRESSANT MEDICATION taken to relieve the symptoms of DEPRESSION. Desipramine and other tricyclic antidepressants act on the brain's neurotransmitters but also affect the EXTRAPYRAMIDAL SYSTEM, the nerve network that carries signals from the BASAL GANGLIA to the muscles of movement. These drugs can cause Parkinson's symptoms such as TREMOR and BRADYKINESIA to worsen and can cause TARDIVE DYSKINESIA (abnormal, involuntary movements that appear with long-term use of a tricyclic antidepressant. Desipramine is available under the brand name Norpramin as well as in generic form.

Tricyclic antidepressants cannot be taken at the same time as MONOAMINE OXIDASE INHIBITOR (MAOI) MEDICATIONS, which may be prescribed to treat depression or as neuroprotective therapy. Desipramine and other tricyclic antidepressants can cause drowsiness as they are central nervous system (CNS) depressants and can intensify the effect of ANTICHOLINERGIC MEDICATIONS being taken at the same time. Desipramine can interact with a number of other drugs, most notably (in addition to those already mentioned) oral contraceptives (birth control pills) or hormone replacement therapy (HRT); medications for gastroesophageal reflux disorder (GERD) such as cimetidine (Tagamet) and ranitidine (Zantac); benzodiazepine drugs such as alprazolam (Xanax) and diazepam (Valium); and thyroid hormones taken to treat hypothyroidism.

See also ANTI-PARKINSON'S MEDICATIONS; SELECTIVE SEROTONIN REUPTAKE INHIBITOR (SSRI) MEDICATIONS.

Desyrel   See TRAZODONE.

dexterity, mental   The ability to concentrate to quickly perform cognitive functions such as reasoning and analytical thinking. Mental dexterity, an element of cognitive function, diminishes as Parkinson's disease progresses. Clinicians test mental dexterity by asking the person to repeat sequences of numbers or words, identify the missing elements in sequences, and perform mathematical functions such as sequential subtraction or addition. More extensive cognitive testing can measure levels of cognitive impairment more thoroughly, but these simple tests can give an accurate assessment of how quickly a person can think and respond.

Activities that exercise mental dexterity such as reading, analytical problem solving (math problems or word puzzles), memory games, dialogue, and debate, and other tasks, help people to preserve cognitive ability. Once these functions are lost, it is difficult if not impossible to restore. OCCUPATIONAL THERAPY can sometimes offer exercises and activities that help. Medications such as donepezil and rivastigmine taken to improve cognitive functions temporarily improve mental dexterity, along with other cognitive functions, in some people with Parkinson's, but their effectiveness varies widely.

See also BRADYPHRENIA; COGNITIVE IMPAIRMENT; MEMORY IMPAIRMENT; QUALITY OF LIFE.

dexterity, physical The ability to perform tasks that require fine motor skills using the fingers and hands. This ability gradually diminishes in Parkinson's disease. An early indicator of Parkinson's is difficulty in performing repetitious tasks that require dexterity, such as tapping the fingers in sequence. The loss of dexterity typically is asymmetrical (unilateral or single-sided), or more pronounced on one side of the body than the other. The person may not notice a problem if the loss affects the nondominant hand. When dexterity loss is minimal, as in the early stages of Parkinson's, compensation occurs without conscious awareness. The person may shift to the nonaffected hand for tasks such as fastening buttons or picking up change. Loss of dexterity affects handwriting, causing the characteristic MICROGRAPHIA, a small, cramped writing style, that is sometimes the first sign that dexterity is reduced. Hand–eye coordination is another dimension of dexterity that suffers in Parkinson's when the disease affects control of eye muscles.

As do other motor symptoms of Parkinson's, dexterity progressively worsens as the disease progresses. Treatment with ANTI-PARKINSON'S MEDICATIONS to some extent but not entirely restores dexterity as it improves other symptoms such as TREMORS and BRADYKINESIA, but loss of dexterity remains an obvious and frustrating problem for people with Parkinsons's. As treatment becomes less effective in controlling tremors, those that affect the hands further compound the loss of dexterity. Any activity that exercises dexterity, such as typing or putting together jigsaw puzzles, keeps fine motor ability at a higher level than inactivity. Switching to large-diameter pencils and pens and printing instead of writing in script can compensate for micrographia. Occupational therapy can teach adaptive methods and strengthening exercises.

See also ADAPTIVE EQUIPMENT AND ASSIST DEVICES; COMPUTER, PERSONAL; COORDINATION; DIAGNOSING PARKINSON'S; EARLY SYMPTOMS; EYE MOVEMENTS.

diagnosing Parkinson's The process of diagnosing Parkinson's is a challenge for both physicians and those who have the disease. As there is no definitive clinical test either to confirm or rule out Parkinson's, for many people diagnosis is a painstaking assessment of symptoms and circumstances. Because the symptoms and the course of the disease are highly variable, the doctor may suspect Parkinson's immediately or not even consider it until other potential explanations for the symptoms turn out to be false leads. Approximately 25 percent of Parkinson's diagnoses are incorrect— false positive or false negative.

There are four cardinal, or classic, symptoms of Parkinson's disease:

- Resting TREMOR, predominantly asymmetrical
- BRADYKINESIA, predominantly asymmetrical
- RIGIDITY, predominantly asymmetrical
- POSTURAL INSTABILITY, including the stooped position characteristic of Parkinson's disease

When all four of these symptoms are present the diagnosis is nearly certain, and most people who have Parkinson's for an extended time eventually have all four of these symptoms. But one in five people who have Parkinson's does not, at least initially, have tremors, which are the most common symptoms that cause people to seek medical attention. And the vast majority of those who have tremors do not have Parkinson's disease; many instead have the far more common and usually less debilitating condition ESSENTIAL TREMOR (sometimes called benign essential tremor or familial essential tremor). Although the classic presentation of symptoms is asymmetrical (affecting one side exclusively or predominantly), about a third of people have symptoms on both sides. STROKE can produce the same one-sided presentation of symptoms as does classic Parkinson's, although generally a COMPUTED TOMOGRAPHY (CT) SCAN or MAGNETIC RESONANCE IMAGING (MRI) can determine whether a stroke has occurred.

Because Parkinson's is a disease that primarily affects people older than age 60 and its risk increases with age, older people with some or even all of the cardinal symptoms often also have other medical problems that mask or confuse the clinical picture. When cognitive impairment and memory impairment are present in older people, doctors often make a diagnosis of ALZHEIMER'S DISEASE, another NEURODEGENERATIVE condition for which there is no conclusive clinical test (except autopsy after death). As there is a strong correlation between Alzheimer's and Parkinson's—misdiagnosis between them is common.

The risk increases with age for numerous other conditions that can cause some of the same symptoms as Parkinson's, including those that are not neurological such as endocrine disorders (the most common of which is hypothyroidism) and clinical DEPRESSION. Some studies suggest, in fact, that depression is an early symptom of Parkinson's disease that manifests itself in response to the beginnings of DOPAMINERGIC neuron deterioration—the progressive loss of dopamine-producing nerve cells in the BRAIN that is the foundation of Parkinson's disease.

Younger people are at far greater risk for numerous other CONDITIONS SIMILAR TO PARKINSON'S such as MULTIPLE SCLEROSIS, AMYOTROPHIC LATERAL SCLEROSIS (ALS, also called Lou Gehrig's disease), and LESIONS or tumors involving the BASAL GANGLIA, cerebellum, or brainstem. As all of these conditions have differ-

ent treatments and prognoses, and for some such as tumors time can be critical, doctors focus attention on determining whether any of these conditions is the cause of the symptoms in younger people before shifting their thinking to consider the possibility of Parkinson's. Further complicating the clinical picture is the tendency for EARLY-ONSET PARKINSON'S to have primary vague or less conventional symptoms, such as VISION PROBLEMS or frequent FALLS without a sense of balance difficulty.

Clinical Assessment

Most commonly the diagnostic journey begins with a PRIMARY CARE PHYSICIAN and concludes with a neurologist (physician who specializes in conditions of the brain and nervous system). The primary care physician's examination should include a careful and complete medical history, general physical examination, general laboratory tests such as blood chemical and thyroid hormone levels, assessment of any medications the person is taking that could be causing the symptoms, and general NEUROLOGICAL EXAMINATION including basic cognitive function assessment such as the MINI-MENTAL STATUS EVALUATION (MMSE). At this point the doctor's main mission is to gather as much clinical evidence as possible to begin the process of affirming or ruling out the likelihood of any of the potential causes of the symptoms. When the clinical findings point to a neurological problem, the primary care physician turns over the diagnostic process to a neurologist.

The neurologist conducts further and more extensive procedures to evaluate neurological and cognitive status. They may but do not always include tests such as COMPUTED TOMOGRAPHY (CT) SCAN, MAGNETIC RESONANCE IMAGING (MRI), POSITRON EMISSION TOMOGRAPHY (PET) scan, SINGLE PHOTON EMISSION COMPUTED TOMOGRAPHY (SPECT) scan. These high-tech imaging procedures are mostly used to rule out other causes for symptoms, though PET or SPECT may provide evidence of brain changes that suggest Parkinson's they cannot supply a conclusive diagnosis of Parkinson's and their findings rarely alter treatment options or recommendations. Numerous visits, sometimes to several neurologists with specific subspecialties such as movement disorders or neurodegenerative conditions, over the course of months to years, may be required before a diagnosis of Parkinson's can be made.

Often the diagnosing neurologist becomes the treating physician when the diagnosis of Parkinson's is made and continues to provide medical care for the course of the disease. When Parkinson's is mild and the person has multiple health problems, as often is the case for elderly people, the primary care physician may resume overall medical management with regular consultation with the neurologist regarding ANTI-PARKINSON'S MEDICATIONS and other neurological treatment issues. Many people, especially those who are older, have a number of doctors involved in different aspects of their medical care.

Challenges for the Person with Parkinson's

For doctors, diagnosing Parkinson's is a clinical puzzle to be solved. For the person with symptoms, the diagnostic journey often feels like a nightmare. People who are seeking medical attention because they have symptoms are worried and often frightened; they know they probably have a serious medical problem, and not knowing what the problem is generates considerable anxiety. People whose doctors discover their symptoms during examination for other conditions suddenly find themselves confronting a potential medical crisis. It is frustrating, in a time when medical technology creates the expectation that diagnosis will be prompt and conclusive and treatment will be curative or at least end symptoms, to be in a situation in which technology is of little help and there are far more questions than answers.

Early symptoms of Parkinson's often are vague. A finger may twitch when the hand is at rest or project itself in an odd position seemingly of its own volition. A person may have a general sense that something is not quite right with movement but be unable to describe what is happening. SLEEP DISTURBANCES are also common early in Parkinson's but often are attributed to causes such as STRESS. Symptoms such as muscle spasms and even RESTLESS LEG SYNDROME have many potential causes. And because symptoms are highly variable, they may not be apparent when the person tries to demonstrate them to family members or

even the doctor. Other people may believe the person is making up the symptoms, and the person may begin to feel that he or she is becoming crazy. Some people even seek, or are referred for, psychiatric treatment before it is clear that their symptoms are real and neurological in origin. As well, it is easy for the person to ignore or deny symptoms for quite some time, usually until they begin to interfere with regular activities and compensatory adjustments no longer accommodate the symptoms.

The Next Steps

Once the diagnosis of Parkinson's seems conclusive, the neurologist determines the stage of the disease on the basis of evidence of neurological damage, an assessment of ACTIVITIES OF DAILY LIVING (ADLs) capability, and overt symptoms. The most commonly used tools for the STAGING OF PARKINSON'S DISEASE are the HOEHN AND YAHR STAGE SCALE and the UNIFIED PARKINSON'S DISEASE RATING SCALE (UPDRS), both of which incorporate comprehensive physical, emotional, and social evaluations. These tools help to determine the appropriate course of treatment with ANTI-PARKINSON'S MEDICATIONS and SUPPORTIVE THERAPIES such as PHYSICAL THERAPY, OCCUPATIONAL THERAPY, and speech/language therapy.

Many people want to obtain SECOND OPINION consultations to affirm the diagnosis. Most doctors fully support obtaining a second opinion when the diagnosis is a condition, like Parkinson's, that has such significant implications. An accurate diagnosis is essential for appropriate treatment. By the time most people receive a diagnosis, however, they have already had evaluations by a number of specialists. Unless there is reason to doubt the diagnosis or there is a specialist with unique expertise in treating Parkinson's, additional consultations are not likely to have much benefit. Because the diagnosis of Parkinson's is a considerable shock for most people, even if it is expected, some people react with protracted denial and consult specialist after specialist in the hope that one of them will give a different diagnosis. Ultimately this process creates more frustration for the person as well as for family members, and it often delays treatment that affects the course of the disease.

See also CLINICAL RESEARCH STUDIES; DENIAL AND ACCEPTANCE; PARKINSON'S DISEASE, CAUSES OF; THERAPEUTIC WINDOW; TREATMENT ALGORITHM.

diazepam A BENZODIAZEPINE drug taken to relieve ANXIETY, muscle spasms, insomnia, and DYSTONIA. The commonly prescribed brand name version of this drug is Valium. Diazepam takes effect quickly, is relatively short-acting, and often causes mild to moderate drowsiness. The drowsiness generally, although not always, wears off after the drug is used for six to eight weeks. Some people also experience CONFUSION and DISORIENTATION with diazepam and other benzodiazepines. Switching to a different benzodiazepine drug often eliminates these reactions. As other benzodiazepine drugs are, diazepam is a CENTRAL NERVOUS SYSTEM (CNS) DEPRESSANT that works by slowing nerve responses in the muscles throughout the body. It also has some addictive qualities and becomes less effective the longer it is taken, requiring larger doses to obtain the same level of relief.

See also ALPRAZOLAM; CLONAZEPAM; LORAZEPAM; MYOCLONUS; RESTLESS LEG SYNDROME.

dietitian, registered An expert in nutrition who has specialized education and training and has passed a national examination. Registered dietitians can provide nutritional assessment and counseling to help people plan meals to meet general and unique nutritional needs that arise in the course of degenerative health conditions. A registered dietitian has the designation *R.D.* after his or her name. Many practitioners call themselves nutritionists but are not registered dietitians. In most states there are no established qualifications for nutritionists; however, the qualifications for registered dietitians are the same in all states as the registration requirements are established at the national level.

See also COOKING; FOODS TO EAT; FOODS TO AVOID; KITCHEN EFFICIENCY; NUTRITION AND DIET.

diffuse Lewy body disease Degenerative dementia in combination with parkinsonism that results from the presence of Lewy bodies throughout the brain. A LEWY BODY is an accumulation of certain proteins within NEURONS that disrupt their normal functions. Lewy bodies, which only can be detected by autopsy after death, are characteristically present in the SUBSTANTIA NIGRA and other structures of the BASAL GANGLIA in people with Parkinson's disease and are present in other parts of the brain in Lewy body DEMENTIA. Some researchers believe that Parkinson's disease and Lewy body dementia are each components of diffuse Lewy body disease that is manifested as one, the other, or both in different people. Scientists do not yet know what causes Lewy bodies to form or how, precisely, they interfere with neuron function.

See also ALPHA-SYNUCLEIN GENE; ALZHEIMER'S DISEASE; CONDITIONS SIMILAR TO PARKINSON'S; PARKINSON'S DISEASE, CAUSES OF.

dihydrophenylalanine (DOPA) See 3,4-DIHYDROXYPHENYLALANINE (DOPA).

dihydroxyphenylacetic acid (DOPAC) See 3,4-DIHYDROXYPHENYLACETIC ACID (DOPAC).

diphenhydramine An ANTIHISTAMINE MEDICATION taken for its ANTICHOLINERGIC effects to relieve mild TREMORS and rigidity or to act as a mild SLEEP MEDICATION. Diphenhydramine is available as an over-the-counter drug in numerous generic forms and as the brand name product Benadryl; the person with Parkinson's should not take it unless directed to do so by the physician who is managing care of the Parkinson's. Diphenhydramine also has a drying effect on mucous membranes, which helps to reduce DROOLING. This drug's primary side effect is drowsiness, which is desirable when diphenhydramine is being taken as a sleep aid.

See also ANTI-PARKINSON'S MEDICATIONS; TREATMENT ALGORITHM.

disorientation No knowledge of people, places, current time and date, and similar information. Disorientation can be transient and infrequent, as in sudden awakening from sleep, or progressive and permanent, as in DEMENTIA. When disorientation is fleeting, the person quickly establishes a sense of environment and setting. Gently talking with the person can help this process and calm the person if the experience is alarming to him or her. When disorientation exists as a function of dementia, the person typically does not know that his or her orientation is incorrect so efforts to reorient him or her can cause confusion. The disorientation of dementia is often distressing to loved ones because the person may not recognize them. Some ANTI-PARKINSON'S MEDICATIONS can cause CONFUSION and disorientation, as can other conditions affecting brain function such as stroke, transient ischemic attacks (TIAs), and ALZHEIMER'S DISEASE.

See also AGING; DELIRIUM; DELUSIONS; MEDICATION MANAGEMENT; MEDICATION SIDE EFFECTS.

dizziness A sensation of unsteadiness, spinning (true vertigo), lightheadedness, or faintness (presyncope). The cause of unsteadiness or otherwise hard to define dizziness is unclear and sometimes may be induced by anxiety. Vertigo is from dysfunction of the vetibular mechanisms of the inner ear or brainstem. Pre-syncopal dizziness occurs from dysfunction of the autonomic nervous system in which nerve impulses from the BRAINSTEM instigate a variety of physiological responses in the body that cause the unpleasant feelings associated with dizziness. Dizziness can occur for numerous reasons. The most common are ORTHOSTATIC HYPOTENSION, in which the blood pressure suddenly drops when a person stands up from a sitting or lying position, and as a side effect of medication. Dizziness often accompanies nausea or fainting and can affect balance and sensory perception.

Occasional dizziness is common and usually has no health significance. Frequent or persistent dizziness suggests an underlying problem that requires further medical attention. Many of the ANTI-PARKINSON'S MEDICATIONS can cause dizziness, so this possibility is the first line of evaluation for the person with Parkinson's. Common culprits are ANTIANXIETY, antispasmodic (muscle relaxant), and DOPAMINE AGONIST MEDICATIONS. Sometimes different drugs within these classifications work equally well to control the Parkinson's symptoms but produce less severe dizziness or fewer other side effects. ANTIHISTAMINE MEDICATIONS have the opposite effect in that they tend to diminish dizziness.

Some people experience dizziness and nausea after taking a LEVODOPA dose. Persistent or extended dizziness can be a symptom of transient ischemic attacks (TIAs) or ministrokes, so this possibility should be evaluated in older people who are at increased risk for such problems.

The balance disturbances of Parkinson's disease result from the dysfunction of the BASAL GANGLIA, cerebellum, and other BRAIN structures involved in movement and the corresponding inability of the muscles to respond to nerve signals that would otherwise make the myriad adjustments necessary to maintain balance, not from damage to the balance mechanisms of the inner ear. Vertigo requires further investigation as many of its causes are treatable and are not related to the Parkinson's.

As most dizziness is brief and self-limiting, the best approach to treatment is to give the body time to restore equilibrium. The balance problems and DYSKINESIAS of Parkinson's increase the risk of falls with dizziness. Pausing for a few moments when rising is a good way to do this, particularly sitting for a few moments before rising to a standing position. Any further treatment depends on the cause of the dizziness.

See also MEDICATION SIDE EFFECTS; POSTURAL INSTABILITY; TREATMENT ALGORITHM.

do not resuscitate (DNR) orders Written instructions to health care providers stating the desire that should a person have a respiratory or cardiac crisis, there be no "heroic" efforts made to revive him or her. When there is a progressive, neurodegenerative condition such as Parkinson's, cardiopulmonary resuscitation (CPR) and other revival efforts typically are not very successful and can cause considerable trauma. Although all adults should have their resuscitation preferences on file with their health care providers in the form of a living will or other ADVANCE DIRECTIVE, such instructions are particularly important when disease is present. If they are not, health care providers are bound in most situations to take whatever efforts are necessary to revive the person in the event of cardiac or respiratory arrest (heart attack or cessation of breathing). There are generally three levels of resuscitation in the event of a health crisis:

Resuscitation Level	Means
Full resuscitation (full code)	Health care providers do everything possible to save the person's life, including cardiac compressions and assisted breathing (CPR), defibrillation (shocking of the heart into a normal rhythm), and mechanical ventilation (use of a breathing machine)
Partial or limited resuscitation (partial code)	Definitions of this are widely variable, and often the specific options are agreed upon in detail between the physician and either the person with Parkinson's or the person speaking on their behalf, but commonly this means that health care providers perform CPR or CPR and defibrillation, but a mechanical ventilator (breathing machine) is not used
No resuscitation (no code or DNR)	Health care providers take no action for revival

DNR orders should be part of a person's advance directives and on file with all health care providers (such as doctors, hospitals, and LONG-TERM CARE FACILITIES) who are likely to provide care for the person. If the person has a durable power of medical attorney (DPMA), the designated representative also should have a copy of DNR instructions as well as other advance directives. The person can change DNR orders at any time, to any level. When the person is incapable of making DNR decisions the DPMA representative or a family member may be asked to make the DNR decision at the time of crisis; which adds to the trauma of the situation.

In general, family members cannot change an already existing DNR directive as long as the person was deemed capable of understanding the full meaning of that decision at the time he or she made it. A DNR order should always include the information that the person has Parkinson's disease, particularly when the person with Parkinson's is younger, so there is no question about the order's validity if the person's regular health care providers are not present when the crisis occurs.

Resuscitation orders, no matter what level, apply only to situations in which the heart or breathing stops. In very rare circumstances, a person's physician could deem such interventions medically futile and place a DNR order without the person's or their representative's express approval; this usually requires special procedures to be followed, sometimes including legal action. The person continues to receive all other medical treatment, including ANTI-PARKINSON'S MEDICATIONS, hydration and nutrition, and treatment for other conditions that may arise such as infections unless there are advance directives that address these conditions. A person or representative may decide to forgo any treatment; people who are either very near death or very debilitated may choose to receive just treatments aimed at comfort if desired, and this may result in their transfer to a hospice.

See also HOSPICE; HOSPITALIZATION; LEGAL CONCERNS; MEDICAL MANAGEMENT; PLANNING FOR THE FUTURE.

doctor visits   Medical appointments, which can be traumatic and unsettling experiences for the person with Parkinson's. Being prepared for each visit streamlines the process and gives the person (or caregiver) a stronger sense of being in control. People with Parkinson's may consult numerous doctors and specialists before receiving a diagnosis and continue to see multiple doctors for different aspects of care after diagnosis. In a disease like Parkinson's in which the treatment regimen is challenging and ever-changing, it is easy to feel "swept into" the system. Many people feel rushed and uncomfortable during doctor visits. The following suggestions can help make visits less stressful and more productive for both patient and doctor:

• Request copies of all medical test results and records each time there is an office visit or procedure and take the copies when consulting a different specialist. Typically, the specialist receives a summary statement and copies of relevant test findings from the referring doctor, but this is not a complete "trail" and may lack information the specialist would find helpful.

- Ask the referring doctor to explain why he or she is making a referral to a specialist and what the specialist is expected to do.
- Take the complete medical record to any doctor's visit when it has been more than three months since the previous visit or when there have been visits to other doctors since the last visit.
- Keep an updated list of medications and take it to all doctor visits. Write the name of the drug, amount taken, time taken, and notes about any unusual effects the drug has.
- Write (or have someone write) questions and take them to the visit. Show the list to the doctor or go through it question by question to make sure each concern gets attention.

In the early stages of Parkinson's the person often is capable of going to doctor visits alone and may choose to do so because it is more convenient. However, it is generally helpful that someone who is close to the person go along to doctor's visits as well, particularly when that person is or will be helping with care. This caregiver or loved one can remember key concerns for the doctor to address, take notes during the visit, and raise questions about various matters. As the Parkinson's progresses, the person will need assistance going to doctor visits, an established pattern makes this transition smoother for both the person with Parkinson's and the caregiver.

See also ADJUSTING TO LIVING WITH PARKINSON'S; COPING WITH DIAGNOSIS OF PARKINSON'S; COPING WITH ONGOING CARE OF PARKINSON'S; DIAGNOSING PARKINSON'S; INDEPENDENCE; MEDICAL MANAGEMENT; RECORD KEEPING.

domperidone A peripheral DOPAMINE RECEPTOR AGONIST drug taken in addition to LEVODOPA or DOPAMINE AGONIST MEDICATIONS to relieve the nausea that these ANTI-PARKINSON'S MEDICATIONS, particularly APOMORPHINE administered as a RECOVERY DRUG, can cause. By binding with DOPAMINE RECEPTORS in the body (but not with those in the brain because it cannot cross the BLOOD-BRAIN BARRIER), domperidone blocks the receptors from binding with dopamine that enters the body's general cir-

culation as levodopa is metabolized after its entry into the bloodstream. This blocking prevents the circulating dopamine from causing unpleasant side effects such as nausea. Motilium is the brand name form of domperidone available in Australia, New Zealand, Great Britain, and Canada. Its safety is well proven; it is even available directly to the public over the counter in Britain. However, domperidone has not been approved by the U.S. Food and Drug Administration (FDA) (largely due to hesitancy by its manufacturer to undergo the high expense of the FDA approval process given the existing competition in the U.S. market), but it is available from a few compounding pharmacies in the U.S.

See also NAUSEA.

donepezil An ACETYLCHOLINESTERASE INHIBITOR MEDICATION (brand name Aricept) that prevents the action of the enzyme ACETYLCHOLINESTERASE from metabolizing ACETYLCHOLINE, a NEUROTRANSMITTER in the BRAIN that is key to COGNITIVE FUNCTION. This drug is approved in the United States for treating the DEMENTIA of ALZHEIMER'S DISEASE. Doctors sometimes prescribe it to treat dementia in Parkinson's disease as well, on the premise that there appears to be a strong correlation in the disease processes. Not all who have either form of dementia who take donepezil experience improved cognitive function, and so far there is no way to assess who is likely to benefit. Side effects are uncommon; when they occur, they may include nausea, diarrhea, headache, DIZZINESS, and SLEEP DISTURBANCES. Rivastigmine has the most evidence of both its usefulness and safety in people with parkinsonism, and hence is currently the acetylcholinesterase inhibitor of first choice of Parkinson's experts for treating dementia.

See also COGNITIVE IMPAIRMENT; NEUROCHEMISTRY; OFF-LABEL DRUG; OPEN-LABEL DRUG STUDY.

dopa decarboxylase **(DDC)** An enzyme in the brain that converts, or metabolizes, the amino acid 3,4-DIHYDROXYPHENYLALANINE (DOPA) and LEVODOPA to DOPAMINE, the NEUROTRANSMITTER essential for facilitating nerve signals in the structures of the BASAL GANGLIA that direct COORDINATION and smooth movement. Peripherally (in the body), DDC acts quickly to metabolize the ANTI-PARKINSON'S MEDICATION levodopa. Because of this action, levodopa doses must be much greater than the amount of levodopa the brain needs, to allow enough levodopa to survive DDC action peripherally and reach the brain. However, this method puts high concentrations of dopamine into peripheral circulation, causing such unpleasant side effects as nausea and lightheadedness.

dopa decarboxylase inhibitor (DDCI) ANTI-PARKINSON'S MEDICATION that blocks the action of the enzyme DOPA DECARBOXYLASE (DDC). Its purpose is to block peripheral metabolism of LEVODOPA to DOPAMINE, allowing a greater concentration of levodopa to reach the brain for conversion to dopamine there. As this process reduces the concentration of peripheral dopamine in the bloodstream, it allows the administration of a lower dose of levodopa, which mitigates the unpleasant side effects of high peripheral dopamine levels such as NAUSEA and lightheadedness. There are two DDCIs currently available; they are always taken with levodopa (generally in a one-to-four ratio of DDCI to levodopa). CARBIDOPA is taken with levodopa in the combination drug SINEMET (also available as the brand name Atamet and in generic forms). Most people require about 75 milligrams a day of carbidopa to prevent the peripheral conversion of levodopa to dopamine; some people require more. It is for this reason that carbidopa/levodopa 10/100 tablets should be avoided in most patients and reserved for only those who require eight or more tablets a day. BENSERAZIDE is taken with levodopa in the combination drug Madopar.

See also ENTAPACONE.

dopamine   A NEUROTRANSMITTER that facilitates communication among central (BRAIN) and peripheral (body) NEURONS. Dopamine is present in many body tissues; it is most highly concentrated in the brain and is essential for the brain functions that direct smooth, coordinated movement. Dopamine circulates as a fluid throughout the brain. The SUBSTANTIA NIGRA, a small, darkly pigmented structure of the BASAL GANGLIA, produces most of the brain's dopamine. Other brain structures that produce dopamine in much smaller quantities include the STRIATUM, cerebellum, THALAMUS, and hypothalamus.

Dopamine Synthesis (Manufacture)

Dopamine belongs to the chemical family of CATECHOLAMINES. Other catecholamines in the human body include epinephrine and NOREPINEPHRINE. Dopaminergic neurons in the brain synthesize, or manufacture, dopamine from its base ingredients, the amino acids TYROSINE and dihydroxyphenylalanine (DOPA). This is a continuous, on-demand process. Once the neurons release dopamine, enzymes in the brain quickly metabolize it.

The brain makes its own supply of dopamine because it needs significantly higher quantities than does the rest of the body. Dopamine molecules cannot cross the BLOOD-BRAIN BARRIER, which maintains the separation between peripheral and central dopamine supplies. In the brain, dopamine exists in balance with two other neurotransmitters, ACETYLCHOLINE and serotonin. Changing the balance of these key neurotransmitters alters brain function. A small structure located in each carotid artery in the neck, the CAROTID BODY, produces dopamine for peripheral circulation. There is no difference chemically between central and peripheral dopamine.

Dopamine and Parkinson's Disease

In Parkinson's disease cells in the substantia nigra die, reducing the body's dopamine production. Researchers believe symptoms begin to become apparent only after roughly when 80 percent of the substantia nigra's cells have died and progress as cells continue to die. As these cells die, the level of dopamine the substantia nigra can produce correspondingly declines. Communication among neurons becomes disrupted, interfering with the brain's ability to control the body's movement. The results are the TREMORS, BRADYKINESIA, RIGIDITY, and other symptoms characteristic of Parkinson's disease.

Researchers discovered the relationship between dopamine and Parkinson's disease in the 1960s; discovery in turn led to the development of drugs that attempt to restore the brain's level of dopamine.

Such drugs relieve the symptoms of Parkinson's disease in most people diagnosed with the condition, decreasing efficacy, decreasing duration of action (on-off phenomena), and dyskinesias tend to develop as these drugs are taken chronically over time. This appears to be the consequence of substantia nigra cells continuing to die, leaving less surviving cells to convert dopamine precursors such as levodopa to dopamine. Researchers do not yet know what causes these cells to die or how to prevent them from dying. Much research focuses on ways either to replace these cells or to alter their genetic structures to change the timing of their death, whereas conventional treatment attempts to increase dopamine levels.

Dopamine as Treatment for Parkinson's

Although the goal in treating Parkinson's disease is to restore a more normal amount of dopamine in the brain, dopamine itself, which is available as an injectable drug, cannot do this. Giving dopamine directly stimulates the heart and other cardiovascular activity (and is in fact a treatment for cardiac arrest, or heart attack) but does not increase the level of dopamine in the brain because dopamine molecules cannot cross the blood-brain barrier either into or out of the brain. Transporting dopamine to the brain requires delivering it in precursor form as levodopa. Levodopa molecules can cross the blood-brain barrier, although they are quickly metabolized when they enter the peripheral (body) bloodstream. So other treatment strategies for Parkinson's focus on extending the time dopamine is available to neurons. Dopamine is metabolized rapidly in central (brain) circulation as well, which is one reason that the brain manufactures so much of it under normal circumstances.

Other Dopamine Actions

Recent studies suggest that dopamine overactivity reduces the sensitivity of the pleasure centers in the brain, contributing to problems such as drug addiction and obesity (use of food as the trigger for activating the brain's pleasure centers). Dopamine overactivity also contributes to psychotic illnesses such as SCHIZOPHRENIA and PARANOIA and is believed to have a role in attention deficit disorder

(ADD) and related conditions. Many ANTIPSYCHOTIC MEDICATIONS are DOPAMINE ANTAGONISTS that act selectively on specific dopamine receptors. Peripheral dopamine affects heart activity and emotional response. The ADRENAL MEDULLA converts peripheral dopamine to epinephrine and norepinephrine.

See also ANTI-PARKINSON'S MEDICATIONS; CATECHOL-O-METHYLTRANSFERASE; DOPA DECARBOXYLASE; DOPAMINE AGONIST MEDICATIONS; MEDICATION MANAGEMENT; PARKINSON'S DISEASE, CAUSES OF.

dopamine agonist medications   Drugs that have chemical structures that are similar in chemical structure to DOPAMINE and therefore can bind selectively to a DOPAMINE RECEPTOR. Dopamine agonists have molecular structures that enable them to cross the BLOOD-BRAIN BARRIER, whereas dopamine itself cannot. As well, dopamine agonists are similar enough to dopamine that they can substitute for it in a limited fashion, facilitating neuronal communication as dopamine would.

Endogenous dopamine (dopamine that is synthesized entirely within the body) binds with dopamine receptors in ways that scientists do not yet fully understand and probably with receptors that are as yet unidentified. Among the identified dopamine receptors, D1–D5, D1 and D2 were the first targets for dopamine agonist drugs as these were the first demonstrated to be involved in neuron activity related to movement. The first dopamine agonist drugs, BROMOCRIPTINE and PERGOLIDE, are formulations of the chemical substance ergot alkaloids. These drugs work well as both monotherapy in early disease and as one of the ADJUNCT THERAPIES to levodopa treatment in moderate to advanced disease, as the dopamine that levodopa produces seems to enhance receptor binding. Side effects, largely due to the ergot alkaloids, are common, and many people cannot tolerate these drugs.

Recent research suggests that D3 and D4 may play equally important roles in movement, and new drugs target them as well. These drugs, PRAMIPEXOLE and ROPINIROLE, are not derived from ergot alkaloids and so have fewer side effects as well as a broader range of receptor binding. These drugs show great promise as MONOTHERAPY in early

Parkinson's, some studies showing them to be as effective as levodopa at this stage. In mid- to late Parkinson's, however, pramipexole and ropinirole can no longer keep symptoms in check and work better as adjunct therapy to levodopa.

Dopamine Agonist	Receptor Binding				
	D1	D2	D3	D4	D5
Bromocriptine (Parlodel)	Strong	Weak	None	None	None
Pergolide (Permax)	Strong	Strong	None	None	None
Pramipexole (Mirapex)	None	Strong	Strong	Weak	None
Ropinirole (Requip)	None	Strong	Strong	Weak	None

Apart from their role in treatment for Parkinson's disease, dopamine agonists are sometimes used to treat erectile dysfunction as the dopamine receptors in the brain also affect the sensation of pleasure. It is believed that dopamine agonists increase the desire for sexual activity (libido).

See also DOPAMINE PRECURSOR; INTIMACY; SEXUALITY.

dopamine autoreceptor   See DOPAMINE RECEPTOR.

dopamine deficiency   A state in which there is an inadequate amount of DOPAMINE present in the brain to conduct proper NEUROTRANSMITTER functions. This deficiency affects movement, as in Parkinson's disease, and is believed to contribute to psychotic disorders and addiction. The primary cause of dopamine deficiency is the death of DOPAMINERGIC NEURONS in the brain, which is progressive in Parkinson's disease. Researchers do not know for certain what causes dopaminergic neurons to die.

See also ANTI-PARKINSON'S MEDICATIONS; APOPTOSIS; DOPAMINE DEGRADATION; DOPAMINE RECEPTOR; DOPAMINERGIC MEDICATIONS.

dopamine degradation   The natural process by which central and peripheral enzymes metabolize DOPAMINE, breaking it down into other chemical components. One strategy in treating Parkinson's

is to delay dopamine degradation by blocking the actions of these enzymes, primarily CATECHOL-O-METHYLTRANSFERASE (COMT) and DOPA DECARBOXYLASE (DDC). MONOAMINE OXIDASE also plays a role. ANTI-PARKINSON'S MEDICATIONS that attempt to do this are the COMT inhibitor medications TOLCAPONE and ENTACAPONE, which act centrally (in the brain), and the DOPA DECARBOXYLASE INHIBITORS (DDCIs) CARBIDOPA and BENSERAZIDE, which act peripherally (in the body) to preserve levodopa to allow more levodopa to cross the BLOOD-BRAIN BARRIER. The inhibitors monoamine oxidase-B (MAOI)-B SELEGILINE and rasagiline are also sometimes effective in extending dopamine's effectiveness.

See also AMANTADINE; APOPTOSIS; MONOAMINE OXIDASE INHIBITOR (MAOI) MEDICATION; NEUROPROTECTIVE THERAPIES.

dopamine precursor   A substance that can be converted into DOPAMINE in the body. The only dopamine precursor currently in use is LEVODOPA, which, as is dopamine, is an AMINO ACID. Levodopa's molecular structure is such that it can cross the BLOOD-BRAIN BARRIER. Once levodopa enters the brain, interactions with various enzymes convert levodopa to dopamine. Nearly everyone who has Parkinson's disease ultimately takes levodopa, as this is currently the most effective means to replace depleted dopamine supplies in the brain.

See also ANTI-PARKINSON'S MEDICATIONS; DOPAMINE AGONIST MEDICATIONS; DOPAMINE RECEPTOR; TREATMENT ALGORITHM.

dopamine receptor   A molecular structure on a cell that can receive, or bind with, the molecular structure of the NEUROTRANSMITTER DOPAMINE. Functionally a receptor is analogous to an electrical wall outlet—it is there and ready to activate the device that plugs into it, as long as the inserted plug configuration matches the openings in the outlet. Different configurations restrict access; in the wall outlet analogy, for example, the plug and outlet for 110-volt current differ from those for 220-volt current. Neurotransmitter binding functions similarly, in that each neurotransmitter has a different molecular structure and can only "plug in" to a matching receptor to complete the circuit and allow nerve impulses to travel through.

There are five identified types of dopamine receptors, labeled D1 through D5. Within each type are various subtypes, designated according to the functions that dopamine binding permits. DOPAMINE AGONIST MEDICATIONS specifically target these receptors. The continued stimulation of dopamine receptors by dopamine agonist medications appears to desensitize them overtime: That is, the number of receptors diminishes, and those that remain require a higher level of the dopamine agonist for effective binding. Researchers do not know why this happens.

See also AMANTADINE; ANTI-PARKINSON'S MEDICATIONS; DOPAMINE DEGRADATION.

dopamine transporter (DAT) Molecular structure that collects the AMINO ACID components that remain after DOPAMINE is metabolized. DATs return these amino acid components to DOPAMINERGIC NEURONS, where they are stored and eventually recycled into fresh supplies of dopamine. DATs are the focus of research scientists who are striving to further unravel the mysteries of dopamine synthesis and binding.

See also DOPAMINE RECEPTOR.

dopamine-producing cells See DOPAMINERGIC NEURONS.

dopaminergic medications ANTI-PARKINSON'S MEDICATIONS that convert to or act in the same way as DOPAMINE in the BRAIN. There are two kinds of dopaminergic drugs, DOPAMINE AGONIST MEDICATIONS and DOPAMINE PRECURSOR drugs. Dopaminergic medications have numerous potential side effects, the most common of which are NAUSEA, sleepiness, lightheadedness, and DYSKINESIA. They also can affect thinking (sometimes decreasing the ability to concentrate) and can cause hallucinations in people who have at least mild dementialike symptoms. Their effectiveness diminishes as Parkinson's disease progresses.

See also AMANTADINE; ANTICHOLINERGIC MEDICATIONS; CATECHOL-O-METHYLTRANSFERASE (COMT)

INHIBITOR; MONOAMINE OXIDASE INHIBITOR (MAOI) MEDICATION.

dopaminergic neurons Nerve cells that produce DOPAMINE. These are present in the brain and throughout the body. In Parkinson's disease, the dopaminergic neurons in the SUBSTANTIA NIGRA die off, diminishing the amount of dopamine that is available to function as a NEUROTRANSMITTER in facilitating conduction of nerve signals related to movement. DOPAMINERGIC MEDICATIONS simulate dopamine production either by activating dopamine receptors or by delivering LEVODOPA, an AMINO ACID that can cross the BLOOD-BRAIN BARRIER and is metabolized to dopamine in the BRAIN.

See also ANTI-PARKINSON'S MEDICATIONS.

Dopar See LEVODOPA.

DOPASCAN See 2 BETA-CARBOXYMETHOLOXY-3 BETA (4-IODOPHENYL) TROPANE (BETA-CIT).

Dostinex See CABERGOLINE.

dressing The actions of putting on and taking off clothing, which become increasingly challenging as Parkinson's progresses. TREMORS, BRADYKINESIA, and diminished DEXTERITY make grasping and manipulating closures such as buttons and zippers difficult. Even pulling on pants and shirts can become a struggle. Some basic adjustments can streamline the process:

• Choose items of clothing that easily pull on and off such as pants and skirts with elastic waists, shirts and blouses with snaps or hook-and-loop fasteners, and slip-on shoes.

• Lay out items of clothing in the order in which they will be put on. Sit on the edge of the bed or on a chair to dress, rather than trying to BALANCE while standing.

• Allow plenty of time for dressing and undressing.

• Focus consciously on each step of the dressing process.

- If early morning is an OFF-STATE, wait until ANTI-PARKINSON'S MEDICATIONS control symptoms before attempting to dress.

Dressing is a function of INDEPENDENCE for which most people resist assistance until they have no other choice. Caregivers and family members can make the process easier by remaining calm, maintaining a sense of humor, and offering but not forcing assistance.

See also ADAPTIVE EQUIPMENT AND ASSIST DEVICES; ADJUSTING TO LIVING WITH PARKINSON'S; CLOTHING; COORDINATION; COPING WITH ONGOING CARE OF PARKINSON'S; DAILY LIVING CHALLENGES; TASK SIMPLIFICATION.

driving   Operating a motor vehicle is a function that requires COORDINATION, DEXTERITY, and mental alertness. As Parkinson's disease progresses, its symptoms impair these abilities and driving becomes difficult as well as unsafe. TREMORS, BRADYKINESIA and other DYSKINESIAS can make movement erratic and unpredictable, particularly when ANTI-PARKINSON'S MEDICATIONS begin to lose their effectiveness. Many people with Parkinson's experience BLEPHAROSPASMS (muscle spasms affecting the eyelids), changes in COLOR PERCEPTION, and other VISION PROBLEMS that make driving risky or dangerous for them.

Because driving is a key marker of independence for most adults, giving it up is not easy. Doing so also publicly acknowledges that the person has a health problem. Often the person with Parkinson's resists, placing family members in the position of intervening. This may involve withholding car keys and taking other measures to restrict access to vehicles. Some families find it necessary to file a report with the state driver's licensing agency to force the person with Parkinson's to have his or her driving skills reevaluated. Often, but not always, this is a successful remedy that puts the "blame" on a third party rather than on family members. Sometimes, however, the person is able to pass the required driving ability tests and then feels confident about his or her driving skills. If this happens, family members often need to involve the person's physician to provide another objective opinion, as well as additional input to the state licensing authority to help it make the determination of whether a person should keep their driving privileges. Sometimes an evaluation by an occupational therapist is useful to document problems with reaction time or visual processing abilities in order to provide objective data on which to base the decision.

The most effective approach for all involved is to discuss the matter of driving before it becomes a problem. The progression of Parkinson's disease is inevitable, and anyone who drives will eventually face the decision of when to stop. Family members and the person with Parkinson's can get input from the doctor and then establish guidelines to identify when the person is no longer capable of performing the functions necessary for safe driving. This should include an assessment of symptoms that persist even with treatment, coordination and balance problems, times and patterns of the WEARING-OFF STATE, medications that cause drowsiness, and any issues with DAYTIME SLEEPINESS or insomnia. Keeping the driving decision objective in this manner makes it more clearly a matter of safety rather than an issue of diminished independence.

See also COGNITIVE IMPAIRMENT; DENIAL AND ACCEPTANCE; GOING PUBLIC.

drooling   Saliva accumulates when the muscles of the face, mouth, and throat become impaired, interfering with SWALLOWING. When this happens, the pooled saliva drips from the mouth. The clinical term for drooling is *sialorrhea*. Drooling is more prevalent at night when there is naturally less tendency to swallow. Even though drooling is uncontrollable, the person with Parkinson's often finds it embarrassing. Moisture that is allowed to remain around the mouth can cause chapping and soreness, so it is important to keep saliva wiped from the face.

The ANTICHOLINERGIC MEDICATIONS taken to treat TREMORS and other neuromuscular symptoms of Parkinson's sometimes help by drying out mucous membranes, thus reducing the volume of saliva. sublingual atropine slows saliva production. Injections of botulinum toxin into the salivary glands also has been studied. Although such treatments lessen problems with drooling, they can produce the opposite problem, DRY MOUTH. A certain amount of saliva is necessary to mix with food for proper chewing and swallowing, so when saliva volume is reduced, the risk of swallowing problems, including choking, increases. Sufficient saliva also is important for maintaining oral health. In early Parkinson's the person can make a conscious effort to swallow regularly and frequently, to prevent saliva from pooling. A speech-language therapist can assess the swallowing process and offer exercises and suggestions to maintain good swallowing function for as long as possible.

See also DENTAL CARE AND HYGIENE; DYSARTHRIA; DYSPHAGIA; HYGIENE; SPEECH.

drug "holiday"   A planned, intentional interruption of medication therapy, also called a structured treatment interruption (STI). The premise is that this interruption gives the person with Parkinson's and his or her physician the opportunity to see a comprehensive representation of Parkinson's symptoms by removing any "masking" that ANTI-PARKINSON'S MEDICATIONS may provide. A drug holiday generally is considered when a person is taking multiple medications and is not receiving complete symptom relief. It is a controversial method, as some experts believe this gives the person's body a chance to clear out all drugs and start "fresh" with a new treatment regimen and others believe that suddenly depriving the brain of chemicals it has begun to depend on risks an intense surge of symptoms that then may become difficult to return under control.

A person with Parkinson's who is considering a drug holiday should make sure he or she fully understands what to expect and should attempt this method only when close observation is available (many experts recommend hospitalization) so that immediate medical attention is always available. Withdrawing anti-Parkinson's medications can leave the person nearly paralyzed, depending on the extent of DOPAMINERGIC NEURON loss and DOPAMINE DEPLETION in the BRAIN. Difficulty in swallowing and breathing can produce a potentially life-threatening problem that must be addressed on an urgent basis. Patients on a large

dose of dopaminergic medications also bear some risk of the onset of severe muscle rigidity, fever, and autonomic disturbances, such as a very volatile blood pressure (so-called neuroleptic malignant syndrome, or occulogyric crises in cases where tonic eye deviation is prominent) with an abrupt cessation of medications.

Even after the person's system is purged of all drugs, the person does not return to a state of DE NOVO PARKINSON'S. Once treatment has been started, it creates irreversible changes in the dopamine network. For most people with Parkinson's whose disease is in the middle to late stages (the point at which a drug holiday typically is considered), resumption of medication is more likely to entail a return to a full-scale regimen than a gradual reintroduction of drugs.

See also MEDICATION MANAGEMENT; THERAPEUTIC WINDOW; TREATMENT ALGORITHM.

drug-induced Parkinson's   Parkinson's symptoms that are side effects of medications, particularly ANTIPSYCHOTIC DRUGS such as HALOPERIDOL and chlorpromazine, and some nausea and gastric motility medications such as prochlor perazine, promethazine, and metoclopramide. Such drugs are DOPAMINE ANTAGONISTS; that means that they block dopamine from binding with DOPAMINE RECEPTORS to reduce the amount of dopamine circulating in the BRAIN. Many older people receive treatment with these drugs for DEMENTIA and related symptoms, then begin to show symptoms of Parkinson's after taking them. Stopping the drugs generally ends the Parkinson's symptoms. Drug-induced Parkinson's is nearly always reversible and not considered true Parkinson's disease. Treatment with ANTI-PARKINSON'S MEDICATIONS typically does not resolve symptoms as would be expected, therefore strongly suggesting that the underlying cause of the symptoms is something other than Parkinson's disease. Particularly in the elderly, medications and drug interactions are often overlooked as the cause of Parkinson's-like symptoms.

See also 1-METHYL-4-PHENYL-1,2,3,6-TETRAHY-DROPYRIDINE; CONDITIONS SIMILAR TO PARKINSON'S; DIAGNOSING PARKINSON'S; PSYCHOSIS.

drug interactions, adverse   See MEDICATION MANAGEMENT.

dry mouth   A condition in which there is a reduced amount of saliva in the mouth. Many of the ANTIPARKINSON'S MEDICATIONS, particularly the ANTICHOLINERGIC MEDICATIONS and the ANTIHISTAMINE MEDICATIONS, restrict secretions of the mucous membranes (tissues that line the mouth) and inhibit saliva production. This effect causes the tissues of the mouth to become dry and sometimes painful. Difficulty in chewing and swallowing increases, establishing conditions in which infections (including dental problems such as cavities) can flourish. Rinsing the mouth frequently with water helps to clear debris and bacteria and to moisten the tissues of the mouth. Lemon and glycerin swabs, available in drug stores, can soothe sore lips and gums.

See also DENTAL CARE AND HYGIENE; DROOLING; SWALLOWING.

durable power of attorney for health care (DPHC)   See ADVANCE DIRECTIVES.

dysarthria, hypokinetic   Difficulties with speech that are the result of BRADYKINESIA involving the muscles of the mouth, throat, and chest (breathing). *Hypokinetic* means "undermoving." This is the speech problem characteristic of Parkinson's disease, which typically includes changes in voice quality, volume, and modulation. The person with Parkinson's may take more time to form words. Speech therapy can help the person learn techniques for breath control and other ways to improve speech.

See also COGNITIVE IMPAIRMENT.

dysequilibrium   See BALANCE.

dyskinesia   Movement that is involuntary and abnormal and that generally results from a neurological injury or disorder. Though most commonly used in reference to abnormal extra movements, technically abnormal reduction in movement also could be classified as dyskinesia. There are many kinds of dyskinesias, some of which are characteristic of particular neurological disorders.

See also AKINESIA; ATHETOSIS; BLEPHAROSPASM; BRADYKINESIA; CHOREA; DYSTONIA; LEVODOPA; MOVEMENT; MOVEMENT DISORDERS; MUSCLE SPASMS; MYOCLONUS; TREMOR.

dyskinesia, levodopa-induced   See LEVODOPA.

Type of Dyskinesia	Description	Characteristic of
Akinesia	Inability to move, freezing	Parkinson's disease
Athetosis	Slow, rhythmic, repetitive writhing	Parkinson's disease (dopaminergic medication side effect), Huntington's disease, cerebral palsy, side effect of antipsychotic medications
Blepharospasm	Contraction of the muscles of the eyelids	Parkinson's disease (often as dopaminergic medications wear off), infection of the eyelid
Bradykinesia	Slowness of movement, including start hesitation and freezing	Parkinson's disease
Chorea	Writhing, dancelike movements	Huntington's disease, side effect of anti-Parkinson's medications
Dystonia	Muscle rigidity and stiffness	Torticollis, stroke, Parkinson's disease (often as dopaminergic medications wear off)
Myoclonus	Jerking spasms of the arm or leg	Rare side effect of anti-Parkinson's medications, PSP, MSA
Spasms	Twitching, stiffness, and jerking	Various disorders
Tic	Repeated contractions of the same muscles	Various disorders
Tremor	Rapid, fluttery movements	Parkinson's disease, essential tremor

dysphagia Difficulty in swallowing. Difficulty arises when RIGIDITY and BRADYKINESIA affect the muscles of the mouth, tongue, and throat. A diminished level of saliva, which can be a side effect of ANTI-PARKINSON'S MEDICATIONS, restricts the ability to chew food properly, making swallowing even more difficult. Choking becomes a significant risk. A speech or swallow therapist can perform a swallowing assessment that isolates the specific parts of the swallowing process that present most problems and teach the person with Parkinson's methods for working around those problem areas. In late stage Parkinson's, it is often difficult for the person to swallow even his or her own saliva. Nutrition becomes a serious concern as well, as often the person is not able to eat regular foods.

See also FOOD PREPARATION; FOODS TO AVOID; FOODS TO EAT; HEIMLICH MANEUVER; SWALLOWING.

dysphasia Difficulty with spoken language that may take the form of difficulty understanding speech (receptive dysphasia) or difficulty with finding the words to say (expressive dysphasia). More severe deficits that make one virtually unable to either speak or to understand speech are termed aphasia. Dysphasia is a COGNITIVE IMPAIRMENT that occurs with a number of neurological conditions such as stroke, transient ischemic attacks (TIAs) or ministrokes, ALZHEIMER'S DISEASE, and Parkinson's disease. Expressive dysphasia generally occurs in the later stages of Parkinson's and tends to be more pronounced during OFF-STATE episodes. Treatment with ANTI-PARKINSON'S MEDICATIONS usually relieves dysphasia to the extent that it improves other symptoms including neuromuscular function and COGNITIVE FUNCTION. Dysphasia is often frustrating for the person with Parkinson's, who knows he or she can not find or is not using the correct word. Patience and compassion from family members and friends help the person to feel more comfortable with this symptom. Sometimes the person can write the word but not speak it.

dystonia Muscle rigidity or stiffness that can prevent movement, force the body into unusual positions, and cause painful muscle spasms. Dystonia can be an IDIOPATHIC movement disorder (exist alone without apparent cause) or a symptom of other MOVEMENT DISORDERS such as Parkinson's disease. In either circumstance, it probably represents dysfunction of the BASAL GANGLIA. In Parkinson's, this damage is the death of DOPAMINERGIC NEURONS with resulting depletion of dopamine. Occasionally dystonia affecting an extremity (often a foot) is one of the first symptoms of Parkinson's. Dystonia tends to worsen as the disease progresses. Sometimes dystonia takes the form of rhythmic, repetitious movement, such as of the lips or tongue.

See also DOPAMINE; DYSKINESIAS; MOVEMENT; MYOCLONUS; POSTURAL DYSFUNCTION.

early menopause   See MENOPAUSE.

early morning off-medication dyskinesia   See OFF-STATE.

early symptoms   See PARKINSON'S DISEASE.

early-onset Parkinson's   Parkinson's disease that develops in a person before the age of 40 (or 50 in some studies and references). About 5 to 10 percent of people with Parkinson's have early-onset disease. A person's age at diagnosis significantly affects a number of aspects of the disease, including severity of symptoms, rate of progression of symptoms, and treatment decisions. Early-onset Parkinson's is sometimes called young-onset Parkinson's or less commonly juvenile Parkinson's. Although Parkinson's disease in people younger than age 20 is rare, people in their early teens have been diagnosed with the disease. In young people, a diagnosis of Parkinson's is a result of ruling out all other possible diagnoses and monitoring the progression of symptoms over time. As with classic IDIOPATHIC Parkinson's, LEVODOPA response (use of levodopa relieves symptoms) provides the strongest evidence that the diagnosis is indeed early-onset Parkinson's.

Genetic Factors

Some scientists believe that most early-onset Parkinson's has a significant genetic component and have identified connections to a number of GENE MUTATIONS, particularly to a group of genes called PARKIN GENES. Currently identified parkin gene mutations are very rare except in very early (before age 30) onset. A number of genes appear implicated at present, and research is exploring links to others. Studies vary widely as to the per-

cent of people who have early-onset Parkinson's and have other family members who have Parkinson's disease, but around 25 percent is commonly quoted. However, people with idiopathic Parkinson's disease sometimes also have gene mutations, so evidence of the genetic connection is far from conclusive. As with other types of Parkinson's, a combination of genetic and environmental factors is the probable cause of early-onset Parkinson's. Much research remains necessary to decipher the Parkinson's puzzle.

Symptoms

Symptoms in early-onset Parkinson's tend to be less severe and less conclusive than in idiopathic Parkinson's. In about half of those ultimately diagnosed with early-onset Parkinson's, a seemingly isolated symptom such as painful muscle spasms in one muscle group, most commonly a foot or finger, causes the person to seek medical attention. People with early-onset Parkinson's are also far more likely to have depression than are people with classic Parkinson's, as well as to seek treatment for it. Further examination reveals subtle symptoms that are also characteristic of Parkinson's such as slight problems with BALANCE and FOOT DRAG. Although TREMORS are the most characteristic symptom in classic Parkinson's, only about 40 percent of people with early-onset Parkinson's have tremors. BRADYKINESIA, another of the CARDINAL SYMPTOMS in classic Parkinson's, is even less common in early-onset Parkinson's.

With the caveat that the course of Parkinson's is inconsistent and impossible to predict, generally early-onset Parkinson's tends to progress more slowly than classic Parkinson's. A person with early-onset Parkinson's often can enjoy decades in which ANTI-PARKINSON'S MEDICATIONS keep symptoms in check. However, the undesired DYSKINESIAS that occur as side effects of anti-Parkinson's medications tend to manifest themselves earlier in the medication regimen, making it necessary to try different medication combinations to keep both symptoms and side effects under control. So although people with early-onset Parkinson's can experience long periods without noticeable symptoms, it also requires more medical diligence to manage the medication regimen that makes this possible.

The progression of Parkinson's is sometimes rapid and aggressive in younger people with the disease. As best scientists understand at present, this characteristic is attributable to the unpredictability of Parkinson's, rather than a response related to age. Classic Parkinson's can as well progress on a sharp curve, as symptoms become severe enough to cause significant impairment quite early in the disease. This remains yet another of the unknowns about Parkinson's that researchers hope to unravel as they learn more about the disease as well as the neurochemical functions of the brain.

The Levodopa Debate

LEVODOPA, the medication most potent in treating Parkinson's disease at present, commonly induces the onset of motor complications after a few years. With ADJUNCT THERAPIES that incorporate additional medications, treatment can generally keep symptoms in reasonable control for a few decades. In people who are in their 70s or 80s when Parkinson's is diagnosed, this is less of a concern because levodopa in combination with adjunct therapies using other ANTI-PARKINSON'S MEDICATIONS can adequately control the symptoms of Parkinson's for the remainder of their lives.

When Parkinson's disease is diagnosed in people who are in their 30s, 40s, 50s, and most people in their 60s, this is not as likely to be the case; their life expectancy exceeds the expected timeframe for the development of significant motor complications from levodopa. As Parkinson's progresses, it takes increasingly higher doses of levodopa to produce the same level of symptom relief. Eventually these higher dosages of levodopa produce undesired side effects such as DYSKINESIAS and fluctuating response and, because of the continuing

depletion of DOPAMINERGIC NEURONS in the brain, can no longer accommodate the brain's need for DOPAMINE. As well, these side effects tend to occur earlier in the course of levodopa treatment than for people with classic Parkinson's, creating the need for innovative MEDICATION MANAGEMENT earlier in the course of treatment.

Innovative Treatment Approaches

People with early-onset Parkinson's challenge doctors to attempt innovative treatment approaches that traditionally have not been necessary in older people who have classic Parkinson's. The overall increasing vigor and life expectancy of the average person in their 50s, 60s, and even 70s, as well as young onset patients, has led most movement disorders experts to argue for treatment algorithms using other agents prior to using levodopa as a means of delaying levodopa associated motor complications. Most knowledgeable physicians would strongly consider using dopamine agonists as the initial treatment, deferring to levodopa when the person with Parkinson's has some decrease in cognition or other factors that would make dopamine agonists too risky.

Younger people sometimes respond differently to conventional treatment regimens than older people with classic Parkinson's and often feel they have little to lose by trying new approaches or treatments. People with early-onset Parkinson's often benefit from seeking treatment through health care facilities and providers linked with research programs. It is critical for every person who considers any investigational treatment, particularly one that is invasive such as surgery, to understand fully the potential risks as well as the possible benefits.

Career and Work Decisions

Many people in their 40s and 50s not only are still working, but also are enjoying the most productive years of their careers. The variable nature of Parkinson's disease makes prediction of how and when symptoms will affect work difficult. It is important to evaluate symptoms and work responsibilities at the time of diagnosis and continually as symptoms change. For some people, the changes will be slow and have little effect on job tasks. For other people, the changes whether slow or quick will have significant impact on work responsibilities. As well, medications taken to treat Parkinson's disease can affect various aspects of functionability, such as mental alertness and fine motor control. Most of the changes due to medication are positive as these drugs hold symptoms in check.

The decision whether to continue working is individual and personal and takes into consideration many factors beyond the ability to continue doing the work. When the person with Parkinson's is the primary income source for the family, he or she likely also provides for the family's health insurance and related needs as employment benefits. Leaving work, in most cases, means giving up these benefits. It is important to make work and career decisions carefully. Most people find that their colleagues are supportive and concerned and want to do as much as possible to allow the person with Parkinson's to continue working.

Many people who are still working when they learn they have Parkinson's disease find that the AMERICANS WITH DISABILITIES ACT (ADA) protects their employment rights. The ADA requires qualifying employers to make reasonable workplace accommodations to allow employees to fulfill the essential requirements of the job. The interpretation and implementation of the ADA vary widely and often are the subject of lawsuits. As well, some classifications of employers are exempt. Some people choose not to notify their employer of their diagnosis, reserving that option until symptoms become apparent. It is important for the person with Parkinson's disease to fully understand the employment requirements of his or her job and organization and to comply with any obligations to notify the employer of health conditions.

Effects on Families

Parkinson's disease at any age has a significant effect on loved ones, particularly immediate family members who might find themselves taking on the role of caregiver. When the person is young, family responsibilities may be more significant. There may be young children still at home, as well as responsibility for aging parents. Younger people with

Parkinson's often struggle with decisions about how much and when to tell children, parents, friends, and coworkers. When treatment succeeds in suppressing symptoms, younger people tend to be reluctant to let others know that they have Parkinson's. Just as having Parkinson's changes life for the person who has it, it changes the perceptions of others. As well, the element of uncertainty in the initial diagnosis is somewhat higher with early-onset Parkinson's that manifests just one or two of the classic symptoms even with positive response to levodopa treatment, often causing the person to feel reluctant to share information with others that could prove false.

It is difficult for family members to confront and accept an illness that typically affects older people. Children, especially teenagers, may not understand the involuntary nature of symptoms and find them embarrassing, particularly in public settings or around their friends. Even though this response is normal, it creates difficulties for the person with Parkinson's, who also may feel embarrassed by his or her lack of control over symptoms. Medical experts encourage families to be open and honest, as is age-appropriate, in discussing Parkinson's disease with children, so children understand that Parkinson's is a disease for which the parent takes medicine but that the parent will still (and often unpredictably) sometimes have problems.

Children often want to know whether the affected parent is going to die of Parkinson's; parents can honestly answer this question with "no" as Parkinson's itself seldom causes death. The child's age and maturity, in combination with the degree to which symptoms affect the parent's abilities, determine what other details are necessary. This is generally an evolving situation, as children are growing up and maturing as the Parkinson's progresses and acquire capacity for deeper understanding as the parent's symptoms become less controllable. SUPPORT GROUPS can be helpful resources for parents who are not sure how to discuss the subject with their children.

Health Care Implications

People with early-onset Parkinson's are decades from qualifying for MEDICARE, the government-funded health care program for seniors, unlike those with classic Parkinson's who are in their 60s, 70s, or 80s at the time of diagnosis. This difference has significant ramifications in terms of health care and MEDICAL INSURANCE. For those who receive health insurance through their job this often becomes a key factor in decisions about whether to remain employed, particularly when the person's employment also provides medical insurance for other family members. ANTI-PARKINSON'S MEDICATIONS and other treatments are expensive. The typical person with Parkinson's disease may need $2,000 to $6,000 of medications a year just to treat the Parkinson's. Costs for doctors' visits and related care can add substantially to this expense.

Most medical insurance covers most of the care-related costs and at least some of the cost of drugs; some plans do not cover drugs. It is crucial to fully understand medical insurance coverage limitations and restrictions when considering any changes that affect insurance status, such as retirement or change of jobs. The best source for information is the insurance company that issues the medical plan. All states have some form of medical assistance programs, known generally as MEDICAID, for people who have no other medical insurance options and meet the program's qualifications. Every state also has an insurance commissioner's office that can provide information and assistance about an insurer's legal obligations related to coverage of health care expenses.

Typically, the person with early-onset Parkinson's has no greater risk for other health problems in the early and mid stages of the disease than does a person of similar age who does not have Parkinson's and so is no more likely to need health care services. The exception is the risk of injuries caused by falls, which increases when BALANCE problems and GAIT DISTURBANCES are among the prominent symptoms. In the later stages of Parkinson's, extensive limitations on movement create increased risk for health problems such as pneumonia and other infections that increase the need for health care services.

See also ALPHA-SYNUCLEIN GENE; CAREGIVING; CLINICAL RESEARCH TRIAL; DENIAL AND ACCEPTANCE; EMBARRASSMENT; ESTATE PLANNING; FAMILY RELATION-SHIPS; FINANCIAL PLANNING; GENE THERAPY; LIFESTYLE FACTORS; LONG-TERM CARE INSURANCE; MARRIAGE RELATIONSHIP; PARKINSONISM; PLANNING FOR THE FUTURE; QUALITY OF LIFE; PREGNANCY; WORKPLACE ADAPTATIONS TO ACCOMMODATE PARKINSON'S; WORKPLACE RELATIONSHIPS.

eating The physical act of consuming nourishment, which becomes difficult for people with Parkinson's as the disease progresses to involve the muscles of the mouth and throat, making chewing and swallowing difficult. As ANTI-PARKINSON'S MEDICATIONS become less effective in controlling symptoms in the later stages of Parkinson's, most people need assistance with eating and drinking. If the muscles of the mouth and throat are severely affected, it often becomes necessary to decide whether to provide nutritional support through a FEEDING TUBE. As well, the person's tastes and food preferences often change as Parkinson's progresses, and those changes may limit what the person is willing to eat. Certain kinds of foods affect the EFFICACY of ANTI-PARKINSON'S MEDICATIONS, sometimes making it necessary to change the diet when medication regimens change.

TREMORS and BRADYKINESIA (slowed movements) affect fine motor control, limiting the ability to hold and use eating utensils. As a result, mealtimes can be messy events that are frustrating and embarrassing to the person with Parkinson's. Problems with chewing and SWALLOWING are common in mid to late Parkinson's. RIGIDITY and DYSKINESIAS affecting the muscles of the face, mouth, tongue, and throat can create difficulty keeping food in the mouth. People experiencing DRY MOUTH as a side effect of ANTICHOLINERGIC MEDICATIONS may not produce enough saliva to moisten food adequately as they are chewing it; the result is a potentially serious choking hazard when they swallow. Even small quantities or pieces of food can become stuck in the throat when saliva is in short supply. Some people can overcome these problems for a time by taking a drink before putting food into the mouth and by consciously focusing effort on the functions of chewing and swallowing. It is a good idea for family members, caregivers, and others who share meals with the person with Parkinson's to know how to do the HEIMLICH MANEUVER, a technique for quickly dislodging pieces of food that become stuck in the airway.

Impaired intestinal mobility (slowed PERISTAL-SIS), a consequence of bradykinesia that affects the smooth muscle tissues of the intestinal tract, causes the digestive system to function much more slowly than normal, with resulting intestinal discomfort and constipation. Some of the anti-Parkinson's medications, particularly anticholinergics, can exacerbate this problem. Drinking plenty of fluids and walking can help reduce the severity of constipation but are not always easy in the later stages of Parkinson's, in which GAIT DISTURBANCES and neuromuscular symptoms make movement difficult. Dehydration is a serious concern for many people with Parkinson's, as drinking becomes as difficult as eating.

Helping the person with Parkinson's to eat nutritiously balanced meals is both important and challenging. The need to accept help with eating represents a significant loss of INDEPENDENCE and can create much distress. Caregivers and family members can make the process easier by doing as much as possible to support the functions and abilities the person with Parkinson's still has. Support can include providing utensils with oversized handles, plates with distinct edges or compartments, and lidded drinking cups with straws and choosing foods that can be cut before serving to make putting the pieces onto a fork or spoon easier.

Challenges of eating often prevent people with Parkinson's from socializing by eating out with family and friends. Many of the same approaches that work at home are useful in restaurants. Order food items that are already bite-size when possible. If it is necessary to cut the person's food, do so discreetly, such as in the guise of sampling. Straws can make drinking easier. Having extra napkins handy makes it possible to clean up any spills quickly and without drawing attention to them. As with many of Parkinson's symptoms, maintaining a sense of humor and compassion about the situations those symptoms can create is often helpful.

See also ADAPTIVE EQUIPMENT AND ASSIST DEVICES; ADVANCE DIRECTIVES; CAREGIVING; COOKING; DYSPHA-GIA; EMBARRASSMENT; FOOD PREPARATION; FOODS TO AVOID; FOODS TO EAT; KITCHEN EFFICIENCY; NUTRITION AND DIET; PARENTERAL NUTRITION.

edema Fluid (water) retention that causes swelling. Edema is a common side effect of several DOPAMINE AGONIST MEDICATIONS taken to relieve the motor symptoms of Parkinson's disease, in particular PERGOLIDE (Permax), PRAMIPEXOLE (Mirapex), and ROPINEROLE (Requip). Most often, edema is mild and most noticeable in the ankles and feet, although it often affects the hands and sometimes the face as well. Mild edema is not usually a health problem and may not even be apparent to the person with Parkinson's. Edema significant enough to cause shoes or rings to become tight requires a doctor's attention to confirm that it is not a symptom of other health problems such as heart disease, liver disease, and kidney disease. If it is a side effect of medications, a neurologist's input often is helpful in making the decision as to whether the motor benefits of the medication outweigh the irritation of having the edema. Walking, standing for a few minutes during periods of prolonged sitting, and elevating the legs and feet when sitting help minimize edema.

See also ANTI-PARKINSON'S MEDICATIONS; HEART DISEASE AND PARKINSON'S; MEDICATION MANAGEMENT.

efficacy A medication's ability to control symptoms or eliminate a disease state.

Elavil See AMITRIPTYLINE.

Eldepryl See SELEGILINE.

Eldercare Locator The U.S. Administration on Aging sponsors a free information and referral service that provides connections to programs and assistance for senior citizens throughout the United States. Established in 1991, this service is telephone- and Internet-based. Telephone hours are Monday through Friday, 9:00 A.M. to 8:00 P.M., Eastern time, when information specialists answer calls and provide assistance. The Eldercare Locator website is available 24 hours a day, seven days a week. The Eldercare Locator contact is: (800) 677-1116 or http://www.eldercare.gov

The Eldercare Locator provides information by state or local area about services such as:

- Alzheimer's assistance and hotlines
- Adult day care, respite care, and long-term care
- MEALS ON WHEELS and other home-delivery meal services
- Housing needs and options
- Senior transportation services
- Home health care and hospice care
- Financial and legal guidance

Eldercare Locator services are available to anyone who calls, at no charge. The toll-free number and the website can provide assistance for TTD/TTY (hearing-impaired) calls.

See also ASSISTED LIVING FACILITY; CARE MANAGEMENT AND PLANNING; LIFESTYLE FACTORS; LONG-TERM CARE FACILITY; SOCIAL INTERACTION.

electroconvulsive therapy (ECT) A treatment for severe or recurring depression in which a mild electrical current discharged into the brain disrupts the brain's natural electrophysiological functions. This disruption also causes muscle contractions throughout the body (convulsions). A psychiatrist or neurologist performs ECT under carefully controlled circumstances, usually in a hospital setting. The person receives sedation and muscle relaxants as well as oxygen to make sure the brain has adequate oxygenation during the procedure. The electrical current affects numerous NEUROTRANSMITTERS in the brain, including DOPAMINE, GAMMA-AMINOBUTYRIC ACID (GABA), serotonin, and NOREPINEPHRINE.

ECT is particularly effective in relieving depression related to Parkinson's disease and at the same time greatly reduces RIGIDITY and DYSTONIA to improve muscle control and function. Why this happens is not clear, but scientists believe it is related to ECT's effects on dopamine. ECT is presently an INVESTIGATIONAL TREATMENT for motor symptoms of Parkinson's disease that do

not respond to medications. ECT carries many risks including seizures and cardiac arrhythmias. An obsolete term for ECT is *shock therapy.* ECT typically consists of a series of treatments given over several weeks. Most people experience marked improvement after three to five treatments. The antidepressant and motor effects in people with Parkinson's disease continue six months to two years.

See also ANTIDEPRESSANT MEDICATIONS; MENTAL STATUS; NEUROCHEMISTRY.

electroencephalogram (EEG) A recording of the brain's electrical activity made primarily to rule out other causes of the symptoms of Parkinson's disease. In the person with Parkinson's the EEG result is generally normal, although some people have a diffuse slowing of electrical activity (slowing throughout the brain rather than in just one area) and disturbed patterns during sleep. Most neurological conditions that cause changes in the brain's electrical activity alter specific kinds of activity or generate characteristic patterns. An EEG cannot diagnose Parkinson's either to confirm or rule out the disease but becomes one of numerous clinical tools that help doctors differentiate, or distinguish, Parkinson's from other neurological conditions.

A neurologist is most likely to request an EEG when the person's symptoms are not clear-cut or when the person is younger than age 50. CLINICAL RESEARCH TRIALS often include EEG among the range of measures used to evaluate INVESTIGATIONAL TREATMENTS and drugs, however. The objective to provide the greatest amount of data possible for researchers, as well as to make sure the treatment or drug is not causing adverse effects in the brain's functions. A neurosurgeon may request an EEG before a surgical procedure such as deep brain stimulation (DBS), PALLIDOTOMY, and THALAMOTOMY.

A routine EEG takes about an hour. The neurologist may request that the person limit sleep before the EEG. Sleep deprivation ensures that samples of awake, drowsy, and asleep states can all be obtained. This is important because the transition from awake to asleep often accentuates certain kinds of brain disturbances, particularly those of many seizure disorders. During an EEG, a technician applies electrodes to specific locations on the scalp and forehead with a conductive glue. There is no discomfort. The person lies on bed in a darkened room (and can fall asleep) while a machine receives the electrical signals from the electrodes and outputs them onto graph paper to create a visual representation. The neurologist then interprets the patterns.

See also COMPUTED TOMOGRAPHY (CT) SCAN; MAGNETIC RESONANCE IMAGING; NEUROLOGICAL EXAMINATION.

electromyogram (EMG)   A recording of the electrical activity in muscles. An EMG can record electrical activity through surface ELECTRODES applied on the skin or through fine needle electrodes inserted into muscle groups to measure the electrical impulses within them. Some people experience slight discomfort with the needle electrodes, but they provide much more information and are the standard of care for diagnostic examinations. Skin electrodes provide only very gross information about muscle activity and are largely relegated to interoperative monitoring, sleep monitoring, EEG monitoring, or other situations in which only gross information about whether a muscle is active is all that is required. The electrodes convey electrical signals to an amplification unit that converts the signals to visual patterns, which then display on a screen called an oscilloscope, or to audio signals, which transmit as sounds. Some amplification units present both visual and audio signals and can generate a print copy of the readings.

During an EMG the technician tells the person to perform movements to activate the muscle group and records electrical activity at reset. Completing a typical EMG takes about 30 minutes to an hour, depending on the muscle groups tested. The doctor may order an EMG for muscle groups where there are spasms or tremors. Sometimes EMG is incorporated as an element of more comprehensive musculoskeletal function testing such as GAIT ANALYSIS or before and after surgery such as PALLIDOTOMY or THALAMOTOMY to assess the surgery's effectiveness objectively.

Many neuromuscular disorders have uniquely characteristic EMG patterns, which help to rule them out as the cause of symptoms. Differences can exist in the amplitude, frequency, and rhythm of electrical activity. In Parkinson's disease, the EMG is normal except for the rhythmic alternating pattern of contraction and relaxation in opposing muscles affected by tremor. Hence, EMGs are rarely done unless to rule out other disorders. Other neuromuscular disorders show different patterns that may include combinations of increased or decreased activity during rest, extension, or contraction. For Parkinson's disease, EMG, like other diagnostic tests, may provide one piece of the overall picture and not a definitive diagnosis.

See also BODY SCHEME; CONDITIONS SIMILAR TO PARKINSON'S; DIAGNOSING PARKINSON'S; NERVE CONDUCTION STUDIES.

electrophysiologic studies   Tests that measure the electrical activity of body functions. These tests, which are primarily diagnostic, include:

Electrophysiologic Test	Measures Electrical Activity of . . .
electrocardiogram (ECG)	the heart
electroencephalogram (EEG)	the brain
electromyogram (EMG)	muscle groups
nerve conduction studies	nerves and muscles (in response to electrical stimulation)

See also DIAGNOSING PARKINSON'S; ELECTROENCEPHALOGRAM (EEG); ELECTROMYOGRAM (EMG); NERVE CONDUCTION STUDIES; NEUROLOGICAL EXAMINATION.

embarrassment   Many people with Parkinson's find the attention that its symptoms draws from other people uncomfortable and unpleasant. The erratic, lurching gait common in the middle to late stages of Parkinson's sometimes causes the misimpression that the person with Parkinson's is intoxicated. Slowness to respond, physically and mentally, and rigidity of the facial muscles that causes the classic, expressionless masked face can make the person with Parkinson's appear to be uninterested or to be ignoring other people. These aspects of Parkinson's are frustrating to the person with the disease; feeling the need to explain them to others, especially those who know nothing about Parkinson's disease, compounds the FRUSTRATION. The symptoms of Parkinson's disease can be particularly distressing for younger people with EARLY-ONSET PARKINSON'S DISEASE, who find that symptoms such as TREMORS draw attention even when they do not interfere with everyday activities.

Embarrassment causes many people with Parkinson's to withdraw from social activities and to resist going to public places such as shopping malls. This reaction leads to a sense of isolation and often to DEPRESSION. Friends and family can help by encouraging the person with Parkinson's to venture out when crowds are likely to be light and ANTI-PARKINSON'S MEDICATIONS are at peak effectiveness and by planning outings to minimize difficult situations. Keeping a sense of humor and trying to stay calm when symptoms do manifest in public can help to overcome feelings of ANXIETY that arise.

See also ADJUSTING TO LIVING WITH PARKINSON'S; COMPASSION; EMPATHY; SOCIAL INTERACTION.

embryonic stem cell   See STEM CELL.

embryonic stem cell research   See STEM CELL.

embryonic stem cell therapy   See STEM CELL.

emotions   Emotions are significant factors in Parkinson's disease in several ways. Primarily, Parkinson's evokes deep emotional response in people who are diagnosed with the disease as well as in family members and friends. It can be emotionally devastating to learn that a loved one has a progressive, debilitating disease—the news is life-changing for everyone involved. Grief, anger, despair, disbelief, frustration, pity, and self-pity are common emotional responses both at first and throughout the course of the disease.

As Parkinson's progresses, the person becomes less able to demonstrate emotion appropriately. This inability is partly due to the disease's effect on the muscles of the face, which prevents the person from generating the facial expressions associated with emotional expression. The "masked face" of Parkinson's makes the person appear to feel no emotion, when in fact his or her emotions are intense. As well, the person with Parkinson's may feel JOY and happiness yet cry, causing others to believe he or she is sad or upset. Softening of the voice often decreases its range of emotional tone, and later difficulty in speaking, another facet of the disease's progression, can further foster misunderstanding. COMPASSION, EMPATHY, and honest communication are essential.

DOPAMINE, the NEUROTRANSMITTER that becomes depleted in Parkinson's with the result that the disease's motor symptoms are manifested, also has functions in the brain related to mood and emotion. Researchers believe that neurons in the CEREBRUM, the part of the brain responsible for thought, memory, and emotion, become overly sensitive to dopamine in states of substance abuse and addiction. There also is evidence that dopamine plays a role in mental illnesses such as schizophrenia and personality disorders, and many ANTIPSYCHOTIC MEDICATIONS suppress dopamine response. Doctors know that the actions of ANTIPSYCHOTIC MEDICATIONS worsen the symptoms of Parkinson's disease and can create Parkinson's-like symptoms in people who take the drugs who do not have Parkinson's disease.

Researchers do not yet know how dopamine depletion in the BASAL GANGLIA, the brain's control center for movement, relates to dopamine production and activity in other parts of the brain. Dopamine levels seem to remain relatively normal in the cerebrum even as they drop precipitously low in the basal ganglia. Yet ANTI-PARKINSON'S MEDICATIONS, especially LEVODOPA, that attempt to boost dopamine levels in the SUBSTANTIA NIGRA and other key parts of the basal ganglia often have pronounced effects on emotion. Many people with Parkinson's disease experience MOOD SWINGS that span the gamut from euphoria to complete despondence in the space of just a few hours—about the cycle of a drug's effectiveness. Scientists are just beginning to unravel the functions and interrelationships of neurotransmitters in the brain, and although they know certain drugs produce certain effects, they do not always know why they do. Extensive research continues in these areas.

Emotional upsets also tend to worsen physical symptoms. The stress of a trip to a store or a visit by friends or family can precipitate GAIT DISTURBANCES and intensify symptoms such as TREMORS and BRADYKINESIA. Many people with Parkinson's learn to identify the circumstances that create emotional stress and adjust their medication dosages to bolster their coverage. Taking a levodopa dose shortly before such a stress-inducing event often can minimize its adverse effects on motor symptoms.

See also DENIAL AND ACCEPTANCE; EMBARRASSMENT; MEDICATION MANAGEMENT; PARKINSON'S PERSONALITY; PSYCHOSOCIAL FACTORS; SUPPORT GROUPS.

empathy   The ability to understand what another person is experiencing. Caregivers often are unsure how to respond to a loved one's difficulties as Parkinson's disease progresses. With Parkinson's, empathy requires learning as much as possible about the disease and its effects on the person who has it. This knowledge enables the caregiver to approach difficult situations with COMPASSION and honesty. With empathy, Parkinson's can draw out love and patience. Without empathy, Parkinson's is likely instead to generate FRUSTRATION and pity, affecting the person who has Parkinson's as well as those who provide care and support. These responses are the hallmark of sympathy, of feeling sorry for someone, and have little positive effect on anyone.

It is far more productive, as well as emotionally satisfying, to be direct and compassionate in acknowledging the deteriorations that are taking place. This attitude helps the person with Parkinson's as well as caregivers. If a loved one has trouble speaking and finding the right words, sympathy may generate the response of ignoring the person's efforts to communicate or talking about the person in the third person as if he or she is not present. This is emotionally devastating to the person with Parkinson's, certainly, and to the caregiver. Empathy allows the honest response "I know you know what you are trying to say, but I do not understand. We will work together to figure it out." This

response empowers both people to look for solutions, drawing them closer instead of further separating them. It also frees both people to be open, with compassion and caring, about their feelings and frustrations without becoming negative toward one another.

See also ANXIETY; CAREGIVER WELL-BEING; COPING WITH ONGOING CARE OF PARKINSON'S; DEPRESSION; EMBARRASSMENT; OPTIMISM; SUPPORT GROUPS.

end of life care and decisions   Planning for the end of life is not a prospect people welcome, yet it is one of the most important facets of managing a chronic, degenerative disease such as Parkinson's. Many people begin to think about matters such as ESTATE PLANNING when they become middle aged, but most postpone discussion or consideration of decisions about end of life care until a health crisis makes apparent the need to address these significant issues. Every adult, regardless of age and health status, should have ADVANCE DIRECTIVES that specify his or her desires about resuscitative actions, life-extending measures such as artificial feeding, and who should make medical decisions should he or she become incapacitated and unable to do so. It is prudent to discuss these desires with spouses, partners, and family members to minimize misunderstandings and disagreements. Loved ones may find it hard to accept a desire to refuse lifesaving measures such as cardiopulmonary resuscitation (CPR); it is good to have these concerns out in the open.

Older people generally have already given some thought to their preferences, if only because they are likely to have had health care experiences in which they have been questioned about them or because they have experienced the death of friends and family members. Most hospitals routinely incorporate discussion of advance directives in presurgery consultations and offer standardized forms to be completed and signed (and notarized, if required). Requirements vary by state. Other end of life care decisions relate more to the desired experience of dying. Some people are adamant about spending the end of life at home, and others want to have the best medical care right until the end. These are very personal matters and preferences, and every effort should be made to honor them.

Parkinson's disease is not itself fatal for most people who have it, although it can set the stage for the health problems that ultimately do result in loss of life. Many older people with Parkinson's disease may die of nonrelated conditions such as heart failure or of pneumonia that develops as a result of aspirated food or drink. People with EARLY-ONSET PARKINSON'S may find that the symptoms progress to the point where they cause complete physical incapacitation. Even at the time of diagnosis, when the person is feeling relatively well and ANTI-PARKINSON'S MEDICATIONS are effective at holding symptoms at bay, the person should consider his or her preferences and begin discussing them with family members. This course is not giving up hope that there are yet many years of life to enjoy, but rather considering the options and making choices and decisions about them while there is opportunity to do so. This method makes the process easier for everyone and helps to assure that all family members are clear about the person's wishes.

See also DENIAL AND ACCEPTANCE; HOSPICE; FINANCIAL PLANNING; PALLIATIVE CARE; PLANNING FOR THE FUTURE.

endotoxin A protein-based poison that gram-negative bacteria produce that is part of the bacterium's cell wall. Endotoxins generate an inflammatory response. In some people with Parkinson's disease swelling occurs in the brain tissues. Some researchers suspect that endotoxins are indirectly responsible by interfering with the actions of substances such as GLUTATHIONE that prevent damage from FREE RADICALS and have found associations of several of them with Parkinson's. Research to explore these connections continues. A common endotoxin (*not* implicated in Parkinson's disease) is *Escherichia coli* O:157, a food-borne bacterium that causes intestinal hemorrhage and can cause kidney failure.

See also EXOTOXIN; NEUROTOXIN.

entacapone A CATECHOL-*O*-METHYLTRANSFERASE (COMT) INHIBITOR MEDICATION taken as one of the ADJUNCT THERAPIES to increase the length of time LEVODOPA stays in an active form in the bloodstream. This increased interval allows more levodopa to pass across the BLOOD-BRAIN BARRIER to be converted to DOPAMINE in the brain. It works by preventing the action of the ENZYME COMT, which metabolizes levodopa as it enters the bloodstream and metabolizes dopamine throughout the body including the BRAIN. The U.S. Food and Drug Administration (FDA) approved entacapone for use in 1999; it is marketed as the brand name product Comtan. A combination of carbidopa, levodopa, and entacapone in one pill has been approved and will be marketed as Stalevo starting in fall of 2003. Among entacapone's potential side effects are gastrointestinal discomfort, diarrhea, and DYSKINESIAS. It also discolors the urine to an orangish color. Though less potent than its similar predecessor, tolcapone, entacapone has none of tolcapone's risk of acute liver toxicity.

See also ANTI-PARKINSON'S MEDICATIONS; MEDICATION MANAGEMENT; TOLCAPONE.

environmental toxins See CHEMICAL TOXINS.

environmental triggers Factors such as CHEMICAL TOXINS or changes in metabolic processes that contribute to the development of Parkinson's disease. Most researchers believe that a combination of genetic and environmental factors causes the depletion of DOPAMINERGIC NEURONS, leading to Parkinson's disease. Much interest currently focuses on the role of environmental factors, as the majority of people with IDIOPATHIC Parkinson's have no evidence of GENE MUTATIONS that would predispose them to (make them more likely to develop) the disease.

See also 1-METHYL-4-PHENYL-1,2,3,6-TETRAHYDROXYPYRIDINE; ACERULOPLASMINEMIA; COMPLEX I; GENETIC PREDISPOSITION; MITOCHONDRIAL DYSFUNCTION; NEUROPROTECTIVE EFFECT; NEUROTROPHIC FACTORS.

enzyme A natural protein that aids in metabolizing (breaking down) or synthesizing (combining together) other substances in the body but is not itself altered during the chemical reactions that take place. There are six categories of enzymes, all of which act in different ways:

- Oxidoreductase
- Transferase
- Hydrolase
- Lyase
- Isomerase
- Ligase

Various enzymes play roles in Parkinson's disease. Among them are

- CATECHOL-O-METHYLTRANSFERASE (COMT), which metabolizes levodopa in the bloodstream and other parts of the body and metabolizes levodopa in the brain
- DOPA DECARBOXYLASE (DDC), which metabolizes levodopa in the bloodstream and dopamine in the brain and other parts of the body
- MONOAMINE OXIDASE (MAO), which affects the metabolism of monoamine neurotransmitters such as serotonin and dopamine in the brain

Some ANTI-PARKINSON'S MEDICATIONS target the actions of these enzymes, to inhibit them and thereby extend the time the proteins upon which the enzymes act remain present and active.

See also CATECHOL-O-METHYLTRANSFERASE (COMT) INHIBITOR; COENZYME Q-10; DOPA DECARBOXYLASE (DDC) INHIBITOR; MONOAMINE OXIDASE INHIBITOR.

Epworth Sleepiness Scale (ESS) A brief, self-rated assessment of the extent to which drowsiness and sleepiness interfere with normal daily activities. The ESS is widely used as a preliminary tool for determining whether individuals have sleep disturbances. DAYTIME SLEEPINESS is common in people with Parkinson's, particularly in the middle and later stages of the disease. The ESS consists of eight situations for which a person rates his or her likelihood of falling asleep on a scale of 0 to 3 (0 = never, 1 = slight chance, 2 = moderate chance, 3 = nearly certain). The eight situations are:

- Sitting and reading
- Watching television
- Sitting passively in a public place such as a theater or a meeting
- Sitting as a passenger in a car for an hour without a break
- Lying down to rest in the afternoon
- Sitting and talking to someone
- Sitting quietly after lunch (with no alcohol)
- In a car stopped in traffic

A total score of 10 or higher suggests that there are sleep problems and bears further investigation. As Parkinson's disease progresses, sleep disturbances become increasingly common. They may result from an inability to change position, painful dystonias, RESTLESS LEG SYNDROME (RLS), and other factors. As much as is practical, treatment focuses on eliminating the causes of sleep problems.

See also SECONDARY SYMPTOMS.

equilibrium A state of being in BALANCE. Delays in muscle response cause disturbances in physical equilibrium in a person with Parkinson's disease, as the body is unable to respond appropriately to adjust to changes in posture and movement. Consequently, the body is continually attempting to compensate for actions of flexion and extension among muscle groups. Regular, consistent exercise helps to maintain balance and strength, improving equilibrium.

See also EXERCISE AND ACTIVITY; FALLS; GAIT DISTURBANCES; OCCUPATIONAL THERAPY; PHYSICAL THERAPY; POSTURAL INSTABILITY.

erectile dysfunction See SEXUAL DYSFUNCTION.

ergot-derived medications Drugs, also called ergot alkaloids, that function as DOPAMINE AGONISTS to activate DOPAMINE RECEPTORS in the BASAL GANGLIA and other parts of the BRAIN involved in MOTOR FUNCTION. Scientists do not understand the precise mechanism through which this process occurs. These drugs have other effects on the body including suppression of the hormone prolactin, leading to their use as fertility drugs by women (to initiate ovulation and the menstrual cycle). Ergot is a naturally occurring fungus that grows on rye. It is highly toxic in its natural form and throughout history has been responsible for much illness and death that resulted from eating foods made with contaminated grains. Modern processing methods prevent this contamination today.

Ergot is a strong vasoconstrictor: That is, it causes the blood vessels to narrow and stiffen. This reaction can lead to a rapid surge in blood pressure with increased risk for stroke or heart attack. Therefore, people with cardiovascular disease such as coronary artery disease or a history of heart attack (myocardial infarction) or stroke generally should not use ergot-derived medications. Modern ergot-derived medications are synthesized in the laboratory. Ergot-derived medications commonly used to treat Parkinson's disease include BROMOCRIPTINE (Parlodel), PERGOLIDE (Permax), and lisuride (Revanil). These medications may be taken as monotherapy in early disease and ADJUNCT THERAPIES to allow lower dosages of levodopa in mid to late Parkinson's disease. Common side effects include nausea, confusion, and hallucinations. Less common but more serious side effects include headache and lightheadedness, which may indicate high blood pressure. They also carry some risk of causing fibrotic scarring reactions in various organs.

See also AMANTADINE; ANTI-PARKINSON'S MEDICATIONS; PRAMIPEXOLE; ROPINIROLE.

essential tremor   A common NEURODEGENERATIVE disorder of fast, involuntary, and rhythmic movements that primarily affects people older than age 50, although it can start early in midlife (and in rare circumstances, in early adulthood or even adolescence). Other terms for this condition are FAMILIAL TREMOR (when it has a hereditary component) and *benign essential tremor*. The classic symptoms of essential tremor include:

- Intentional tremor (tremor that worsens with reaching or other directed movement)
- Postural tremor (tremor that worsens while holding a non-resting position such as the arms extended)
- Symmetric symptoms (tremors that affect both sides fairly evenly, although tremor may be more pronounced on the dominant side)
- Head involvement that produces a side-to-side motion, as if signaling "no"
- Tremors disappear during sleep

It is sometimes difficult to distinguish between essential tremor and Parkinson's disease when tremor is the primary symptom. The most significant differentiating factor is whether the tremors are most pronounced during activity or at rest. The tremors of Parkinson's disease are usually most prominent at rest and tend to diminish or cease with activity. The tremors of essential tremor intensify during activity and diminish at rest. Other tremor characteristics further support the diagnosis.

Essential tremor progresses slowly, as symptoms typically emerge over several decades. In some

Tremor Characteristic	Essential Tremor	Tremor of Parkinson's Disease
Body parts affected	Hands, feet, head, usually symmetrical; can involve voice, full limbs, and trunk in later stages of the disease	Hand/arm, foot/leg, usually asymmetrical; jaw later in the course of the disease
Handwriting	Shaky but normal size	Very small, cramped lettering (micrographia)
Intentional tremor (activity)	Yes	No
Muscle group involvement	Agonist/antagonist (opposing)	Agonist/antagonist (opposing)
Postural tremor	Yes	No
Rate	Moderately fast, 6–12 Hz	Slow, 4–8 Hz
Resting tremor	No	Yes

people, symptoms may be present for several months or even a few years and then seem to disappear for several years before reemerging. The longer a person has essential tremor the more severe the symptoms tend to become, although for most people symptoms are not as debilitating as are the symptoms of Parkinson's disease. When essential tremor is mild enough that it does not interfere with the person's ability to manage the regular ACTIVITIES OF DAILY LIVING, treatment is not necessary. Propanolol (such as the brand name drug Inderal), a BETA-ADRENERGIC (BLOCKER) ANTAGONIST medication, relieves symptoms for many people who have moderate tremor. An anticonvulsive medication, primidone, taken alone or in combination with propanolol, is effective for moderate to severe symptoms, though it tends to be sedating. Other anticonvulsants including topiramate (Topamax), lamotrigine (Lamictal), and possibly gabapentin (Neurontin) may be useful. The antipsychotic clozapine (Clozaril) has been found useful in a randomized controlled trial as well as open label trials. The antidepressant mirtazapine (Remeron) has also been reported to help in an open label trial. Some people also experience relief from antianxiety medications such as BENZODIAZEPINES (DIAZEPAM, ALPRAZOLAM) paroxitine (Paxil), and buspirone (BuSpar). Botulinum toxin injections have been found to be potentially helpful in open label studies, but often with resultant muscle weakness. Occasionally essential tremor symptoms do not respond to medications; in that case surgery such as deep brain stimulation (DBS) of the thalamus or THALAMOTOMY may be an option.

Although researchers estimate that essential tremor is about 10 times more common than Parkinson's disease, they know less about what causes it. Unlike Parkinson's disease, essential tremor appears to involve no NEUROTRANSMITTER depletion or other detectable change in brain function. However, the same parts of the brain—especially the motor THALAMUS—appear to be involved in generating tremor activity, as deep brain stimulation or ABLATION to these areas can end the tremors. About half of people who have essential tremor have a family history of the disease, in which case doctors call the condition familial. In the late 1990s scientists isolated several GENE MUTATIONS that appear to be present in people who have the familial form. This discovery prompts hope that GENE THERAPY will allow more effective treatment in the future.

See also CONDITIONS SIMILAR TO PARKINSON'S; DIAGNOSING PARKINSON'S.

estate planning   Creation of a legally binding plan for managing assets during life and distributing them after death. When appropriate plans have not been made, state laws make such determinations. There are many factors to consider, including ways to protect assets until death so they are available to meet the family's needs. Each person's situation is unique, and the person or the family should consult an attorney who specializes in estate planning to make sure to cover all salient points. It is important that the person with Parkinson's begin estate planning earlier rather than postponing it, as the course of Parkinson's disease is unpredictable and can include symptoms such as DEMENTIA that interfere with judgment as well as the ability to make legally binding decisions and sign legal documents.

Probate

Probate is the process in which courts approve and verify the distribution of assets. Each state has its own probate structure. Although probate is largely a matter of paperwork, the procedures are complex and time-consuming. As well, there are considerable expenses. Most people hire attorneys specializing in probate to handle the estate. Probating an estate can take several months to a year. There are numerous ways to keep parts or all of an estate out of the probate process; an attorney specializing in estate planning can provide the best guidance for individual circumstances.

Wills

A will is a written, signed, and witnessed document that specifies a person's intentions for distribution of property after death. A will also can stipulate guardianship for dependent children. Wills are the most common estate planning tools, and many people use standard forms available in stationery stores or over the Internet. This approach is usually inadequate for anyone who owns property or has dependent children, as a generic template is not specific enough to suit all individual needs and circumstances.

Nearly everyone who is considering a will should discuss his or her needs and possible options with an attorney who specializes in estate planning. For many people, other options such as living trusts provide better protection of assets and interests. At the very least, the person needs to find out what procedures apply in his or her state with regard to probating wills (filing them, reading them, and following their stipulations) and who should have copies. Wills become public record once they are filed for probate.

In some states a will can be probated within days of death; other states have longer timelines. It is also important to know the state procedures for matters such as sealing bank safe deposit boxes. Some people keep their will in a safe deposit box, considering it the most secure location, but in some states the box is sealed at the person's death and a court order is required to unseal it, unnecessarily complicating the probate process. For this reason, too, it is a good idea to specify funeral and burial preferences elsewhere; writing them into the will is not likely to assure they will be followed.

Living Trusts

A living trust is a popular and easy method for avoiding probate. It provides for asset management during life as well as distribution of assets after death. A living trust transfers ownership of property and other assets to a trust that is under the control of a trustee. The person who establishes the trust also can be the trustee, retaining full control of all assets. At death, the designated beneficiary becomes the trustee. Living trusts are most effective for people who are in midlife and have fairly significant assets. An attorney specializing in estate planning can help determine whether a living trust is an appropriate tool.

Life Insurance

Most people who do not already have life insurance at the time they are diagnosed with Parkinson's disease are not likely to obtain coverage. Life insurance, as does all insurance, requires the person to pay premiums on a set schedule for a predetermined payout if the person dies while the policy is in effect. There are several kinds of life insurance; what is appropriate depends on individual circumstances. A licensed independent insurance agent is a good source for information about assessing life insurance needs. It is always prudent to compare the benefits and costs of various policies.

Not everyone needs life insurance. Although many older people have it because they purchased it when they were younger, life insurance primarily benefits people who are responsible for supporting dependent children or a spouse. The primary advantage of life insurance is that it provides immediate cash to the person or persons named as beneficiaries. Usually life insurance payments are exempt from taxes; such an exemption varies, however, and an attorney is the best source of information.

Long-Term Care Insurance

Long-term care insurance pays for residential care in a long-term care facility (nursing home). There are various plans with different deductibles and coverages; it is crucial to understand all the restrictions and limitations as well as the benefits fully. Most plans have some sort of qualification process; people with a high probability of needing long-term care services, such as those already diagnosed with DEGENERATIVE CONDITION such as ALZHEIMER'S DISEASE or Parkinson's disease, are less likely to qualify.

Accommodating Medicaid Requirements

Each state has its own forms of health care and long-term care assistance, but all have in common their income-based qualifications. Medicaid regulations are complex and sometimes difficult to interpret and apply to a person's individual circumstances. It is wise for anyone with assets to consult an attorney who is familiar with Medicaid procedures before committing to himself or herself to any estate planning. Otherwise, families can find themselves being forced to use assets they thought were protected to cover health care and other expenses.

Funeral Arrangements

For many people, a funeral trust is the most logical means of paying for funeral arrangements. Banks can help establish such a trust, in which the money is held in reserve specifically to cover funeral expenses. This money typically is exempt from Medicaid spend-down requirements, however, this exemption varies among states. Another option is a prepaid funeral plan. This involves paying in full for the cost of the funeral; payment is then placed into a trust. When the person dies, the funeral arrangements that were selected and purchased are provided; even if the cost for them at the time of death would have been more, there are no additional charges. It is important to choose carefully when purchasing a prepaid funeral. If the funeral home goes out of business, the money could be lost.

At the very least, the person should state his or her wishes regarding funeral services, including burial versus cremation, in writing. At least one family member should have a copy of these instructions. Because weeks or months may pass before a will is opened and read, do not use a will to convey funeral and burial instructions.

Taxes

The most compelling reason to consult an attorney about estate planning is to protect assets as much as possible from taxes. There are local and state probate and estate taxes. The U.S. Congress repealed the federal estate tax in 2001, but on a graduated scale that will not end federal estate taxes until 2011, unless Congress enacts an extension or new legislation. Again, it is best to consult an attorney who specializes in estate planning to determine how best to shelter assets and to know what taxes will apply so the estate is prepared to pay them. Although many people worry about the federal estate tax, it applies only to those whose estate is worth more than $1 million (increasing to $3 million by 2010).

Choosing an Executor

The executor of an estate is a person trusted and designated to make sure the intentions of the person are honored and followed. The person chosen as executor should know this and should agree to take on this responsibility. There are no qualifica-tions or restrictions for who can serve as executor; the person can be a beneficiary of the estate. Typically, an executor is someone who is familiar with the person's financial affairs and who will be capable of handling the details of executing the estate's documents.

See also FINANCIAL PLANNING; MEDICARE; PLANNING FOR THE FUTURE; RECORD KEEPING.

estrogen   The predominant HORMONE responsible for female secondary sexual characteristics. The ovaries produce most of the estrogen in a woman's body. Estrogen levels are at their peak in women between menarche (the start of menstruation) and MENOPAUSE (the end of menstruation). For many years, health experts believed estrogen had a protective effect on a woman's brain, helping to stave off many NEURODEGENERATIVE disorders including ALZHEIMER'S DISEASE, DEMENTIA, and Parkinson's disease. Numerous studies through the decades provided the basis for this presumption, showing that these diseases are far more common in women whose estrogen level was low, such as after menopause or surgical menopause (removal of the ovaries). This appeared consistent regardless of the woman's age. Women past menopause who had hormone replacement therapy (HRT) or estrogen replacement therapy (ERT) seemed to lower their risk for neurodegenerative disorders to near normal.

Studies in 2001 and 2002 cast serious doubt on this premise, as they did not conclusively demonstrate that estrogen provides any NEUROPROTECTIVE EFFECT. Further, these studies showed an alarming increase in the rate of heart disease and estrogen-driven cancers involving the breast and the uterus among women taking ERT (estrogen alone) or HRT (estrogen in combination with progesterone). Further research is needed to explore the connections between estrogen and the brain and estrogen's role in preventing degenerative diseases that affect the brain. A woman should base her decision whether to have ERT or HRT on other considerations than their potential to prevent Parkinson's disease and other neurodegenerative conditions.

See also ACCELERATED AGING; AGING; ANTIOXIDANTS; APOPTOSIS; DOPAMINE DEGRADATION; NEUROTROPHIC FACTORS; NEUROPROTECTIVE THERAPIES.

ethopropazine An ANTICHOLINERGIC MEDICATION taken as one of the ADJUNCT THERAPIES to reduce the motor symptoms of Parkinson's disease, primarily TREMORS and rigidity. It works by countering the effect of ACETYLCHOLINE, a NEUROTRANSMITTER that stimulates muscle activity. Ethopropazine is available in the United States as the brand name product Pardidol. Side effects can include drowsiness, dry mouth, confusion, hallucinations, and visual disturbances.

See also ANTI-PARKINSON'S MEDICATIONS; BENZTROPINE; MEDICATION MANAGEMENT; TRIHEXYPHENIDYL.

evening primrose oil An ANTIOXIDANT that contains the essential fatty acid gamma-linolenic acid (GLA), a substance the body cannot manufacture and must derive from dietary sources. Some people with Parkinson's disease find that taking evening primrose oil helps reduce symptoms such as TREMORS. Researchers believe this effect occurs because evening primrose oil, made by pressing the oil content from the plant's seeds, contains TRYPTOPHAN. This AMINO ACID is a precursor for SEROTONIN, a NEUROTRANSMITTER. There is some evidence that tryptophan extends the effectiveness of LEVODOPA. However, as an amino acid it can also interfere with the absorption of levodopa from the intestine into the bloodstream, so it may make sense to avoid taking it within an hour or two of any levodopa dose. It is a good idea to discuss with a physician or pharmacist the potential benefits and risks of taking evening primrose oil along with ANTI-PARKINSON'S MEDICATIONS.

See also ACETYLCHOLINE; ALTERNATIVE THERAPIES; ANTIOXIDANT THERAPY; CATECHOLAMINES; DOPAMINE; FAVA BEANS; FOODS TO AVOID; FOODS TO EAT; NEUROPROTECTIVE THERAPIES; NUTRITION AND DIET; PROTEIN RESTRICTIONS, DIETARY.

excessive daytime sleepiness (EDS) See DAYTIME SLEEPINESS.

excitotoxin An AMINO ACID–based substance that causes overstimulation of neurotransmitter receptors in the brain, resulting in NEURON death. Most excitotoxins enter the body as food additives. There are about 70 identified excitotoxins, one of the most common of which is glutamate (found in foods as the flavor enhancer monosodium glutamate [MSG]). Injuries to the brain, such as from trauma or stroke, also cause the release of excitatory neurotransmitters (neurotransmitters that stimulate, as opposed to suppress, neuron activity) that then function as excitotoxins: That is, when they are present in the brain at abnormally high levels, their actions are toxic and they result in cell death. Researchers believe that excitotoxins cause cell death by causing the cell to release excess calcium; intensification of the cell's metabolism results. This in turn causes the cell to deplete its protein resources, at which point the cell can no longer survive.

Some scientists believe that excitotoxins provide the environmental impetus that sets in motion the events that cause neurodegenerative conditions such as ALZHEIMER'S DISEASE, AMYOTROPHIC LATERAL SCLEROSIS (ALS), MULTIPLE SCLEROSIS, and Parkinson's disease to develop. Glutamate, although as yet not directly implicated as having a role in Parkinson's disease, is present in areas of the brain affected by Parkinson's, including the STRIATUM and SUBTHALAMIC NUCLEUS (STN). Much research remains to be done in this area before scientists will fully understand the role of excitotoxins. Some researchers recommend that as much as possible, people with Parkinson's avoid processed foods, which commonly contain excitotoxins as flavor enhancers.

See also CHEMICAL TOXINS; FOODS TO AVOID; NUTRITION AND DIET; ENDOTOXINS; ENVIRONMENTAL TRIGGERS; GLUTAMATE; PARKINSON'S DISEASE, CAUSES OF.

exercise and activity Remaining as physically active as possible helps to maintain physical functions, improving COORDINATION and BALANCE. The adage "Use or lose it" is particularly applicable to people with Parkinson's disease. Numerous studies demonstrate that people who follow a regular and consistent exercise regimen, such as WALKING for 30 minutes each day, are able to maintain control of voluntary movement more effectively and longer into the course of the disease than those who do not have much physical activity. As well, most people enjoy being out and about, even if that just means walking around the block or around the yard. Physical activity is also good for relieving STRESS and improving mood.

Walking is the best form of physical exercise for most people with Parkinson's disease because it exercises nearly all of the body's muscle groups without putting much strain on the body. It helps the person to maintain eye-to-body coordination, which is essential for balance and coordination of movement. And it also presents an ideal opportunity to spend time with a loved one. Even when their Parkinson's becomes fairly advanced, most people can still take short walks. It is important to take appropriate safety precautions; a person whose stability is unreliable should use a WALKING AID and walk with a companion.

People who are having on–off fluctuations can, through experimentation, learn to time periods of physical activity with their medication dosages so they are least likely to have problems such as freezing of gait. Such planning makes the activities more enjoyable as well as more effective. It also is important to plan the time for walks and other physical activities so there is no sense of a need to rush through them to get to something else.

Additionally, a PHYSICAL THERAPIST or OCCUPATIONAL THERAPIST might recommend specific exercises and activities to strengthen certain muscle groups or to teach different muscle groups to take over for those that are more severely affected by the symptoms of Parkinson's disease. They can be especially beneficial in addressing GAIT DISTURBANCES and fine motor movements such as those involving the hands and fingers. Exercises may include working with light weights or resistance devices such as bands. Activities that call on fine motor control, such as putting together jigsaw puzzles, are not physically strenuous but nonetheless help to keep neuromuscular paths as open as possible.

See also EQUILIBRIUM; GAIT; MEDICATION MANAGEMENT; QUALITY OF LIFE.

exotoxin　A poison that gram-positive and gram-negative bacteria produce and release into the body that interferes with the functions of other cells.

Botulinum A is a paralytic exotoxin injected into muscles to control dystonias (abnormal sustained muscle contractions) and possibly TREMORS; these problems may occur in people with Parkinson's and may do not respond to ANTI-PARKINSON'S MEDICATIONS. Under controlled circumstances, exotoxins cause serious and sometimes fatal infections. Botulism is an infection that results from botulinum exotoxin found in improperly canned foods, which can cause widespread paralysis that interferes with movement as well as breathing. Other common exotoxins include those that produce infections, including cholera, pertussis (whooping cough), diptheria, and anthrax.

See also BLEPHAROSPASM; BOTULINUM TOXIN THERAPY; ENDOTOXIN; NEUROTOXIN.

experimental drug　See INVESTIGATIONAL NEW DRUG.

extrapyramidal symptom rating scale　(ESRS) An objective measurement system to assess the extent of damage to the EXTRAPYRAMIDAL SYSTEM and the MOTOR FUNCTIONS that it controls. The ESRS consists of 12 multipart items, four of which are general neurological assessments and eight of which are specific to the symptoms of Parkinson's disease, rated on a scale of 1 to 7 of severity of their effect on the person. The higher the score, the more severely the symptoms affect function. The ESRS is one of several clinical assessment tools that physicians and researchers use to gauge the effectiveness of ANTI-PARKINSON'S MEDICATIONS and other treatments.

See also ACTIVITIES OF DAILY LIVING; HOEHN AND YAHR STAGE SCALE; INSTRUMENTAL ACTIVITIES OF DAILY LIVING; PARKINSON'S IMPACT SCALE; QUALITY OF LIFE; SICKNESS IMPACT SCALE; STAGING OF PARKINSON'S DISEASE.

extrapyramidal system　A functional division of the NERVOUS SYSTEM that isolates the structures and processes of the BASAL GANGLIA (caudate nucleus, putamen, STRIATUM, PALLIDUM, subthalamic nucleus, and SUBSTANTIA NIGRA) and the THALAMUS as they exist within the BRAINSTEM and the cortex (outer layer) of the cerebrum. This is the structure of the nervous system, along with the PYRAMIDAL PATHWAY and cerebellar pathways, that controls motor functions and voluntary or intentional movement. The extrapyramidal system is so named because it is beyond, or outside, the pyramidal pathway (the triangular-shaped nerve structures that convey nerve messages directly from the cortex to the body). Physically these structures often intertwine; the distinctions between them are primarily functional. Damage to the extrapyramidal system, such as that which occurs with the depletion of DOPAMINERGIC NEURONS and DOPAMINE that characterizes Parkinson's disease, results in neuromuscular disturbances.

See also BRAIN; CONDITIONS SIMILAR TO PARKINSON'S; CORTICOBASAL DEGENERATION; GAIT DISTURBANCES; HUNTINGTON'S DISEASE; LESIONS; MOVEMENT; MULTIPLE SCLEROSIS; MULTIPLE SYSTEM ATROPHY; MUSCULAR DYSTROPHY; PROGRESSIVE SUPRANUCLEAR PALSY.

eye movements   The ability to control the movements of the eyes becomes impaired as Parkinson's disease progresses. TREMORS and BRADYKINESIA (slowed movement) can affect the muscles that move the eyes. This effect creates visual disturbances as the eyes cannot move quickly enough to capture and transmit visual cues from the environment to the brain appropriately. Nerve messages from the brain to the eye become delayed and distorted, which in turn distorts visual perception due to the mismatch between where the eyes are pointing and where the brain thinks they are pointing.

Neuromuscular symptoms that affect the muscles of the eyelids affect the eye's ability to maintain adequate lubrication. RIGIDITY affecting the lower eyelid causes it to distort and stiffen, reducing its ability to retain tears. Spasms that affect the muscles of the eyelids (BLEPHAROSPASMS) are common and can cause the eyes to remain closed for extended periods. These problems reduce the frequency of blinking, thereby causing the eye to become dry and irritated and contributing to blurriness of vision. Limited eye movement also creates problems with BALANCE, which relies on the close integration of visual signals and neuromuscular signals that control MOVEMENT. This impairment lessens the person's ability to make adjustments in movement, increasing the risk of falls. This same delay of response to visual stimuli creates difficulty for the person with Parkinson's in focusing the eyes for functions such as reading. One eye may focus adequately and the other be unable to respond, creating problems such as double vision or BLURRY VISION.

As with other motor symptoms of Parkinson's, making a conscious effort to use the eye muscles helps to keep them as functional as possible and to protect the eye from irritation and injury. Most people in the mid stages of Parkinson's, when eye movement disturbances tend to become more prominent, can intentionally blink and move their eyes. Up and down motion becomes restricted more quickly and more severely than side to side motion; an ophthalmologist (physician who specializes in eye conditions) or a PHYSICAL THERAPIST may be able to recommend exercises to help maintain muscle function related to the eyes for as long as possible. Artificial tears can help to keep the eyes well lubricated, rinsing out debris such as dust that can scratch the cornea and other surfaces of the eye.

See also BLINK RATE; COLOR PERCEPTION; GAIT DISTURBANCE.

facial expressions   See HYPOMIMIA.

facies   See HYPOMIMIA.

falls   The motor symptoms, GAIT DISTURBANCES, and POSTURAL INSTABILITY typical of Parkinson's make falls a common source of injury for people with the disease. As well, many ANTI-PARKINSON'S MEDICATIONS contribute to unsteadiness, particularly those that cause DROWSINESS, DIZZINESS, or ORTHOSTATIC HYPOTENSION (a sudden drop in blood pressure when rising from lying down). Falls are most likely to occur during changes in position— from sitting to standing, from standing to walking, when changing direction during movement, and from walking to sitting. Situations in which the person with Parkinson's is getting in and out of bed, a car, and the shower present high risk for loss of BALANCE and falling.

The person may realize that a fall is imminent but be unable to prevent it or may be unaware of a potential fall until it is under way, too late to prevent it. Because the motor symptoms of Parkinson's disease impair normal reflexive actions to "break" the fall, such as extending an arm or curling to land with minimal harm to the body, even minor falls can result in injuries such as cuts, bruises, and fractures. Head injuries, even those that appear minor, can have serious consequences, as can falls that take place in the shower or bath. Any head injury that results in loss of consciousness, however brief, requires follow-up, at least by telephone, with the doctor. Family members should know basic first aid including cardiopulmonary resuscitation (CPR).

Measures to reduce the risk of falling are fairly simple. In and around the home,

- Remove throw rugs, including those in the bathroom (and bath mats). Their edges, even when fastened down with carpet tape, tend to catch feet that drag and WALKING AIDS such as canes or walkers.

- Arrange furniture so there are clear and wide paths of travel through every room that allow the person with Parkinson's to walk without concern for bumping into things and comfortably make a U-turn. End tables and coffee tables are often obstacles to sitting in a chair or on a couch.

- Remove or block wheels and casters from chairs, especially those in rooms with hard surface (noncarpeted) floors. Have at least one chair in every room that is sturdy, is steady (does not rock or swivel), has arms, and has a seating surface that is 32 to 36 inches from the floor.

- Run telephone, television cable, electrical cords, and extension cords along baseboards or walls and secure them in place with construction staples such as those staple guns use (straddle the cable or cord with the staple; do not puncture it) or with heavy-duty tape.

- Make sure all interior areas, including hallways and closets, have good lighting. For areas not already wired with fixtures, use battery-operated lights that mount (usually with adhesive patches or small screws) on a wall or ceiling. Choose styles that have easy-to-operate switches; some are turned on and off by pushing the main part of the light.

- Use motion-activated lights in driveways, garages, entry doors, and even basements; there are styles that incorporate the motion sensor into the bulb unit and are screwed into a standard light fixture.

- Install appropriate ADAPTIVE EQUIPMENT AND ASSIST DEVICES such as hand railings in bathrooms and hallways, lever-style door handles and light switches, and slip-resistant grips in showers and tubs.

As well, there are precautions the person with Parkinson's disease can take to reduce the risk of falls further. The most effective is to be aware of fluctuations in motor functions that are related to medication dosages. Falls are most likely to happen when medications are wearing off and motor response is unpredictable. Other precautions include

- When walking, make a conscious effort to lift each foot cleanly off the floor and then place it down again rather than letting it shuffle or drag. Although this activity becomes more difficult as Parkinson's progresses, such purposeful focus helps to improve balance and mobility.

- Plan for directional changes, and allow enough time and space to conduct them. If it appears the space is too small or constrained, stop to consider the options and then select the one that is safest. Ask for help!

- Turn on the lights before entering a room, even if it is not completely dark. Being able to see clearly helps spatial orientation (judging distance and depth of field) and compensates for postural instability.

- Wear closed, flat-heeled shoes with somewhat smooth soles (not rubberized) and clothing that fits comfortably but is not so loose as to pose a tripping hazard or to be caught on furniture or cabinets.

- Sit down to dress and undress, including when putting on or taking off shirts or blouses. The action of pulling clothing over the head is disorienting and disrupts balance.

When falls do occur, follow a head-to-toe pattern to check for injuries immediately, and then later (such as at bedtime) if the fall seemed substantial. Pain that continues more than 10 or 15 minutes after the fall bears further investigation, if

only a telephone call to the doctor. Cuts that gape or do not stop bleeding in a few minutes or injuries that cause the person to resist using an extremity require prompt medical attention. People with Parkinson's disease often are reluctant to tell family members of falls and other mishaps for fear that doing so will prompt further curtailment of their activities. Low-key reactions in these matters encourage openness about them. It is also a good idea for the caregiver to be observant about fresh bruises, cuts, and other signs of falls.

See also ADJUSTING TO LIVING WITH PARKINSON'S; AMBULATION; BATHING AND BATHROOM ORGANIZATION; BEDROOM COMFORT; BODY SCHEME; COMPASSION; COOKING; HOME SAFETY; KITCHEN EFFICIENCY; POSITION CHANGES.

familial predisposition to Parkinson's   See GENETIC PREDISPOSITION.

family history   Information about medical problems through as many generations as possible on both sides of the family. Family history can be important in establishing possible hereditary connections for many health conditions including those that are similar to Parkinson's at the onset such as ESSENTIAL TREMOR and HUNTINGTON'S DISEASE. Researchers do not yet fully understand the genetic links of Parkinson's disease, although they know such connections exist.

It is only in recent years that doctors have been able to differentiate diagnoses of many NEURODEGENERATIVE diseases, so a family history may relates to general symptoms rather than being specific for conditions such as Parkinson's disease or ALZHEIMER'S DISEASE, which appear to have some connections and coexist frequently. Parkinson's disease was once called the "shaking palsy," and an untold number of people who had Alzheimer's disease were instead diagnosed as having what was called "senile dementia." It is important to establish written records of family health problems, including descriptions of symptoms and behavior as well as diagnoses.

At present, a family history of Parkinson's disease has little influence on diagnosis or treatment, although it does alert physicians to look more closely at the possibility of PARKINSON'S DISEASE, particularly EARLY-ONSET PARKINSON'S. With continuing advances in genetics and GENE THERAPY, this condition could quickly change. In any case early diagnosis leads to early treatment, which yields the best PROGNOSIS and prospects for desirable QUALITY OF LIFE.

See also ALPHA-SYNUCLEIN GENE; CHEMICAL TOXINS; EARLY-ONSET PARKINSON'S; ENVIRONMENTAL TRIGGERS; PARKIN GENE; UBIQUITIN.

family relationships   Chronic, degenerative conditions such as Parkinson's disease affect the entire family, not just the person with the disease. Roles and relationships among family members change as the condition progresses and the needs of the person with Parkinson's increase. Most families struggle with the challenges of these changes. It is difficult, to say the least, to watch a loved one follow the path of a degenerative disease. The ways in which family members meet these challenges, however, can draw them together rather than tear them apart. HUMOR, COMPASSION, and EMPATHY are crucial in shifting focus from a progression of loss to the possibilities that remain.

Often a spouse or an adult child becomes the primary caregiver for the person with Parkinson's. For a person with Parkinson's who has been the head of the family it is difficult to cede control to others. It is also difficult for other family members, particularly adult children, to step into taking control. Maintaining a position of collaboration in which the situation is a partnership can help everyone take a positive view of the changing circumstances. The person with Parkinson's and family members should discuss crucial aspects of future care, such as ASSISTED LIVING FACILITIES and ADVANCE DIRECTIVES, as early as possible in the course of the disease so that everyone involved clearly understands the preferences of the person who has Parkinson's.

This is not an easy dialogue to initiate, but postponing it does not make it easier. Early on, the person with Parkinson's should make, and be fully supported by family members in making, decisions about the future from treatment options to end of life care, unless there are reasons to question the person's ability to make informed choices. The person's capacity to make them takes a tremendous burden off both him or her and family members who would otherwise have to face such decisions without the participation of their loved one. This process is more stressful in the end and can lead to disagreements, hard feelings, and guilt among family members.

The challenges that Parkinson's imposes on families are not easy to confront and often cause considerable frustration. This is normal and natural. Despite best intentions, not all families are able to approach the situation collaboratively. Sometimes unresolved family issues get in the way. Family members may have different concepts of what it means to be involved in the person's care or may themselves be emotionally unable to cope with the challenges of the disease and the changes that are taking place in their parent or spouse. SUPPORT GROUPS provide safe forums for sharing experiences and learning from those of other families and caregivers.

See also ADJUSTING TO LIVING WITH PARKINSON'S; CAREGIVER WELL-BEING; COPING WITH ONGOING CARE OF PARKINSON'S; DAILY LIVING CHALLENGES; EARLY-ONSET PARKINSON'S; END OF LIFE CARE AND DECISIONS; ESTATE PLANNING; GOING PUBLIC; GRIEF; HONESTY; JOY; LIFESTYLE FACTORS; MARRIAGE RELATIONSHIP; PARENT/CHILD RELATIONSHIPS; PLANNING FOR THE FUTURE; STRESS; STRESS REDUCTION TECHNIQUES.

fat, dietary   See NUTRITION AND DIET.

fatigue   A feeling of persistent weariness, heaviness, or lack of energy. Fatigue is a common problem for people with Parkinson's and may be a symptom or a consequence of the disease. RESTLESS LEG SYNDROME (RLS) and other SLEEP DISTURBANCES can lead to inadequate sleep. ANTI-PARKINSON'S MEDICATIONS can interfere with sleep or cause feelings of tiredness. Sometimes adjusting the timing of dosages or the combinations of drugs can relieve some of the fatigue as well as make it easier to sleep at night. SLEEP MEDICATIONS also help the person to fall asleep and stay asleep to get adequate rest.

As Parkinson's progresses, physical movement takes more intense concentration and effort.

BRADYKINESIA makes the legs feel heavy, and once-simple actions such as walking across a room to turn on the television become major undertakings. TREMORS and cramps can leave muscles sore and tired. It is helpful to plan outings and activities such as shopping or traveling for times when energy levels are highest and to allow for brief resting periods to prevent total exhaustion. NUTRITION AND DIET are also factors; eating several small meals spread out through the day can help to provide more consistent nutritional energy.

When fatigue persists despite efforts to relieve it (such as assuring adequate sleep), it is important to look for common physical causes that are easy to treat. These include hypothyroidism (underactive thyroid), ANEMIA (insufficient oxygen in the blood), and vitamin B_{12} deficiency. These health conditions become increasingly common with age, but the focus on treating the symptoms of Parkinson's makes it easy to overlook them or to attribute their symptoms to the Parkinson's or anti-Parkinson's medications.

See BEDROOM COMFORT; DAYTIME SLEEPINESS; DAY–NIGHT REVERSAL; EXERCISE AND ACTIVITY; NUTRITIONAL SUPPLEMENTS.

fava bean   A legume that is a natural source of LEVODOPA, the DOPAMINE precursor taken to treat the symptoms of Parkinson's disease. When ingested, levodopa becomes converted to dopamine in the body and in the brain. Fava beans also are called faba beans, broad beans, long beans, and horse beans; the scientific name for this legume is *Vicia faba*. Fava beans are popular in dishes and recipes of the Mediterranean and the Middle East, where fava beans grow in abundance. Known as broad beans in Europe, fava beans are also common in Central European dishes.

Some people advocate eating fava beans as a means of stabilizing levodopa levels in the bloodstream and helping to reduce the fluctuating response that becomes a problem with long-term levodopa treatment. However, the levodopa content of fava beans depends on the growing conditions of the beans, their freshness at the time of preparation, and their preparation. Variations in levodopa concentration are considerable even when growing and preparation conditions are controlled. The beans contain measurable quantities of levodopa; the pods and stems contain the highest amounts. Some fava bean products combine beans, pods, and stems cooked and mashed together into a paste.

Typically, a half-cup of fava beans contains enough levodopa to affect the levodopa levels of a person who is taking levodopa as an ANTI-PARKINSON'S MEDICATION. However, it is difficult to consume enough fava beans consistently or to obtain a consistent level of levodopa, to substitute eating them for taking the drug form of levodopa. Fava beans should never be used as a substitute for medication. The human digestive system does not handle large amounts of legumes very easily or efficiently; they are very fibrous and typically cause digestive problems that include flatulence (gas) and constipation. Because of the body's difficulty in digesting large amounts of legumes the absorption of levodopa from fava beans would be inconsistent and unpredictable. The protein content of fava beans also makes the amount of levodopa that is absorbed into the bloodstream somewhat variable.

A person with Parkinson's who is considering eating fava beans to supplement levodopa should first discuss this idea with his or her physician; the side effects of excessive levels of peripheral levodopa are unpleasant and can create other health problems including heart arrhythmias (irregular heartbeat). Many doctors are willing to try alternative treatment approaches, particularly when the effectiveness of conventional treatments begins to diminish, and adjust the anti-Parkinson's medication regimen to accommodate the increased levodopa the fava beans will provide. For best results, start with small amounts of well-cooked fava beans and increase the quantity gradually, to allow the digestive system to adjust. It will probably be necessary to continue adjusting the medication regimen, just as if adding another of the ADJUNCT THERAPIES, until there is a good balance between the anti-Parkinson's medications and the fava beans.

Some people, mostly those of Mediterranean descent, have a rare deficiency of the enzyme glucose-6-phosphate dehydrogenase (G6PD), which is necessary to metabolize levodopa. When this deficiency exists, eating fava beans or taking levodopa as a medication may produce a reaction called favism in which hemolytic anemia (premature destruction of red blood cells) develops. Many people with a G6PD deficiency can tolerate a certain dose of levodopa (either via medication or fava bean) before this reaction becomes manifest, so it is important for people with Parkinson's to promptly report potential side effects to their neurologist (or other physician managing their Parkinson's medications) when starting or increasing their dose of levodopa. This disorder is potentially serious, as it affects the ability of the blood to transport oxygen and can cause blood clots that result in heart attack or stroke, but all problems from this condition rapidly vanish with cessation or reduction in the amount of levodopa taken/consumed. This reaction was named *favism* because it has been known for centuries among people who regularly consume fava beans, although it is of course a relatively new phenomenon in relation to taking levodopa as a drug. A blood test called a Coombs test can detect whether G6PD deficiency is present. People with G6PD deficiency cannot take levodopa in any form, as a medication or through diet.

Fava beans should be purchased when they are "green" young beans (before they have developed the "strings" characteristic of mature legumes), and boiled in a small amount of water until they are tender or even almost mushy—about 10 to 15 minutes for a half-cup. Some supermarkets carry fava beans, and most will order them on request. Specialty stores such as health food markets often have fava beans in stock. Green fava beans have the highest levels of levodopa and cook to tenderness; older beans are tough and chewy. Fava beans, as are other legumes, are a good source of many vitamins and minerals including vitamin C, iron, and magnesium.

See also NUTRITION AND DIET; PROTEIN; PROTEIN RESTRICTIONS, DIETARY.

fear   A strong feeling of apprehension. Fear can be an appropriate reaction to a situation that represents potential danger, evoking the body's "flight or fight" response to get out of harm's way quickly.

A person may react with fear to the memory of the situation or to anticipation that the situation may occur again. A person with Parkinson's often fears situations in which symptoms such as inability to move draw attention and create EMBARRASSMENT. This fear typically follows at least one experience in which this happened, as an intense emotional response that causes the person to go to all lengths to avoid the situation.

Sometimes the fear of a potential event is well founded, such as the fear of falling. For the person with Parkinson's the risk of falling is very high, and the consequences can be serious. So the person may avoid circumstances in which a fall is more likely to happen, such as walking in dim lighting or on uneven surfaces. The downside is that fear often prevents people with Parkinson's from going out. Fear also intensifies symptoms of Parkinson's such as BRADYKINESIA (slowed movements), start hesitation and freezing of gait (inability to move), festination (rapid, uncontrolled steps), and other GAIT DISTURBANCES. Using a walking aid, allowing adequate time, and having a walking companion are ways to help lessen these fears.

There is also an element of fear about Parkinson's disease itself and what will happen as it progresses. As there is no predictable course the disease follows, after diagnosis there is great uncertainty that generates understandable worry. Talking about concerns and fears helps to put them in perspective. PLANNING FOR THE FUTURE also helps to allay fears about matters such as health care decisions, LONG-TERM CARE FACILITIES, and END OF LIFE CARE AND DECISIONS.

It is reasonable to have concerns and fears about what will happen, but it is also important to enjoy life as much as possible. Worrying about something, such as whether the person will become wheelchair-bound, does not prevent it and often prevents the person from focusing on and enjoying the abilities that he or she still has. Turning fear into constructive action, such as taking a trip planned for a later time early in the course of Parkinson's instead, helps to shift attention from the negative to the positive.

See also ANXIETY; DEPRESSION; FAMILY RELATIONSHIPS; LIVING WITH PARKINSON'S; SOCIAL INTERACTION.

feeding tube A small, thin, flexible tube passed through the nose and down the throat into the stomach (nasogastric [NG] tube) or the duodenum (nasoduodenal tube), through which liquified nutritional supplements are given. When there appears to be long-term need for a feeding tube, as when there are problems with SWALLOWING or obtaining adequate nutrition through EATING but the person's condition is otherwise stable, doctors sometimes surgically insert a tube through a small abdominal incision directly into the stomach or small intestine. This is commonly called a percutaneous endogastric (PEG) tube even though the gut end almost always is in the small intestine rather than the stomach. The point at which the tube passes through the skin can be covered with a small cap called a button and uncovered at times of feeding. This approach is less conspicuous, although it carries the risk of infection as it involves a wound (the incision). The person can still eat by mouth, if he or she chooses, with any of these tubes in place.

People often dread the idea of "tube feeding" or "artificial feeding" as extending life beyond the point at which it has enjoyable quality. This need not be the case, and in most situations family members and often the person with Parkinson's disease are able to discuss and decide whether this intervention is desired. However, it is important to make decisions in advance about supportive nutrition at the end of life, so the person's desires are known and followed. It is emotionally difficult to make the decision to stop nutritional support once it has been started, so it is to everyone's advantage to be clear about when and whether that should be considered. The purpose of nutritional support is to maintain the health of the body's systems, not to prolong life beyond the body's capability to sustain it.

There are many reasons that a person might not receive adequate nutrition through regular eating. The physical mechanisms of eating become difficult when Parkinson's affects the muscles of the mouth and throat. It is difficult for the person to CHEW and swallow, and the likelihood of aspiration (food particle's being sucked into the trachea or lungs) increases.

BRADYKINESIA (slowed muscle movement) also can affect GASTRIC MOTILITY (the rate at which food leaves the stomach) and PERISTALSIS (movement of food through the intestinal tract), such that even though the person is eating sufficient amounts of food the body is not appropriately digesting it and inadequate nutrition results. Some people find the option of using a surgical feeding tube preferable to being fed by others, as it is less conspicuous.

See also ADVANCE DIRECTIVES; END OF LIFE CARE AND DECISIONS; HEIMLICH MANEUVER; NUTRITION AND DIET; PALLIATIVE CARE; PARENTERAL NUTRITION; SWALLOWING.

feet The BRADYKINESIA (slowness of movement) and RIGIDITY (muscle stiffness) of Parkinson's disease often cause a perception that the feet have become separate entities that function independently. Although these symptoms affect the muscles of the legs and trunk as well, their effect seems centered in the feet. People commonly describe GAIT DISTURBANCES such as start hesitation and FREEZING OF GAIT as a feeling of having "magnetic feet" or feet that are glued to the floor. Even with intense concentration, the person often cannot force the feet to make the movements necessary to initiate or resume walking. Although the person may feel his or her leg muscles contract as though the legs are moving, the feet do not go anywhere. During walking the feet often feel heavy, as if considerable effort is required to pick each one up and put it back down again. Symptoms such as foot drag, in which the foot scuffles along the walking surface, and shuffling are common. As well, being unable to move the feet affects balance.

The focus on the feet is partly physiological, as a function of the disease process. Parkinson's disease results from depletion of DOPAMINE, the NEUROTRANSMITTER that facilitates nerve signals to control movement, in the BRAIN. The feet are at the end of the neuromuscular chain of command, so to speak. When there are delays in transmitting nerve signals along this chain, as is the essence of Parkinson's disease, the signals often are distorted and fragmented by the time they reach the end of the chain. As a result, the lowest level of response takes place. For reasons researchers do not fully understand, people with EARLY-ONSET PARKINSON'S (those who are age 40 or younger at diagnosis) often experience painful foot DYSTONIAS (intense cramping and distorted positions). Although these can occur throughout the course of the disease, they tend to happen with increasing frequency in the middle and late stages and are most likely during OFF-STATE periods (when the effectiveness of ANTI-PARKINSON'S MEDICATIONS is at its lowest level) such as early in the morning.

Some people with Parkinson's find that an effective approach to countering these disturbances in neuromuscular communication is to focus consciously on the sequence of actions of the entire body during walking, from ARM SWING and trunk movement to leg extension from the hip and knee. Although researchers believe there is no physical change in the transmission of nerve signals as a result of such effort, it does shift focus away from worry and fear about freezing and other gait disturbances to emphasize and visualize the desired movements. This restores a sense of control and confidence. Conscious effort to lift each foot completely from the walking surface and then to place it down with the next forward step helps to make focus on the feet proactive and positive. However, concentrating on the feet during an episode of freezing is more likely to extend the episode, creating ANXIETY and FRUSTRATION.

Some anti-Parkinson's medications can cause edema, or swelling, that is most noticeable in the feet and ankles. This condition usually is painless, and the person or caregiver notices it at the end of the day. It results from an accumulation of fluid. Other health conditions that become more common with increasing age, such as congestive heart failure and kidney problems, can cause edema. Sitting for long periods and sitting with the legs crossed at the knee also can cause edema. Occasional edema is common; edema that persists should be evaluated by a doctor. Taking frequent short walks and sitting with the legs and feet elevated help reduce the swelling.

See also AMBULATION; GAIT DISTURBANCE; SHOES; WALKING.

festination   See GAIT DISTURBANCE.

fetal dopaminergic brain cell transplant   An INVESTIGATIONAL TREATMENT in which DOPAMINE-producing BRAIN cells taken from aborted human fetuses are transplanted into the brain of a person with Parkinson's disease. Once the fetal cells "take," they grow and reproduce, eventually restoring enough dopaminergic neurons to replace those lost to Parkinson's disease. This treatment is highly controversial for ethical reasons; some people consider it inappropriate to use cells and tissue that result from abortions. In this procedure, the donor cells are extracted from fetal brain tissue, prepared in a solution, and injected into a catheter that is carefully threaded into the STRIATUM and SUBSTANTIA NIGRA of the person with Parkinson's. This procedure "seeds" this area of the brain that is essential to movement with cells that will readily infiltrate the brain and begin producing dopamine.

Although the first fetal dopaminergic brain cell transplants were done in Sweden in 1987, this procedure remains highly experimental. The number of patients who have received transplants is small, and the results so far have ranged from amazing to disappointing. This inconsistency is one reason the procedure remains experimental. Some people have experienced 10 or more years without any symptoms of Parkinson's and have apparently normal dopaminergic function, as measured by imaging techniques such as SINGLE PHOTON EMISSION COMPUTED TOMOGRAPHY (SPECT) or MAGNETIC RESONANCE IMAGING (MRI) within the striatum and substantia nigra. In other people the transplanted cells did not seed and grow, providing little to no relief of symptoms.

In two large well-designed studies in the United States, the vast majority of patients did not benefit from the surgery, though a few did benefit. As for the complication of "run away" DYSKINESIAS, though these abnormal involuntary fidgety movements commonly develop as a side effect of peaking levodopa levels in people with longstanding Parkinson's, roughly one in six people who had the surgery had these movements all the waking day, even when they were off of all ANTI-PARKINSON'S MEDICATIONS. Such results have led to a virtual moratorium on fetal cell transplantation studies in humans in the United States.

The procedure's controversial nature further limits research studies, particularly in the United States where abortion and a fetus's "right to life" are hotly debated; with current techniques, the procedure requires roughly four aborted fetuses to provide the cells necessary for one transplant. Researchers differ in their views of the viability of fetal dopaminergic brain cell transplants for treating Parkinson's; even among those who support research in this area, many believe there are more effective ways to obtain the same result. One such method is FETAL PORCINE BRAIN CELL TRANSPLANT, in which the dopaminergic brain cells are taken from pig embryos. Porcine tissue is closely related to human tissue and is already used in other transplant applications such as growth of heart valves.

See also ALLOGRAFT; BIOETHICS; CLINICAL RESEARCH STUDIES; NEURAL GRAFT; XENOGRAFT.

fetal porcine brain cell transplant   An investigational treatment in which dopaminergic brain cells are taken from the brain of fetal pigs and transplanted into the BRAIN of a person with Parkinson's disease. This procedure is being explored as an alternative to FETAL DOPAMINERGIC BRAIN CELL TRANSPLANT, which is highly controversial because the cells used for transplant are taken from aborted human fetuses. As with fetal human dopaminergic brain cell transplant, the donor cells are extracted from the brain tissue of the porcine fetus, prepared in a solution, and injected into a catheter that is carefully threaded into the STRIATUM and SUBSTANTIA NIGRA of the person with Parkinson's, where they seed and reproduce.

Although the numbers of people who have received this highly experimental treatment are small, fetal porcine brain cell transplant appears to be at least as successful as fetal human dopaminergic brain cell transplant. It may also have fewer risks, particularly of cross-infection from the donor, as porcine pathogens do not transfer to humans. Research continues to explore this and other NEURAL GRAFT possibilities.

See also ALLOGRAFT; BIOETHICS; CLINICAL RESEARCH STUDIES; XENOGRAFT.

fiber, dietary   See NUTRITION AND DIET.

financial planning   A process of balancing resources with anticipated expenses in looking at potential future needs. Although Parkinson's disease is a medical condition, it affects every aspect of a person's life. However modest a family's resources, it is essential to plan, as early as possible, for future needs. Expenses, direct and indirect, can be overwhelming. ANTI-PARKINSON'S MEDICATIONS can cost $500 a month or more. Residence in a retirement community or an assisted living facility can cost $3,000 a month or more; long-term care facilities are even more costly. Even when a family member serves as full-time caregiver so the person with Parkinson's remains in the home, there are numerous costs associated with transportation to doctor appointments, special items such as protective undergarments and nutritional supplements, adaptive equipment and assist devices, and perhaps loss of income if the caregiver has given up or cannot take a paying job.

Each family's circumstances and needs are unique. Yet nearly every family needs to make adjustments to accommodate both short-term and long-term expenses. Factors to consider include:

- What is the age of the person with Parkinson's, and to what extent is he or she responsible for the family's financial status? A person who is still working is likely making significant contributions to the family's income. In EARLY-ONSET PARKINSON'S, the person may still be in a career-building phase.

- How significantly do the symptoms of Parkinson's disease affect the person's abilities? If still employed, can he or she continue to work? If not, how close is he or she to retirement? What, if any, consequences are attached to early retirement, such as reduced payments or loss of insurance?

- Are there dependent children living at home? What are their needs? How will those needs be met if the person with Parkinson's is the family's primary wage earner? If a spouse works outside the home, who provides care for the person with Parkinson's?

- What benefits are available to help pay for medical expenses? The care that the person with

Parkinson's requires becomes more extensive and expensive as the disease progresses. MEDICAL INSURANCE or MEDICARE, for those who have either, covers most of the initial expense of evaluation and diagnostic testing as well as the costs of much of the ongoing care. Some people also qualify for other medical benefits such as those of the Veterans Administration (VA) (veteran's benefits for those who were honorably discharged from military service). Many benefit plans do not pay for prescription drugs or pay nominal amounts for them. This means that many people must pay for ANTI-PARKINSON'S MEDICATIONS, which can be quite expensive.

• What physical challenges exist, such as stairs, for the person with Parkinson's in the current place of residence? How feasible is it to make any necessary modifications as the disease progresses?

• How will the family accommodate the person's need for extensive assistance with the ACTIVITIES OF DAILY LIVING (ADLs), should that need arise? Does the family have the resources to pay for in-home care, assisted living, or long-term care?

• How can the family preserve resources and still meet the needs of the person with Parkinson's? How will the family accommodate MEDICAID spend-down requirements, if that becomes necessary?

A qualified financial consultant can help families identify their resources as well as potential expenses, which often include aspects that families do not consider such as ESTATE PLANNING, tax issues, wills, and funeral arrangements. It is important to choose a consultant who has no vested interest in the decisions the family makes and can present an objective assessment of the family's situation and workable solutions for potential problems. Support groups, senior centers, and social service organizations (many of which are not-for-profit organizations and charge minimal fees for their services) are good resources.

See also ADAPTIVE EQUIPMENT AND ASSIST DEVICES; ESTATE PLANNING; INDEPENDENCE; LONG-TERM CARE INSURANCE; PLANNING FOR THE FUTURE; PRESCRIPTION ASSISTANCE PROGRAMS.

fluctuating phenomenon (fluctuating response) The inconsistency in symptom relief from ANTI-PARKINSON'S MEDICATIONS that develops as a person takes the medications over an extended period and as the Parkinson's progresses. This dual dynamic is the result of progressive depletion of DOPAMINERGIC NEURONS, and consequently of DOPAMINE (a neurotransmitter with key responsibilities for conveying nerve signals related to movement) in the brain and of the resistance remaining dopaminergic neurons develop to LEVODOPA, the drug that is currently the cornerstone of treatment regimens for Parkinson's disease, after this medication is taken for years. Increasingly higher doses of levodopa are required to produce an effect on symptoms; unpleasant side effects, which include NAUSEA and DYSTONIA (severe muscle rigidity, distortion, and cramping), result.

Within the fluctuating phenomenon there is an ON-STATE, during which medications hold symptoms at bay, and an OFF-STATE, during which symptoms are prominent and uncontrolled. In addition to motor symptoms, other symptoms such as mood swings, anxiety, and depression tend to be manifested or to intensify during an OFF-STATE. Doctors attempt to moderate fluctuations by manipulating ADJUNCT THERAPIES—trying different drugs or changes in medication combinations, dosages, and timing. Medications that are most effective for this purpose are DOPAMINE AGONIST MEDICATIONS such as PERGOLIDE, PRAMIPEXOLE, and ROPINIROLE. COMT inhibitors are also useful in extending the duration of levodopa's effect and smoothing out response. Dyskinesias, both choreiform involuntary fidgeting movements (most commonly during the first part of the on-state when the levodopa levels in the brain are peaking) and dystonic involuntary muscle cramping (usually as levodopa levels are falling and the off-state is starting), are also common manifestations of fluctuating phenomena, and amantadine is often helpful in alleviating them. If one of these drugs is not effective, another may be, so it is worth juggling them around to try to find a successful combination. Such multidrug therapies for fluctuations typically require further adjustments over the ensuing months and years as symptoms progress.

Some pharmaceutical companies are experimenting with anti-Parkinson's medications such as a dopamine agonist (rotigotine) that can be delivered via transdermal (skin) patch (sometimes erroneously referred to as a dopamine or Sinemet patch). This arrangement allows steady, consistent, and long-term absorption of the drug without interference from digestive factors such as foods and slowed gastric mobility and peristalsis, all of which influence the rate and amount of an oral drug's absorption. However, at present this method of medication delivery remains investigational.

Other factors that contribute to fluctuations in symptom control include the kinds of foods eaten and the times of meals relative to medication dosage times, stress, sleep quality, and tiredness or FATIGUE. In the early stages of the disease, most people with Parkinson's take medications, particularly levodopa, with meals to offset the nausea these drugs can cause. But protein, iron, and other nutrients can affect the amount of levodopa that enters the bloodstream. By mid to late Parkinson's, most people find it necessary to shift to taking levodopa and other anti-Parkinson's medications on an empty stomach (an hour before or two to three hours after meals) to increase their absorption, and to take additional medications for nausea, if that is a problem. This often helps, at least for a short time, to extend the effectiveness of the medications.

For many people with Parkinson's, the fluctuating phenomenon has an element of predictability in that on-states and off-states clearly follow medication dosage schedules. For other people, and in the later stages of Parkinson's, fluctuations can be unpredictable and extreme, taking the person from immobility to a nearly symptom-free condition in the space of a few minutes without apparent pattern. Intense EMOTIONS also can precipitate off-state episodes.

The fluctuating phenomenon is among the most frustrating and challenging aspects of Parkinson's disease for most people with Parkinson's as well as loved ones and caregivers, particularly when it is unpredictable. During off-state episodes, the person with Parkinson's can be essentially immobilized and unable to perform even the most basic ACTIVITIES OF DAILY LIVING (ADLs). The extent to which fluctuating phenomenon occurs is one of the key measures in the STAGING OF PARKINSON'S (assessing the level of the disease's progression) and in evaluating the level of disability the disease is causing.

See also ADJUSTING TO LIVING WITH PARKINSON'S; COPING WITH ONGOING CARE OF PARKINSON'S; FOODS TO AVOID; FOODS TO EAT; HOEHN AND YAHR STAGE SCALE; INVESTIGATIONAL NEW DRUG; NUTRITION AND DIET; RESCUE DRUG; SLEEP DISTURBANCES; TREATMENT ALGORITHMS; UNIFIED PARKINSON'S DISEASE RATING SCALE; WEARING-OFF EFFECT.

fluoxetine An ANTIDEPRESSANT MEDICATION better known by its trade name, Prozac. Fluoxetine is a SELECTIVE SEROTONIN REUPTAKE INHIBITOR (SSRI) that works by preventing neurons from reabsorbing serotonin, a NEUROTRANSMITTER that affects brain activity related to mood and emotion. It extends the length of time and amount of serotonin available in the brain, easing symptoms of DEPRESSION. Fluoxetine was the first of the SSRIs to gain U.S. Food and Drug Administration (FDA) approval, in 1987. It is now available in a once-a-week product (Prozac Weekly) and in generic formulations of the regular form. Fluoxetine can cause DROWSINESS, NAUSEA, DRY MOUTH, and AGITATION in some people. Fluoxetine also is now approved for use in treating obsessive-compulsive disorder and the eating disorder bulimia.

See also ANXIETY; PSYCHOSOCIAL FACTORS; PSYCHOTHERAPY.

flurazepam A SLEEP MEDICATION in the BENZODIAZEPINE family, commonly known by its trade name, Dalmane, that is chemically related to DIAZEPAM (Valium) and ALPRAZOLAM (Xanax). Its primary use is to cause drowsiness and maintain sleep. Some people become tolerant to its effects with long-term use. Flurazepam also has addictive qualities. It can enhance the DROWSINESS effect of ANTI-PARKINSON'S MEDICATIONS, but because flurazepam is taken before bedtime this effect is not usually a problem. Side effects are uncommon; they can include NAUSEA, headache, DIZZINESS, and DISORIENTATION. When taking this or any medication for sleep, use extra caution when getting up during the night to go to the bathroom. It is a good idea to sit on the edge of the bed for a minute or two to become oriented and to make sure there is no dizziness or other response that could affect balance when walking.

See also ANTIHISTAMINE MEDICATIONS; BEDROOM COMFORT; SLEEP DISTURBANCES.

food preparation Methods for fixing foods that make EATING, CHEWING, and SWALLOWING easier and reduce the risks of choking and aspiration (entry of food particles into the lungs, which can cause pneumonia). Classic symptoms of Parkinson's such as BRADYKINESIA (slowed muscle movement), RIGIDITY (muscle stiffness), and TREMORS (involuntary, rhythmic, repetitive movements) often affect the face, mouth, and throat as the disease progresses. As well, these symptoms affect fine motor control of the fingers and hands, making grasping and manipulation of eating utensils difficult. As a result, the person's ability to prepare as well as eat food is affected.

Food preparation needs change as the Parkinson's progresses. In the early stages of the disease, the person with Parkinson's may have little or no trouble eating his or her usual foods. It is still prudent for the person to cut food items into smaller bite sizes, to reduce the risk of choking. As the disease enters its mid stages, swallowing becomes more of a challenge for many people with Parkinson's. It is easier and safer for them to eat foods that are soft, such as well-cooked or mashed potatoes, and cooked rather than raw vegetables. In the later stages of Parkinson's, the person may have difficulty in swallowing anything other than pureed foods and liquids. Such foods should have no lumps or chunks.

See also COOKING; EATING; FEEDING TUBE; FOODS TO AVOID; FOODS TO EAT; KITCHEN EFFICIENCY; NUTRITION AND DIET; PARENTERAL NUTRITION; PROTEIN; PROTEIN RESTRICTIONS, DIETARY.

foods to avoid Certain foods interfere with the action of ANTI-PARKINSON'S MEDICATIONS or exacerbate symptoms such as slowed GASTRIC MOTILITY, slowed PERISTALSIS, and CONSTIPATION. It is important for the person with Parkinson's disease to eat

a nutritiously balanced diet, and avoiding foods that can cause problems helps to keep symptoms and discomforts in check. In the early stages of Parkinson's, most people have little difficulty eating their favorite foods, although this period provides the ideal opportunity to shift toward a more healthful diet by replacing high-fat foods with fruits, vegetables, and whole grain products. This diet aids the digestive process, helping to minimize problems such as constipation.

Food interference becomes more of a concern as Parkinson's progresses, and foods that are high on the list of those to avoid are those that are high in protein (such as meats, dry beans, nuts, and dairy products). During digestion, dietary protein competes with LEVODOPA, the primary anti-Parkinson medication, for absorption from the intestine. Levodopa is an AMINO ACID, as are proteins (digestion breaks down proteins into their component amino acids). The body can only absorb so many amino acids at one time, and it is not selective in how it does so. When the amino acid "quota" is met, the intestine simply stops absorbing amino acid.

This is not so much of a problem in the early stages of Parkinson's as levodopa dosages are fairly low and amino acid competition is slight. As symptoms progress and the person requires increasingly higher amounts of levodopa, however, the circumstances change. By the mid stages of Parkinson's, or when fluctuations in symptoms begin to appear, most doctors recommend restricting protein to the minimum and shifting most protein-rich foods to the evening meal (levodopa doses are structured to be highest during waking hours for maximal effectiveness in controlling symptoms).

Other foods to avoid are those that are likely to contribute to problems such as gastric reflux and constipation. Gastric reflux, in which acid and stomach contents leak back into the esophagus, is a common problem in people with Parkinson's as the disease affects the functioning of the smooth muscle tissues of the stomach. This effect slows stomach function and gastric motility (movement of food from the stomach into the intestine). To compensate, the stomach increases acid production. Foods most likely to exacerbate gastric reflux include tomatoes and tomato sauce, citrus fruits, caffeine (coffee, tea, and colas), alcoholic beverages, garlic, and chocolate. Other foods may also create problems; each person has unique "triggers" for gastric reflux and should avoid them as much as possible. Cigarette smoking also contributes to gastric reflux because of nicotine's effect on smooth muscle function.

Although fiber is important to proper bowel function, when peristalsis (intestinal movement) is slowed, as is the case in Parkinson's disease, presence of too much fiber can slow digestion even further. Foods that are high in fiber include whole grains and whole grain products, fruits, and vegetables. Most people learn through experimentation what is the appropriate balance of these foods in their diet, information that is essential for good nutrition.

Foods to Avoid or Eat in Minimal Amounts	Reason
Meat, chicken, dairy products (milk, cheese, ice cream)	Interfere with levodopa absorption
Lentils, legumes (dry beans), nuts	Interfere with levodopa absorption
Clams, shrimp, red meat, beef liver	Can interfere with absorption; potential for high iron levels to be deposited in the brain
Tomatoes and tomato sauce, citrus fruits, caffeine (coffee, tea, and colas), alcoholic beverages, garlic, chocolate	Precipitate or exacerbate gastric reflux
Legumes, bran	Can cause constipation
Foods containing excess vitamin B_6	Interferes with levodopa absorption

See also ACERULOPLASMINEMIA; EATING; EXERCISE AND ACTIVITY; NUTRITION AND DIET; PROTEIN RESTRICTIONS, DIETARY.

foods to eat   There are no foods demonstrated to improve the symptoms of Parkinson's disease or to prevent its development. Many people believe a diet high in ANTIOXIDANTS, which are found naturally in foods such as raw fruits and vegetables, helps to stave off degenerative conditions by reducing the levels of FREE RADICALS (destructive molecules) in the body. Although there is some

evidence that the antioxidant COENZYME Q-10 is effective in neutralizing free radicals, the benefit of this action to the person with Parkinson's is not clear, as researchers do not yet understand the roles, if any, free radicals play in the development and progression of Parkinson's disease. One of the largest CLINICAL RESEARCH STUDIES to study the effectiveness of antioxidants, the DATATOP (Deprenyl and Tocopherol Antioxidative Therapy for Parkinson's Disease) study found no scientific evidence that tocopherol (the active ingredient of vitamin E, an antioxidant) had any effect on the symptoms of Parkinson's.

Nonetheless, it is important that people with Parkinson's disease include a wide variety of fruits and vegetables in their diet, not because they supply antioxidants but because they are rich in necessary nutrients. Maintaining good nutrition becomes an increasing challenge as Parkinson's progresses, so establishing a solid nutritional base is important. Some people advocate eating FAVA BEANS as a means for leveling out the peaks and valleys of LEVODOPA dosages. This legume, also called the broad bean, is naturally high in levodopa. However, legumes also are high in PROTEIN, which competes with levodopa for absorption into the bloodstream from the intestine. It is a good idea to consult a doctor before adding fava beans to the diet on a regular basis, as they may necessitate adjustment of the levodopa dose.

See also EATING; EXERCISE AND ACTIVITY; NUTRITION AND DIET; PROTEIN RESTRICTIONS, DIETARY.

foot drag   See GAIT DISTURBANCE.

Fox, Michael J.   A well-known Canadian actor diagnosed with EARLY-ONSET PARKINSON'S disease at age 31. Fox began acting as a teen and is best known for his starring roles in several popular television situation comedies including NBC's *Family Ties* (1982–89) and ABC's *Spin City* (1996–2000), the last two seasons of which were filmed after Fox publicly announced his Parkinson's diagnosis. Fox also starred in a number of movies including the successful *Back to the Future* comedies and the drama *Bright Lights, Big City*.

Although Fox concealed his diagnosis from the public for eight years, since GOING PUBLIC he has become one of the most visible and outspoken advocates for research supporting the search for a cure. His appearance before the U.S. Congress to testify in support of increased funding for Parkinson's research was dramatic as he presented himself during an OFF-STATE to demonstrate the full effects of the disease for legislators. He has made similar appearances in television interviews.

Fox started the MICHAEL J. FOX FOUNDATION FOR PARKINSON'S RESEARCH in 2000 to raise public awareness of Parkinson's disease and money for research. The organization's website, www.michaeljfox.org, provides information about Parkinson's disease, CLINICAL RESEARCH STUDIES that are recruiting participants or are under way, results of completed studies, innovative treatment approaches, and more information about Fox himself.

See also ALI, MUHAMMAD; MORRIS K. UDALL PARKINSON'S RESEARCH ACT; RENO, JANET; UDALL, MORRIS K.; WHITE, MAURICE.

free radical   A normal molecular by-product of metabolism. Free radicals are so named because their molecular structure is unstable, leaving them "free" to bind with any other molecule that is "open." Such binding creates unusual chemical structures that the body cannot use and that prevent other molecules that are hijacked by them from meeting the body's needs. Many scientists believe this action disrupts body functions and processes to the extent that, over time, it causes damage that leaves cells vulnerable to diseases such as cancer and NEURODEGENERATIVE CONDITIONS such as ALZHEIMER'S DISEASE, AMYOTROPHIC LATERAL SCLEROSIS (ALS), and Parkinson's disease.

In health, cells produce a natural chemical called COMPLEX I that alters free radicals to prevent them from binding with other molecules. Other chemical substances called ANTIOXIDANTS then can bind to the free radicals in processes that allow them to pass from the body as waste. In a chronic condition such as Parkinson's disease, the amount of complex I the cells produce decreases. Scientists are uncertain whether this effect is a cause or a consequence of the disease but believe that in either case the drop in complex I level contributes to the disease's development. Recent studies suggest that COENZYME Q-10, an antioxidant found in many fruits and vegetables as well as available as a NUTRITIONAL SUPPLEMENT, is effective in reducing the numbers of free radicals. Free radicals alone probably do not account for disease development but instead interact with various other factors such as genetic predisposition and environmental circumstances to allow a disease state to establish itself. Free radical damage appears to be cumulative: That is, it becomes more extensive and more likely to result in disease over an extended period, probably decades.

See also APOPTOSIS; COENZYME Q-10; COMPLEX I; LIPOPOLYSACCHARIDES; MITOCHONDRIAL DYSFUNCTION; MITOCHONDRIAL ELECTRON TRANSPORT CHAIN; NUTRITION AND DIET; PARKINSON'S DISEASE, CAUSES OF.

freezing of gait (FOG)   See GAIT DISTURBANCE.

frequent urination   See URINARY FREQUENCY.

frequent voiding schedule   A structured schedule for urination established to help prevent bladder leaks and URINARY URGENCY. INCONTINENCE (the inability to hold urine) is a common problem of aging as well as of Parkinson's disease. Typically a frequent voiding schedule is every two hours while awake. Maintaining the schedule on outings such as shopping requires careful planning, and it is important to make every effort to do so. This process helps to minimize the person's worries about leaks and accidents; worrying makes the urgency worse. When nighttime incontinence is a problem, the schedule includes urinating immediately before going to bed and getting up every three to four hours throughout the night to empty the bladder. It is important to balance nighttime voiding schedules with sleep patterns so the person receives adequate rest.

Urinary tract infections are more common in people with incontinence, especially women, and can cause urgency. When urinary urgency continues despite a frequent voiding schedule, the doctor should test a urine sample for bacteria to determine whether an infection is present. Treating the infection with antibiotics often ends the urgency. If no infection is present, there are medications such as oxybutynin (Ditropan) or tolterodine (Detrol) that may be helpful in reducing bladder urgency that persists despite frequent voiding, but they do carry some risk of side effects.

See also UNDERGARMENTS, PROTECTIVE; URINARY RETENTION.

friendships Close associations with others that are important to emotional health and for a sense of well-being. For many people, friends are like extended family and it is sometimes easier to share worries and concerns with them than with family members. Yet friendships form for various reasons, and sometimes the common interests that bind friends disappear as Parkinson's progresses. Friends who enjoyed playing golf together, for example, may struggle to find other common activities that the person with Parkinson's can still do.

However close friends are, it is sometimes difficult for them to know how to respond to the challenge of a life-changing condition such as Parkinson's disease. It is important to remember that despite the changes the person's body is experiencing, the essence of the person remains. Common interests are still common interests, even if the person with Parkinson's can no longer participate in them in the same ways. Sometimes there are ways to adapt to the person's changing abilities, such as taking a golf cart instead of walking the course or watching golf on television. Sometimes friends can find other interests in common.

As with other relationships, open and honest communication is essential with friends. The person with Parkinson's needs to make clear his or her limitations and constraints and not pressured to engage in activities that exceed them. This is not always easy, as the person with Parkinson's does not want to prevent friends from enjoying favorite activities. But going along with them and then having a crisis is not beneficial for anyone. For the friend, it is important to pay close attention to the person's state and to ask whether the person is becoming tired or is exceeding his or her abilities.

Friends should learn as much as possible about Parkinson's disease, so they understand what is going on.

As Parkinson's progresses, the symptoms make participating in social activities and events more difficult. This difficulty inherently limits contact with friends and can cause the person with Parkinson's to feel isolated and lonely. Friends can help by making short visits. It is not necessary to entertain the person; generally just the shared companionship is very meaningful. Sometimes just sitting together is enough. Friends may also offer to stay with the person so the caregiver can get away for a while or help with tasks around the house that are not getting done. As it progresses, Parkinson's disease demands more attention and time, leaving little of either for routine chores. Friends who can recognize what needs to be done and pitch in to get it done can make all the difference.

See also ADJUSTING TO LIVING WITH PARKINSON'S; COMPASSION; EMPATHY; MARRIAGE RELATIONSHIP; PARENT/CHILD RELATIONSHIPS; SOCIAL INTERACTIONS; WORKPLACE RELATIONSHIPS.

frustration A strong feeling of annoyance or irritability about being prevented from doing things or forced to do them or a sense of lack of control over events and circumstances that the person feels should be within his or her ability to control. Persistent frustration can lead to ANGER, ANXIETY, and DEPRESSION. Parkinson's creates much frustration in people who have the disease, as its motor symptoms prevent them from performing the common and essential functions of everyday life and independence. Limbs that will not move, feet that feel frozen to the floor, eyes that do not focus, fingers that do not grip, words that evade recall—these are the hallmark characteristics of Parkinson's disease, and they entail the actions of voluntary movement. Yet for the person with Parkinson's, there is nothing voluntary about them. They simply do not happen and therefore interfere with activities once taken for granted.

Frustration is a difficult emotion to manage. It requires accepting the loss of control over things that are important and focusing on things that are still possible. The inconsistent response to treatment and the progressive nature of Parkinson's disease thwart these adaptive approaches. They are moving targets, which create their own level of frustration. It helps to share fears and worries with friends and family members, who sometimes can offer suggestions for working around impairments to allow the person to regain a sense of control. Support groups are also excellent resources. Frustration is also a challenge for caregivers, who must constantly readjust to the changing condition and capabilities of the person with Parkinson's.

As much as is possible and practical, it is important for the person with Parkinson's to maintain control over his or her environment and personal functions. Often doing so requires readjusting expectations. ADAPTIVE EQUIPMENT AND ASSIST DEVICES can extend INDEPENDENCE. Other efforts such as organizing bedrooms, bathrooms, and kitchens to accommodate the person's changing physical capabilities can allow the person to more effectively manage the ACTIVITIES OF DAILY LIVING (ADLs). Patience, too, is important. The person needs more time to do things as the Parkinson's progresses, and trying to force or rush them invariably makes the situation worse. Making a conscious effort to focus on the positives and what the person can do helps to keep circumstances in perspective.

See also ADJUSTING TO LIVING WITH PARKINSON'S; BATHING AND BATHROOM ORGANIZATION; COMPASSION; COPING WITH ONGOING CARE OF PARKINSON'S; EMOTIONS; EMPATHY; HUMOR; KITCHEN EFFICIENCY; OPTIMISM.

functional capacity   A person's physical capability to perform tasks. Functional capacity testing, typically performed by a PHYSICAL THERAPIST or an OCCUPATIONAL THERAPIST, provides an objective measure of this capability that is primarily useful for disability insurance or Social Security claims when the person is still of employment age at the time he or she is diagnosed with Parkinson's disease. This is sometimes called work capacity or work capacity testing. Employers may also request such evaluation to determine whether the person qualifies for workplace accommodations under the AMERICANS WITH DISABILITIES ACT (ADA). When a

person wants to continue working, the occupational therapist can use the functional capacity test results to design exercises and activities to improve his or her ability to perform the job's tasks.

In functional capacity testing the person performs a variety of tasks under controlled circumstances. The therapist assesses the person's ability to perform each task and then provides an overall evaluation of the person's physical capacity. Disability insurance companies and the Social Security Administration have specific parameters that functional capacity testing must include; therapists who are qualified to perform the testing are familiar with these. A person's functional capacity rating varies according to the requirements of the job. For example, a person with moderate BRADYKINESIA (slowed movement) and mild GAIT DISTURBANCES will probably lack the functional capacity to work in a job that requires lifting and carrying, although he or she may be capable of work that requires sitting at a desk.

See also ACTIVITIES OF DAILY LIVING; INSTRUMENTAL ACTIVITIES OF DAILY LIVING; WORKPLACE ADAPTATIONS TO ACCOMMODATE PARKINSON'S.

functional imaging studies   Sophisticated radiological and nuclear medicine procedures that allow doctors and researchers to visualize the changes in activity patterns within the brain; these changes may be due to diseases such as Parkinson's disease, but some techniques are sensitive enough to map the changes involved in a particular movement or mental activity in people with no brain pathology. Although there are presently no tests that can conclusively diagnose Parkinson's disease, functional imaging studies allow doctors to rule out other possible causes of the symptoms of Parkinson's disease such as tumors or other neurodegenerative disorders that have distinctive patterns of change in the brain's physiological processes.

Commonly used functional imaging studies include POSITRON EMISSION TOMOGRAPHY (PET) and SINGLE PHOTON EMISSION COMPUTED TOMOGRAPHY (SPECT). Notably, the PET technique that holds the most promise for usefulness in the diagnosis and staging of Parkinson's (using flurodopa as the radiolabeled tracer) is very difficult to perform and, hence, is only available at a handful of centers in the world. In research settings, other imaging techniques use different radioisotopes such as 2 BETA-CARBOXYMETHOLOXY-3-BETA (4-IODOPHENYL) TROPANE (DOPASCAN), currently in phase III clinical trials in the United States, that allow researchers to measure the density of DOPAMINERGIC NEURONS in the brain as a means of assessing the rate and extent of their loss. Another rare functional imaging technique that does not require radioactive agents is functional MAGNETIC RESONANCE IMAGING (MRI), a very sensitive and specialized technique that is different than standard MRI which only shows anatomy and not function.

See also BIOMARKERS; CLINICAL RESEARCH STUDIES; DIAGNOSING PARKINSON'S.

GABA   See GAMMA-AMINOBUTYRIC ACID (GABA).

GAD   See GLUTAMIC ACID DECARBOXYLASE (GAD).

gait   The pattern of movements in walking. Gait requires proper functioning and integration of the NERVOUS SYSTEM and the musculoskeletal system. Injury or dysfunction of either interferes with normal gait. The nature of the GAIT DISTURBANCE is key to diagnosing neuromuscular disorders. Gait analysis is an essential element of a NEUROLOGICAL EXAMINATION. In natural or normal gait, the movements of walking are smooth and coordinated, with opposing but comparable ARM SWING and LEG STRIDE. When the right leg steps forward, the left arm swings forward and the right arm swings back. When the left leg steps forward, the right arm swings forward and the left arm swings back. As the heel of the forward leg makes contact with the walking surface, the toe of the back leg is releasing from such contact. As contact of the forward foot rolls from heel to toe, the back foot clears contact and the back leg begins to swing forward.

For counterbalance, the shoulders and the hips also rotate opposite one another, clockwise or counterclockwise, during walking. The shoulders follow the arm swing, rotating counterclockwise when the right arm is forward and clockwise when the left arm is forward. Similarly, the hips follow the leg extension, rotating counterclockwise when the right leg is extended and clockwise when the left leg is extended. These movements are all continuous and synchronized, occurring without hesitation or exaggeration.

Gait Characteristic	Normal	In Parkinson's
Arm swing	Proportionate to stride	Minimal to nonexistent
Posture	Torso upright	Bent forward at waist
Stance (stationary)	Can stand without losing balance or moving when feet are close together	Difficult to stand still or to maintain balance unless feet are at least shoulder-width apart
Starting	Smooth and coordinated with no hesitation	Often pronounced, and sometimes extended, hesitation
Step	Each foot cleanly clears the walking surface; heel of forward foot goes down as toe of back foot pushes up	Steps are short and shuffling; toes might overlap heels; high-stepping; might drag one or both feet
Stopping	Smooth and coordinated with no hesitation	Often unable to stop for several steps after being asked; might lose balance when stopping
Stride	Moderate length (2 to 3 feet); consistent pace and cadence; can smoothly change stride and pace upon request	Short (6 to 10 inches); pace slow and without cadence; often cannot change stride or pace when asked; tends to gain momentum and lose control
Turning	Smooth and coordinated with no hesitation; typically initiated from pivot on ball of foot	Often stops before turning or loses balance; shortened, quick, shuffling steps

The moment at which the toe of one foot and the heel of the other foot are both in contact with the surface, called the stance phase of gait, is a crucial point in the gait cycle. During the stance phase the body transfers weight from the back leg to the forward leg, known in biochemical terms as load response. It requires BALANCE, stability, coordination, and strength. The actions of motion are called the stride phase of gait. A third component of gait is the stationary phase, during which the person stands still with both feet in full (heel to toe) contact with the surface.

When gait is normal, the body maintains EQUILIBRIUM upright and from side to side, both during movement (the stride and stance phases of gait) and while standing still (the stationary phase of gait). In a person with Parkinson's disease, nearly all characteristics of gait become altered in a typical and often pronounced pattern of gait disturbances. Muscle RIGIDITY and TREMORS further restrict movement and control of motion. Treatment with ANTI-PARKINSON'S MEDICATIONS to augment the brain's supply of DOPAMINE can restore movement and gait to near-normal in the early and mid stages of the disease in most people with Parkinson's.

Clinical Gait Analysis

Clinical gait analysis is primarily observational and generally provides enough information for a NEUROLOGIST or other clinician to suspect or confirm (and sometimes to rule out) a diagnosis of Parkinson's disease. It is part of a typical neurological examination or functional assessment. To conduct a clinical gait analysis, the clinician asks the person to walk a short distance and observes movements as the person walks away and then walks back.

Gait disturbances characteristic of Parkinson's include short, shuffling steps; limited or nonexistent arm swing; foot drag; high-stepping; and hesitation when starting, stopping, or turning. The clinician may also ask the person to repeat the process; walking the same distance only on the toes and then only on the heels. People with Parkinson's may find it easy to, or tend to, walk on their toes but difficult to walk only on their heels. The clinician also observes the person for balance, swaying from side to side, upper body movement, and any evidence of hemiplegic gait (swinging the leg out to the side during forward movement) that might suggest damage to parts of the brain other than those that are typical in Parkinson's disease (such as from stroke).

Instrumental Gait Analysis

Instrumental gait analysis uses videotaping, ELECTROPHYSIOLOGIC STUDIES, computerized modeling, and other methods to provide in-depth assessment of motor skills and movement dysfunctions. Such analysis helps to pinpoint areas of difficulty so that a physical therapist, occupational therapist, or physiatrist (physician specializing in rehabilitative medicine) can develop an individualized program of exercises to help compensate for already lost function and to preserve remaining function as long as possible. This analysis is particularly useful in EARLY-ONSET PARKINSON'S, in the early stages of Parkinson's, and when gait disturbances do not follow a typical pattern. Such techniques are also very useful in research since it provides data from numerous measurements that more readily lends itself to further analysis for small improvements than the more subjective (and less readily converted to numbers) clinical gait exam.

See also BALANCE; CONDITIONS SIMILAR TO PARKINSON'S; DYSKINESIA; ELECTROMYOGRAPHY; MOBILITY; MOBILITY AIDS; MOVEMENT; POSTURAL DYSFUNCTION; POSTURAL INSTABILITY; POSTURAL RIGHTING REFLEX; POSTURE, STOOPING; PROPRIOCEPTION; WALKING.

gait disturbance A deviation from the normal pattern of movement in walking. A number of gait disturbances characterize Parkinson's disease. These all result from the disruption of communication among the neurons in the BRAIN related to movement, caused by the depletion of the NEUROTRANSMITTER DOPAMINE. As with other symptoms of Parkinson's, gait disturbances affect people in different and various ways. One person with Parkinson's may have severe and numerous gait disturbances as early symptoms while another has barely perceptible problems until much later in the course of the disease; gait problems severe enough to cause falls very early (within the first two years of symptoms) raises questions as whether another form of parkinsonism, such as progressive supranuclear palsy or multisystem atrophy, may be the correct diagnosis. A person with Parkinson's may have one gait disturbance or multiple problems with walking. ANTI-PARKINSON'S MEDICATIONS can control gait disturbances for most people during the early and mid stages of the disease, although in later stages these symptoms typically "break through" during OFF-STATE EPISODES, when the medications, particularly levodopa, are not effective. There is a general feeling that levodopa may be a slightly more effective medication for gait and balance problems than even high doses of dopamine agonists.

Gait disturbances ultimately affect everyone whose Parkinson's becomes moderate to advanced as the brain's ability to direct the functions of movement continues to deteriorate. The way this takes place varies greatly among individuals. A particular gait disturbance may become progressively more severe, or additional disturbances may develop. Freezing of gait, start hesitation, and shuffling are the most prevalent gait disturbances in Parkinson's. Although these symptoms are involuntary, it does often help for the person to focus conscious attention and effort on the functions of movement. Because these functions have always occurred automatically (without conscious awareness), learning to focus in this way is frustrating, especially at first, for many people with Parkinson's. As well, there is a point at which the damage from the Parkinson's becomes extensive enough that it is no longer possible to "will" the body into movement.

Changing Direction (Turning)

Changing direction, or turning, becomes a challenge for many people with Parkinson's and is a function of movement during which the risk for falling is high. In natural or normal movement, changing direction takes place as a pivoting action. In the stance phase of the gait cycle the foot plants, and the body shifts not only its weight but its direction of travel. This sequence of motions requires balance, equilibrium, and coordination—all of which deteriorate as Parkinson's disease progresses. The person with Parkinson's attempts to accommodate the loss of these abilities by using small, shuffling steps to move in an arc when changing

direction. This gait has the appearance of walking around an unseen obstacle. As the Parkinson's becomes more severe, and during OFF-STATE episodes in which ANTI-PARKINSON'S MEDICATIONS cannot control movement, the span of this arc becomes wider and wider. Effort to shorten this span often results in loss of balance and falling.

Sometimes the person with Parkinson's attempts to stop and then change direction. Often, however, this is no easier a combination of movements and results in other gait disturbances such as stop hesitation (difficulty in stopping) and start hesitation (difficulty in beginning the next movement). Movement specialists recommend that the person with Parkinson's attempt to overcome turning challenges by planning directional changes and making them in a U-turn style, allowing for an adequate approach and wide arc or turning radius to minimize balance loss. This action, like other movement accommodations, requires focus and concentration.

Festination

The Latin origin of the word *festination* means "to hasten," as a person with this gait disturbance appears to do. A festinating gait consists of short, increasingly rapid steps with a marked forward lean, as though the person is about to break into a run. This is an involuntary attempt to restore balance, but it instead shifts the body's center of gravity increasingly farther from center. It is very difficult for the person with Parkinson's to stop moving when festination occurs, and often he or she falls. Festination often begins when the person is attempting to change direction or to stop; it is a combination of gait disturbances and postural instability. walking aids such as a walker, walking stick, or cane can help to prevent festination.

Foot Drag

People with Parkinson's often drag one foot or sometimes both feet, depending on whether movement dysfunctions are unilateral (primarily affect one side) or bilateral (affect both sides). Foot drag involves both MOTOR and PROPRIOCEPTION dysfunctions. The DOPAMINE depletion that characterizes Parkinson's disease causes distortion in the movement signals from the brain to muscles that results in BRADYKINESIA and incomplete motions. As well, the body's sense of orientation and placement becomes distorted as sensory signals from the muscles to the BRAIN also encounter disruption. Foot drag raises the risk of injury because it increases the likelihood of stumbling and falling. The person with Parkinson's can help overcome mild to moderate foot drag by consciously concentrating on lifting each foot completely from the surface with every step. This effort also improves shuffling, another gait disturbance common in Parkinson's.

Freezing of Gait

Freezing when walking or attempting to walk, in which the person with Parkinson's temporarily cannot move, is one of the most frustrating and common gait disturbances of Parkinson's disease. Freezing of gait (FOG) is sometimes called "magnetic feet" as the person with Parkinson's feels that his or her feet are stuck in place. Other terms for FOG include gait hesitation and stop hesitation. It is most likely to occur when there is a change in the walking surface, such as going from a carpeted room to a tiled floor or approaching stairs, and at the point of the change, such as a threshold. This tendency suggests that there is a visual component of FOG.

Although FOG occurs because of the disruption of nerve signals from the BASAL GANGLIA and other structures in the brain that direct movement, scientists do not fully understand the mechanisms of how it takes place. FOG likely represents dysfunctions of the motor–sensory feedback loop, in which signals back to the brain from the muscles are distorted as well. Some people with Parkinson's experience FOG during off-state episodes, and others experience FOG regardless of their medication cycles. Anxiety about walking can increase the frequency of freezing episodes. The duration of a freeze varies from a few seconds to as long as several minutes.

People with Parkinson's deal with FOG in various ways, from waiting it out to concentrating on the intended movement to thinking about something entirely different. One of the most effective techniques for many people is to anticipate points at which FOG is likely, such as surface transitions, and approach them as though they are tangible

obstacles that must be stepped over. Consciously raising the foot in a high step and "reaching" it over the imagined obstacle then seem to circumvent the freeze. Marching or thinking about dancing to a rhythmic beat are also techniques to break out of a freezing episode. Changes in the environment, including removing carpet or rugs in favor of tile or hardwood floors, and removing clutter around the home to make rooms seem more open are often effective in reducing freezing as well.

Retropulsion/Pulsion

Retropulsion is the tendency to step back; pulsion (sometimes called antepulsion) is the tendency to step forward when bumped or bumping into an object. A person with normal gait may take a step or two; a person with Parkinson's takes an uncontrolled number of steps. This is a function of impairments to balance and motor skills (muscle control). Retropulsion or pulsion can also occur at points of transition during movement, such as initiating walking, changing direction, and stopping. Retropulsion and pulsion events often end with falls as the person loses control of movement. Walking aids reduce the risk for these gait disturbances.

Shuffling Gait

Walking stooped forward with short, shuffling steps is perhaps the most distinctive gait disturbance of Parkinson's. In this gait, the person's feet barely clear the surface when walking, or one or both feet may drag. Heel and toe typically overlap, sometimes to the extent that the feet barely clear each other and forward progress is very slow. There is minimal to no arm swing. This shuffling gait is a combination of postural instability, rigidity (increased muscle tone), and impaired movement. In the early and mid stages of Parkinson's disease, anti-Parkinson's medications typically eliminate this gait disturbance and the person appears to walk almost normally. The difference can be striking, and apparent within 20 to 30 minutes of a levodopa dose.

Start-and-Stop Hesitation

Start-and-stop hesitations are manifestations of freezing of gait that occur at the beginning or end of walking. In start hesitation, the person with Parkinson's is in position to walk but cannot initiate movement. Stop hesitation occurs when the person is walking and suddenly stops, or freezes. Start hesitation is common during change of direction when walking, if the person stops before turning. The same approaches for overcoming FOG are often effective for start and stop hesitation. Most important is patience, both to the person with Parkinson's and to others.

Techniques for Accommodating or Overcoming Gait Disturbances

Even though walking appears to be a conscious act and concentration can overcome some of the challenges people with Parkinson's face, the gait disturbances that characterize Parkinson's disease are involuntary. Physical therapy and occupational therapy can teach methods for overcoming or compensating for gait disturbances. Remaining as physically active as possible helps to maintain independent mobility for as long as possible.

People with Parkinson's who have pronounced gait disturbances often are uncomfortable in public, afraid that they may fall and worried that others will not understand that their mobility problems are beyond their ability to control. People with Parkinson's-related gait disturbances who can view their situations with HUMOR find it easier to deal with the challenges. Maintaining a POSITIVE OUTLOOK allows the person with Parkinson's to explore creative, even if unusual, solutions to common but frustrating gait problems such as start hesitation and freezing. Some people scold or cajole their feet, for example, as though they are recalcitrant children, or sing or recite favorite poems during FOG episodes. This method helps to relieve anxiety for the person with Parkinson's as well as for others present. As the person with Parkinson's knows all too well, directing frustration at the situation only prolongs and intensifies it.

When gait disturbances occur in early or mid-stage Parkinson's, adjusting the ANTI-PARKINSON'S MEDICATIONS regimen often corrects them. This may mean changing doses or dosage times or trying different drugs or different combinations. In later stages of the disease when anti-Parkinson's medications are losing their effectiveness, such

adjustments are less likely to often do help. For some people, especially those with EARLY-ONSET PARKINSON'S who are younger and have few or no other health disorders, surgery such as DEEP BRAIN STIMULATION (DBS) or PALLIDOTOMY becomes a viable option and can improve not only gait but other motor Parkinson's symptoms such as TREMORS. Because motor system deterioration continues as the Parkinson's progresses, however, these approaches do not produce permanent relief.

See also BODY SCHEME; COGWHEELING; EMBARRASSMENT; HOPE FOR A PARKINSON'S CURE; LEAD PIPE RESISTANCE; MOVEMENT DISORDER.

galantamine An acetylcholinesterase inhibitor medication taken to improve COGNITIVE FUNCTION. At present, this drug has U.S. Food and Drug Administration (FDA) approval in the United States for treating DEMENTIA of ALZHEIMER'S DISEASE and is in clinical trials to explore its effectiveness for treating vascular (multiinfarct) dementias. Galantamine and other acetylcholinesterase inhibitors appear to improve memory and cognition in some people who have dementia of Parkinson's disease as well according to a number of published case reports. Not all people with dementia who take these drugs, whether the dementia's origin is Alzheimer's or Parkinson's, experience cognitive improvement. Researchers do not know why some people respond and others do not.

As do other drugs in this classification, galantamine works by preventing the action of ACETYLCHOLINESTERASE, an enzyme in the BRAIN that metabolizes ACETYLCHOLINE. This NEUROTRANSMITTER plays a key role in cognitive functions and becomes depleted in people who have Alzheimer's disease. Such a depletion does not affect people with Parkinson's disease unless they also have Alzheimer's, as is the case for about one in four. The depletion of DOPAMINE, the neurotransmitter of functions in the BASAL GANGLIA and other parts of the brain related to movement, does affect the balance between dopamine and acetylcholine; some researchers believe that their imbalance contributes to Parkinson's dementia and perhaps explains why acetylcholinesterase inhibitors can be effective. Other researchers believe the connections between Alzheimer's disease and Parkinson's disease are more intricate and complex than scientists presently understand and that these drugs are effective for people who have either condition because of these connections.

There is some evidence that galantamine also activates nicotinic receptors in the brain, which are selected ACETYLCHOLINE receptors in certain parts of the brain that also are receptive to NICOTINE. When nicotine binds with these receptors, it produces an intensified effect that enhances memory and other cognitive functions. Although galantamine does not contain nicotine, it appears capable of binding with nicotinic receptors in the same way. This mimics the action of NICOTINE, a stimulant chemical that exists in small amounts in a number of foods and in much larger amounts in tobacco.

Galantamine derives from a substance first extracted from the bulbs of certain daffodils and lilies and in the United States is sold as a prescription drug under the brand name Reminyl. Side effects that can arise from taking galantamine include DIZZINESS, nausea, vomiting, and, in some people, weight loss (believed to be a function of galantamine's activation of nicotinic receptors).

See also DONEPEZIL; OPEN-LABEL DRUG; RIVASTIGMINE; TACRINE.

gamma-aminobutyric acid (GABA) An AMINO ACID that functions as an inhibitory NEUROTRANSMITTER in the BRAIN. GABA reduces the sensitivity of muscle cells to nerve stimulation, decreasing muscle movement. It appears that the amount of GABA present in the brain decreases in Parkinson's disease, particularly in the subthalamic nucleus (STN), possibly contributing to symptoms such as TREMORS, RESTLESS LEG SYNDROME, and LEVODOPA-induced DYSKINESIA and DYSTONIA. The drug BACLOFEN (common brand name Lioresal), a GABA AGONIST taken to relieve these symptoms, binds with GABA receptors and mimics the action of GABA. However, there is also some evidence that GABA functions to an extent as a DOPAMINE ANTAGONIST, blocking the effect of this neurotrans-

mitter, which is already depleted in Parkinson's. The result would be worsening of symptoms such as BRADYKINESIA. Research continues to explore the role of GABA and other amino acids in MOVEMENT DISORDERS.

See also GENE THERAPY.

ganglion A cluster of NEURONS and related structures, often with specialized functions. The BASAL GANGLIA, located in the BRAIN, are a number of such clusters that each have functions, some overlapping and some distinct, related to movement. Most ganglia are outside the brain and are named for their locations or functions. For example, a dorsal root ganglion is the base of a nerve in the spinal cord, and an autonomic ganglion is a nerve cluster that is part of the autonomic NERVOUS SYSTEM.

gastric motility Movement of the gastrointestinal system. Parkinson's disease affects the action of smooth (involuntary) muscle tissue such as that of the digestive system. Many people with moderate to advanced Parkinson's have DYSPHAGIA (difficulty in swallowing) and chronic CONSTIPATION, which reflect the slowed activity of the muscles responsible for moving food down the esophagus and through the intestines and colon. Researchers believe this occurs in part as a result of the imbalance between DOPAMINE and ACETYLCHOLINE, two NEUROTRANSMITTERS integral to movement. It also is likely that the overall reduction in movement further slows the gastrointestinal tract; walking and physical activity are traditionally recommended for gastrointestinal problems such as constipation. As Parkinson's erodes the ability to walk, physical activity becomes challenging if not impossible.

As well, many of the ANTI-PARKINSON'S MEDICATIONS taken to treat the disease's motor symptoms adversely affect the gastrointestinal tract, causing many of the same problems and compounding their effects. As dopamine depletion in the brain progresses in advancing Parkinson's disease, the imbalance between dopamine and acetylcholine deepens. Although there is no increase in the amount of acetylcholine, its actions intensify because there is less dopamine to counteract them. A key therapeutic line of attack in Parkinson's disease employs the ANTICHOLINERGIC MEDICATIONS, taken to reduce the action of acetylcholine in the brain. However, they also reduce acetylcholine levels peripherally (elsewhere in the body). This effect slows muscle response and activity throughout the body, helping to reduce TREMORS and rigidity. Although the slowing is an intended therapeutic effect from the standpoint of the motor symptoms of Parkinson's, it also has unintended and undesired effects on other muscle action.

See also CISAPRIDE.

gene   The basic unit of heredity. Genes can act alone or in combinations with other genes to determine the multitude of characteristics that determine an individual's physical characteristics, from eye and hair color to the presence of or predisposition for certain diseases. Each individual gene, among the tens of thousands of them in the human body, carries just a small fragment of a hereditary message. Genes align in specific sequences on chromosomes, forming the cellular structures that determine the ways genetic information is manifested. The alignment follows the same sequence for each repetition of the same chromosome throughout the body. The consistency of the repetition contributes to a particular trait's presentation.

At present, scientists believe that it is a combination of GENETIC PREDISPOSITION and ENVIRONMENTAL TRIGGERS that converges to allow Parkinson's disease to develop. Although researchers have discovered a number of GENE MUTATIONS in some people with Parkinson's, the extent to which genes influence the development of Parkinson's remains unknown. About 15 percent of people with Parkinson's also have a close relative, such as a parent or sibling, who also has Parkinson's. A few limited studies of identical twins in which one twin has Parkinson's disease indicate that the other twin does not seem to have any greater tendency to development of the disease than the general population when the twins are older than age 50 but is more likely also to

have Parkinson's when the twins are younger than age 50. Most scientists believe that rather than a single causative factor or event, a convergence of genetic and environmental factors allows Parkinson's disease to develop, although genetic factors may be the key factor in many young onset cases.

Although a couple of genetic mutations have been associated with Parkinson's disease, no defect seems to reliably cause the disease: many people with the suspect genes never develop Parkinson's. Genetic testing is generally available only in research settings, is expensive, and in people with Parkinson's disease does not provide conclusive evidence of the disease's presence or absence. As yet, genetic testing does not yield information that makes the course of treatment any different, nor provide information that is of much value for reproductive counseling.

See also APOPTOSIS; AUTOSOMAL DOMINANT INHERITANCE; AUTOSOMAL RECESSIVE INHERITANCE; BIOETHICS; CHROMOSOMES LINKED TO PARKINSON'S DISEASE; GENE THERAPY; HOPE FOR A PARKINSON'S CURE; HUMAN GENOME PROJECT; PARKINSON'S DISEASE, CAUSES OF.

gene mapping   The process of identifying the location of specific GENES on their chromosomes or deoxyribonucleic (DNA) molecules. Gene mapping uses complex scientific procedures and follows precise methodologies. Gene mapping can be specific for certain traits or diseases, such as ALZHEIMER'S DISEASE or Parkinson's disease. It can also be broad-based and general, as in the HUMAN GENOME PROJECT to identify and locate all the genes in the human body. Gene mapping is essential for understanding the genetic, or hereditary, connections of various diseases and perhaps eventual gene therapies to correct genetic mutations.

See also CHROMOSOMES LINKED TO PARKINSON'S DISEASE.

gene mutation   A change that takes place within the structure of a GENE, altering its hereditary message. A mutation may be neutral, beneficial, or harmful and may be transmitted (passed on within families) or acquired (the consequence of damage such as caused by radiation or exposure to toxins).

Genetic mutations can establish the foundation for specific diseases and conditions or can have broad health implications.

A number of gene mutations have been implicated in Parkinson's disease. Mutations of the ALPHA-SYNUCLEIN GENE and the PARKIN GENE, for example, affect aspects of protein function in the BRAIN. This effect appears to contribute to the development of LEWY BODIES, which are abnormal accumulations of proteins in the brain that are characteristic of Parkinson's disease (detectable only at autopsy). Other genes may play roles in different ways as well. Scientists believe the gene mutations set the stage for development of Parkinson's disease, and then certain environmental events (circumstances that occur within or outside the body) trigger the course of disease. Although researchers know certain gene mutations exist in some people with Parkinson's disease, they do not know the extent to which these same mutations exist in people who do not have Parkinson's disease.

See also CHROMOSOMES LINKED TO PARKINSON'S DISEASE; COMPLEX I; ENVIRONMENTAL TOXINS; ENVIRONMENTAL TRIGGERS; PARKINSON'S DISEASE, CAUSES OF.

gene therapy Treatment that manipulates or alters genetic material within the deoxyribonucleic acid (DNA) structure of cells. At present, gene therapy for Parkinson's holds great promise but is experimental. Current research is exploring ways to use gene therapy to stimulate natural production of DOPAMINE and other brain chemicals involved in movement such as GAMMA-AMINOBUTYRIC ACID (GABA) and glial derived neurotrophic factor (GDNF).

One promising method of delivering altered genetic code to cell DNA involves using as a carrier a virus manipulated to be harmless (called an adeno-associated virus [AAV]). The virus "infects" the targeted cells, delivering the altered genetic material, which then replicates when the cells do. This is the same manner in which a viral "infection" spreads, but by manipulating the virus's contents scientists create a beneficial rather than harmful payload. In this way, researchers hope,

the new cells will eventually take over and will function normally, restoring NEUROTRANSMITTER production and balance.

The first phase I clinical trials testing gene therapy in people with Parkinson's began in the United States in October 2002. It is likely to be several years before researchers know whether the technique produces long-term or even permanent changes. Other gene therapy approaches are likely to target altering mutated genes such as the ALPHA-SYNUCLEIN GENE that are linked to Parkinson's development, hoping to head off the disease before it gets started. Because gene therapy is in its infancy, scientists do not yet understand what risks, both short- and long-term, it poses for people.

See also CLINICAL RESEARCH STUDIES; HOPE FOR A PARKINSON'S CURE; INVESTIGATIONAL TREATMENTS.

genetic predisposition A hereditary tendency toward a condition. Many modern health problems appear to have hereditary components, from certain forms of cancer and heart disease to ALZHEIMER'S DISEASE and Parkinson's disease. Generally a number of other factors, such as NUTRITION or exposure to ENVIRONMENTAL TRIGGERS, must converge to allow a genetically predisposed condition or disease to develop.

A genetic predisposition for a health condition does not make development of the condition inevitable. Having a genetic predisposition differs from having a genetic defect, in which the condition will occur regardless of other factors. A defective, or mutated, gene causes the NEURODEGENERATIVE condition HUNTINGTON'S DISEASE, for example, and every person who has the mutated gene is certain to develop the disease by middle age. Having mutated genes that are linked to conditions such as Parkinson's and Alzheimer's, however, does not alone determine whether the disease will manifest itself.

See also CHROMOSOMES LINKED TO PARKINSON'S DISEASE; COMPLEX I; ENVIRONMENTAL TOXINS; ENVIRONMENTAL TRIGGERS; PARKINSON'S DISEASE, CAUSES OF.

ginger as a treatment for nausea Ginger root is a natural alternative for calming feelings of NAUSEA and queasiness related to ANTI-PARKINSON'S MEDICATIONS. It can be eaten fresh or in crystallized form as prepared for use in cooking. Fresh ginger root can be boiled into a tea, and ground ginger can be dissolved in water. Health food stores also sell ground ginger in capsule form, which may be difficult to swallow for the person with Parkinson's disease. It takes 20 to 30 minutes to feel the effect. Ginger has no side effects and can be taken with any medication, making it a safe alternative to conventional antinausea medications. Not everyone gains relief from ginger, however, or can tolerate the taste. Many grocery stores carry fresh ginger root in the produce department, and nearly all carry ground or crystallized ginger in the seasoning section of the store. Ginger also helps to reduce intestinal gas (flatulence).

See also MEDICATION MANAGEMENT; MEDICATION SIDE EFFECTS.

glaucoma, treatment with Parkinson's   Glaucoma is a condition in which the pressure within the eye increases, threatening vision. Glaucoma can be acute, coming on suddenly and often without any symptoms, or chronic, developing slowly over time with gradual loss of vision. The risk for glaucoma rises with age and is most prevalent among those also at greatest risk for Parkinson's because of their age. A family history of glaucoma further increases the risk. A number of ANTI-PARKINSON'S MEDICATIONS can further increase intraocular pressure. Most notable for this are LEVODOPA, taken to relieve BRADYKINESIA, and ANTICHOLINERGIC MEDICATIONS such as BENZTROPINE and biperiden, taken to relieve TREMORS. Anticholinergics can cause acute (sudden-onset) glaucoma, particularly in people with a family history of narrow angle glaucoma (in which an excess of aqueous humor does not drain properly from the inner eye). People who already have narrow angle glaucoma should not take anticholinergic medications or LEVODOPA. People who have open, or wide, angle glaucoma (roughly 90 percent of people with glaucoma) can take anti-Parkinson's medications as long as the glaucoma is well controlled and frequently monitored. People with narrow angle glaucoma are usually told so by the eye doctor due to their needing to be instructed as to medications they should avoid. A diagnosis of simply "glaucoma" can be assumed to be open-angle glaucoma, but one's optometrist or ophthalmologist should be consulted prior to taking anticholinergics or levodopa if there is any question as to the diagnosis.

See also BLEPHAROSPASM; COLOR PERCEPTION; EYE MOVEMENTS; VISION PROBLEMS.

glial derived neurotrophic factor (GDNF)   See NEUROTROPHIC FACTORS.

globus pallidus   See PALLIDUM.

glutamate   An AMINO ACID in the BRAIN that functions as an excitatory NEUROTRANSMITTER. Glutamate stimulates the general activity of neurons within the brain that contain glutamate receptors (molecular structures that can bind with, or receive, glutamate). In a healthy brain, the action of DOPAMINE holds glutamate binding in check. As dopamine quantities diminish with the progressive loss of DOPAMINERGIC NEURONS, glutamate binding increases. Scientists believe this process accelerates cell death and the progression of Parkinson's disease. Drugs called GLUTAMATE ANTAGONISTS inhibit, or block, the action of glutamate and are being investigated for a number of neurologic conditions.

See also APOPTOSIS; PARKINSON'S DISEASE, CAUSES OF.

glutamate antagonist   A drug that blocks the action of GLUTAMATE, an AMINO ACID in the BRAIN that functions as a NEUROTRANSMITTER that stimulates general activity in brain NEURONS, possibly hastening their death and contributing to the progression of Parkinson's disease. Extending a NEURO-PROTECTIVE EFFECT, glutamate antagonists prevent glutamate from binding with glutamate receptors in various neurons. This action also helps to relieve some of the motor symptoms of Parkinson's. The NMDA type of glutamate receptor has attracted the most attention, and clinically available glutamate antagonists block the NMDA type of glutamate receptor.

Glutamate antagonists generally are more effective when taken as one of the ADJUNCT THER-

APIES to LEVODOPA treatment. The exception is AMANTADINE, an antagonist of glutamate taken early in the course of Parkinson's, which often is effective at controlling TREMORS, BRADYKINESIA, and other motor symptoms of Parkinson's for about a year and sometimes as long as three years, delaying the need to begin levodopa. Amantadine also is effective in mid to later stages of Parkinson's as an adjunct therapy to either levodopa or dopamine agonists. Riluzole, a glutamate antagonist that has some evidence that it may prolong survival in amyotrophic lateral sclerosis, is currently being investigated for possible neuroprotective effects in people with Parkinson's. The other glutamate antagonist currently used to treat the symptoms of Parkinson's disease is REMACEMIDE, a drug that first came into use as an ANTISEIZURE MEDICATION.

See also ALPHA-ADENOSINE RECEPTOR; COENZYME Q-10; NEUROPROTECTIVE THERAPIES.

glutamic acid decarboxylase (GAD) An ENZYME produced in the BRAIN that synthesizes GAMMA-AMINOBUTYRIC ACID (GABA), an AMINO ACID that functions as a NEUROTRANSMITTER in the brain to reduce the sensitivity of muscle cells to nerve stimulation. GABA level decreases with DOPAMINE DEPLETION, which researchers believe contributes to the TREMORS and BRADYKINESIA characteristic of Parkinson's disease. Increasing the brain's production of GAD consequently increases the action of GABA, helping to reduce motor symptoms and normalize movement. Researchers are experimenting with injecting the GAD gene, transported via an engineered virus structure, directly into the SUBTHALAMIC NUCLEUS (STN). The STN is a component of the BASAL GANGLIA that produces much of the brain's GABA. GAD gene injection appears to "turn on" the STN's production of GABA. The U.S. Food and Drug Administration (FDA) approved the first PHASE I CLINICAL RESEARCH STUDIES involving a small group of human volunteers, all younger than age 65 with advanced Parkinson's disease that no longer responds to other treatments, in late 2002.

See also GENE THERAPY; INVESTIGATIONAL TREATMENTS.

glutathione An ANTIOXIDANT that clears the by-products of DOPAMINE metabolism from the BRAIN. The action of glutathione becomes impaired in Parkinson's disease as well as in other NEURODEGENERATIVE conditions such as ALZHEIMER'S DISEASE and AMYOTROPHIC LATERAL SCLEROSIS (ALS), allowing these by-products to accumulate in the brain as FREE RADICALS that can do further cell damage. There also seem to be correlations between exposure to pesticides and certain metals such as mercury and lowered glutathione levels. Some doctors believe nutritional supplements that contain antioxidants such as cysteine can help boost glutathione levels in the brain. Small research studies in which people with DE NOVO PARKINSON'S DISEASE received intravenous injections of glutathione showed promising improvement in motor symptoms, but the findings were inconclusive. Hence most experts feel that it is premature to offer intravenous glutathione as a therapy until more convincing evidence appears. Orally ingested glutathione pills do not appear to have any effect on the brain levels of glutathione. The glutathione nasal spray does seem to get across the blood-brain barrier, but there are no studies regarding its usefulness in people with Parkinson's.

See also MONOAMINE OXIDASE; NEUROPROTECTIVE EFFECT; NEUROPROTECTIVE THERAPIES.

going public The decision to inform others of a diagnosis of Parkinson's disease. Most people do not care to have the details of their health conditions made public regardless of what those conditions are, yet Parkinson's puts those who have it in an uncomfortable position in which it is fairly obvious, particularly in middle and later stages of the disease, that something is wrong. Many people, especially those who have EARLY-ONSET PARKINSON'S or are still employed at the time of diagnosis, choose to share their diagnosis only with close friends and family members until the progression of symptoms makes it impossible to suppress the truth longer. Some people choose to alter their lifestyles to avoid situations in which others can observe their symptoms, opting to forgo social events and activities at which surfacing symptoms would be apparent to others present. This is a deeply personal decision for each individual.

In jobs and career fields that require fine motor skills and other abilities that degenerate as Parkinson's progresses, a Parkinson's diagnosis has far-reaching consequences. In others, it is both possible and practical to make workplace accommodations that allow the person to continue performing job tasks. The person with Parkinson's may choose to inform a boss or supervisor of the diagnosis and to keep the information private from other employees. DRIVING is often an early issue; the point at which driving is no longer safe varies from individual to individual. As driving is such a common dimension of life nearly everywhere in the United States, giving it up nearly always requires the person to go public about the reason.

For many people, the decision finally to go public about their Parkinson's is a great relief. It is difficult enough to cope with the challenges of the disease; trying to keep those challenges hidden can become overwhelmingly stressful. Family members, friends, and coworkers often are supportive and encouraging despite the person's worries about their response. Odds are, most of them have suspected that there was a problem and are relieved to know what the problem really is. Sometimes, too, letting others in on the situation opens doors to helpful information and suggestions.

In recent years a number of public figures have acknowledged that they have Parkinson's disease, among them former heavyweight boxing champion MUHAMMAD ALI, actor turned activist MICHAEL J. FOX, former U.S. attorney general JANET RENO, and the singer MAURICE WHITE. They have increased public awareness and understanding of Parkinson's disease in general, making it easier for other people with Parkinson's also to go public.

See ADJUSTING TO LIVING WITH PARKINSON'S; AMERICANS WITH DISABILITIES ACT; COPING WITH A DIAGNOSIS OF PARKINSON'S; DENIAL AND ACCEPTANCE; WORKPLACE ADAPTATIONS TO ACCOMMODATE PARKINSON'S; WORKPLACE RELATIONSHIPS.

goniometer A device that can measure the RANGE OF MOTION of a joint, sometimes called an arthrometer. This measurement is useful in assessing neuromuscular status for planning PHYSICAL THERAPY, OCCUPATIONAL THERAPY, and REHABILITATION THERAPY interventions to improve POSTURAL INSTABILITY and MOBILITY. Such interventions can help the person with Parkinson's to remain as physically active and independent as possible.

See also ELECTROMYOGRAPHY; ELECTROPHYSIOLOGIC STUDIES.

gray matter See BRAIN.

grief A profound feeling of loss and sadness. In many respects, Parkinson's disease is a progression of losses: physical, emotional, and lifestyle losses for the person with Parkinson's as well for caregivers, family members, and other loved ones. It is natural to mourn these losses, to wish that they had not happened or were not happening, and to feel frustration and anger about them. For many people with Parkinson's and those who are close to them, it often seems that no sooner do they adapt to one set of challenging circumstances than another arises to take its place. The ups and downs of the disease's course and symptoms make it difficult to adjust and sometimes to know how to feel. Unlike in other situations of loss, such as the death of a loved one, the losses of Parkinson's seem to cascade endlessly.

Although Parkinson's disease is itself seldom fatal, it changes forever the lives of those who have it as well as the lives of loved ones. It is important to acknowledge grief and to accept that it is valid and appropriate to feel sadness and loss with Parkinson's disease. In doing so, it becomes possible to begin shifting focus from loss to appreciating and enjoying the present, and even, as difficult as it is, looking forward to the future. There is life beyond Parkinson's, even though it often seems that all of life revolves around the disease and its demands and uncertainties. Sharing feelings with others, such as through SUPPORT GROUPS, helps to put fears and worries in context. For many people, part of the loss they are grieving is the communication, partnership, and INTIMACY they had before Parkinson's. Finding other people to talk to does not compensate for this loss, of course, and does not make the grief end, but it can make dealing with it easier.

See also CAREGIVER WELL-BEING; DENIAL AND ACCEPTANCE; DEPRESSION; EMOTIONS; JOY; MARRIAGE RELATIONSHIP; PARENT/CHILD RELATIONSHIPS; PSYCHOTHERAPY; QUALITY OF LIFE; STRESS.

Guam Amyotrophic Lateral Sclerosis-Parkinsonism Dementia Complex (Guam ALS-PDC) A NEURODEGENERATIVE disease, also known as Lytico-Bodig, that affects about one percent of native residents of Guam (the indigenous Chamorro population), typically manifested in late midlife. In Guam ALS-PDC the person has parkinsonism, Alzheimer's dementia, and AMYOTROPHIC LATERAL SCLEROSIS (Lou Gehrig's disease) concurrently and typically eventually shows symptoms of all three, although one or two may be more prominent at onset or throughout the course of the disease. Scientists do not know why this complex of disease occurs in this particular population but believe that because it seems to occur *only* in this population there are strong genetic (hereditary) factors, though there have been strong arguments that an environmental agent may be the culprit.

In its early stages Guam ALS-PDC is sometimes misdiagnosed as one of its component diseases, although the true nature of the condition becomes obvious within a few years as the degeneration progresses rapidly. Damage to the BRAIN often also includes the tangles and plaques of ALZHEIMER'S DISEASE, giving rise to the belief that this disease involves extensive and complex deterioration affecting nearly all of the brain. Treatment attempts to manage the symptoms but is not very effective. Plaques, tangles, and protein deposits characteristic of Parkinson's, Alzheimer's, and ALS are widespread throughout the brain at autopsy.

See also CONDITIONS SIMILAR TO PARKINSON'S; GENE MUTATIONS; GENETIC PREDISPOSITION; PROGRESSIVE SUPRANUCLEAR PALSY.

Hallervorden–Spatz syndrome The most common, though now discouraged name for a rare, usually inherited MOVEMENT DISORDER caused by an abnormal accumulation of iron in the BASAL GANGLIA and other parts of the brain that control movement, which destroys the cells. The syndrome is named after the two German researchers who first identified it in 1922 but the well-documented unethical actions of Dr. Hallervorden, and perhaps Dr. Spatz as well, during the Nazi era have led to popular efforts to rename the disorder. In medical circles today, it is more properly called neurodegeneration with brain iron accumulation type 1 (NBIA-1) or neuroaxonal dystrophy. Recent genetic discoveries have led many in the direction of considering this to be a syndrome (cluster of diseases with a nearly identical clinical picture) that can be split into more specific diseases, based upon the genetic defect. About 50 percent of patients with this syndrome have PKAN (pantothenate kinase associated neurodegeneration), caused by a defect of the gene PANK2, which causes a deficiency of the enzyme pantothenate kinase. NBIA-1 is considered a PARKINSONISM: That is, it affects the same parts of the brain in the same ways and its symptoms mimic those of Parkinson's disease. Occasionally NBIA-1 occurs sporadically (as a random genetic defect that is not familial), though the usual form is AUTOSOMAL RECESSIVE and can easily appear sporadic unless there are affected siblings: only one in four offspring of unaffected parents who both carry the defect will have the disease. There also are components of NBIA-1 that are similar to ALZHEIMER'S DISEASE.

The Pathology of NBIA-1

Symptoms typically begin in childhood or early adolescence and progressively worsen over a period of about 10 years. They include BRADYKINE-SIA (slowed movement), TREMORS (involuntary, repetitive movements), CHOREOATHETOSIS (rhythmic, writing movements), DYSTONIA (abnormal fixed postures), SPASTICITY (abnormal tightening of the muscles), RIGIDITY (continuous resistance of the muscles to relaxing), and GAIT DISTURBANCES (changes in the movements related to walking). COGNITIVE DYSFUNCTION and DEMENTIA rapidly follow as these neuromuscular symptoms progress. Unlike Parkinson's, NBIA-1 is fatal. ANTI-PARKINSON'S MEDICATIONS, including LEVODOPA, and drugs taken to treat HUNTINGTON'S DISEASE, another hereditary movement disorder, can provide symptom relief early in the course of the disease but are not very effective by mid and later stages.

Why NBIA-1 Interests Researchers in Parkinson's Disease

NBIA-1 contains pathological components (symptoms and progression of the disease process) that are very similar to those of both Parkinson's and Alzheimer's, bolstering the belief that there is a connection between Parkinson's and Alzheimer's and possibly with other neurodegenerative conditions. The loss of DOPAMINERGIC NEURONS and other cellular structures (such as glial cells and myelinated fiber clusters) in NBIA-1 is so severe and so rapid that FUNCTIONAL IMAGING STUDIES such as MAGNETIC RESONANCE IMAGING (MRI) show that rather than shrinking, as occurs with Parkinson's, the SUBSTANTIA NIGRA and the STRIATUM appear filled with holes. There are also pervasive LEWY BODIES with high ALPHA-SYNUCLEIN content throughout the basal ganglia, another hallmark of Parkinson's disease (detectable only at autopsy). Neurofibrillary tangles containing TAU, the hallmark of ALZHEIMER'S DISEASE (also detectable only at autopsy), are present as well, reinforcing the perception many researchers have that there are pathological connections between Alzheimer's and Parkinson's.

In recent years scientists have isolated several GENE MUTATIONS that appear responsible for NBIA-1 and suspect that there are others that act in concert to cause the development of the syndrome. These involve different genes than those isolated for either Alzheimer's disease or Parkinson's disease. Yet many of the mutations isolated among these diseases have in common that they have roles in enzyme–protein functions that are essential for cell activities. Disrupting these functions results in cell dysfunction and death. Figuring out how to correct or overcome the effect of the mutations could take researchers to the cure for these diseases. Because there has not yet been a known case of NBIA-1 in which there were not gene mutations, it appears that environmental factors may play little to no role in this syndrome (as in HUNTINGTON'S DISEASE). As most scientists believe that interactions among genetic and environmental factors cause the development of both Parkinson's and Alzheimer's, this aspect of NBIA-1 is particularly intriguing.

See also ACERULOPLASMINEMIA; ALPHA-SYNUCLEIN GENE; AMYOTROPHIC LATERAL SCLEROSIS; CONDITIONS SIMILAR TO PARKINSON'S; GENE MAPPING; GENE THERAPY; GENETIC PREDISPOSITION; HUMAN GENOME PROJECT; IRON; MULTIPLE SCLEROSIS; PARKIN GENE.

hallucination A sensory perception of an event that is not really occurring. Hallucinations can affect any or all of the five physical senses (sight, hearing, touch, taste, smell). Hallucinations, usually visual, are common in Parkinson's and can be side effects of ANTI-PARKINSON'S MEDICATIONS, particularly DOPAMINERGIC MEDICATIONS such as LEVODOPA and DOPAMINE AGONIST MEDICATIONS such as BROMOCRIPTINE and ROPINIROLE. Hallucinations also can be an indication that the symptoms of Parkinson's are progressing to include COGNITIVE IMPAIRMENT (loss of reasoning and intellectual skills), DELUSIONS (the belief that something is true although it is not), and DEMENTIA.

It is common to consider illusions, hallucinations, and delusions to be the same phenomenon, but they are not. They arise from different causes. An illusion involves a faulty perception of real sensory inputs. A mirage, such as the appearance of a puddle in the distance on a desert highway, is a common example of a visual illusion. Illusions are typically fleeting, but they may be prolonged and may be precursors of hallucinations. Increased illusions seem to be related to the changes in sensory processing (especially vision) that accompany Parkinson's disease and anti-Parkinson's medications.

A hallucination results when the brain creates a perception that something exists when there really is nothing there, such as seeing imaginary people in an empty space or hearing voices in a quiet room. In Parkinson's, sleep deprivation, anti-Parkinson's medications, and the presence of Lewy bodies in the cerebral hemispheres all increase the risk of hallucinations.

A delusion is a disruption of thought processes; the person may believe there is an intruder in the house although he or she sees or hears nothing to support such a belief. In Parkinson's, it appears to have similar risk factors as hallucinations; suggesting a common link of both being due to imbalances in neurotransmitters.

Hallucinations tend to be more distressing for the person who is having them than for others, because the person having them does not know whether what appear to be physical stimuli are real, whereas others do know they are not. People having delusions, on the other hand, do not even question the veracity of their perceptions because they have no awareness that those perceptions may be inaccurate.

Observation can sometimes help to identify whether hallucinations are a side effect of medications or a manifestation of disease processes. Hallucinations related to medications are more likely to occur in some consistent relationship to taking the medication, often at the time of its peak effectiveness. When a medication is the suspected cause of hallucinations, changing to another drug or changing the times the drug is taken can sometimes put an end to this side effect. Hallucinations generally are harmless unless they cause the person to feel undue anxiety or to react to them in ways that put the person or others in harm's way. Hallucinations and delusions are symptoms that most Parkinson's stage scales, such as the UNIFIED PARKINSON'S DIS-EASE RATING SCALE (UPDRS) use to assess the progression and severity of symptoms.

See also MEDICATION MANAGEMENT; MEMORY; MENTAL STATUS; NEUROCHEMISTRY; NEUROPSYCHIATRY.

haloperidol A powerful ANTIPSYCHOTIC MEDICATION, sometimes called a neuroleptic, taken to relieve the symptoms of PSYCHOSIS, SCHIZOPHRENIA, and DEMENTIA. The drug is available in the United States in generic forms as well as the brand name product Haldol. There are very few circumstances in which someone with Parkinson's disease should take haloperidol; the drug is noted for its significant side effects which include DYSTONIA (extreme muscle stiffness and distortion) and DYSKINESIA (involuntary movements). These side effects are so predictable that neurologists often use haloperidol to treat the CHOREIFORM DYSKINESIAS (involuntary, rhythmic, writhing movements) that characterize HUNTINGTON'S DISEASE, another NEURODEGENERATIVE DISORDER.

People in the later stages of ALZHEIMER'S DISEASE may be prescribed haloperidol as a means of mitigating the symptoms of dementia. As the coexistence of Parkinson's disease is fairly common in Alzheimer's disease, this medication can bring out motor symptoms of Parkinson's that have previously gone unrecognized because they were mild relative to the symptoms of Alzheimer's. It can be difficult to distinguish whether the motor symptoms are side effects of the haloperidol or are emerging symptoms of Parkinson's. Even stopping the haloperidol does not always provide a conclusive diagnosis, as it is well known that occasionally the parkinsonism and other motor effects that antipsychotic medications cause are irreversible (permanent). Involuntary movements (usually of the tongue and mouth) caused by antipsychotic medications are often permanent, a condition known as TARDIVE DYSKINESIA.

Haloperidol was one of the first medications available to treat schizophrenia and other serious psychotic illnesses, and it is very effective for this purpose. Other, newer medications are likely to be more effective for treating the agitated behavior often associated with dementia in diseases such as

Parkinson's and Alzheimer's. Atypical antipsychotics, especially quetiapine (Seroquel) and clozapine (Clozaril), are safer choices in people with Parkinson's. Another useful class of medications are the ACETYLCHOLINESTERASE INHIBITORS; among those currently available in the United States are DONEPEZIL (Aricept), GALANTAMINE (Reminyl), RIVASTIGMINE (Exelon), and TACRINE (Cognex). They enhance the actions of ACETYLCHOLINE, a NEUROTRANSMITTER primarily involved in brain activity related to COGNITIVE FUNCTION. Despite acetylcholine also having effect on muscle activity, these medications, with the exception of tacrine, have no significant motor side effects in people with Parkinson's. For this reason, tacrine should be avoided in lieu of the others in people with Parkinson's.

See also COGNITIVE IMPAIRMENT; MEDICATION MANAGEMENT; MEDICATION SIDE EFFECTS; MEMORY; MENTAL STATUS; NEUROCHEMISTRY; NEUROPSYCHIATRY.

Hamilton Depression Rating Scale A series of questions that a health care professional, such as a physician, psychologist, neurologist, or psychiatrist, asks of a person to assess the severity of clinical DEPRESSION. There are 21 questions that address these general areas:

• Mood and feelings such as sadness and guilt
• Thoughts of suicide
• Insomnia
• Work and everyday activities
• Anxiety and agitation
• Physical symptoms such as tiredness and discomforts
• Psychiatric disturbances such as paranoia and obsessive/compulsive behavior

A person's score helps the clinician to determine the most appropriate methods of treatment and to assess the effectiveness of treatment over time. The Hamilton Depression Rating Scale has been in use since 1967 and remains a standard assessment tool for evaluating depression. Because a portion of the Hamilton Depression Rating Scale deals with physical symptoms that Parkinson's disease often masks, it should be just one facet of diagnosis and treatment for depression in people who have Parkinson's disease.

See also ANTIDEPRESSANT MEDICATIONS; BECK DEPRESSION INVENTORY; EMOTIONS; MEDICATION SIDE EFFECTS; MENTAL STATUS; PSYCHOTHERAPY.

hand-to-eye coordination   The ability to adjust motor movements in response to visual information. People with Parkinson's often have trouble with hand-to-eye coordination. Motor symptoms such as TREMORS, BRADYKINESIA, and deterioration of fine motor skills contribute significantly, and visual disturbances further compound the difficulties. BLEPHAROSPASM (muscle spasm of the eyelids) and RIGIDITY affecting the muscles that control eye movements interfere with focus and with synchronized eye movement, both of which are essential for depth perception. Poor hand-to-eye coordination affects many everyday functions and interferes with activities from preparing and eating foods to getting dressed. A physical therapist or an occupational therapist can develop exercises to help maintain eye-to-hand coordination. Activities such as playing cards and board games are also effective and can be more enjoyable than performing exercises.

See also COORDINATION; DEXTERITY, PHYSICAL; VISION PROBLEMS.

handwriting   See MICROGRAPHIA.

hearing loss   Damage, through injury or degeneration, that affects the structures of the ear or the nerve conduction pathways between the ear and the BRAIN and results in the inability to interpret auditory signals. There is no association between hearing loss and Parkinson's disease except that they are both more common with age. Age-related degeneration is the most common cause of hearing loss; a third of adults older than the age of 65 have some degree of hearing impairment. Regular screening that measures the ear's ability to transmit sound is the most effective way to detect hearing loss, as most people are adept at compensating for hearing impairment until it becomes severe. The person with hearing loss might not be aware that he or she does not hear properly.

Hearing loss interferes with communication, causing misunderstandings and confusion. This loss becomes particularly challenging for the person with Parkinson's, as many of the symptoms make the person not to be responding or paying attention. These are also common characteristics of hearing loss. Anyone older than age 65 who has Parkinson's should have his or her hearing tested. Hearing aids can provide partial to complete restoration of hearing ability for many people with hearing loss. Other people can learn alternate methods of communication. It is helpful for caregivers to know that there is a hearing impairment, so they can use approaches such as writing instructions for the person or making certain to confirm that the person understands what is being communicated. Hearing impairments are commonly related to AGING or other factors such as noise exposure.

heart disease and Parkinson's   Heart disease and Parkinson's disease often coexist in older people who have Parkinson's, as both are more likely to develop later in life. Heart disease covers a broad spectrum of conditions including hypertension (high blood pressure), coronary artery disease, and congestive heart failure. Presence of any other health problems in conjunction with Parkinson's disease complicates treatment for any and all health conditions, as there are numerous potential interactions among medications. Lifestyle factors such as exercise that are beneficial for heart disease are also beneficial for Parkinson's disease, for as long as motor functions permit. The person with Parkinson's disease does not appear to have any greater risk for heart disease than the person who does not have it, although recent research suggests that whatever mechanism is responsible for the death of DOPAMINERGIC NEURONS in the BRAIN as Parkinson's progresses may also affect the heart.

Dopamine and the Heart

Some research suggests that as Parkinson's progresses, the numbers of ADRENERGIC NEURONS in the heart fall. Dopamine is a precursor to epinephrine and NOREPINEPHRINE, neurotransmitters that affect heart activity. The relationships among these events are not yet clear, although scientists believe that Parkinson's disease affects body systems other than the BRAIN. One possible explanation is that the same mechanism that causes the death of dopaminergic neurons in the brain also affects similar neurons throughout the body; dopamine and epinephrine can activate the same receptors. Another possible explanation looks to the dopamine replacement regimen of treatment that is currently the standard approach to relieving the symptoms of Parkinson's, particularly LEVODOPA therapy. Peripheral levodopa—that which enters the bloodstream from a levodopa dose—becomes quickly converted to DOPAMINE. This process can have a number of effects on the cardiovascular system, including an increase in heart rate and blood pressure. The exposure over time to these elevations and fluctuations in peripheral dopamine levels could suppress the actions of the heart's adrenergic neurons, causing their numbers to diminish as they are not needed. Recent research also suggests that levodopa may increase the amount of the amino acid homocysteine, a possible risk factor for heart attack and stroke, but this research is far too preliminary to support routine folic acid supplementation (to lower homocysteine levels) for people on levodopa. Much research remains to be done to unravel these and other mysteries of Parkinson's disease.

Adrenergic Agonists and Antagonists

Some ANTI-PARKINSON'S MEDICATIONS taken to relieve TREMORS act either to stimulate or to suppress adrenergic response. This action can affect blood pressure and heart rate. Many commonly prescribed antihypertensive medications (drugs that lower elevated levels of blood pressure) are adrenergic antagonists, commonly referred to as alpha- or beta-blockers. These medications inhibit or block the actions of epinephrine; decreased activity from epinephrine helps to relax muscle tissue including the smooth muscle tissues of the walls of the arteries and of the heart. Adrenergic antagonists are also taken to treat urinary retention from enlargement of the prostate gland that is common in older men.

Adrenergic agonists have the opposite action, binding with adrenergic receptors to mimic epinephrine. These drugs cause smooth muscle tissues to contract and stiffen, increasing blood pressure. They may be taken to treat heart failure or certain arrhythmias (irregularities in the heartbeat). Doctors may prescribe an adrenergic agonist for a person with Parkinson's disease to treat erectile dysfunction or ORTHOSTATIC HYPOTENSION (blood pressure that drops with changes in position).

Interactions between Heart Medications and Anti-Parkinson's Medications

The possible interactions between anti-Parkinson's medications and medications taken to treat heart conditions are too numerous to cite and vary with the combinations of medications taken. Medications can interfere with the actions of each other by increasing effectiveness, decreasing effectiveness, or negating effectiveness. Whenever there is a change in medications, whether anti-Parkinson's or heart, the prescribing doctor should review all of the medications the person with Parkinson's is taking to make sure that adverse interactions are not likely to result.

See also MEDICATION MANAGEMENT; MEDICATION SIDE EFFECTS.

Heimlich maneuver   An emergency action to relieve choking. Introduced by the physician Henry J. Heimlich, M.D., in 1974, the Heimlich maneuver uses subdiaphragmatic pressure—a quick, upward thrust just below the diaphragm—to dislodge objects that are blocking the trachea (windpipe) or throat. Because choking is a significant risk for people with Parkinson's, especially in the middle to later stages of the disease, all caregivers and family members should learn how to perform the Heimlich maneuver. This is taught in most basic first-aid classes and as part of cardiopulmonary resuscitation (CPR). The basic steps of the Heimlich maneuver are as follows:

- From behind, wrap your arms around the person.
- Hold your fists together just below the person's ribs and give a quick upward thrust (do not squeeze).
- Repeat until the object dislodges.

A person who is choking may cough or gasp or may make no sound at all. The hallmark test for whether a person is truly choking or is, as he or she may attempt to convey, beyond the crisis, is to ask the person to speak. If the person cannot speak, he or she is still choking and needs immediate help. Choking happens most often during eating, usually because the person swallows a piece of food that is too large to go down the throat. For people who have problems SWALLOWING, which occur in Parkinson's disease, even small or liquified foods can become lodged in the throat. Immediate action is imperative. Small food particles and liquids sometimes pass down the trachea and into the lungs, where they can cause infection that leads to pneumonia. Family members and caregivers should keep a close watch on the person for several days after a choking episode to observe early signs of infection such as fever. If there is any concern that food remains lodged in the throat, a doctor should check the person.

See also DYSPHAGIA; EATING; FOOD PREPARATION.

herbal remedies   See ALTERNATIVE THERAPIES.

hereditary   The traits and characteristics of a person that are genetic in origin; they are also called familial or said to "run in the family." Some characteristics that appear to be genetic are instead environmental, the result of shared lifestyle factors among family members, or are activated by ENVIRONMENTAL TRIGGERS. These might range from exposure to CHEMICAL TOXINS to dietary habits. Most scientists believe there are both hereditary, or genetic, and environmental aspects of NEURODEGENERATIVE CONDITIONS such as Parkinson's disease and ALZHEIMER'S DISEASE.

When Parkinson's disease "runs in the family," there are usually several individuals who have it but most family members do not. When there is a family history of Parkinson's disease, researchers say that there is a GENETIC PREDISPOSITION for Parkinson's disease in the family. This contrasts with MOVEMENT DISORDERS such as HUNTINGTON'S DISEASE, in which anyone who has the gene mutation for the disease will develop the disease and

environmental factors are inconsequential to the disease process.

See also AUTOSOMAL DOMINANT INHERITANCE; AUTOSOMAL RECESSIVE INHERITANCE; DIAGNOSING PARKINSON'S; ENVIRONMENTAL TRIGGERS; GENE MAPPING; GENE MUTATIONS; GENE THERAPY; HETEROGENEITY; HUMAN GENOME PROJECT; PARKINSON'S DISEASE, CAUSES OF.

heredity and Parkinson's   See GENETIC PREDISPOSITION.

heterogeneity   Presence of different characteristics, in contrast to homogeneity, in which characteristics are the same in each sample or case. One of the key challenges in identifying the causes of, and designing effective treatments for, Parkinson's disease is its heterogeneous nature: Although there are common symptoms that nearly everyone who has the disease experiences, the combinations and progression of those symptoms make the course of disease uniquely individual. It is not much of an exaggeration to say that no two people with Parkinson's have the same experience of the disease.

Within the context of GENE MUTATIONS, Parkinson's disease is also considered heterogeneous because any of several known mutations may be present. As well, none of these mutations is specific to Parkinson's disease; all can be found, singly or in differing combinations, in other neuromuscular disorders. The ALPHA-SYNUCLEIN GENE mutation is present in LEWY BODY DISEASE, for example. Whether this means there are as yet unknown connections among these disorders or the mutations have broad-based implications is one of the many dimensions that researchers continue to explore. Scientists are fairly certain that other genes that contribute to the development of Parkinson's are not far from being discovered and hope that these discoveries will lead to an understanding of how the various genetic factors shape Parkinson's.

See also AUTOSOMAL DOMINANT INHERITANCE; AUTOSOMAL RECESSIVE INHERITANCE; GENE MAPPING; GENE THERAPY; GENETIC PREDISPOSITION; TREATMENT ALGORITHMS.

high-stepping   See GAIT DISTURBANCE.

Hoehn and Yahr stage scale   One of the assessment tools doctors use to evaluate the progression of symptoms and the extent of disability that results from them for the person with Parkinson's disease. Developed in 1967 by the physicians Margaret Hoehn and Melvin Yahr, this scale primarily assesses MOBILITY and MOTOR FUNCTION. The scale designates five stages of Parkinson's disease.

Stage	Extent of Disease Impairment	Degree of Mobility
HOEHN AND YAHR STAGE SCALE FOR PARKINSON'S DISEASE		
I	Unilateral symptoms	No difficulty walking: normal stride, step, and change of direction
II	Bilateral symptoms	No difficulty walking: normal stride, step, and change of direction
III	Bilateral symptoms with postural instability	Minor difficulty walking: shortened stride, slight foot drag, may freeze, extra step with change of direction
IV	Bilateral symptoms with significantly impaired movement	Moderate difficulty walking: shuffling stride, pronounced foot drag, frequent freezes, several extra steps with change of direction
V	Bilateral symptoms with extremely impaired movement	Great difficulty walking: only with assistance uses walker or wheelchair for mobility

Unlike rating scales for diseases such as cancer, the Hoehn and Yahr stage scale and similar assessment tools do not project the likely progression of symptoms or success of treatment. Parkinson's stage scales only indicate the current level, relative to the full spectrum of the disease, of a person's symptoms. The higher the stage, the more significantly the Parkinson's affects the person's ability to function.

Many people with Parkinson's move back and forth among the stages, particularly in the midcourse of the disease. As well, the person's rating may be stage V during an OFF-STATE (at the end of a medication dose's effectiveness) and stage II during an ON-STATE.

See also ACTIVITIES OF DAILY LIVING; INSTRUMENTAL ACTIVITIES OF DAILY LIVING; PARKINSON'S IMPACT SCALE; STAGING OF PARKINSON'S DISEASE.

home health care   Professional nursing services that provide medical care in the home setting, such as for people recovering from surgery, injury, and illness. A home health nurse may perform dressing changes and wound care, maintenance of intravenous or parenteral lines, medication and blood pressure checks, diabetes checks and care, and similar services. Home health care is for the person who is not quite sick enough to be in the hospital or skilled nursing facility but who needs a fairly high level of medical care and is homebound. Other health care professionals who may provide home health care include physical therapists and occupational therapists. Many MEDICAL INSURANCE plans, including MEDICARE, pay for a certain level of home health care ordered by a doctor, under certain conditions.

Many home health agencies also provide PERSONAL CARE ASSISTANCE, such as help with bathing and eating, as a separate service that is different from home health care. Personal care assistance generally is not covered by medical insurance, although some LONG-TERM CARE INSURANCE plans may include payment for certain services.

See also HOSPICE; HOSPITALIZATION; LONG-TERM CARE FACILITY; SKILLED NURSING FACILITY (SNF).

home safety   The physical home environment is fraught with hazards for the person with Parkinson's disease. As a result of neuromuscular symptoms that limit movement and mobility even common structures such as stairs can present dangerous obstacles. Most people choose a place of residence based on various factors that typically have little relation to ability to maneuver through the house or apartment without full mobility. Many older people live in the home they have occupied for most of their adult years, the home where perhaps they raised their family. They are so accustomed to the "lay of the land" within the home that the floor plan, furnishings, and other elements of the home's environment do not appear hazardous, yet they can create hazards for the person with Parkinson's. A comprehensive home safety inventory can help to identify potential hazards and possible solutions.

Entryways and Doors

The entry to a house or an apartment can present a number of hazards for a person who has mobility problems. Take an objective look at entryways from the outside. There should be a clear and unobstructed path from the driveway, sidewalk, or street to the home's door.

- Foliage such as hedges and shrubs is attractive but can present actual or perceived obstacles. Trim foliage so branches do not hang over sidewalks and stair railings.

- Many houses have double doors, a screen or storm door, and a security door. Do these doors open in the same direction or in opposing directions? Double doors can be difficult for someone with impaired coordination to manage; consider removing the screen or storm door.

- Are there cracks, uneven sections, or breaks in sidewalks or steps? These present tripping hazards for a person with Parkinson's who may shuffle or drag the feet when walking.

- Where the car is parked, is there enough room to open the car door completely to get in and out? Is there a clear path around the car and to the entry?

- Are entryways, driveways, and garages brightly lit at night? Lights that are activated by motion sensors assure that lighting is available whenever someone is present. Lights should be on (or available if motion-activated) during times of marginal daylight, such as early morning and early evening, as these are times when visibility is diminished.

- If the home is an apartment, are common areas well lit and properly maintained? Elevator buttons should be easy to activate, and elevator doors should stay open long enough to allow someone moving slowly to enter. The building manager can adjust the timing if necessary.

- If the person with Parkinson's uses a wheelchair or a walker, are sidewalks and doorways wide enough for it? If not, how can they be modified? If there are steps, is there a way to construct a ramp? Sometimes it is necessary to use a different entry.

Interior Doorways, Hallways, and Stairs

Most interior doorways are 30 inches across, not wide enough to accommodate a wheelchair, and can be tricky with a walking aid such as a walker. Narrow spaces such as doorways may also trigger freezing of gait. Some doorways can be widened; for others, the structure of the house or placement of walls makes this impractical. Hallways are generally at least four feet wide, usually wide enough for clear passage. However, long hallways feel narrower, even if they are not; this feeling of narrowness can cause freezing. Bright lighting can help offset this perception. Make sure hallways and stairs have sturdy railings on both sides. If the main living areas are on one level and bedrooms are on another, are there ways to rearrange rooms so the person with Parkinson's can remain most of the time on one level? At the very least, climbing up and down stairs takes energy and concentration. When GAIT DISTURBANCES and BRADYKINESIA are prominent symptoms, they can make it impossible for the person to maneuver steps.

Electrical Access

Often electrical outlets are behind furniture. This is not a problem when lamps, televisions, stereos, and the like, are plugged into them, as these items generally stay plugged in. As well, this arrangement keeps cords safely out of tripping range. Reaching behind a couch or under a table to plug in a vacuum cleaner or other limited use device can be a risky proposition. Removing covers that plug into the outlets, such as those designed to prevent small children (including grandchildren) from experimenting with electricity, can be difficult for someone who has limited dexterity.

- Run electrical cords under furniture and along baseboards as much as possible, and fasten them down if they can stray into a common path of travel. Use extension cords, if necessary, to eliminate exposed cords that present tripping hazards.

- Use extension cords to provide access if furniture arrangements block outlets.

Furniture and Décor

The deep, soft cushions of the sofa that were once so comfortable now present a challenge for the person with Parkinson's who has BALANCE problems. Many people with Parkinson's have difficulty moving from standing to sitting or sitting to standing. Sofas and chairs with firm seating surfaces and chairs that have arms but do not rock or swivel offer the safest seating options.

Many people display photos, collectibles, and other items on end tables, coffee tables, and shelves. These arrangements can present obstacles for the person with Parkinson's, whose slowed movements and difficulty in changing direction can result in bumping into such displays. The person with Parkinson's may be injured or be distressed about breaking items. Plant stands and hanging planters can also create hazards. Consider placing shelves and plants along walls that are away from common travel paths or displaying favorite items in rooms that are less frequently used.

Room Arrangements

What is the traffic pattern through commonly used rooms? Must people wind their way around and between items of furniture? Although this process may be second nature for other family members (and may have been for the person with Parkinson's before motor symptoms began to interfere with mobility), it can now present an obstacle course. Try to arrange furniture so there are wide paths of travel, preferably through the center of the room rather than along a wall if practical. People with Parkinson's are especially sensitive to feeling "trapped" in areas that are too confined for them to maneuver for changes in direction, such as turning around. This trapped feeling can lead to freezing and falls. In commonly used areas, there should be adequate room to allow the person to make a U-turn.

Some rooms, such as kitchens and bathrooms, are difficult to rearrange because items such as cabinets, counters, fixtures, and appliances are in fixed locations. As much as possible, keep countertops and floors free of clutter. Remove throw rugs, even from bathrooms.

Appliances

Most household appliances such as microwave ovens and coffee makers are designed for ease of use and have large or touch-sensitive controls. Controls for major appliances such as stoves, ovens, and dishwashers vary considerably. Many stoves have knobs that must be pushed in and turned simultaneously to safeguard against accidentally turning on a burner; these can be difficult for the person with Parkinson's to manage.

- Some toasters and toaster ovens use small sliding levers for light–dark toast settings; these are designed to be difficult to manipulate so bumping them does not cause them to move. Leave the settings at the preferences of the person with Parkinson's; other family members can change them for their own use and then change them back.

- Leave frequently used appliances accessible and plugged in, ready to use, if this arrangement is practical. In kitchens, make sure items on countertops do not block access to electrical outlets.

- Consider hand-held electric can openers that are lightweight and require minimal manipulation. Countertop or mounted can openers can require dexterity and strength to maneuver and hold cans in place.

- Do refrigerator doors open completely? Are interior drawers and trays easy to open and close?

Laundry Facilities

Where are the clothes washer and dryer? Laundry facilities that are in the basement or the garage may require maneuvering up and down steps or through doors. Interior laundry rooms are generally safer, although they may be small and used for storage as well as laundry.

- The most popular washing machines are those that load at the top; the most popular dryers load at the front. If practical, consider putting a table between the washer and the dryer for clothes that go into and out of the washer. This arrangement reduces the need to bend.

- Put a chair at the table so the person with Parkinson's can sit down to move wet clothes from the table to the dryer.

- Are there general settings on the washer and the dryer that typically are safe for most of the laundry the person with Parkinson's might do? If so, leave the machines on these settings. Some machines have touch-sensitive controls; others have push buttons or push-and-turn dials that may be difficult for someone with limited dexterity and coordination to operate.

Floor Coverings

Throw rugs and area rugs pose significant tripping hazards for people with Parkinson's and cause many falls. The shuffled steps and foot drag that are common GAIT DISTURBANCES make catching the feet on the edge of or becoming entangled in a rug easy. Rugs also catch walking aids such as canes. Long-pile and textured carpets are also difficult walking surfaces for people with Parkinson's. If practical, replace them with short-pile carpet or leave the floor uncarpeted.

Lighting

Subdued lighting is wonderful for making a room feel comfortable and cozy, but it makes walking difficult for the person with Parkinson's who has vision problems. Bright, but not glaring, lighting is best in areas such as hallways, kitchens, and bathrooms. Bedrooms, living rooms, and other common areas should have variable lighting that can be bright for walking and dimmed when the person is seated.

- Replace conventional light switches with broad toggle switches that are easy to activate.

- Consider lights that are turned on automatically, such as at darkness, or through motion sensors.

Water, Faucets, and Fixtures

The most important safety factor in bathrooms and kitchens is hot water temperature. To reduce the risk of scalding and burns from water that is too hot, keep the hot water heater set no higher than 140 degrees. This temperature is hot enough to satisfy the person who enjoys a hot shower or bath but is below the point that can cause damage to skin and tissues. Most faucets have knobs that turn, push, or pull. These can be difficult for someone with limited coordination and dexterity to operate. Replace them with lever-style controls that move smoothly and freely.

See also BATHING AND BATHROOM ORGANIZATION; BEDROOM COMFORT; KITCHEN EFFICIENCY.

homovanillic acid (HVA) See 3-METHOXY-4-HYDROXYPHENYLACETIC ACID.

honesty The actions of telling what is true, guided by kindness, COMPASSION, and EMPATHY. No one likes or wants to see a loved one suffer, and family members often make every effort to protect loved ones from what they perceive as harsh truths. Yet most people appreciate knowing the full seriousness of a situation, even when the information is unpleasant. It is much easier to prepare for the known that for the unknown. Although most people with Parkinson's live the remainder of their natural lives as the disease is seldom fatal, Parkinson's changes the course and quality of life for everyone who has it. Facing challenges together, rather than pretending they do not exist, is ultimately more satisfying to the person with Parkinson's as well as to family members and friends. Honesty can acknowledge the negative but emphasize the positive.

See also ADJUSTING TO LIVING WITH PARKINSON'S; EMOTIONS; EMPATHY; FAMILY RELATIONSHIPS; FRUSTRATION; JOY; LONELINESS; MARRIAGE RELATIONSHIP; OPTIMISM.

hope for a Parkinson's cure Current research holds great promise that discoveries about the causes and mechanisms of Parkinson's will soon result in treatments that can permanently end the loss of DOPAMINERGIC NEURONS that is the foundation of the disease and restore full neuromuscular function.

Much of the most promising research is in the area of GENE THERAPY. Several GENES have been identified as having roles in Parkinson's disease, although the precise nature of those roles, and what activates them, remains a mystery. The HUMAN GENOME PROJECT has contributed much knowledge and information that is helping researchers to unravel the mysteries of the genetic components of Parkinson's. Gene therapy could target GENE MUTATIONS, reversing or neutralizing their deleterious effects.

Research involving stem cells, which have the capability to function as any kind of cell depending on the tissues in which they reside, also shows great promise. Stem cells transplanted into the BASAL GANGLIA of people with Parkinson's can "take root" and reproduce as dopaminergic neurons, replacing those lost to the disease process of Parkinson's and restoring DOPAMINE production and function to near-normal. In some people, these INVESTIGATIONAL TREATMENTS have put Parkinson's disease in apparent remission for as long as 10 years. Researchers are currently trying to improve the existing somewhat low success rate and bothersome complication rate of the last large randomized trial of fetal stem cell implantation in humans.

Other treatments currently under investigation include transplantation of mature dopaminegic cells from donors and infusion of neuronal growth factors into the brain. Although it is likely that treatments arising from these research studies are still years or even a decade from becoming practical treatments for all people with Parkinson's, the findings are exciting for researchers and people with Parkinson's alike.

New medications, particularly new DOPAMINE AGONISTS that act as DOPAMINE does but without the side effects that are common with LEVODOPA and earlier dopamine agonists, appear to offer extended relief of symptoms as well as some evidence of their slowing the disease. The newer dopamine agonists have largely replaced levodopa as the treatment of choice for initial therapy in Parkinson's disease in most people.

The public advocacy of people such as former heavyweight boxing champion MUHAMMAD ALI and actor MICHAEL J. FOX has done much to increase awareness of Parkinson's disease and to generate and renew interest in research to find its causes, more effective treatments, and an eventual cure. As the "faces" of this neurodegenerative disease, they have put it before the public.

See also ALPHA-SYNUCLEIN GENE; CHROMOSOMES LINKED TO PARKINSON'S DISEASE; COMPLEX I; ENVIRONMENTAL TOXINS; ENVIRONMENTAL TRIGGERS; GENE MAPPING; PARKIN GENE; PARKINSON'S DISEASE, CAUSES OF.

hormone   A chemical that certain cells within the body produce, that affects the functions of other cells that have receptors for the hormone. There are numerous hormones in the body, some of which, such as EPINEPHRINE and NOREPINEPHRINE, are NEUROTRANSMITTERS. Hormones regulate cell activities that control body functions. There has been a long-held belief that ESTROGEN, the hormone primarily responsible for female secondary sex characteristics, offered a NEUROPROTECTIVE benefit for women. Recent studies, among the most extensive ever done, negate this belief.

See also MENOPAUSE.

Hornykiewicz, Oleh   The neurologist and researcher at the Brain Research Institute of Vienna University Medical School who, in 1960, analyzed brains of people who had died of various causes and discovered that the brains of people with Parkinson's disease had substantially lower levels of DOPAMINE than did the brains of people who did not have Parkinson's disease. Hornykiewicz proposed dopamine replacement therapy as a treatment for Parkinson's disease and in 1961 reported the first successful use of LEVODOPA for that purpose. Modern neurologists and researchers consider Hornykiewicz's work to be the foundation for current treatment approaches as well as the platform for subsequent research.

Hornykiewicz's work followed the discovery in the late 1950s by the neuroscientist Arvid Carlsson at the University of Gothenberg in Sweden that dopamine is an independent neurotransmitter in the brain and identified its crucial role in nerve signals related to movement. Before Carlsson's discovery, scientists believed dopamine was just a precursor for the neurotransmitters epinephrine and NOREPINEPHRINE. Carlsson also discovered that the naturally occurring amino acid levodopa is converted to dopamine in the body.

In 2000, Hornykiewicz was at the center of a controversy over the awarding of the 2000 Nobel Prize in physiology or medicine, which was awarded to Carlsson and two other neuroscientists, the Americans Paul Greengard and Eric Kandel. The three were recognized for their work in understanding the roles of neurotransmitters, and Carlsson was honored for the significance of his work in understanding and treating Parkinson's disease. Although Carlsson's recognition was well deserved, neuroscientists around the world believed that the Nobel committee had slighted Hornykiewicz and 250 of them signed an open letter describing the significance of Hornykiewicz's work. The letter was published in several professional journals.

hospice Medical, emotional, psychological, and spiritual support at the end of life. Hospice exists as a collection of structured services intended to provide comfort and dignity during the last stages of life. Hospice workers include nurses and nurses' aides, personal care assistants, spiritual personnel such as chaplains, nutritionists, massage therapists, bereavement counselors, social workers, and often people who volunteer their services to fulfill whatever needs the person and family have. Although some hospitals have inpatient hospice units, most hospice services are provided on an outpatient basis so people can remain in the comfort and familiarity of their homes. Hospice services are generally available to people who are expected to live six months or less and to their families. Most doctors, hospitals, and senior organizations are familiar with local hospice resources and can make recommendations or, in the case of doctors, referrals.

Medicare pays for hospice services with no deductible or copayments in most situations. There

are qualification requirements that vary with the person's diagnosis, prognosis, and other factors. Generally the doctor must refer the person for hospice care and document, in writing, the person's diagnosis and prognosis (the person's terminal condition and expectation of living six months or less). Hospice providers are knowledgeable about the current requirements (which are subject to change as Medicare procedures change) and can guide families through the proper procedures. It is sometimes difficult for the person with Parkinson's disease to qualify for hospice services under Medicare. The person's physical and mental condition can become severely debilitated, yet the body remains strong.

See also ADVANCE DIRECTIVES; CARE MANAGEMENT AND PLANNING; COMPASSION; EMPATHY; END OF LIFE CARE AND DECISIONS; GRIEF; HOME HEALTH CARE; HONESTY; HOSPITALIZATION; PALLIATIVE CARE; SUPPORTIVE THERAPIES.

hospitalization Medical treatment and care received during admission for an overnight stay to a hospital. With advances in outpatient surgery and treatment options such as home health care, hospitalization is becoming increasingly less common. Most often, people with Parkinson's are hospitalized for other reasons such as surgery, illness, or injury. It is important, yet sometimes challenging, to receive appropriate attention for the aspects of Parkinson's that hospital staff might not view as relevant to treatment of the condition for which the person is hospitalized. This includes schedules for ANTI-PARKINSON'S MEDICATIONS, any special dietary schedules, RANGE OF MOTION exercises, and regular activity such as WALKING. The higher the level of assistance the person with Parkinson's requires, the more difficult meeting these needs usually is. This is partly because hospital care typically is narrowly focused on the person's medical condition and treatment rather than on the person as a whole, and partly because hospital staff generally do not have great depth of knowledge about Parkinson's disease.

To the extent that it is practical, the person's neurologist should be in contact with the physician responsible for the person's care in the hospital (known as the attending physician) to ensure proper consideration of Parkinson's disease care issues. Some hospitals permit a family member or regular caregiver to administer ANTI-PARKINSON'S MEDICATIONS, if the attending physician gives a written order authorizing it. This helps maintain the person's medication schedule with minimal disruption. Some hospitals do not allow this and require that their personnel administer any and all medications; the policy depends on how the hospital's view of the potential liability for any errors that might take place. In either case, it is important for the attending physician (and ideally the patient or the caregiver acting in an advocate role) to monitor other medications being given, and to consult with the person's neurologist when necessary, to make sure they do not interfere with the anti-Parkinson's medications, including anesthetics and medications for pain relief. If the hospitalization is planned, such as a scheduled surgery, often it is possible to work out with the hospital's dietitian a meal plan that meets the person's needs such as PROTEIN RESTRICTIONS, or to supply the foods the person regularly eats. Again, this requires the attending physician's order.

Being in the hospital can be a frightening experience for the person with Parkinson's, particularly if he or she experiences fluctuating symptoms and the ON–OFF STATE that increase dependence on others for routine activities such as toileting or has symptoms that include COGNITIVE DYSFUNCTION, MEMORY LOSS, or DEMENTIA. Hospitalization often is disorienting under the best of circumstances. If possible, family members and friends can take turns staying with the person so someone familiar is always there. When the person is released to go home from the hospital, check with the doctor about whether HOME HEALTH CARE is appropriate. People who return home with wound dressings (such as after surgery), casts for fractured bones, or other medical care needs often qualify for home health care services in which health care professionals such as nurses and physical therapists go to the home to provide medical care.

Typically, a person with Parkinson's disease is not hospitalized unless there is no other way to provide needed medical treatment. Regardless of the reason for hospitalization, make sure the admitting physician has a copy of the person's ADVANCE DIRECTIVES. In many hospitals this is part of the routine admission procedure. The family member or caregiver who will be spending most time with the person during the hospitalization should have a copy of the advance directives as well, so there are never any questions as to what actions are appropriate should a medical crisis occur.

See also CARE MANAGEMENT AND PLANNING; FLUCTUATING PHENOMENON; MEDICATION MANAGEMENT.

human embryonic stem cell therapy   See STEM CELL.

Human Genome Project   An extensive effort to identify the 30,000 to 35,000 genes and establish the sequences of the nearly 3 billion chemical structures that constitute human deoxyribonucleic acid (DNA) and to store and analyze the data with the expectation of using the resulting information to advance research into the causes and treatments of diseases. Although primarily supported by the U.S. Department of Energy and National Human Genome Research Institute and the National Institutes of Health, the Human Genome Project incorporates the work of scientists around the world. The project started in 1990 and completed the full human genome sequence in April 2003, two years ahead of schedule. Already the project has produced numerous significant findings leading to the discovery of genes responsible for or linked to conditions such as Parkinson's disease and ALZHEIMER'S DISEASE. The Human Genome Project's website at www.genome.gov provides updates and analyses of project findings.

See also BIOETHICS; GENE MAPPING; GENE THERAPY.

humor   The ability to find good-natured amusement in difficult or potentially embarrassing situations. Humor helps people to see the good in each other and in the circumstances they share and creates a bond of collaboration. Humor is not about making fun of, but finding the fun in, events. Laughter is good medicine, as the saying goes, and helps people to feel better about themselves and their situations.

See also COMPASSION; EMBARRASSMENT; EMOTIONS; EMPATHY; JOY; OPTIMISM.

Huntington's disease   An inherited NEURODEGENERATIVE disease characterized by motor symptoms such as CHOREA (writhing, dancelike movements) and DYSTONIA (rigid and distorted muscles) and by COGNITIVE DYSFUNCTION and MEMORY LOSS. Symptoms tend to begin in early midlife and can be confused with the symptoms of Parkinson's in their early stages, depending on which appear first. However, the progression of symptoms makes it quickly apparent that the condition is not Parkinson's, and a genetic analysis provides the confirming diagnosis.

Huntington's disease results from a GENETIC MUTATION; in everyone who has the mutation the disease will develop. The GENE for Huntington's was discovered in 1993 and is autosomal dominant. If one parent has Huntington's, each child has a 50–50 chance of also having the gene for the disease. Although the vast majority of people with Huntington's have a clear family history of it passing from generation to generation, occasional cases may present due to newly occurring mutations (usually during the creation of the father's sperm) or in cases where one or both parents died young (before symptoms could occur) or where there is mistaken paternity. Only people with the gene mutation can develop the disease; unlike Parkinson's, Huntington's does not seem to have an environmental component. Huntington's disease progresses until all voluntary abilities deteriorate, rendering the person virtually motionless. It is ultimately fatal. Some ANTI-PARKINSON'S MEDICATIONS can relieve symptoms early in the course of Huntington's, but as yet there is no effective treatment for the disease.

For more information, contact

Huntington's Disease Society of America
158 West 29th Street, 7th Floor
New York, NY 10001-5300
(800) 345-HDSA
http://www.hdsa.org

See also AUTOSOMAL DOMINANT INHERITANCE; CONDITIONS SIMILAR TO PARKINSON'S; GENE THERAPY; MULTIPLE SCLEROSIS; MUSCULAR DYSTROPHY.

hygiene   Personal cleanliness becomes an increasing challenge as Parkinson's disease progresses. Basic activities such as toileting, bathing, brushing teeth, and personal grooming (shaving, combing hair, applying deodorant) require COORDINATION and DEXTERITY. For as long as possible, encourage the person to handle or participate in personal hygiene. Make this easy by keeping hygiene items within easy reach and allowing adequate time for the person to perform personal hygiene functions without feeling hurried or half-finished.

Symptoms such as excessive drooling and sweating, both of which are common in the middle to later stages of Parkinson's, require diligent attention to make sure they do not cause health problems. Persistent moisture irritates the skin, creating discomfort and leaving it vulnerable to bacterial infection. Incontinence, urinary or stool, also can be a problem that requires diligent attention. Multiple clothing changes throughout the day may be necessary. Cleanliness is important to prevent infection, as well as to reduce problems such as unpleasant odors.

It also contributes greatly to a person's SELF-IMAGE and SELF-ESTEEM to be clean and presentable; everyone appreciates looking and feeling his or her best, even under less than ideal circumstances. Even though the person with Parkinson's may be unable to manage personal hygiene tasks without considerable assistance, he or she likely remains very aware of appearance and presence. It is a difficult loss of INDEPENDENCE to become unable to take care of personal needs; COMPASSION and EMPATHY are very important. As much as possible, respect the person's privacy when providing assistance with personal hygiene.

See also ACTIVITIES OF DAILY LIVING; ADAPTIVE EQUIPMENT AND ASSIST DEVICES; BATHING AND BATHROOM ORGANIZATION; DRESSING; FREQUENT VOIDING SCHEDULE; UNDERGARMENTS, PROTECTIVE.

hypokinesis   A term infrequently used for BRADYKINESIA that refers to the slowed muscle response and movement characteristic of Parkinson's disease.

hypomimia   The clinical term for the composite of symptoms that includes reduced facial movements, slowed eye movements, slowed blinking, and reduced facial expression. These symptoms occur as Parkinson's disease affects the muscles that control facial movement. In composite, these symptoms give the false impression that the person with Parkinson's is emotionless and uninterested. Hypomimia is one of the more frustrating manifestations of Parkinson's disease as much of human interaction and communication relies on facial expressions. People who do not understand that such an expression is not within the person's control find it confusing and distressing. Even family members and friends who are frequently with the person who has Parkinson's sometimes find it disconcerting. It is important to remember that the person feels and wants to express his or her emotions but is unable to do so.

See also BLEPHAROSPASMS; BLINK RATE; EMOTIONS.

hypophonia   Reduced VOICE volume and strength that develops when Parkinson's disease affects the muscles that control the vocal cords. The vocal cords also sometimes become thinned. A soft, sometimes whispery voice is often one of the earliest symptoms of Parkinson's, although this connection does not become apparent until more definitive symptoms such as TREMORS (involuntary, rhythmic movements) and BRADYKINESIA (slowed movements) appear. Generally hypophonia improves with ANTI-PARKINSON'S MEDICATIONS, as do other motor symptoms. SPEECH THERAPY can help the person with Parkinson's to develop techniques that increase voice volume. Hypophonia sometimes occurs as a side effect of surgical treatments for Parkinson's such as PALLIDOTOMY or THALAMOTOMY, as a result of damage to areas of the brain that are involved in functions related to SPEECH.

Hypophonia often coexists with DYSARTHRIA, in which there are changes in speech quality, modulation, and rate. The bradykinesia that slows the muscles of movement can also slow those involved with speech. The person may start talking and then pause for an inappropriately long time before resuming or speak in rapid bursts in which words rush out in a jumble of sounds that are difficult to understand. Modulation changes include flatness of tone that makes the voice sound emotionless. DYSPHASIA (difficulty in finding the right words) and COGNITIVE DYSFUNCTION can further complicate spoken communication.

See also BREATH CONTROL.

hypotension   Low blood pressure. ORTHOSTATIC HYPOTENSION, a drop in blood pressure when changing positions from lying to sitting and standing, is a common side effect of many ANTI-PARKINSON'S MEDICATIONS and can be caused by Parkinson's (or especially a similar disease, MULTI-SYSTEMATROPHY [MSA]). Hypotension also may be an IDIOPATHIC condition. Symptoms of hypotension include dizziness, lightheadedness, and a feeling that the room is spinning. Hypotension can affect balance. When hypotension persists without apparent relation to medications, a cardiologist should examine the person for possible heart problems.

See also HEART DISEASE AND PARKINSON'S.

hypotension, orthostatic   A drop in blood pressure that occurs with a change in position, most commonly from lying down to standing up and sometimes from sitting to standing. Orthostatic HYPOTENSION is a common side effect of many ANTI-PARKINSON'S MEDICATIONS, and can be caused by Parkinson's (or especially a similar disease, MULTIPLE SYSTEM ATROPHY [MSA]). These medications and conditions can affect the functioning of smooth muscle tissue, which allows the walls of the arteries to relax. This effect reduces the pressure blood encounters as it travels through them, lowering blood pressure. The primary action of BETA-ADRENERGIC ANTAGONIST (BLOCKER) MEDICATIONS, sometimes taken to relieve TREMORS, is to lower blood pressure by causing arteries to relax (blocking the actions of epinephrine, which causes arteries to contract). Some ANTIDEPRESSANT MEDICATIONS also can cause orthostatic hypotension.

Because orthostatic hypotension is common with anti-Parkinson's medications, it is a good idea for the person with Parkinson's to develop the habit of pausing before standing up from a sitting position and sitting for a few moments after rising from a lying position. This adjustment allows the mechanisms that regulate the body's blood pres-sure to restore appropriate blood pressure, reducing the risk of FALLING. Orthostatic hypotension sometimes is called postural hypotension.

See also HEART DISEASE AND PARKINSON'S.

iceberg phenomenon The belief of many scientists that far more people have Parkinson's disease than are diagnosed. In 2001 the National Institute of Neurological Disorders and Stroke (NINDS), an agency of the National Institutes of Health (NIH), reported the perception among researchers that there are as many as 20 people who have Parkinson's for each person who is diagnosed. Several factors contribute to this perception:

- Autopsies performed for various reasons show that as many as 15 percent of people older than age 75 have Lewy bodies in their brain although they did not show any symptoms of Parkinson's disease before death. The presence of Lewy bodies, which are only detectable through examination of brain tissue at autopsy, has long been considered classic and definitive evidence of a Parkinson's diagnosis.

- There has been a three- to fourfold increase in the number of people younger than age 40 who are diagnosed with Parkinson's disease since the early 1990s. The majority of those with EARLY-ONSET PARKINSON'S have minor symptoms that, before recent breakthroughs in understanding the mechanisms of Parkinson's, likely would not have been identified as suggestive of this "disease of the elderly."

- Researchers are learning more about the health effects of ENVIRONMENTAL TOXINS such as pesticides and herbicides, including their possible complicity in diseases such as Parkinson's. Scientists can induce Parkinson's-like symptoms in lab rats, for example, by injecting them with the common pesticide rotenone, which is an ingredient of a wide range of products from flea and tick controls for pets to garden insecti-

cides. Exposure to these substances remains widespread.

- Parkinson's disease is incorrectly diagnosed in about one in five people, maybe more. As researchers learn more about how and why Parkinson's disease develops, diagnostic techniques will become more precise.

- The U.S. population is aging, as more people are living longer. Some scientists believe that as longevity extends, the intricate interplay between the multiple and varied causes of Parkinson's disease and the natural aging process means that eventually anyone who lives long enough will develop the symptoms of Parkinson's.

At present, Parkinson's disease is the third most common NEURODEGENERATIVE disorder among adults in the United States, yet many people do not know of it until it affects someone close to them.

See also CHEMICAL TOXINS; ENVIRONMENTAL TRIGGERS; LEWY BODY; DIAGNOSING PARKINSON'S.

idiopathic Without obvious cause or explanation; also often referred to as "of unknown etiology." The word itself means "individual disease." Most cases of Parkinson's disease, about 85 percent, are idiopathic. Although researchers widely believe that it is an interaction of genetic and environmental factors that sets Parkinson's disease in motion, as yet they do not fully understand the nature of these factors. About 15 percent of people with Parkinson's have one or more close family members (parents, grandparents, siblings, aunts, uncles) who also have the disease. In such cases, the disease is considered familial—that is, it has hereditary components that are passed on genetically.

The designation of what is considered idiopathic changes as researchers learn more about the causes of diseases such as Parkinson's.

See also ENVIRONMENTAL TRIGGERS; GENETIC PREDISPOSITION; PARKINSON'S DISEASE, CAUSES OF; DIAGNOSING PARKINSON'S.

imipramine An ANTIDEPRESSANT MEDICATION. Imipramine belongs to the family of drugs called TRICYCLIC ANTIDEPRESSANTS. It was one of the first antidepressants to receive U.S. Food and Drug Administration (FDA) approval and was first released as the brand name drug Tofranil in 1959. Imipramine and other tricyclic antidepressants have mild to moderate ANTICHOLINERGIC effects and can contribute to reduced GASTRIC MOTILITY. Other possible side effects include ORTHOSTATIC HYPOTENSION (a drop in blood pressure on arising from lying down), which is a common side effect of many ANTI-PARKINSON'S MEDICATIONS, and multiple drug interactions including with many of the medications taken to treat the symptoms of Parkinson's. As well, these drugs cannot be taken in conjunction with MONOAMINE OXIDASE INHIBITOR (MAOI) MEDICATIONS. The MAOI SELEGILINE is a common anti-Parkinson's medication. Generally, doctors avoid prescribing imipramine and other tricyclic antidepressants for people with Parkinson's disease because another family of antidepressants, the SELECTIVE SEROTONIN REUPTAKE INHIBITORS (SSRIs), effectively treat most mild to moderate DEPRESSION with fewer potential side effects.

See also MEDICATION SIDE EFFECTS.

Inappropriate Sleep Composite Score (ISCS) questionnaire A structured series of questions to help measure whether a person is getting adequate and appropriate sleep. Researchers at the University of Manitoba in Winnipeg, Canada, developed the ISCS specifically to address issues of DAYTIME SLEEPINESS in people with Parkinson's disease who take DOPAMINE AGONIST MEDICATIONS. The questionnaire incorporates questions about nighttime sleep quality, episodes of drowsiness during the day, and falling asleep during activities and questions about ANTI-PARKINSON'S MEDICATIONS, other medications, and symptoms of Parkinson's to help determine whether a person with Parkinson's is at risk for falling asleep while driving. Although the ISCS provides valuable information about these matters, in itself it cannot provide a complete picture of a person's sleep quality or likelihood for falling asleep during critical activities such as driving.

See also EPWORTH SLEEPINESS SCALE; INSOMNIA; MULTIPLE SLEEP LATENCY TEST; SLEEP DISTURBANCES.

incontinence The inability to retain urine or feces. In the person with Parkinson's, this usually results from the loss of muscle control of the sphincter muscles in the bladder and rectum, typically in later stages of the disease. Urinary incontinence is much more common than fecal incontinence among people with Parkinson's disease, partly because impaired GASTRIC MOTILITY causes CONSTIPATION. Although sometimes the incontinence is complete (the person has no ability to retain), in most people with Parkinson's incontinence is episodic (happens occasionally) or partial (happens when the bladder is full). The most common form of incontinence in people with Parkinson's is urge incontinence, also known as overactive bladder, in which the sensation of the need to urinate comes on suddenly and abruptly. Stress incontinence, in which the bladder leaks urine during coughing, sneezing, and laughing, is also common and is more common in women than in men. Overflow incontinence, in which the bladder fills and may reflexively empty without any perception of a need to urinate, is much less common in Parkinson's and typically only occurs in very late stages of LEWY BODY DISEASE or Parkinson's coexisting with ALZHEIMER'S DISEASE.

Incontinence is also more likely in older people, as diminished muscle tone and strength occur with aging, and is not necessarily connected to Parkinson's. Infections, inflammation of the bladder (cystitis), bladder spasms, and scarring from abdominal surgeries can cause incontinence, as can structural damage resulting from pregnancy and childbirth in women and prostatitis (infection and inflammation of the prostate gland) and benign prostatic hypertrophy (BPH), enlargement of the prostate gland, in men. In men, urinary incontinence also can be a symptom of prostate cancer. When incontinence occurs regularly, it should be evaluated by a physician.

There are a number of methods for treating incontinence. Nonmedical interventions include

- Doing exercises to strengthen the pelvic muscles (such as Kegel exercises)

- Following a frequent voiding schedule to prevent the bladder from overfilling

- Emptying the bladder completely when urinating

- Wearing absorbent pads or underwear (made in styles for men and for women)

- For men, wearing an external catheter that fits over the penis as a condom does

- Taking medications such as tolterodine (Detrol) or oxybutynin (Ditropan) that reduce URINARY URGENCY (the sensation that the bladder is full although it is not)

- Having surgery, as a treatment of final resort, to strengthen and repair weakened or damaged muscles in the pelvic area

Worry about incontinence tends to make it worse. Taking as many precautions as possible to reduce the likelihood of "accidents," such as voiding before going on a drive of any distance and using the bathroom whenever one is available while shopping and participating in other social activities, can relieve some of the anxiety. When incontinence is a consistent problem, it is helpful to take along a change of clothing whenever traveling any distance from home. Although people with Parkinson's often are embarrassed by incontinence, it is no more within their ability to control it than are symptoms such as TREMORS and GAIT DISTURBANCES. In the later stages of Parkinson's or in a person who also has ALZHEIMER'S DISEASE, incontinence may be a function of COGNITIVE IMPAIRMENT in which the person no longer knows what to do for toileting tasks and requires extensive assistance with them as well as with other matters of personal hygiene.

See also ACTIVITIES OF DAILY LIVING; BATHING AND BATHROOM ORGANIZATION; EMBARRASSMENT; URINARY RETENTION.

independence The ability to maintain a lifestyle with minimal assistance from others. Independence is an important element of life for all adults. Most people with Parkinson's disease are able to maintain independent living for a considerable period after diagnosis, provided they are not otherwise debilitated. As Parkinson's progresses, however, it threatens and, in most people with the disease, eventually overtakes independence.

Treatment for Parkinson's should focus on two dimensions of intervention, medical therapies (primarily ANTI-PARKINSON'S MEDICATIONS) to control the symptoms and lifestyle adaptations to maintain independence. PHYSICAL THERAPY and OCCUPATIONAL THERAPY can teach ways to cope with diminishing physical capabilities, including techniques for improving mobility and accommodating symptoms. ADAPTIVE EQUIPMENT AND ASSIST DEVICES also extend independence.

Changes in the level of independence are important in monitoring the progression of Parkinson's. Clinicians use a number of measurement tools to do this; the most commonly used are the generalized ACTIVITIES OF DAILY LIVING (ADLs) assessment, the SCHWAB AND ENGLAND SCALE OF CAPACITY FOR DAILY LIVING, and the SICKNESS IMPACT PROFILE (SIP). Assessments specifically for Parkinson's disease that incorporate measures of independence include the HOEHN AND YAHR STAGE SCALE, the UNIFIED PARKINSON'S DISEASE RATING SCALE (UPDRS), the PARKINSON'S DISEASE QUALITY OF LIFE QUESTIONNAIRE (PDQL), and the parkinson's measure of impact scale (PMIS).

Equally important are the observations of family members and caregivers, as well as the person's own assessment of functional capability. This is often a considerable challenge, as a key focus of adapting to living with Parkinson's is learning how to accommodate its symptoms. The more adept the person with Parkinson's is at doing so, the more difficult it can be for loved ones to determine when physical and cognitive skills have become impaired enough to interfere with independence. Always the overriding concern must be for the safety and well-being of the person with Parkinson's as well as for others who might be affected by the person's actions.

Until the late stages of the disease, the level of independence can vary considerably with the effect of anti-Parkinson's medications as well as other, less unpredictable factors. This variability makes it difficult to make decisions about care needs. One day the person with Parkinson's may seem nearly normal and the next day be unable to get out of bed without assistance. Because the course of Parkinson's is unique for each individual, determining when it is time to consider care assistance and alternative living arrangements is difficult. Planning for these circumstances before the need for them arises makes the decision easier for all involved.

See also BATHING AND BATHROOM ORGANIZATION; BEDROOM COMFORT; CHANGING ROLES; COOKING; DRIVING; INSTRUMENTAL ACTIVITIES OF DAILY LIVING; KITCHEN EFFICIENCY; MARRIAGE RELATIONSHIP; PARENT/CHILD RELATIONSHIPS; PLANNING FOR THE FUTURE; QUALITY OF LIFE; WORKPLACE ADAPTATIONS TO ACCOMMODATE PARKINSON'S.

informed consent Granting of permission for treatment procedures such as SURGERY or for participation in CLINICAL RESEARCH STUDIES AND INVESTIGATIVE TREATMENTS, which is based on a comprehensive explanation and disclosure of potential benefits and risks. It is essential to have a full and complete understanding of what will be done and what are all of the known possible complications and problems. There is always the potential for previously unknown complications as well. Informed consent for research studies should also include information about the right to leave the study and to return to conventional treatment.

A person's signature on an informed consent document generally acknowledges understanding and acceptance of the risks and benefits identified, and the document constitutes a legal record. An informed consent document for participation in clinical research trials and investigative treatments should include an explanation of what medical

care and other responsibilities the clinical investigator or facility sponsoring the research will provide if adverse results do occur.

See also ADVANCE DIRECTIVES; HOSPITALIZATION; INVESTIGATIONAL NEW DRUG; LEGAL CONCERNS; RANDOMIZED DOUBLE-BLIND STUDY.

insomnia See SLEEP DISTURBANCES.

instrumental activities of daily living (IADLs) Activities and tasks that a person performs daily or routinely that are related to independent living, extending beyond the measurement of the basic functions necessary for daily living. Regular ACTIVITIES OF DAILY LIVING (ADLs) include functions such as toileting, bathing, dressing, eating, and performing other essential self-care tasks. IADLs measure a person's ability to manage more complex tasks such as using the telephone, typing or using the computer, shopping, doing laundry, and performing similar activities. The IADL questionnaire is short and concise, asking the person with Parkinson's (or the caregiver) to rate his or her capabilities to perform tasks in eight areas.

Fine motor control is often among the earlier losses that Parkinson's disease causes, making many previously common tasks increasingly difficult. ADAPTIVE EQUIPMENT AND ASSIST DEVICES such as large button telephones and adaptive accommodations for equipment such as computers can extend the person's ability to continue using these items.

See also ADJUSTING TO LIVING WITH PARKINSON'S; INDEPENDENCE.

insurance, health See MEDICAL INSURANCE.

insurance, long-term care See LONG-TERM CARE INSURANCE.

intimacy Personal closeness between loved ones. Although intimacy often alludes to the relationship between spouses or life partners and embraces sexual intimacy, it also more broadly encompasses any relationship in which there is deep sharing of feelings and emotion. Parkinson's disease challenges intimacy in a number of ways. It often is difficult for loved ones and the person with Parkinson's to share their worries, fears, and emotions with each other about what the diagnosis means for them as individuals and within their relationships. As Parkinson's progresses relationships change, further affecting the ability to share and connect on an intimate level, physically in a marriage or partnership as well as emotionally.

See also EMOTIONS; MARRIAGE RELATIONSHIP; SELF-ESTEEM; SEXUALITY.

intrathecal baclofen therapy (IBT)   A method of infusing the antispasmodic medication BACLOFEN directly into the thecal sac of the spinal cord (the sheath that surrounds the spinal cord) using an implanted pump. IBT is a treatment more commonly used in neurodegenerative conditions such as MULTIPLE SCLEROSIS in which the disease process attacks the tissues that insulate NEURONS. The loss of this protective covering causes neurons to deliver their signals erratically and uncontrolled, causing debilitating and painful MUSCLE SPASMS. IBT is rarely used for some people with Parkinson's disease who have severe DYSTONIA (muscle RIGIDITY) and muscle spasms that are not relieved by any other means.

The method involves surgery to implant a small pump into a pouch of skin, usually in the abdomen, from which a small catheter runs under the skin and into the thecal sac. The pump is programmed to deliver precise and consistent amounts of baclofen (Lioresal) into the cerebrospinal fluid that surrounds the SPINAL CORD and BRAIN. Baclofen interrupts nerve signals as they leave the spinal cord, preventing them from activating peripheral muscle response. The drug also acts as a GAMMA-AMINOBUTYRIC ACID (GABA) AGONIST, stimulating the brain's production of GABA. This effect slows the action of ACETYLCHOLINE, a NEUROTRANSMITTER with central (brain) and peripheral (body) functions related to movement.

IBT allows a much higher concentration of baclofen to have direct contact with spinal neurons than could otherwise be achieved; the amount of oral baclofen that would be necessary to achieve this same concentration would produce intolerable side effects (such as severe nausea and drowsiness). Because IBT requires surgery, it carries risks of infection and other complications similar to those of other surgical treatments for Parkinson's disease such as DEEP BRAIN STIMULATION (DBS), PALLIDOTOMY, and THALOTOMY.

investigational new drug (IND)   A regulatory classification that exempts a drug that has not yet received U.S. Food and Drug Administration (FDA) approval for sale and distribution from U.S. regulations restricting it from being transported across state lines. Such an exemption is necessary to allow researchers in different facilities across the country to test a newly developed drug in phase III CLINICAL PHARMACOLOGY TRIALS. There are three circumstances under which the FDA's Center for Drug Evaluation and Research (CDER) can approve a drug for IND status:

- Research use for phase III clinical trials in which the drug will be given to selected people who have the condition the drug is intended to treat, under strict FDA-approved protocols (procedural guidelines)

- Emergency use when there is an urgent need to use the drug, when a person does not meet a protocol's criteria or there is no protocol yet but the person would clearly benefit from the drug

- Treatment use, usually restricted to serious conditions, when phase III clinical tests show the drug offers clear benefit but the clinical trial is not yet completed or while FDA approval is pending and approval is expected

There are numerous requirements that must be satisfied before the FDA will approve an IND application, which differ with the drug and its intended use. The CEDR's website, www.fda.gov/cedr, provides comprehensive information about these requirements, applicable federal laws, and the IND application process.

investigational treatments   Therapeutic approaches that have not yet been determined to be effective or safe but that demonstrate potential to be. Investigational treatments may employ new drugs and products or new applications of existing medications and devices. At any given time, there are hundreds of approved CLINICAL RESEARCH STUDIES in various stages under way throughout the United States. The NATIONAL INSTITUTES OF HEALTH funds or otherwise supports many and diverse research studies. Private organizations that want to promote Parkinson's research, such as the MICHAEL J. FOX FOUNDATION and the PARKINSON STUDY GROUP, and companies that are developing new treatments, such as pharmaceutical manufacturers, also sponsor research.

Investigational treatments are the therapeutic applications of drugs, devices, or techniques that have passed phase I (testing in healthy volunteers to determine metabolism and safety) of clinical research trials. They are ready for phase II (testing in a limited number of volunteers who have Parkinson's and are not obtaining relief from their symptoms through conventional treatments to gain an idea of the effectiveness and a confirmation of safety) or phase III (broader testing in people with Parkinson's who would be among the treatment's targeted patient population were it approved for use) testing. Most investigational treatments have shown great promise to the extent that they already have undergone testing, but their complete benefits and risks are not yet fully apparent.

Anyone considering an investigational treatment should receive fully informed consent information and discuss the investigational treatment with his or her regular physician. Often it is the physician who suggests considering the investigational treatment. It is crucial to learn as much as possible about the treatment before agreeing to try it. Some treatments, such as surgery, produce permanent results or can cause permanent harm. Other investigational treatments produce temporary results, and any adverse effects they produce are also temporary.

See also GENE THERAPY; TREATMENT ALGORITHM.

iron A mineral that the body uses for various functions including formation of hemoglobin to transport oxygen in the blood. Most people can get as much iron as their body needs from the foods they eat, although menstruating women with heavy flow can become iron-deficient (a condition called anemia). The body's ability to extract iron, as well as other nutrients, from dietary sources diminishes with increasing age so physicians often advise older people to take an iron supplement, usually in the form of a multiple vitamin and mineral formula. However, iron supplements interfere with the absorption of LEVODOPA, the most potent ANTIPARKINSON MEDICATION.

Most people with Parkinson's disease who are taking levodopa should not have iron supplements, either alone or in multiple mineral formulas. If iron supplementation is necessary, timing the levodopa and supplement dosages to be administered at the maximal number of hours apart reduces the level of interference. People taking levodopa also should not eat foods high in iron within several hours of taking a levodopa dose. Foods high in iron include green vegetables, red meat, fish (particularly canned tuna), shrimp, shellfish, and legumes (pinto beans, kidney beans, garbanzo beans, navy beans). Many breads, cereals, and pastas are fortified with minerals including iron. A rare genetic disorder called ACERULOPLASMINEMIA, in which the body cannot metabolize iron, causes a form of PARKINSONISM. In aceruloplasminemia, iron accumulates in the neurons of the BASAL GANGLIA, blocking their actions and causing impaired motor function.

See also FOODS TO AVOID; NUTRITION AND DIET; NUTRITIONAL SUPPLEMENTS; VITAMINS.

J

John Paul II   The world leader of the Roman Catholic Church whose Parkinson's disease became apparent in the 1990s. Although official comment about his health status is limited, the pope illustrates the TREMORS, BRADYKINESIA, and soft, faltering SPEECH characteristic of Parkinson's disease. The pope's insistence on maintaining an intense schedule of public appearances despite his health challenges has been inspiring to millions of people around the world who have Parkinson's disease.

See also ALI, MUHAMMAD; FOX, MICHAEL J.; RENO, JANET; WHITE, MAURICE.

joy   The ability to take pleasure in the events of everyday life. When chronic illness strikes, it rearranges life's priorities. The moment in which the doctor delivers the diagnosis of Parkinson's disease becomes a pivot on which the direction of life suddenly swings. The focus shifts from daily details to "Let's get this under control." All planning for the future centers on medications and therapeutic interventions. Even when the diagnosis was suspected, having the suspicion confirmed is a shock. After all, Parkinson's is a progressive NEURODEGENERATIVE disease whose unpredictable course confounds people's expectations for the last decades of life. When the diagnosis is a bombshell, as it often is in EARLY-ONSET PARKINSON'S, the sense of loss can be overwhelming. It is difficult, to say the least, to find joy in the midst of such turmoil.

Yet joy is an essential element of human existence. It gives life meaning and value. People engage in activities and relationships for the happiness and pleasure they yield. Even in the face of adversity, it is possible—and crucial—to seek and experience joy. For most people with Parkinson's, the circumstances of daily life change slowly to accommodate the disease's gradual progression of symptoms. Life takes on a new perspective, certainly, but ANTI-PARKINSON'S MEDICATIONS and SUPPORTIVE THERAPIES can keep symptoms and their disruptions under control for years and sometimes decades.

To make the most of this time it is important to remain as active as possible, and to feel free—as well as entitled—to experience joy. Numerous studies show that people do better, and feel better about themselves and life in general, when their outlook is positive. For each individual who has Parkinson's, the course of the disease is unpredictable. Finding the positive, the good, and the joy in life is perhaps the most effective way to remain in control of living.

See also ADJUSTING TO LIVING WITH PARKINSON'S; COMPASSION; DEPRESSION; FOX, MICHAEL J.; GRIEF; HOPE FOR A PARKINSON'S CURE; PLANNING FOR THE FUTURE.

kinesia paradoxica Sudden and unexpected movement, usually walking and sometimes running, that affects a person with Parkinson's disease. Kinesia paradoxica can occur after the person has experienced freezing of gait or when the person is intentionally standing still. Researchers believe kinesia paradoxica and freezing are related dysfunctions that result from deterioration and damage within the BASAL GANGLIA and other structures of the BRAIN involved with movement.

There is some speculation that kinesia paradoxica and other gait disturbances are related to dysfunctions of vision. In Parkinson's disease, BRADYKINESIA often affects the muscles that control eye movement. The effect distorts the process of collecting visual information, with the result that visual signals are garbled by the time they reach the visual interpretation centers in the brain. During normal movement, there is a close interplay between vision and motor adjustments. The eye sees an obstacle, it sends the signal to the brain, the brain "notifies" the cerebellum, and the cerebellum initiates the sequence of responses and movements necessary to avoid the obstacle. Such a sequence typically takes less than a second. In conditions such as Parkinson's in which neuromuscular communication is altered, the sequence may unfold in segments, incompletely, or not at all.

GAIT DISTURBANCES such as freezing and start hesitation are more likely to occur when there is a change in the walking surface, such as when going from carpet to tile. As well, kinesia paradoxica is more likely to occur when the person's eyes are following a moving object. Stairs, stepping over a line, having floor tile lines perpendicular to the gait path, or a bouncing ball all may inexplicably allow a person with Parkinson's who has "frozen" to step easily. People who use the technique of envisioning themselves stepping over an imaginary line on the floor to break free during a freezing episode may in fact be activating an episode of kinesia paradoxica. In kinesia paradoxica, the person usually begins walking or running at a constant pace, rather than at the continuously accelerating pace of FESTINATION. Another form of kinesia paradoxica is the unexpected and usually temporary return of mobility in a person who has been unable to walk, such as when a person with Parkinson's has been restricted to a wheelchair and suddenly gets up and walks.

kitchen efficiency Organizing the kitchen to facilitate safe and convenient FOOD PREPARATION. Being able to cook and prepare foods is a key measure of independence. For the person with Parkinson's, as the disease progresses many tasks that once required little thought begin to require considerable effort. It becomes difficult to reach up or bend down. As well, TREMORS and other symptoms make use of utensils, especially knives, and kitchen appliances such as can openers, difficult. A few simple measures can make the kitchen more efficient for the person with Parkinson's:

- Rearrange cupboards and drawers to put commonly used items within easy reach.
- Label or otherwise identify commonly used seasonings and spices. Write the names in printed block letters on self-adhesive labels, for example.
- Leave regularly used appliances, such as electric can openers, on the countertop and plugged in, so they are ready to use.
- Forgo throw rugs and other potential falling hazards. Make sure there is clear and uncluttered access to counters, stove, sink, and refrigerator.

- Use a self-contained floor mop, which has detergent in a dispenser, to make cleaning up minor spills easier.

- Prepare commonly used foods in advance, and store them in single-serving quantities.

- Use carton holders with handles for cartons of milk and orange juice to make them easier to pick up and pour.

- Place burner covers over stove burners when the stove is not in use.

- Inventory cupboards, refrigerator, and freezer weekly to check for outdated food items as well as to make sure necessary or desired food items are available.

As the Parkinson's progresses, it is important for family members or caregivers to monitor the person's ability to manage kitchen tasks safely. Sharing these tasks can be a way to spend time together that is enjoyable as well as productive and helps to maintain the person's sense of INDEPENDENCE.

See also ADJUSTING TO LIVING WITH PARKINSON'S; COOKING.

Klonopin   See CLONAZEPAM.

lap buddy   A thick flat cushion that fits over a person's lap and under the armrests of a wheelchair. This device helps to keep the person properly positioned in the wheelchair and provides a surface to support reading materials and other items. A person with normal cognitive abilities and moderate physical COORDINATION can easily remove the device, which may or may not have notches to help hold it in place. However, for a person with impaired function or motor skills the lap buddy serves as a light RESTRAINT to keep him or her from getting out of the wheelchair unassisted, as a means of reducing the risk of injury from FALLS. Many states regulate the use of RESTRAINTS of any kind, including devices that have other uses such as the lap buddy, in LONG-TERM CARE FACILITIES, as do credentialing organizations.

See also CARE MANAGEMENT AND PLANNING; COGNITIVE FUNCTION; COGNITIVE IMPAIRMENT; COPING WITH ONGOING CARE OF PARKINSON'S; LONG-TERM CARE.

Larodopa   See LEVODOPA.

L-dopa   See LEVODOPA.

lead pipe resistance   An early symptom of Parkinson's disease in which the muscles of a limb stiffen and resist passive movement (attempt by another person to manipulate the arm or leg when the person relaxes the limb). It gets its name from both the fact that it gives smooth constant resistance no matter how fast or slow the limb is moved and the perception that the limb is heavy and nonresponsive, "like a lead pipe." Lead pipe resistance is typically what a neurologist

looks for as a sign of rigidity. Another form of passive resistance in people with Parkinson's is common COGWHEELING, in which the muscles move in a ratcheting motion and that neurologists recognize as being tied to tremor. Both cogwheel and lead pipe resistance result from the same damage to the EXTRAPYRAMIDAL SYSTEM, the network of nerves that conveys signals between the BASAL GANGLIA and the muscles. The person with Parkinson's often does not notice this resistance but may perceive aching and stiffness in the arm or leg. It is apparent to the doctor examining the person, however.

As can cogwheeling, lead pipe resistance can affect any muscle group on either side of a joint and is most commonly detected at the ankle, knee, wrist, and elbow. It is most often an ASYMMETRICAL, or one-sided, symptom. As Parkinson's progresses, the delays and confusion in the nerve communication between the brain and the muscles expand beyond symptoms such as lead pipe resistance and cogwheeling to become GAIT DISTURBANCES such as start hesitation and freezing of gait. The kind of rigidity that marks lead pipe resistance can be a symptom of other neurological conditions such as tumors of the basal ganglia; FUNCTIONAL IMAGING STUDIES such as MAGNETIC RESONANCE IMAGING (MRI) can identify these other conditions.

See also BALANCE; BRADYKINESIA; CARDINAL SYMPTOMS; DIAGNOSING PARKINSON'S; GAIT; POSTURAL INSTABILITY; TREMORS.

leg stride   The movement of the leg during WALKING. In normal stride, the walking movement begins from the hip and extends through the toe with each segment of the leg moving smoothly in a flowing sequence. When the forward step starts, the leg extends from the thigh to swing the entire leg ahead. When the heel contacts the floor, the knee bends and the lower leg pulls back. The typical reach during a normal walking pace is about 30 inches. For counterbalance, the arm on the opposite side swings forward with the leg stride; the right leg and the left arm move forward together as the left leg and the right arm move back. The shoulders and trunk also twist, further stabilizing the body during motion. The movements require a complex interaction of neurological and muscular events, although they take place without conscious thought or attention.

Parkinson's disease interferes with this interaction. As DOPAMINE levels decline, communication among NEURONS in the BRAIN becomes jumbled. Motor function reflects this confusion in alterations in GAIT, particularly leg stride. Starting with hip extension, the leg swing begins to shorten as the stride begins. This motion draws up the entire stride, and walking reach (the distance between the back foot and the forward foot) lessens. All joints in the leg—hip, knee, ankle—move shorter distances. Leg stride correspondingly slows, so the pace of walking decreases as well. The feet overlap when walking, shortening the reach of each step. Shuffling is an extreme form of stride shortening in which a foot may only move even less than an inch with each attempt to step forward. As Parkinson's progresses, leg stride diminishes to the shuffle that is characteristic of the disease. Correspondingly, arm swing and trunk movements also diminish, and the person appears to be walking in small steps that begin at the knees.

ANTI-PARKINSON'S MEDICATIONS that replace dopamine in the brain, such as DOPAMINE AGONISTS (which activate dopamine receptors in the brain in much the same way as does dopamine) and LEVODOPA (which is converted to dopamine in the brain), improve leg stride to normal or near-normal in early to middle stages of Parkinson's. Dopamine agonists are less potent than levodopa in improving gait. The ability of these medications to restore motor function wanes as DOPAMINERGIC NEURON degeneration continues, and gait disturbances such as festination (short, rapid steps) and freezing gait become more prominent.

See also ARM SWING; GAIT DISTURBANCE; POSTURAL INSTABILITY.

legal concerns As Parkinson's disease is a progressive, neurodegenerative condition that eventually limits a person's ability to take care of himself or herself, people with Parkinson's disease and their families face numerous legal concerns as disease advances. Families often must make decisions about how the person with Parkinson's will live, in matters related to

- Medical and health care needs and services
- Money management and financial matters
- Living arrangements

It is difficult for the person with Parkinson's to give up independence, and it is not easy for families to make decisions that take away independence. Families' knowledge that the decisions they are making are consistent with their loved one's wishes provides comfort and security. Families must work out key details in advance of the need to implement them. It is important to determine these details before there is any question about the person's competence to make decisions about them. Many families are able to handle financial and living arrangement matters informally, particularly when the person with Parkinson's is elderly and may already be accustomed to a spouse's or an adult child's managing such affairs. As the person with Parkinson's becomes less able to function independently, particularly when MENTAL STATUS and COGNITIVE IMPAIRMENT are factors, it is important that there be formal structures in place to allow a family member or trusted friend to make decisions on the person's behalf. If they are not, the courts may be forced to intervene and impose them by appointing someone to represent and protect the person's best interests.

Sometimes family members disagree about the appropriate actions to take on a loved one's behalf. It is important to know what are the lines of authority within the state of residence, as these vary among states. In most states, the spouse is the first line of authority, followed by adult children or siblings if there are no children. A few states recognize domestic partners, such as couples who have same-sex relationships or live together but are not married, as having the same status as spouses. Documents such as advance directives and durable power of attorney for asset management can help to avert clashes over these matters. Because there are significant consequences with regard to these matters, it is a good idea to consider consulting an attorney before preparing and signing documents. Attorneys who specialize in elder law or estate planning are particularly well versed in the full spectrum of needs.

Advance Directives

All adults should create ADVANCE DIRECTIVES. These are documents, most commonly a living will and a durable power of attorney for health care (DPHC), that detail the person's preferences and desires regarding medical decisions and treatment should the person become incapacitated and unable to articulate them. These documents pertain to matters such as resuscitation, "heroic efforts" to sustain life such as mechanical ventilation (breathing machine), and end of life nutritional support. The DPHC appoints a person, known as the agent, to represent the person in medical decisions.

The requirements for preparing advance directives vary among states; most hospitals, doctors' offices, and senior organizations or centers have informational brochures about applicable regulations and procedures. In many states, generic forms are available for people to fill out, modify as desired, and sign. Each doctor who provides care for the person with Parkinson's should have a copy of the person's advance directives, as should each hospital where the person receives care. As well, the person designated as the agent through a DPHC should have a copy available at all times.

Durable Power of Attorney for Asset Management

A durable power of attorney for asset management, sometimes called a durable power of attorney for finances or just a durable power of attorney, is a document that appoints an agent to handle the person's financial actions and decisions. It can be conditional (also called springing), becoming active only if the person becomes incapacitated, or imme-

diate (also called fixed), activated when it is signed. If conditional, the document should establish the circumstances under which the person will be considered incapacitated, such as on hospitalization or entry into a long-term care facility. Many families find that an immediate or fixed durable power of attorney for asset management allows the greatest flexibility, although it requires a high level of trust between the person with Parkinson's and other family members. Again, it is a good idea to consult an attorney about the most appropriate way to structure a durable power of attorney for asset management.

Conservatorship

In a conservatorship, a court appoints an individual to become responsible for managing an incapacitated person's affairs. This becomes necessary when such arrangements have not been made before the person's incapacitation. The appointed conservator, under supervision of the court, may oversee only financial matters (a conservator of the estate) or all decisions including residence and medical care (a conservator of the person). The conservator can be, and often is, a family member or close friend. However, he or she may not be the individual the person with Parkinson's, or even other family members, would have chosen. Although conservatorship is intended to protect the interests and assets of the incapacitated person, many people view it as intrusive and restrictive. The court approves all decisions and transactions. The conservator must report regularly to the court to account for all actions. Conservatorship is a complex legal process that requires an attorney's assistance.

In some states a conservator is called a guardian, although typically guardianship refers to legal responsibility for a minor child.

Medicaid

Many families find they are unable to manage the expenses of a prolonged degenerative health condition such as Parkinson's disease without running out of resources. The state-funded MEDICAID program is designed to provide assistance when this occurs. All states have different structures and requirements for their Medicaid programs; in general, Medicaid requires depletion of assets before a person qualifies. There are many ways for a person to protect key assets, such as home ownership, to maintain a reasonable standard of living for family members while qualifying for assistance. It is important to consult an attorney who specializes in Medicaid issues and estate planning to make sure transfers of property and other matters are handled appropriately. If they are not, the person with Parkinson's may not meet Medicaid requirements.

See also ACTIVITIES OF DAILY LIVING; ADJUSTING TO LIVING WITH PARKINSON'S; AMERICANS WITH DISABILITIES ACT; LONG-TERM CARE INSURANCE; MEDICAL INSURANCE; MEDICARE; MEMORY LOSS; MONEY MANAGEMENT, DAILY; PLANNING FOR THE FUTURE; RECORD KEEPING.

lesion   A break in the continuity of tissue. A lesion often is a tumor or scar. Sometimes motor symptoms arise from lesions in the BASAL GANGLIA or along the PYRAMIDAL PATHWAY. Imaging studies such as MAGNETIC RESONANCE IMAGING (MRI) usually can detect lesions. When symptoms leave doubt as to whether a disorder is Parkinson's disease, doctors often order such tests to rule out lesions as the cause of the symptoms. Test results that are negative for lesions do not provide confirmation of a Parkinson's diagnosis but may point in that direction.

ABLATION, sometimes called lesioning, is a surgical treatment for Parkinson's disease in which neurosurgeons create lesions in the THALAMUS, PALLIDUM, and other structures of the BRAIN related to movement for the purpose of disrupting nerve signals originating in these areas. As the death of DOPAMINERGIC NEURONS that is the hallmark trait of Parkinson's disease progresses, it causes increasing DOPAMINE depletion. Discontinuity in synaptic communication results, causing chaos and confusion in the nerve transmissions sent to the muscles that result in TREMORS. Ablative lesions reduce the volume of transmissions, easing and sometimes eliminating tremors. However. as Parkinson's progresses the damage in the basal ganglia continues and the jumbling of nerve signals returns.

See also NERVOUS SYSTEM; NEURON; PALLIDOTOMY; THALAMOTOMY.

lesioning   See ABLATION.

levodopa   A naturally occurring AMINO ACID that is a DOPAMINE precursor (substance that becomes dopamine in the body). Dopamine is the NEUROTRANSMITTER crucial for communication among neurons involved with motor function that becomes depleted in Parkinson's disease. Levodopa is synthesized into an oral drug that is the current cornerstone of dopamine REPLACEMENT TREATMENT for Parkinson's disease. Levodopa is almost always taken in combination with a DOPA DECARBOXYLASE INHIBITOR (DDCI) such as CARBIDOPA (Sinemet, Atamet) or BENSERAZIDE (Madopar) to slow peripheral metabolism, which takes place rapidly after levodopa enters the bloodstream. Levodopa is also available as a single drug, generically as levodopa or as the brand name products L-Dopa, Laradopa, and Dopar. However, taking levodopa without a DDCI requires much higher doses and causes much more side effects than combination preparations.

History of Levodopa Treatment

In the late 1950s the Swedish scientist Arvid Carlsson conducted milestone research into the functions and actions of neurotransmitters in the BRAIN. At the time, neurologists knew of dopamine's presence in the brain but believed it functioned only as an EPINEPHRINE precursor, as it did peripherally (in the body). Carlsson postulated that dopamine was itself a neurotransmitter on the basis of his research, in which very high doses of an antihypertensive medication (drug taken to treat high blood pressure), RESERPINE, administered to mice created symptoms similar to those of Parkinson's disease. The brains of the mice showed severe dopamine depletion, and Carlsson suspected a similar process occurred in Parkinson's disease.

In 1960 neuroscientist OLEH HORNYKIEWICZ, a researcher at the Brain Research Institute of Vienna University Medical School, conducted autopsy examinations of the brains of people who had died of various causes and discovered that those who had Parkinson's disease had substantially lower levels of dopamine, confirming Carlsson's assertions about dopamine's role as a neurotransmitter with actions essential to MOTOR FUNCTION. Meanwhile Carlsson and other researchers explored ways to replace diminished dopamine, again working with mice in which they induced the symptoms of Parkinson's with high doses of reserpine. Their efforts to use a synthesized form of naturally occurring dopamine (found in legumes), dihydrophenylalanine or dopa, were unsuccessful as the dopamine molecule is too large to cross the BLOOD-BRAIN BARRIER, and as a result dopa remains in peripheral circulation. Carlsson next tried levodopa, a naturally occurring PRECURSOR to dopamine also found in legumes, and this was successful. The levodopa molecule is small enough to cross the blood-brain barrier, allowing levodopa to enter the brain, where it becomes metabolized to dopamine. Carlsson developed a synthesized form of levodopa as well as a means for measuring its presence in the brain.

Hornykiewicz attempted the treatment on human volunteers with Parkinson's disease and reported success with the method in 1961. In 1967, the U.S. Food and Drug Administration approved levodopa as the first PHARMACOTHERAPY for Parkinson's disease, and levodopa has remained the mainstay of treatment for Parkinson's.

How Levodopa Works

Levodopa is taken as an oral medication and absorbed from the intestinal tract into the bloodstream. As an amino acid, it is absorbed quickly and easily, although the rate and the amount of drug that enter the bloodstream depend on numerous variables including the length of time it takes to move from the stomach to the intestines and the other substances being digested. It is important to note that transport of levodopa from the gut to the blood stream requires the action of protein transporters; this is the reason that eating protein too close to the time that one takes levodopa reduces the amount of levodopa that is absorbed. The enzyme DOPA DECARBOXYLASE rapidly metabolizes levodopa once it enters the bloodstream, so only a fraction of the dose taken actually reaches the brain. The peripheral conversions of levodopa to dopamine and of dopamine to epinephrine and NOREPINEPHRINE cause the unpleasant side effects such as NAUSEA that are common with levodopa treatment. Taking levodopa in combination with a dopa decarboxylase inhibitor such as carbidopa or

benserazide delays levodopa's peripheral metabolism, reducing side effects and allowing more of the levodopa to reach the brain.

Dopa decarboxylase in the brain also metabolizes levodopa to dopamine. Carbidopa cannot cross the blood-brain barrier, however, and so has no effect on this process in the brain. The new supply of dopamine replenishes the brain's dopamine levels, binding with DOPAMINE RECEPTORS (molecules on neurons that "accept" the dopamine molecules) on neurons in the SUBSTANTIA NIGRA, STRIATUM, and other structures of the BASAL GANGLIA that are responsible for motor function. This completes the communication circuit, and for a time neuron activity is normal. Neuron activity begins to deteriorate as the levodopa is used.

Limitations of Levodopa Treatment

Levodopa therapy generally is effective throughout the course of Parkinson's disease, but its use is associated with the onset of motor complications such as dyskinesia and on-off cycling, in which the medication's effects last a shorter and shorter time, as well as slowly decreasing quality of the on response. Some people go without developing many complications for over 20 years, and others begin to show signs of dopamine resistance within two or three years. The lack of a consistent pattern is frustrating to both clinicians and people with Parkinson's. The conventional approach to treating Parkinson's disease is to begin treatment with levodopa agonist monotherapy in younger people or levodopa MONOTHERAPY in elderly people or those with signs of cognitive impairment, when symptoms begin to impact daily function. Dopamine agonist monotherapy is particularly useful to try to delay the onset of motor complications even further by delaying levodopa's entry into the treatment regimen. There is even some evidence in humans that dopamine agonists may slow the progression of Parkinson's. There is some evidence from animal studies that suggest that giving a CATECHOL-O-METHYLTRANSFERASE (COMT) INHIBITOR with levodopa from the initiation of therapy may have benefits in delaying motor complications.

Once dopamine agonists are at their maximum tolerated dose, levodopa is usually added to the regimen. Once ON–OFF STATE fluctuations, DYSKINE-SIA, or DYSTONIA become problems, doctors then add other medications—such as AMANTADINE, ANTI-CHOLINERGIC MEDICATIONS (in young people with no cognitive problems) and CATECHOL-*o*-METHYLTRANS-FERASE (COMT) INHIBITOR MEDICATIONS—as ADJUNCT THERAPIES. These other medications extend the effectiveness of levodopa in various ways.

In the beginning of regular levodopa therapy symptom relief can extend for four hours or longer, but as Parkinson's progresses the effective time diminishes. Controlled release, or sustained release, forms of the medication can help extend the interval when levodopa is available in the bloodstream, which in turn significantly extends the time that levodopa is effective in the brain in early and middle stages of the disease. Controlled release forms have the relative disadvantage of being more variable in both the amount of lev-odopa that is absorbed, as well as the delay between when the medication is taken and when peak absorption occurs. As Parkinson's progresses it takes more levodopa to relieve symptoms, and relief is often incomplete or inconsistent. As well, adverse effects such as dystonia become more common, indicating that the brain is receiving more dopamine than existing dopamine receptors can accept. This creates a different kind of communication chaos among the neurons, overstimulating them and causing them to send a barrage of messages to the muscles that "jam' muscle response. Muscles cramp, spasm, or stiffen and freeze in awkward and often painful positions (dystonia). At this point there is little choice but to reduce the levodopa dosage, thus allowing the symptoms of Parkinson's to emerge.

Researchers believe the diminishing effectiveness of levodopa results from two factors: the continued death of DOPAMINERGIC NEURONS, which deepens the loss of dopamine at baseline, as well as provide less sites for levodopa to be converted to dopamine in the brain; there may also be dampened sensitivity among remaining DOPAMINE RECEPTORS to the action of the replacement dopamine. Researchers presume that the latter indicates that there are subtle but significant differences between endogenous dopamine (dopamine that the brain's dopaminergic neurons produce) and the replacement dopamine the brain metabolizes from levodopa. Some scientists suspect that levodopa, even as it functionally replaces dopamine in the brain, may actually accelerate the loss of dopaminergic neurons as it forces them to utilize energy to convert levodopa to dopamine, hence producing harmful free radicals. This possibility is difficult to assess, as dopamine replacement therapy (levodopa also masks the continuing degeneration of the brain's dopamine-producing mechanisms. Although some cell culture studies and a handful of animal studies support the acceleration of dopaminergic cell loss theory, all human evidence, the bulk of animal evidence, and even lots of cell culture evidence argue that there is no clear effect of levodopa in either accelerating or slowing the loss of dopaminergic neurons. Accordingly, most movement disorders experts believe that levodopa is safe and does not accelerate the course of Parkinson's disease.

Eventually the combination of events results in dopamine resistance, causing erratic response to levodopa therapy, fluctuating on–off state, and side effects such as dystonia and CHOREIFORM DYSKINE-SIA. Other drugs taken as ADJUNCT THERAPIES can help to offset these problems for a short time, but the continuing loss of dopaminergic neurons causes a relentless worsening of symptoms.

Side Effects and Interactions

Levodopa has numerous potential side effects, most of which can be unpleasant but are not harmful. Some side effects, however, can have serious health consequences. Side effects can either diminish or develop when the drug is taken over time. Levodopa also interacts with numerous drugs, interfering with their actions. As well, some drugs interfere with the absorption or action of levodopa.

People who have a condition called FAVISM cannot take levodopa. Favism, which is rare and appears mostly in people of Mediterranean descent, occurs when there is a deficiency of the ENZYME glucose-6-phosphate dehydrogenase (G6PD), which prevents levodopa metabolism. If a person takes levodopa as a medication or eats foods that are natural sources of levodopa (such as FAVA BEANS, also called broad beans or long beans), hemolytic anemia (premature destruction of red

Mild to Moderate Side Effects	Potentially Serious Side Effects	Drugs That Levodopa Interferes With	Drugs That Interfere With Levodopa
Lightheadedness, dry mouth, fatigue headaches	Choreic dyskinesia, dystonia	*Decrease in other drug's action:* digoxin, oral hypoglycemics, metoclopramide	*Decrease in levodopa action:* antacids, tricyclic antidepressants, butyrophenones, clonidine, methionine, papaverine, phenothiazines, phenytoin, propanolol, pyridoxine, thioxanthines
Stomach upset, diarrhea, constipation	Anxiety, depression psychosis, paranoia, dementia	*Increases in other drug's action:* antihypertensives, methyldopa	
	Irregular heartbeat, hypertension		
Weight gain or loss	Hemolytic anemia	*Other interactions:* MAOIs	
Insomnia, nightmares	Agranulocytosis		*Increase in levodopa action:* anticholinergics, furazolidone, metoclopramide
Blurred vision, double vision	Leukopenia		
	Thrombocytopenia		*Other interactions:* MAOIs
Increased tremor, mild dyskinesias	Activation of existing but undiagnosed malignant melanoma		
Excessive sweating			
Orthostatic hypotension			
Unusual breathing patterns			

blood cells) can develop. This condition affects the blood's ability to transport oxygen and can lead to serious health problems. A blood test called the Coombs' test can detect a G6PD deficiency, although a person who is already taking levodopa may have a false-positive test result. Testing for G6PD is most accurate before levodopa therapy begins, and some neurologists do it routinely. Although levodopa is safe for the vast majority of people who also have glaucoma, it can precipitate or exacerbate narrow angle glaucoma.

See also 3,4-DIHYDROXYPHENYLALANINE; ANTI-PARKINSON'S MEDICATIONS; CARE MANAGEMENT AND PLANNING; CONTROLLED RELEASE MEDICATION; FLUC-TUATING PHENOMENON; HOPE FOR A PARKINSON'S CURE; HORNYKIEWICZ, OLEH; MEDICAL MANAGEMENT; MEDICATION MANAGEMENT; MEDICATION SIDE EFFECTS; THERAPEUTIC WINDOW; TREATMENT ALGORITHM.

Lewy body   An abnormal deposit of protein, primarily alpha-synuclein, within a neuron, which is characteristically round and of greater density than the surrounding cell structure. The presence of Lewy bodies in the neurons of the SUBSTANTIA NIGRA, STRIATUM, and other structures of the BASAL GANGLIA is a hallmark trait of Parkinson's disease. At present the only way to detect Lewy bodies is at autopsy after death. Until recently, researchers believed Lewy bodies were unique to Parkinson's disease. However, in people with Parkinson's who have DEMENTIA as well as MOTOR FUNCTION symptoms, Lewy bodies also usually are present in the CEREBRUM (the part of the brain that controls cognitive function). Doctors sometimes diagnose this combination of pathology (brain changes) and symptoms as LEWY BODY DISEASE. In such cases, neither treatments for Parkinson's disease nor treatments for ALZHEIMER'S DISEASE are as effective as would be expected.

The researcher Fritz Lewy was the first to identify and describe, in 1912, the protein deposit structures that now bear his name. Lewy bodies form within the neuron's cytoplasm and when stained for visualization under a microscope look somewhat like a full solar eclipse—a dark brownish sphere in the center of a brighter orange-yellow sphere. A neuron can contain numerous Lewy bodies of varying sizes.

Researchers discovered the ALPHA-SYNUCLEIN GENE in 1997 and discovered mutations in it that are associated with familial Parkinson's disease. This gene controls the processes in which the body manufactures and uses alpha-synuclein, a protein that aids communication among neurons in the brain. The gene mutation allows neurons to produce more alpha-synuclein than is necessary. The excess alpha-synuclein molecules clump together, creating the characteristic deposits. Some researchers believe the deposits eventually "choke" the cell, causing it to die. Lewy body formation is one of the potential causes of Parkinson's disease; some scientists speculate that a concentration of Lewy bodies in the DOPAMINERGIC NEURONS of the basal ganglia initiates the accelerated deaths of these cells, resulting in the DOPAMINE DEPLETION that is the hallmark of Parkinson's disease. Genetic manipulations in flies and in mice demonstrate this sequence of events, but researchers do not yet know whether the same scenario unfolds in people. As well, laboratory research in which scientists exposed rats to high levels of the common pesticide rotenone produced Parkinson's-like symptoms with diffuse Lewy body infiltration. All of these factors point to Lewy bodies as having a role in Parkinson's disease, but the mechanisms of that role remain unclear. Some researchers now believe that Lewy bodies are just attempts to segregate and recycle errant proteins and, hence, are just markers of a natural protective reaction to the abnormal proteins and not destructive.

See also CHEMICAL TOXINS; GENE THERAPY; GENETIC PREDISPOSITION; PESTICIDES AND HERBICIDES; UBIQUITIN.

Lewy body disease A form of DEMENTIA, the symptoms of which resemble those of ALZHEIMER'S DISEASE, that results from LEWY BODY infiltration of BRAIN tissue and in which there are components of MOTOR FUNCTION impairment similar to the symptoms of Parkinson's disease. The condition is sometimes called diffuse Lewy body disease. It generally affects people who are older than age 60, although it can occur in people who are younger. The blend of symptoms makes differentiation of Lewy body disease from Parkinson's disease and Alzheimer's disease difficult.

Pathology and Symptoms of Lewy Body Disease

Lewy body disease resembles a combination of Alzheimer's and Parkinson's, as the person shows some of the classic or hallmark symptoms of each disease but full symptoms for neither disease. As well, Lewy body disease has a faster progression than either Alzheimer's or Parkinson's alone; typically death occurs within 10 to 15 years of the onset of symptoms. Neurologists have established the following diagnostic criteria for Lewy body disease:

- Significant and progressive COGNITIVE IMPAIRMENT including two or more symptoms such as MEMORY LOSS, thought disturbances, loss of analytical reasoning skills, DELUSIONS, and dementia
- Distinctive fluctuations in mental alertness and ability to focus, as the person experiences alternating periods of lucidity and impairment
- Persistent visual HALLUCINATIONS (seeing of objects or people that are not present)
- Frequent, unexplained FALLS or evidence of extrapyramidal symptoms such as the neuromuscular symptoms characteristic of Parkinson's disease
- Unexplained fainting or brief episodes of loss of consciousness

The overlaps with Parkinson's disease and Alzheimer's disease are obvious and make diagnosis difficult. Although at present this distinction makes little difference in the course of any of these diseases, it may in the near future provide further insights into the mechanisms of, and relationships among, all three that lead to more effective treatments.

Treatment of Lewy Body Disease

Treatment, as does diagnosis, remains an area of uncertainty. Medications to treat the symptoms of Alzheimer's disease generally are not effective at relieving dementia or improving COGNITIVE FUNCTION in Lewy body disease. ANTI-PARKINSON'S MEDICATIONS can relieve motor symptoms in those who have them, although the dementia continues to progress.

Doctors commonly prescribe atypical antipsychotic medications (especially QUETIAPINE) for people with moderate to severe Alzheimer's disease, to relieve dementia symptoms. Although doctors know that some people with Alzheimer's experience DYSTONIA (muscles "frozen" in distorted and often painful positions) and other serious motor symptoms as undesired side effects of antipsychotic medications, the reason for the apparent randomness of their incidence has eluded understanding. Researchers know, however, that the presence of Lewy bodies in the CEREBRUM, where they affect cognitive functions, increases the likelihood that they are present throughout the brain including the BASAL GANGLIA, where they affect motor functions. At the least, the diffusion of Lewy bodies into regions of the brain involved with movement compromises the functions of the EXTRAPYRAMIDAL SYSTEM (the network of nerve structures that serves as the viaduct for nerve–muscle communication).

Scientists speculate that little is required to push that compromise into dysfunction, causing motor symptoms to surface. In similar fashion, anti-Parkinson's medications often relieve motor symptoms in people with Lewy body disease but cause the emergence of symptoms of psychosis, for which the treatment of choice would ordinarily be an antipsychotic medication but in Lewy body disease is likely to exacerbate motor symptoms. Attempts to find the appropriate balance of medications to treat all of the symptoms becomes a spiral of frustration as one solution leads to other problems.

One bright spot in treatment is that many people who have symptoms of both Parkinson's and Alzheimer's, but may actually have Lewy body disease, is that symptoms of both diseases respond particularly well to ACETYLCHOLINESTERASE INHIBITOR MEDICATIONS such as rivastigmine (Exelon), DONEPEZIL (Aricept), GALANTAMINE (Reminyl), and TACRINE (Cognex); these are all called cholinesterase inhibitors, which extend the activity of ACETYLCHOLINE in the brain. Acetylcholine is a neurotransmitter with key functions in cognition that becomes depleted in Alzheimer's disease; scientists believe that its depletion is the core cause of the symptoms of Alzheimer's (as dopamine depletion is similarly the core cause of the symptoms of Parkinson's). Doctors typically prescribe acetylcholinesterase inhibitors to improve cognitive function and in doing so for people with Parkinson's who are experiencing cognitive impairment have discovered that these drugs also may improve motor symptoms in some people. Much research remains necessary to explore this effect, however, and at present the U.S. Food and Drug Administration (FDA) has approved acetylcholinesterase inhibitors only to treat cognitive dysfunction in Alzheimer's disease.

Why Lewy Body Disease Interests Parkinson's Disease Researchers

Parkinson's disease and Alzheimer's disease are far likelier to coexist with each other than chance would dictate. When they do, brain autopsy shows TAU plaques (protein-based deposits that lack the specific structure of Lewy bodies) and NEUROFIBRILLARY ENTANGLEMENTS with Alzheimer's disease as well as Lewy body deposits. This overlapping of symptoms and possibly of disease processes not only is part of the reason diagnosis and treatment are so challenging for these symptoms, but also is causing scientists to reconsider the disease definitions. Some researchers believe that people who have symptoms of both Alzheimer's and Parkinson's instead have Lewy body disease.

See also AGITATION; ANXIETY; CONDITIONS SIMILAR TO PARKINSON'S; CORTICOBASAL DEGENERATION; DIAGNOSING PARKINSON'S; EXTRAPYRAMIDAL SYMPTOM RATING SCALE.

lifestyle factors It is important for the person with Parkinson's disease to establish and follow lifestyle habits that support general good health and well-being. These include nutritious diet, regular physical activity and exercise, SOCIAL INTERACTION, and a network of supportive family and friends. For most people with Parkinson's, the years following diagnosis are generally ordinary aside from the ANTI-PARKINSON'S MEDICATIONS they take. The medications keep symptoms under control, sometimes for several decades, and the person generally can enjoy many of the same activities enjoyed before the diagnosis. Attitude and outlook make a significant difference in the way a person experiences Parkinson's disease, and the way Parkinson's affects the experience of living.

- Learn as much as possible about Parkinson's disease and stay informed about research and new findings.
- Follow prescribed medication regimens, including timing of dosages. Discuss concerns and side effects with the neurologist.
- Get enough rest and sleep. Sometimes anti-Parkinson's medications cause SLEEP DISTURBANCES such as insomnia (inability to fall or stay asleep) and disruption of rapid eye movement (REM) sleep; SLEEP MEDICATIONS or relaxation methods such as MEDITATION can help.
- Eat enough and eat the right foods. In the early and middle stages of Parkinson's disease, there are no dietary constraints. (In later Parkinson's stages, many doctors recommend restricting PROTEIN intake to allow maximal LEVODOPA absorption.) If appetite is diminished, eat small meals more frequently. Fruits and vegetables, especially eaten raw, contain valuable ANTIOXIDANTS and nutrients.
- Establish and practice breath control and breathing exercises. They help to keep the voice strong and energy-giving oxygen flowing to cells throughout the body.
- Keep the body active. Every day, move every body part. Learn YOGA postures that gently stretch and open the body, which help to maintain flexibility, strength, and balance and great stress relief. TAI CHI, a form of martial arts that uses slow, flowing, graceful movements, provides another excellent means to keep motor functions at their best.
- Enjoy life! This is an ideal time to reconsider personal priorities and restructure lifestyle to accommodate them. There is no reason for the person with Parkinson's to withdraw from living or from favorite activities as long as medications keep symptoms under control. Most people with Parkinson's can keep working, dri-

ving, traveling, and doing what gives them pleasure.

Although demographics establish Parkinson's as a disease of old age, in reality many people are diagnosed when they are in middle age and live with the disease for 20 years or longer. Lifestyle is a great influence in shaping those years.

See also ADJUSTING TO LIVING WITH PARKINSON'S; COPING WITH ONGOING CARE OF PARKINSON'S; EXERCISE AND ACTIVITY; JOY; MARRIAGE RELATIONSHIP; MEDITATION; OPTIMISM; PLANNING FOR THE FUTURE; PARENT/CHILD RELATIONSHIPS; QUALITY OF LIFE.

lightheadedness   A sensation of DIZZINESS and a feeling of being about to faint or lose consciousness. Lightheadedness is a common symptom of ORTHOSTATIC HYPOTENSION, a drop in blood pressure with a change in position (usually from lying down to sitting or standing). It is a good idea to pause for a few moments when changing position, to let the body stabilize. Lightheadedness is a common, mild, and usually harmless side effect of many ANTI-PARKINSON'S MEDICATIONS. The greatest risk of lightheadedness is loss of balance that causes a fall. Other factors that can cause or contribute to lightheadedness include low blood sugar level that results from inadequate food intake.

See also FALLS; HYPOTENSION, ORTHOSTATIC; MEDICATION SIDE EFFECTS.

lipopolysaccharides   Molecules that contain both lipids (fatty acids) and sugars that are part of the cellular structure of nearly all bacteria. Lipopolysaccharides (LPSs) are present in the healthy body and in health appear to have no harmful effects. Their levels increase when there is any inflammatory response, contributing to increased levels of FREE RADICALS (unstable molecules that scientists believe play a significant role in many disease processes). The DOPAMINERGIC NEURONS of the SUBSTANTIA NIGRA and STRIATUM appear particularly susceptible to lipopolysaccharide damage.

Researchers have been able to create the conditions of Parkinson's disease in laboratory animals by injecting lipopolysaccharides into these areas of the brain (often referred to as the LPS-induced animal model). Dopaminergic neurons quickly die in response, causing disruptions to MOTOR FUNCTION that are identical to the symptoms of Parkinson's. They hope that such studies will increase understanding of environmental influences on the development of Parkinson's disease and help to determine to what extent, if any, reducing exposure to lipopolysaccharides lowers the risk of development of Parkinson's.

See also ANTIOXIDANT; COMPLEX I; ENDOTOXIN; ENVIRONMENTAL TRIGGERS; EXOTOXIN; MITOCHONDRIAL DYSFUNCTION; NEUROPROTECTIVE THERAPIES.

livido reticularis A side effect of some ANTI-PARKINSON'S MEDICATIONS, particularly AMANTADINE (Symmetrel), in which there is a purplish mottling of the skin. It can appear anywhere on the body but is most common on the lower arms and lower legs. The term means "dark-colored network" in reference to the lacelike network of blood vessels under the surface of the skin that causes the appearance of mottling. Livido reticularis can be a symptom of severe illness such as renal crisis (impending kidney failure) and cardiovascular disease, so a doctor should always be consulted with its occurrence.

See also MEDICATION MANAGEMENT; MEDICATION SIDE EFFECTS.

living will See ADVANCE DIRECTIVES.

load response See GAIT.

loneliness Feeling of being isolated and removed from social contact and other people. When Parkinson's disease is in its early stages, it typically does not alter the person's lifestyle. The person can remain active and involved with work, friends, and social activities. As symptoms progress, however, mobility becomes limited. Favorite activities may no longer be possible, and contact with friends must rely on their visits. A person who continues working until symptoms make it necessary to retire or quit loses a strong social network at that time. As well, the person with Parkinson's may find his or her symptoms embarrassing or too challenging to manage in public.

Loneliness arises from the sense of loss that results from these changes. FRIENDSHIPS remain important, however, and are key to overcoming feelings of loneliness. The person with Parkinson's often is reluctant to ask others to visit; caregivers and family members can help by arranging visits that are comfortable for the person with Parkinson's. Often there are other shared activities that friends can enjoy together.

Loneliness also becomes a challenge for caregivers, who often feel isolated by the demands of caring for the person with Parkinson's. It is important for caregivers to find time and ways to maintain their friendships and some level of social interaction. Sometimes a friend can visit the person with Parkinson's and allow the caregiver a brief respite to get away.

See also ADJUSTING TO LIVING WITH PARKINSON'S; CAREGIVER WELL-BEING; DEPRESSION.

long-term care An inclusive term that encompasses a range of health care and related services that a person may need for an extended period. Care may include hiring of health care professionals who provide care in the home, such as home health nurses and physical therapists, or admission to residential care, as in an ASSISTED LIVING FACILITY, a SKILLED NURSING FACILITY (SNF), or a LONG-TERM CARE FACILITY. Although it is a common perception that long-term care relates to care in a residential setting other than the home, more people receive long-term care services at home than in residential care facilities. Home services extend the care options available for those who are partially independent. Private MEDICAL INSURANCE plans and MEDICAID may cover part of the related expenses of in-home services.

See also CARE MANAGEMENT AND PLANNING; HOSPICE; HOSPITALIZATION; MEDICAL MANAGEMENT; MEDICARE; RESPITE CARE.

long-term care facility A residential facility that provides care for people whose physical and health circumstances prevent them from living independently. State agencies accredit or license long-term facilities according to state laws and regulations (including MEDICAID) as well as in compliance with federal MEDICARE regulations. The staff at long-term care facilities include registered nurses, licensed practical nurses (called licensed vocational nurses in some states), certified nursing assistants, physical therapists, occupational therapists, speech pathologists, recreational therapists, dietitians, and other allied health care personnel. Long-term care facilities provide complete care, including personal care and any needed medical treatments. There are no limits to the time a person can remain in a long-term care facility.

The decision to move a person with Parkinson's to a long-term care facility is a difficult and emotional one for families. It requires a candid assessment of the person's abilities, needs, and rate of decline. PLANNING FOR THE FUTURE when the person with Parkinson's can express his or her preferences and participate in care decisions makes the process easier. Planning also allows time to make a careful selection of the facilities that the person and family members consider best suited to the person's needs. Most long-term care facilities have admissions coordinators on staff who can talk with families about care needs, services the facility provides, and financial matters.

Facility Licensing or Certification

All states have licensing requirements for RESIDENTIAL CARE facilities, typically managed through the state's department of health and social services, these requirements vary considerably among states. Choose a facility that meets Medicare and Medicaid standards, regardless of the financial status of the person with Parkinson's, to assure the most consistent level of care. Ask to see documentation of licensing or certification. Also ask the facility as well as the state's licensing agency to review all records for inspections and any disciplinary or censure actions. Additionally, look for a long-term care facility that is certified by an industry organization to meet industry-established standards of care. Finally, check with the local Better Business Bureau and similar organizations to see whether there are complaints about the way the facility does business.

Physical Environment

Visit the long-term care facility several times. It is good to schedule an appointment with the facility's admissions coordinator or director and to have an escorted tour of the facility to see all areas of interest. It is also important to drop by the facility at varying times during the day, to get a sense of the level of activity, efforts and attitude of the staff, and overall operational mode of the facility. These drop-in visits should include a brief look at common areas such as dining rooms as well as walking down corridors where resident rooms are located. Some facilities ask all visitors to check in at the office; if this is the case, someone should be available to walk along on the "tour" if the facility requires this. Be leery of any facility that allows visits only with scheduled appointments.

On visits to facilities, pay attention to

- Cleanliness: Floors, walls, and furniture should look and feel clean. Corridors should be free of clutter such as wheelchairs, walkers, laundry carts, utility carts, and other objects that block clear passage. The facility should smell clean as well.

- Staff attitude and appearance: Do staff smile and greet residents and visitors? How do staff address residents? Are staff neatly dressed and groomed?

- Staff attentiveness: Do all staff appear engaged with resident care? How long do they take to answer call lights?

- Resident appearance: Are residents up in chairs or walking during the main part of the day? or do most residents appear to be lying in bed? Do residents appear clean, appropriately clothed, and comfortable? This is a key reason to visit at different times of the day, to get a sense of the facility's routines and how residents spend their time.

- Activities: What level of organized or structured activities take place during the day? Do staff seem enthusiastic? Do residents actively participate? Are there a variety of activities to meet different interests and needs?

- Meals: Ask to walk through the dining room. Do meals look inviting? Do people appear to be enjoying their food? Are there enough staff to assist residents who need help?

- Medical care: Is it possible to identify staff who are nurses? Are medication and treatment carts attended or left standing in corridors? Do staff wash their hands before and after providing any personal care or services for residents?

Financial Matters

Neither Medicare nor medical insurance pays for a person's stay in a long-term care facility, so it is crucial to consider financial concerns in advance. Costs can range from $40,000 to well over $100,000 a year, depending on the geographic location, the spectrum of services the facility offers, and the person's needs. Because many families soon exhaust their resources, FINANCIAL PLANNING is essential. Each person's circumstances are unique; the long-term care facility's admissions coordinator typically can provide suggestions and recommendations for the most effective management of financial matters, including evaluation of resources, LONG-TERM CARE INSURANCE, and applicable Medicare and Medicaid requirements.

For economic reasons long-term care facilities strive to keep their occupancy high. When it appears that the need for a long-term care setting is imminent, discuss a possible timeline with the facility's admissions coordinator. Although facilities do not reserve space, they can plan to match availability with prospective residents.

See also ASSISTED LIVING FACILITY; HOME HEALTH CARE; HOSPICE; HOSPITALIZATION; RETIREMENT COMMUNITY; SKILLED NURSING FACILITY (SNF).

long-term care insurance An insurance plan to cover some of the expenses of residence and services in a LONG-TERM CARE FACILITY. Some plans also pay for services provided in a person's home. There are many variations on the terms of coverage, including the services that are covered or excluded, deductibles and copayments (out-of-pocket expenses), "trigger events," length of coverage, and number of events the plan allows. It is essential to

know these details before purchasing a long-term care insurance plan. In many cases, it is not possible to get long-term care insurance after a condition such as Parkinson's is diagnosed, and a plan may exclude services related to any medical conditions existing at the time the plan is purchased. Many companies offer long-term care insurance plans among their employee benefit programs. It is important to determine whether there is a conversion option to maintain the plan if employment ends and whether conversion requires qualifying for coverage.

Most long-term care insurance plans are designed to pay what the industry calls a daily benefit allowance. Typically this is a flat amount, although some plans cover a percentage of the facility's actual charges. The plan may cover a certain number of days or specify a fixed total payout. What the plan pays also may be related to other resources, paying against remaining balances. Decisions regarding long-term care insurance, as in other FINANCIAL PLANNING matters, should take into account the person's entire financial picture. As well, it often is valuable to consult an independent insurance agent who has no vested interest in a particular company or plan to compare benefits, costs, limitations, and requirements of long-term care insurance plans, taking into consideration the person's specific needs and circumstances. Medicare and most private medical insurance policies have no benefits for long-term care.

See also CARE MANAGEMENT AND PLANNING; ESTATE PLANNING.

lorazepam An ANTIANXIETY MEDICATION in the benzodiazepine family taken to relieve ANXIETY, distress, and AGITATION. Lorazepam also may help relieve symptoms of Parkinson's disease such as muscle spasms, muscle cramps, RIGIDITY, and DYSTONIA (stiffness and distortions of the muscles). It also is often taken as a sleep medication. In people who take lorazepam, commonly prescribed as the brand name product Ativan, for more than six months a resistance to its effects may develop; in that case another benzodiazepine medication is sometimes effective. All benzodiazepines, including lorazepam, have a risk from mild to moderate of addiction. In general, the longer the length of action of a benzodiazepine, the less the risk of addiction. Lorazepam has a moderately long length of action and a lower risk of addiction than triazolam (Halcion) and alprazolam (Xanax), a similar addiction potential to temazepam (Restoril) and diazepam (Valium), and more addiction potential than clonazepam (Klonopin). Although the benzodiazepines generally all have the same actions and potential side effects, people respond differently to individual drugs within this pharmacological family. The most common side effect of lorazepam is drowsiness, which typically ends after the medication has been taken for two to three weeks.

See also AGITATION; ANXIETY; CLONAZEPAM; DEPRESSION; DIAZEPAM; FLURAZEPAM; MENTAL STATUS; TEMAZEPAM.

macroelectrode   A conductive device that measures the electrical activity in a group of neurons. Macroelectrodes attached to the scalp transmit electrical signals and patterns from the BRAIN during an ELECTROENCEPHALOGRAM (EEG), for example. Neurosurgeons use macroelectrodes to help identify and stimulate (by sending a mild electrical current) regions of the brain during ablative surgery such as DEEP BRAIN STIMULATION (DBS), PALLIDOTOMY or THALAMOTOMY, procedures that insert stimulating electrodes into target areas of the brain create LESIONS (scar tissue) in the PALLIDUM, or lesion the THALAMUS, respectively, to disrupt NEURON activity to lessen parkinsonian symptoms such as TREMORS, RIGIDITY, or BRADYKINESIA.

See also ABLATION; MACROELECTRODE STIMULATION; MICROELECTRODE.

macroelectrode stimulation   A procedure in which a neurosurgeon uses a MACROELECTRODE to stimulate, or activate, specific NEURON clusters to confirm their functions. Different structures in the BRAIN, such as the PALLIDUM, subthalamic nucleus (STN), and the THALAMUS, produce unique patterns of electrical activity. The neurosurgeon uses the responses from macroelectrode stimulation to make sure microelectrodes are in correct position during surgeries such as PALLIDOTOMY, THALAMOTOMY, and DEEP BRAIN STIMULATION (DBS). During these surgeries the person is sedated but awake, so he or she can respond to instructions from the neurosurgeon and provide additional information about any sensations that macroelectrode stimulation produces. Macroelectrode stimulation is painless, although it sometimes evokes responses such as perception of particular tastes or smells or movement of a part of the body. These responses help the neurosurgeon create a "map" of the brain's functional areas.

See also ABLATION; STEREOTAXIS.

Madopar   See BENSERAZIDE.

magnesium   A mineral that is essential to enable cells to produce adenosine triphosphate (ATP), the primary energy source for cell functions. Magnesium enters the body through diet. Along with calcium, magnesium is essential for electrical conductivity among cells, particularly in the BRAIN and NERVOUS SYSTEM and in the heart. There is some evidence that increasing magnesium intake, either through dietary sources or supplementation, enhances NEURON communication in the BRAIN. Magnesium and calcium function in concert to balance cell functions. Calcium carries signals that induce activity; magnesium carries signals that terminate activity. Magnesium also helps maintain bone tissue and has a mild muscle relaxant effect.

A healthy adult who eats nutritiously gets enough magnesium through dietary sources; red meat, whole grains, and dark green vegetables such as broccoli, spinach, beans, and peas are high in magnesium. The person with Parkinson's who eats small amounts of limited foods often does not get enough magnesium (or other vital nutrients) through dietary sources. As well, difficulty in eating, particularly with chewing and swallowing, curbs food choices, as does the protein restriction that becomes important later in LEVODOPA treatment. Many doctors recommend a vitamin supplement that includes magnesium for people whose Parkinson's disease is in the mid to later stages. It is possible, however, to have an excess of magnesium, which can cause health problems such as arrhythmias (irregular heartbeat). Most people should not exceed the recommended dietary allowance (RDA) for magnesium, which is 350 milligrams for an adult, without a doctor's instruction to do so.

See also NUTRITION AND DIET; METABOLIC NEEDS; NUTRITIONAL SUPPLEMENTS.

magnet therapy   See ALTERNATIVE THERAPIES.

magnetic feet   See GAIT DISTURBANCE.

magnetic resonance imaging   (MRI)   A noninvasive method for creating visual images of internal body structures and organs. During an MRI, the person lies flat on a special table that slides inside a large tubelike device. The outer layer of the device contains magnetic coils that surround the body; the inner layer contains radio frequency coils that send and receive radio signals (waves of electromagnetic energy). The MRI's powerful magnets surround the body in a magnetic field that polarizes the hydrogen atoms in the body's tissues, causing them to align uniformly (all in the same direction). Then radio frequency coils send radio signals into the body, to excite the atoms into motion. When the radio signals stop, the atoms realign themselves and in so doing send out electrical signals that transmitters in the radio frequency coils pick up. The coils send these signals to a computer. Various kinds of cells realign at different rates, which the computer translates into visual, and typically three-dimensional, images. MRI produces extraordinarily precise, high-resolution images that are capable of detecting all sorts of problems ranging from muscle and ligament tears to tumors no bigger than a few cells.

MRI's primary value in Parkinson's disease is to rule out other possible causes of symptoms such as brain lesions (tumors), structural anomalies, stroke, and other NEURODEGENERATIVE disorders such as MULTIPLE SCLEROSIS, in which the MRI often can show the demyelinization of neurons that is characteristic of that disease. In late Parkinson's disease MRI sometimes can visualize the loss of DOPAMINERGIC NEURONS in the SUBSTANTIA NIGRA and STRIATUM, visualization serves no therapeutic

purpose and is primarily of interest to researchers studying the ways in which Parkinson's disease progresses.

Researchers have also been looking at ways to obtain more than just information on anatomy (structure) with MRI. In magnetic resonance spectroscopy (MRS) special equipment and techniques allow researchers to look for concentrations of a certain chemical in each little voxel, the small unit of volume of the brain (sometimes as small as cube a few millimeters in each dimension) that is treated as a single unit for computational purposes, which appears to have much promise in the evaluation of possible brain tumors. Another research technique is functional MRI (fMRI) in which special techniques and equipment are used to estimate the amount of blood flow to each area of the brain; fMRI has been used to study Parkinson's disease and the changes in blood flow in different areas of the basal ganglia and brain that occur with ANTIPARKINSON'S MEDICATIONS and DEEP BRAIN STIMULATION (DBS).

There is no special preparation for MRI, and MRI causes no discomfort, although some people do not like the closed-in feeling of being inside the magnetized tube. Sometimes the radiologist injects a contrast agent into a vein, to improve the details of the image. People with magnetic metals implanted in their bodies, such as stainless steel pins or plates used to repair bone fractures or aneurysm clips, or devices such as pacemakers cannot have MRI. Some dental implants contain magnetic metals as well; the radiologist should know of these to make a determination about whether it is safe to proceed with MRI. The magnets of MRI are so powerful that they can move implanted metals. They also can cause any metal object in the room at the time the magnets are activated to fly around, a very dangerous condition. Radiology staff ask that the person remove any and all metal, including bra straps, watches, eyeglasses, and other items. The MRI magnets also demagnetize credit cards. The radiology department should provide a secure place to leave such items.

See also COMPUTED TOMOGRAPHY (CT) SCAN; DIAGNOSING PARKINSON'S; FUNCTIONAL IMAGING STUDIES; MYELIN SHEATH; POSITRON EMISSION TOMOGRAPHY; SINGLE PHOTON EMISSION COMPUTED TOMOGRAPHY.

marriage relationship Diagnosis of a chronic condition such as Parkinson's disease has a significant effect on the relationship between spouses (and nonmarried life partners) in numerous ways. It presents challenges for the partner with Parkinson's as well as the partner who will become caregiver. Meeting these challenges with HONESTY, COMPASSION, and a spirit of collaboration is important.

For many couples, the diagnosis of Parkinson's has little effect on daily living at first or may even improve it as finally there is an explanation for the symptoms the person has been experiencing and the ANTI-PARKINSON'S MEDICATIONS are now keeping those symptoms in check. Work, social activities, family functions, and recreational interests go on as usual. This state can lull partners into believing there is no reason to discuss the possibilities of an uncertain future, as nothing looks especially different. Yet such communication is critical from the onset. It establishes a pattern of open dialogue and sharing that becomes the foundation for the more difficult challenges that lie ahead. As important as it is to continue a normal life, it is essential to prepare for the changes that are part of the overall picture of Parkinson's.

Whichever partner has Parkinson's, the roles of both partners gradually shift. The partner with Parkinson's becomes less able to manage physical tasks, so the caregiver partner takes those over. A key challenge for both partners often is determining when it is time to transition responsibilities. The unpredictable course and daily variations of Parkinson's make it difficult to know when a function, such as driving or paying the bills, is no longer possible. Partners who begin the Parkinson's journey in collaboration are better able to manage these challenges and changes than those who forge ahead with the presumption that when the time comes to express their needs, they will communicate. Unfortunately, the cognitive and physical abilities necessary for such communication are sometimes casualties of Parkinson's.

Most couples sometimes feel intense frustration about the unfairness of the changes Parkinson's forces on the INTIMACY of their relationships. Just as the neurologic degeneration of Parkinson's affects walking and fine motor skills, it also often affects physical intimacy. Actions once nearly automatic, such as holding hands and hugging, can become slow and clumsy. The same neurodegeneration that slows intestinal function can cause erectile dysfunction in a man, impeding the flow of nerve signals and muscle response that permit an erection. The medication sildenafil (Viagra) often is effective in restoring sexual function and does not interact with ANTI-PARKINSON'S MEDICATIONS (however, men who are taking nitrate medications for heart disease cannot use sildenafil).

Patience and humor are important for both partners as they learn how to accommodate these deteriorations and still have a loving, intimate relationship. Most couples who have had satisfying sexual relationships before Parkinson's do not lose desire for each other because of the Parkinson's but may feel uncomfortable or confused about how to express that desire within the constraints that Parkinson's imposes. With open, honest communication and planning, most couples can remain sexually intimate for as long as both partners enjoy the relationship.

Additional challenges can surface when the caregiving partner also has, or develops, health problems, as is more likely to occur among older couples. These problems may require particularly careful planning to meet the caregiving and financial needs for both partners.

See also ADJUSTING TO LIVING WITH PARKINSON'S; CARE MANAGEMENT AND PLANNING; CAREGIVER WELL-BEING; COPING WITH ONGOING CARE OF PARKINSON'S; ESTATE PLANNING; INTIMACY; FAMILY RELATIONSHIPS; FINANCIAL PLANNING; OPTIMISM; PARENT/CHILD RELATIONSHIPS; PREGNANCY; SEXUAL DYSFUNCTION; SEXUALITY.

masked face See HYPOMIMIA.

massage therapy See ALTERNATIVE THERAPIES.

Meals on Wheels A not-for-profit organization of more than 3,200 local programs throughout the United States that prepares and delivers nutritious, hot meals daily to seniors who need such assistance to remain independent. Federal, state, and local funding supports the programs, which also charge a nominal fee (income-adjusted, if necessary) for meals. The program that evolved into Meals on Wheels started in the United States in 1954, modeled after a program that started during World War II in England. Today a substantial level of funding and other support for Meals on Wheels is provided through the U.S. Agency on Aging's Elderly Nutrition Program.

Many local Meals on Wheels programs provide two meals a day, a hot meal and a cold meal, in a single delivery to a senior's home. There are no income restrictions to qualify for services, although people requesting reduced rates may need to provide income verification. Most programs charge $6 to $8 a day; however, cost varies among locations. Generally a person must be 60 years of age or older, although most Wheels on Meals programs also accept younger people who have disabilities, such as those with Parkinson's disease, that prevent them from shopping for groceries and preparing their own meals.

Registered DIETITIANS plan the meals, which are then prepared and packaged in commercial kitchens. Most programs accommodate certain special nutritional requirements, such as low-sodium or diabetic diets. The two meals for each day typically provide two-thirds of the recommended calories and nutritional requirements. Most programs provide meals seven days a week, although some may deliver four meals on Saturdays and forgo Sunday deliveries. Service can be provided to meet temporary needs, such as during recovery from surgery, or long-term needs. Local telephone directories list contact information; in most areas, a phone call is all that is required to establish eligibility and sign up for meals. Local senior and social services organizations also know about services available in their area. Most Wheels on Meals programs can begin service immediately; those in smaller communities may have waiting lists.

See also NUTRITION AND DIET; EATING; METABOLIC NEEDS.

Medicaid A government-funded medical insurance and health care services program for people who do not have other MEDICAL INSURANCE and cannot afford to pay for needed services. There are strict asset-based requirements for qualification. The federal government and state governments formalized the structure of Medicaid in 1965, establishing a system under Title XIX of the Social Security Act for jointly funding state-managed programs. About 36 million Americans, many of them elderly, receive Medicaid support each year. Medicaid is the largest payer for residential long-term care services in the United States, covering about 80 percent of those in long-term care facilities.

Although the federal government establishes the general framework for Medicaid services, each state structures and administers its Medicaid program, setting its own eligibility requirements, benefits levels, and payment structures. Appendix II, Directory of State Medicaid Offices, lists the Medicaid contact information for each state. States have the option of enhancing basic Medicaid services through state-funded benefits and less restrictive eligibility qualifications but must provide the minimal benefits established by federal guidelines to qualify for matching funds to support state services.

Medicaid is a particular concern for people with Parkinson's who are at a point in the disease's progression at which they need more extensive care than a home caregiver can provide and are facing admission to a LONG-TERM CARE FACILITY. Few families have the financial resources to accommodate this need beyond several months to perhaps several years; care in a long-term care facility ranges from $40,000 to more than $100,000 a year, depending on the facility's services and the person's level of need.

General Medicaid Eligibility Requirements

At their most basic level of qualification, Medicaid programs generally tie program eligibility to federal poverty guidelines: That is, to qualify for Medicaid assistance a person can have an income no higher than a certain percentage of the established federal poverty level. Federal economists adjust this level annually, so this aspect of qualification changes from year to year. As well, Medicaid considers a person's assets—any property, tangible or intangible, that the person owns. In certain specified situations, a person may exceed income and asset limits but qualify as "medically needy." There are no requirements related to age; Medicaid serves people of all ages who meet other program qualifications. These qualifications vary widely among states and typically change from year to year. States have broad latitude to use income and resources guidelines that are less restrictive than federal guidelines to establish eligibility for their programs.

General Medicaid Benefits and Services

Medicaid covers a broad base of medical services through basic and enhanced programs. Each state's program is required to cover basic benefits, which include the following:

- Hospital services including inpatient hospitalization, surgery, outpatient care (including emergency department), lab, X-ray, and other diagnostic procedures
- Doctor, nurse practitioner, and medical clinic services
- Care and services in a residential nursing facility (long-term care facility)
- Home health care as an alternative to care in a residential nursing facility
- Family services including family planning and supplies and screenings, early and periodic screening, diagnosis, and treatment (EPSDT) services for family members younger than age 21
- Services for medical and surgical dental needs (but not routine dental prophylaxis)

States determine the benefits, beyond basic benefits, their programs will provide. The federal government provides matching funds to support additional benefits. Common extended benefits often include:

- Routine dental care and prophylaxis
- Optometry services and eyeglasses
- Prescription medications
- Prosthetic devices
- By waiver (specific written permission), services such as home-based care management, personal care, respite care, home health aide, and other needed services

Medicaid programs contract with community providers to provide care and services, and the person receiving Medicaid benefits can choose among them for care. These providers, which include hospitals, doctors, and pharmacies, agree to accept Medicaid payments for services as payment in full. A growing delivery model in state Medicaid programs is managed care, in which people receiving Medicaid agree to receive care through a closed network of providers. This structure helps states to keep greater control over the costs of medical services. In return, the managed care program provides extended benefits such as payment for prescription medications.

Asset Protection and Spend-Down

It is prudent for most people to begin thinking about asset protection early after a diagnosis of Parkinson's disease. Asset protection is a method of legally transferring resources and ownership to others, so they do not become counted against Medicaid eligibility. Asset protection can help assure that at least some of the resources the person with Parkinson's has worked a lifetime to accumulate remain available to support the spouse and family. This is best done with the advice of an attorney who specializes in ESTATE PLANNING or elder law. Spend down is a process of spending assets to reach the qualification mark for Medicaid. Although it serves the purpose of qualifying the person with Parkinson's for Medicaid benefits, usually to pay for the services of a long-term care facility, spend down does not leave many resources for surviving family members.

Medicaid has strict requirements governing spend down procedures. In general, resources used for spend down must be allocated medical expenses; a person cannot gift property or money to relatives to eliminate assets. Income and resource levels are minimal and to a great extent require the person with Parkinson's to deplete savings, possessions of value, and even cash-value life insurance policies. Extensive reforms to Medicaid regulations in 1988 made it possible for a person's spouse to maintain certain assets (such as a home) without jeopardizing his or her spouse's eligibility. However, Medicaid spend down remains a difficult and complex process. Long-term care facilities generally have staff who work with families to help them meet Medicaid qualifications.

The earlier a family begins planning to protect assets, the less traumatic the spend down process is. It is important to begin spend down early enough before the anticipated time of need, as well; Medicaid looks at all asset disbursements in the previous 30-month period to determine whether they are qualifying spend down actions. If they are determined to be nonqualifying, the person must spend an additional amount to compensate. There are ways to establish Medicaid trusts, such as to cover funeral expenses, that can divert assets within Medicaid guidelines. Again, a long-term care facility's representative or a lawyer specializing in elder law can help determine whether this is a prudent action.

Medicare–Medicaid Dual Eligibility

Some people who qualify for Medicare but have limited income and resources are also eligible for at least some Medicaid benefits to help pay for medical expenses. Each program covers certain services the other does not, so that the respective program pays for covered services. One of the most significant differences in this regard for the person with Parkinson's is that Medicaid provides coverage for prescription medications whereas Medicare does not. In situations in which there are overlaps of coverage for services, Medicare pays first and Medicaid pays the balance. Even seniors enrolled in Medicare who do not meet the qualifications for full Medicaid support are sometimes eligible for limited medical benefits through Medicaid as well as partial or complete assistance in paying Medicare Part B premiums.

See also CARE MANAGEMENT AND PLANNING; FINANCIAL PLANNING; LEGAL CONCERNS; MEDICAL INSURANCE.

medical insurance   A privately purchased insurance plan that pays for medical care including hospitalization, surgery, doctor visits, and related services. Each medical insurance plan has specific coverage requirements; many plans have copayments and deductibles (amounts the insured person pays out of pocket). Most medical insurance plans provide at least partial coverage for prescrip-

tion drugs; some do not. Medical care is the most costly consumer expense after housing in the United States. Although medical insurance rates may be $3,500 to $7,000 a year or more, depending on the plan's coverage, a single surgery such as an emergency appendectomy (removal of an infected appendix) costs as much or more. So can a year's worth of ANTI-PARKINSON'S MEDICATIONS.

If there is a single rule that applies to all medical insurance plans, it is to know the plan. Know the benefits, limitations, restrictions, exclusions, copayments, deductibles, grace periods (if any) for premium payments, cancellation procedures, and renewal requirements. Medical insurance complex is a legal contract that deserves careful consideration and thorough review. Yet most people know little more about their medical insurance than its rates and copayments. Even for a group plan through an employer, request a copy of the full medical plan from the employer's benefits coordinator or human resources department. A summary of benefits or benefits brochure, which is what most employers distribute to employees, is not adequate for determining coverage of health conditions as complex as Parkinson's disease. When medical insurance does not cover a service it is the insured person's responsibility to pay the costs, which can quickly become substantial.

Kinds of Medical Insurance Plans

There are a number of different kinds of medical insurance plans. Most fit into one of the following general benefit structures. Some combine structures, such as participating provider plans that also offer fee-for-service coverage (usually at a reduced benefit level). A person always has the right to go outside the benefit structure for care, such as to see a specialist that the plan does not cover, at his or her own expense. It is important to know the ramifications of this, however. If that specialist orders tests, the insurance plan may not cover those tests. Always obtain clarification from the insurance company before going outside the plan's network.

- Managed care organizations or structures: Many medical insurance plans require people to use designated provider networks to receive benefits. Typically a PRIMARY CARE PHYSICIAN oversees a person's medical care and must authorize any specialty referrals. The most common structures are health maintenance organizations (HMOs) and preferred provider organizations (PPOs). A few HMOs across the country are staff model HMOs, meaning they own the hospitals, medical centers, laboratories, and other facilities and hire the providers (doctors, nurses, and other health care professionals). PPOs are community providers who have signed agreements with the insurance company to accept specified payment or reimbursement and to follow the insurance company's procedures and guidelines regarding medical services. Managed care plans may refuse to pay for care provided outside their networks; it is essential to know the requirements for out-of-network and out-of-area (such as when traveling) coverage.

- Fee-for-service plans: These medical insurance plans, sometimes called major medical plans, pay set fees for covered services, and the insured person must pay the difference between the benefit amounts and the charges billed. Typically there is a limit or cap on the total out-of-pocket expenses a person may have to pay in a year. With such a plan, a person often can self-refer to a specialist, if the specialist will accept patients without a referral (many will not).

Obtaining or Maintaining Medical Insurance

Most people who have private medical insurance have it as an employment benefit; the insured person pays part or all of the monthly premiums. Such group medical insurance plans typically offer broad-based coverage. The person and his or her family, if applicable, remain eligible for the plan as long as the person remains employed. There are extensions of coverage and conversion options when ending employment; these generally require the person to pay the full premium, are time-limited, and can affect a person's right to obtain individual medical insurance in the future (see the discussion of HIPAA in the next section). As well, they may apply only under specific circumstances and may not apply if the person retires. Individual medical insurance, which a person purchases independently of employment, typically costs more and covers less. State laws regarding individual medical insurance vary widely, so coverage and rates can differ significantly. Many states offer subsidized medical insurance (different from MEDICAID) for people who meet certain income and other criteria.

Nearly all medical insurance plans renew annually. Benefits, exclusions, restrictions, and rates can, and often do, change at each renewal period. It is important to review the plan carefully at each renewal period. Some plans continue a person's enrollment unless the person files paperwork to withdraw; other plans require new enrollment documents with each renewal period.

Health Insurance Portability and Accountability Act of 1996 (HIPAA)

Important federal legislation is the Health Insurance Portability and Accountability Act of 1996 (HIPAA), which establishes guidelines that medical insurance companies must follow. HIPAA provides important protections for people who have serious or chronic health conditions such as Parkinson's disease. It prevents insurance companies from

- Denying enrollment on the basis of medical conditions (under any circumstances for group medical insurance plans and under specified circumstances for individual medical insurance plans)
- Selectively refusing to cover a particular medical condition (exclusions and limitations must apply to all people who have the same plan)
- Selectively raising one person's premiums
- Denying renewal of the medical insurance plan because of medical conditions

For detailed and updated information about how HIPAA applies in specific situations, contact the U.S. Centers for Medicare and Medicaid Services (CMS):

U.S. Centers for Medicare and Medicaid Services (CMS)
7500 Security Boulevard
Baltimore, MD 21244-1850
877-267-2323 (toll-free)
TDD 866-226-1819 (toll-free)
http://cms.hhs.gov/hipaa/online/

Most states have additional regulations and consumer protections under state extensions of HIPAA, particularly for individual medical insurance plans; the state's office of the insurance commissioner can provide additional information.

Medical insurance is essential for the person with Parkinson's. However, a person who does not have medical insurance at the time of diagnosis may have difficulty finding a plan that will cover expenses related to Parkinson's. Local Parkinson's disease support groups and the AMERICAN PARKINSON'S DISEASE ASSOCIATION can provide information about insurance companies that offer good medical plans for people with Parkinson's disease.

When Retiring

People who are diagnosed with Parkinson's disease while they are still employed often consider early retirement. However, MEDICARE eligibility does not begin until age 65 (with limited exceptions for disability). This restriction can create a significant period during which the person will need a private medical insurance plan. Some employer-sponsored group plans have conversion options; the benefits coordinator can explain these if they exist. These can be expensive and time-limited, although they may be adequate to cover the interval between retirement and eligibility for Medicare.

The benefits coordinator, or retirement planning coordinator if the employer has one, often can help identify other medical insurance options. These may include coverage through a spouse's group medical plan, if the spouse is employed; enrollment in a plan through a membership organization; or purchase of an individual medical insurance plan. An independent insurance agent also can provide advice and recommendations. As well, it can be helpful to talk with other people who have Parkinson's disease who have followed a similar process.

Restrictions and Exclusions

All medical insurance plans have restrictions and exclusions. It is crucial to know what these are and how they apply to specific situations. There are circumstances in which an insurance company may issue an exception; always obtain documentation of the exception, as well as any coverage clarifications, in writing. Common limitations include:

- Preexisting conditions and coverage waivers: Some medical insurance plans exclude coverage for preexisting conditions—medical conditions present at the time the plan begins (or in the previous six months). A preexisting condition exclusion is temporary but can remain in effect for as long as a year. During this time, the medical insurance plan will not pay for any services related to the condition. Some states permit insurance companies to sell individual medical insurance plans with waivers that permanently exclude coverage for preexisting conditions (employer-sponsored group medical plans cannot do this); these are not a good option for the person with Parkinson's disease as medical needs related to Parkinson's increase over time.

- Preauthorization: Most medical insurance plans require advance approval of any major procedure, whether diagnostic or therapeutic. Doctors' offices generally know what services require preauthorization, but it is the insured person who is ultimately responsible to pay for the expenses the medical insurance plan does not cover. It is prudent to check with the insurance company before having any scheduled surgery or hospitalization. Some medical insurance plans also require preauthorization or notification to receive care from providers (sometimes including urgent care and emergency care) who are not members of the plan's network, as when traveling.

- No coverage for investigational or experimental treatments, including drugs: With rare exception, medical insurance plans do not pay for investigational or experimental treatment. Investigational treatments typically are part of CLINICAL RESEARCH STUDIES; in those cases the study should cover all expenses related to the condition under investigation. Doctors sometimes recommend using approved treatments in ways other than those for which they are approved. This is a gray area as far as insurance coverage goes.

- Very limited or no coverage for skilled nursing facility (SNF) and long-term care: Many private medical insurance plans provide limited coverage for admission to a SKILLED NURSING FACILITY (SNF). There are often strict qualifications including preauthorization, and necessities such as prescription drugs may not be covered. Medical insurance sometimes pays for certain long-term care services provided on an outpatient basis, such as HOME HEALTH CARE, but does not pay for residential care in a LONG-TERM CARE FACILITY.

The medical insurance plan's benefits and procedures for specialty care are particularly important for people with Parkinson's disease. Some managed care plans may have limited access to specialists such as neurologists or may require a referral from a primary care physician each time the person consults a neurologist.

See also FINANCIAL PLANNING; MEDICAL MANAGEMENT; PLANNING FOR THE FUTURE.

medical management   Use of methods other than surgery to control symptoms, such as those of Parkinson's disease. These typically include medications (PHARMACOTHERAPY), PHYSICAL THERAPY, OCCUPATIONAL THERAPY, speech therapy, and other therapeutic approaches that target helping the person with Parkinson's to remain as INDEPENDENT and mobile as possible. The most effective approach is for the person with Parkinson's (or the primary caregiver) to work closely with one physician who serves as the point person for medical decisions. Although specialists such as neurologists should be at the forefront of ensuring a proper care plan for Parkinson's disease, it is important that the primary care physician and other specialist physicians who care for the person with Parkinson's disease have good communication with each other. Many conditions such as Parkinson's have many elements that necessitate the involvement of specialists, but steps should be taken to avoid having care become too fragmented. When one physician has a good overview of a person's condition medical management is more likely to remain on track.

See also CARE PLANNING AND MANAGEMENT; MEDICATION MANAGEMENT.

Medicare   A federally funded health insurance program for the elderly in the United States of America. People who have end-stage kidney disease (on kidney dialysis or who have had kidney transplantation surgery) and certain other disabilities also are eligible for Medicare benefits. Administered by the federal Centers for Medicare and Medicaid Services (CMS), Medicare provides medical benefits for more than 40 million Americans.

There are two levels of benefits for Medicare, Part A Hospital Insurance and Part B Medical Insurance. Nearly all Americans are entitled to Medicare Part A when they become age 65, which provides benefits for hospitalization (inpatient care and services). Medicare Part B is available as a purchased option to provide benefits for outpatient care and services. There are no income or asset restrictions for Medicare. The Medicare website, www.medicare.gov, provides comprehensive information about Medicare benefits, premiums, policies, and contact phone numbers by state.

Medicare Part A: Eligibility and Benefits
Americans who are employed pay Social Security taxes that in part support the Medicare system. Those who do so for at least 10 years, and their spouses, are entitled to Medicare Part A at no cost at age 65. People who receive or are eligible to receive Social Security retirement or disability benefits also are eligible. Most people who do not qualify for Medicare Part A at no cost have the option of paying premiums to enroll for coverage. People who have medical insurance coverage through other pension systems and do not pay into Social Security may not be eligible for Medicare. The Social Security Administration fields general Medicare eligibility questions; the toll-free number is 1-800-772-1213.

Medicare Part A pays for defined levels of specified inpatient services within a benefit period, which begins on the first day of hospitalization and ends when 60 days pass without further inpatient services. In general, benefits include

- Up to 90 days in the hospital and medications while in the hospital
- Up to 100 days in a skilled nursing facility (shared payment, called coinsurance, for days 21–100) for rehabilitation and recovery after hospitalization
- Eighty percent of qualifying home health care expenses
- Hospice services

Medicare begins payment after the deductible for the benefit period has been met; deductible levels change each year. Medicare does not pay for custodial care and services in a long-term care facility. There are strict rules for covered services; most providers are diligent about following them, but the person with Medicare or a caregiver should monitor them.

Medicare Part B: Eligibility and Benefits

Only those who have Part A can purchase Part B, and they can do so only during specified enrollment periods. Medicare either deducts monthly premiums from Social Security payments or bills quarterly for them. Benefits include doctor visits, physical therapy, occupational therapy, and other specified outpatient services. Part B has an annual deductible and numerous copayments. As well, there are many exclusions and limitations. A person can receive such services but must pay for them in full.

Medicare Plans

People on Medicare receive medical care and services through community providers (doctors, hospitals, pharmacies, and others). As with private MEDICAL INSURANCE, there are different kinds of plans through which a person can enroll for a year at a time to receive care. A person can change to a different Medicare plan during annual open enrollment.

- Original Medicare Plan (OMP): This is the payment-for-service plan in which everyone is automatically enrolled. Private insurance companies pay Medicare claims to providers, who agree to accept Medicare assignment (Medicare as pay-

ment in full for qualifying services). After Medicare pays its portions, providers bill patients for uncovered services and eligible balances.

- Medicare managed care: The person on Medicare receives medical care and services through a closed network of providers such as a health maintenance organization (HMO) or preferred provider organization (PPO). These networks agree to accept complete Medicare assignment and typically offer more extensive benefits such as routine health screenings and prescription drugs. A Medicare managed care plan has minimal out-of-pocket costs for a person with extensive medical needs, as long as the plan has good access to appropriate specialists. However, such plans are not always available in all areas.

- Private fee-for-service: Medicare pays a set fee for eligible services and the person pays all balances. Although this option offers the widest choice among providers, which may be important to a person with Parkinson's who sees multiple specialists, it entails the highest out-of-pocket expenses.

Help with Medicare and Medical Expenses

Both Part A and Part B have deductibles, coinsurance, and benefit limitations that result in out-of-pocket costs. For the person with Parkinson's who needs significant medical care, these expenses can become substantial. Some people have additional medical insurance that helps to cover some of these expenses. Social Security provides assistance with Medicare Part B premiums for people who meet income and resources guidelines (at or below the federal poverty level). As well, many drug companies offer PRESCRIPTION ASSISTANCE PROGRAMS for seniors who cannot afford to buy their medications.

See also FINANCIAL PLANNING; MEDICAL MANAGEMENT; PLANNING FOR THE FUTURE.

medication management   The need to monitor carefully the ANTI-PARKINSON'S MEDICATIONS that are currently the mainstay of treatment for Parkinson's disease, assuring that they are taken in the correct dosages at the right times. These medications have numerous potential side effects and interactions with each other or with medications taken to treat other health conditions such as heart disease. As well, timing of dosages often is key to maximizing benefit from the medication. Effective medication management provides optimal symptom control.

Dosing is particularly crucial with LEVODOPA, the cornerstone of Parkinson's PHARMACOTHERAPY. Because of this drug's tendency to cause nausea at the beginning of levodopa therapy, some pharmacists and doctors recommend taking it with food. Although this arrangement slightly reduces nausea, it also interferes with the way the body absorbs the levodopa. One common error that many nonneurologists and even some neurologists make is not dosing sufficient carbidopa to avoid levodopa associated nausea; Sinemet 10/100 tablets in particular should not be used as initial therapy (too little daily carbidopa unless at least five to 10 of them are taken in one day), and additional carbidopa (Lodosyn) can be prescribed if necessary. In the disease's early stages the decreased absorption from taking medications with food that contains protein is not so much of a problem as the dosage can be increased to compensate. In later stages, however, increasingly higher dosages are required to relieve symptoms, there is a point at which the person cannot tolerate the dosage and it is necessary to take smaller amounts more frequently and on an empty stomach to maximize absorption. As well, levodopa is most effective within the first hour or two of administration. Many people with Parkinson's find themselves managing dosages to provide the maximal effect for times when they need it most, such as when going out in public or having visitors.

It also is important to accommodate other medications taken to treat Parkinson's as well as other health conditions. As Parkinson's progresses and the person moves from MONOTHERAPY (use of a single drug, usually levodopa, to control symptoms) to ADJUNCT THERAPIES (addition of different drugs to the medication regimen), coordinating the timing of all medications becomes crucial. Some medications must be taken with meals and others on an empty stomach. Some are better taken in the evening or at bedtime. It often becomes necessary to create a schedule of medication dosages and

times. The person with Parkinson's should always have a copy of this schedule and enough medication to cover the next few dosages whenever leaving home, even when he or she intends to be out for a short time.

Medication management can become a challenge in situations such as traveling to different time zones; whether it makes sense to adjust dosage to accommodate time changes depends on how long the person will be in the new time zone. Medication management also becomes challenging if the person needs to be hospitalized for any reason, and in particular for surgery or diagnostic procedures in which preparation requires temporarily withholding food and water. In general most "nothing by mouth" orders before surgeries or procedures make an exception that allows important medications to be taken as usual with water; however, this should be clarified with the physician or dentist who will perform the procedure. If the practitioner performing the procedure demands no medications, communication between that practitioner and the neurologist managing the Parkinson's disease should be facilitated to ensure that no unnecessary harm comes to the person who has Parkinson's. When anti-Parkinson's medications must be interrupted, it is important to make the interruption as brief as possible and to resume the schedule quickly. If one is hospitalized, it is important to carefully review all of the current medications—especially anti-Parkinson's medications—with the admitting physician and remind both the admitting physician and the nursing staff of the importance of receiving anti-Parkinson's medications on schedule. For planned admissions, it may be worthwhile for the person with Parkinson's to bring his or her medications to the hospital and ask the admitting physician to authorize self-administration of the usual anti-Parkinson's medications as a way to avoid the potential delays of relying on a busy nursing staff.

When the person who has Parkinson's disease has cognitive difficulties, a caregiver must oversee or take over medication management. It is always a good idea for someone other than the person with Parkinson's to know the medication schedule. There are numerous aids for managing medications, from simple date- and time-organized pill dispensers to more sophisticated alarm-notification systems. Some people set a wristwatch alarm clock or timer to help them keep track of dosage times.

See also CARE MANAGEMENT AND PLANNING; COPING WITH ONGOING CARE OF PARKINSON'S; DAILY LIVING CHALLENGES; DRUG HOLIDAY; MEDICATION SIDE EFFECTS; TREATMENT ALGORITHM.

medication side effects ANTI-PARKINSON'S MEDICATIONS have many undesired and sometimes unpleasant actions, independently and the result of combination with other medications (drug interac-

COMMON POTENTIAL SIDE EFFECTS OF ANTI-PARKINSON'S MEDICATIONS

Medication Type	Common Medications	Common Side Effects
Adrenergic antagonists (alpha- and beta-blockers)	Alpha: prazosin, clonidine, methyldopa Beta: propanolol, nadolol, metoprolol	Low blood pressure, orthostatic hypotension, erectile dysfunction
Amantadine	Amantadine	Dry mouth, hallucinations, livido reticularis (mottled skin)
Antianxiety medications	Benzodiazepines: alprazolam, diazepam Other: paroxitine, buspirone	Benzodiazepine: drowsiness, dependence, incoordination Other: dizziness, nausea
Anticholinergics	Trihexyphenidyl, benztropine, procyclidine, biperiden	Dry mouth, constipation, vision problems, hallucinations, drowsiness
Antidepressants	Tricyclic: amitriptyline, desipramine, nortriptyline, imipramine SSRI: citalopram, fluoxetine, paroxetine, sertraline MAOI: phenelzine, isocarboxazid, tranylcypromine	Tricyclic: dry mouth, constipation, blurred vision, drowsiness SSRI: headache, nausea, sexual dysfunction MAOI: sudden high blood pressure, interactions with foods containing tyramine, interactions with numerous drugs
Antihistamines	Diphenhydramine	Sleepiness, dry mouth
Antipsychotics	Chlorpromazine, haloperidol, thioridazine, thiothixene, risperidone, clozapine, quetiapine	Sleepiness, dry mouth, constipation, hallucinations, delusions, tardive akathisia, bradykinesia, dyskinesias, significant worsening of Parkinson's symptoms
Cognitive enhancers	Donepezil, tacrine	Headache, dizziness, nausea
COMT inhibitors	Tolcapone, entacapone	Nausea, gastrointestinal distress, dyskinesias (related to extending levodopa's effectiveness); liver damage (tolcapone)
Dopamine agonists	Pergolide, bromocriptine, ropinirole, pramipexole, cabergoline	Drowsiness, orthostatic hypotension, cognitive impairment, dementia, psychosis
Dopaminergics	Levodopa, levodopa/carbidopa (Sinemet, Atamet), levodopa/benserazide (Madopar)	Drowsiness, nausea, dyskinesias, interactions with numerous drugs, orthostatic hypotension, cognitive impairment, hallucinations
MAOI-B inhibitors (neuroprotective therapy)	Selegiline	Nausea, dizziness, confusion, dry mouth, headache, hallucinations, vivid dreams
Muscle relaxants/ antispasmodics	Alprazolam, clonazepam, diazepam	Drowsiness, dizziness, disorientation
Sleep medications	Flurazapam, temazepam	Disorientation, confusion, dependence, sleep disturbances when medication is stopped

tions). These can range from nausea (common with LEVODOPA and DOPAMINE AGONIST MEDICATIONS) and drowsiness (common with ANTIANXIETY MEDICATIONS, ANTIDEPRESSANTS, DOPAMINE AGONISTS, DOPAMINERGICS, and muscle relaxants/antispasmodics) to serious and potentially life-threatening complications such as liver damage (a rare but known side effect of the COMT inhibitor TOLCAPONE) and blood disorders. Side effects that pose potential concerns are called adverse reactions.

People with Parkinson's disease should not take certain medications unless the benefits clearly outweigh the likely side effects. Such medications include most antipsychotics and MAOI antidepressants. Many minor side effects subside after the medication is taken over time; most adverse reactions resolve if the person stops taking the medication. Each time a new medication is introduced or the medication schedule is changed, the pharmacist or neurologist should review all of the medications the person with Parkinson's is taking and discuss any new side effects that may occur. People who use anti-Parkinson's medications should not take any over-the-counter medications, including herbal remedies, without discussing possible side effects and interactions with a pharmacist or neurologist.

See also CARE MANAGEMENT AND PLANNING; COPING WITH ONGOING CARE OF PARKINSON'S; MEDICAL MANAGEMENT; MEDICATION MANAGEMENT; TREATMENT ALGORITHM.

meditation A technique for stress relief. There are many forms of meditation, all of which help to relax and calm the person who practices meditation regularly. One of the simplest forms of meditation is to sit comfortably in a quiet location and concentrate on the breath, to feel and listen to the functions of breathing and the flow of life-giving oxygen to every part, tissue, and cell in the body. The absolute focus on the breath gently pushes worries and thoughts from the mind and creates a sense of physical relaxation. Just five or 10 minutes of this meditative practice done several times a day helps to relieve ANXIETY and AGITATION.

See also BREATH CONTROL; BREATHING EXERCISES; MINDFULNESS; TAI CHI; YOGA.

medulla oblongata See BRAIN.

memory The process of storing and retrieving information in the BRAIN. Memory is a complex interaction of physical and chemical functions in the brain. Although COGNITIVE FUNCTIONS including memory take place in the CEREBRUM, and the components of the so-called Pape's Circuit (most prominently, the bilateral brain structures known as the hippocampi) are critical to storing new memories, the exact processes and brain locations responsible for storing and recalling an individual memory remain unclear. Researchers know that the NEUROTRANSMITTER ACETYLCHOLINE is essential for cognitive function. Medications to improve cognitive function including memory that are effective in people with ALZHEIMER'S DISEASE, in whom acetylcholine becomes depleted in critical areas of the basal forebrain, do not appear to be uniformly successful in people with Parkinson's, in whom acetylcholine levels remain normal but out of balance as a result of DOPAMINE depletion. However, ANTI-PARKINSON'S MEDICATIONS taken to restore dopamine levels in the brain that improve neuromuscular function also improve cognitive function including memory. This finding suggests that there are varied pathways and processes through which memory storage and retrieval take place.

Short-term memory records information needed for immediate use, such as in reading. The brain's capacity for short-term memory is limited; information either moves into long-term memory or is "dumped" from the brain. Long-term memory is the brain's most significant storage and retrieval system. Disturbances with short-term memory can interfere with long-term memory processes. MEMORY IMPAIRMENTS that develop with Parkinson's affect both short-term and long-term memory functions. Activities that exercise memory help to keep it as functional as possible. However, the physical deteriorations that take place in the brain with Parkinson's disease eventually interfere with memory and cognition.

See also COGNITIVE IMPAIRMENT; NEUROPROTECTIVE THERAPIES.

memory impairment A loss of ability to store and retrieve memories. Everyone forgets things from time to time; this is normal. Memory impairment occurs when there is damage to the physical processes of memory storage and retrieval that take place in the BRAIN. Such damage can occur through trauma (head injury), stroke, or NEURODEGENERATIVE diseases (Alzheimer's, Parkinson's, Huntington's) and as a consequence of changes that take place in the brain through normal aging (APOPTOSIS, diminished blood supply due to atherosclerosis or arteriosclerosis). Memory impairment significantly affects COGNITIVE FUNCTION. Some degree of memory impairment is common in the later stages of Parkinson's disease, particularly in older people.

See also COGNITIVE DYSFUNCTION; COPING WITH ONGOING CARE OF PARKINSON'S; DEMENTIA; MEMORY.

menopause   The end of menstruation and of a woman's fertility. At menopause a woman's ovaries significantly reduce the amount of ESTROGEN that they produce, causing numerous changes in her body's hormonal balance. These changes affect body systems in varied ways.

For many years researchers believed estrogen had a NEUROPROTECTIVE effect, helping to prevent development of NEURODEGENERATIVE diseases such as ALZHEIMER'S DISEASE and Parkinson's disease. Some of this belief hinged on perceptions that women who experienced early menopause such as those who had total hysterectomy (surgery to remove the uterus and ovaries) had a higher rate of Parkinson's disease than women who experienced normal menopause, and as a result many doctors encouraged women to take hormone replacement therapy (HRT; estrogen and progesterone in combination) or estrogen replacement therapy (ERT; estrogen alone). NUMEROUS CLINICAL RESEARCH STUDIES have not supported this hypothesis, however.

Most researchers now believe that there is little or no direct correlation between estrogen levels and such diseases, although there remains some debate and research continues in this area. Other studies have demonstrated that long-term HRT or ERT significantly increases a woman's risk for certain forms of breast and uterine cancer, and it does not reduce her risk for heart disease according to

the most recent evidence, causing doctors to revise recommendations about this approach.

See also AGING; HORMONE.

mental status   A comprehensive perspective of a person's state of function with regard to awareness, alertness, confusion, COGNITIVE FUNCTION, reasoning, judgment, EMOTIONS, mood, behavior, thoughts, and SPEECH. Assessing mental status is part of a NEUROLOGICAL EXAMINATION, which may involve any number of assessment tools such as the MINI MENTAL STATUS EXAMINATION (MMSE), general questions and instructions that elicit responses from the person (such as repeating a sequence of numbers or spelling a word backward), and the neurologist's observations.

Mental status can reflect symptoms of Parkinson's disease such as ANXIETY, DEPRESSION, DEMENTIA, cognitive dysfunction, MEMORY IMPAIRMENT, and MOOD SWINGS. Mental status typically changes with events and circumstances and in Parkinson's tends to show a slow but steady decline as the disease progresses. The ways in which mental status changes often provide insights into problems such as MEDICATION SIDE EFFECTS or FLUCTUATING PHENOMENON (ANTI-PARKINSON'S MEDICATIONS are becoming ineffective, causing unpredictable lapses in control of symptoms). COGNITIVE IMPAIRMENTS often improve with anti-Parkinson's medications and worsen when medications wear off, although they can be persistent in the late stages of Parkinson's.

See also NEUROCHEMISTRY; PARANOIA; PARKINSON'S DISEASE QUALITY OF LIFE QUESTIONNAIRE; PSYCHOTHERAPY.

mercury   A metal that is highly toxic to the nervous system at very low levels of exposure. Mercury is one of the world's most common industrial pollutants and is a particular problem when it settles to the bottom of waterways (including the ocean). Some people experience health problems related to mercury through occupational exposure, but most mercury exposure occurs through eating of contaminated fish. According to the U.S. Food and Drug Administration's Center for Food Safety and Applied Nutrition (FDA CFSAN), fish with the highest mercury contamination levels are large long-lived species including tilefish, swordfish, king mackerel, and shark. The fish most commonly eaten in the United States—tuna, pollock, halibut, grouper, and shellfish—typically have low levels of mercury. Although debate continues about the safety of mercury in dental fillings, most health experts believe the level of mercury in dental amalgams is too low to have adverse health effects.

Mercury poisoning causes neurological damage that can include numbness and problems with vision and hearing and has been investigated as a potential cause of Parkinson's disease. Some genetic mutations that interfere with the body's processing of metals such as iron do cause Parkinson's-like diseases. However, these diseases are progressive and neurodegenerative, as is IDIO-PATHIC Parkinson's, whereas the neurological symptoms of mercury poisoning are usually temporary and subside as the body clears itself of excess mercury. As well, they differ from the classic symptoms of Parkinson's. Research continues to investigate the role mercury exposure, as well as exposure to other environmental contaminants, may play in Parkinson's disease, but at present it seems an unlikely cause.

See also ACERULOPLASMINEMIA; CHEMICAL TOXINS; ENVIRONMENTAL TRIGGERS; HALLERVORDEN–SPATZ SYNDROME; PARKINSON'S DISEASE, CAUSES OF.

metabolic needs   People with Parkinson's disease tend to have increased metabolic rates: That is, the body burns more energy at rest than the normal body does. In many people with Parkinson's, tremor or medication induced dyskinesias are readily identifiable causes, but for many others the reasons for this phenomenon are unclear. Many scientists believe it is primarily a manifestation of MITOCHONDRIAL DYSFUNCTION. Mitochondria, small structures within cells, produce the energy sources that cells need to function. The main source is a chemical called adenosine triphosphate (ATP). Researchers suspect that disruptions in the MITOCHONDRIAL ELECTRON TRANSPORT CHAIN known to occur in Parkinson's disease affect many aspects of metabolism.

Metabolic needs increase under numerous circumstances in health, such as during pregnancy and as a result of moderate to strenuous physical activity. The normal mechanism for responding is an increase in appetite, which causes the person to eat more and supply additional calories to the body. The person with Parkinson's has various impediments to this mechanism, including changes in taste that affect preferences and the desire to eat, difficulty with the mechanics of EATING including chewing and swallowing (foods that are nutrient-dense also are more difficult to eat), and slowed gastrointestinal function (as a result of the neuromuscular effects of the Parkinson's and associated degeneration of the autonomic nervous system). Many people acquire a craving for sweets in the later stages of Parkinson's, which some scientists believe is the body's attempt to increase caloric intake to accommodate increased metabolic needs. However, the result is further disruption of metabolic processes because carbohydrates alone cannot supply the body's nutritional needs.

See also GENETIC PREDISPOSITION; MITOCHONDRIAL DYSFUNCTION; NUTRITION AND DIET; PARKINSON'S DISEASE, CAUSES OF.

metoclopramide   A commonly prescribed anti-nausea medication, also taken to treat gastroesophageal reflux disorder (GERD) and sometimes morning sickness in pregnancy. Metoclopramide (Reglan) increases GASTRIC MOTILITY (the rate at which food moves through the stomach and into the intestine). However, it has some DOPAMINE antagonist effect (blocks the actions of dopamine), which can worsen the motor symptoms of Parkinson's disease. It also can generate such symptoms in a person who has not been diagnosed with Parkinson's disease, in which case the symptoms subside when the person stops taking the metoclopramide. Metoclopramide reduces the effectiveness of numerous ANTI-PARKINSON'S MEDICATIONS, particularly LEVODOPA and DOPAMINE AGONIST MEDICATIONS such as BROMOCRIPTINE and PERGOLIDE. People with Parkinson's disease generally should not take metoclopramide.

See also DOPAMINERGIC MEDICATIONS; MEDICATION MANAGEMENT; MEDICATION SIDE EFFECTS.

metoprolol A BETA-ADRENERGIC BLOCKER MEDICA-TION taken to relieve TREMORS and to treat HYPER-TENSION (high blood pressure). ESSENTIAL TREMOR, which is a different condition from Parkinson's disease, typically responds well to metoprolol, whereas the tremor of Parkinson's does not. However, metoprolol is sometimes effective in mid to late stages of Parkinson's disease as one of the ADJUNCT THERAPIES. A common brand name metoprolol product in the United States is Lopressor. LEVODOPA, the standard of PHARMACOTHERAPY (medication treatment) in Parkinson's disease, can intensify the effect of metoprolol and other beta-blockers. Orthostatic hypertension (a drop in blood pressure with change of position) can be a symptom of this interaction.

See also ALPHA-ADRENERGIC BLOCKER; ANTI-PARKINSON'S MEDICATIONS; HYPOTENSION, ORTHOSTA-TIC; TREATMENT ALGORITHM.

Michael J. Fox Foundation for Parkinson's Research A not-for-profit organization established by the actor MICHAEL J. FOX in 2000 that is committed to raising public awareness of Parkinson's disease as well as money and support for research. The website for the Michael J. Fox Foundation for Parkinson's Research, www.michaeljfox.org, provides extensive information about Parkinson's disease including innovative treatment approaches and reports on current and ongoing studies. The foundation funds research through competitive grants and through the Michael J. Fox Foundation Fellowship Program, which awards stipends to researchers and clinicians at some of the nation's leading medical institutions.

Fox's interest in Parkinson's became personal when he was diagnosed with the disease in 1991 at age 31. He made his diagnosis public in 1998 and has since become an outspoken advocate for aggressive research to find a cure for Parkinson's.

See also HOPE FOR A PARKINSON'S CURE; MORRIS K. UDALL PARKINSON'S RESEARCH ACT; MUHAMMAD ALI PARKINSON RESEARCH CENTER; NATIONAL PARKINSON FOUNDATION; PARKINSON STUDY GROUP.

microelectrode A wirelike conductive probe that can transmit the electrical activity of a single neuron. Neurons generate different levels of electrical activity, depending on their location and function. For example, those in the globus PALLIDUS internal (GPi), the site of surgery to ease TREMORS and BRADYKINESIA (PALLIDOTOMY or deep brain stimulation [DBS]), emit a slow, continuous signal. By contrast, neurons in the globus pallidus external (GPe) emit signals in short bursts that become longer as they are closer to the GPi. A technique called MICROELECTRODE RECORDING allows neurosurgeons to use these signals to create a precise map of the structures of the BASAL GANGLIA, which vary somewhat from person to person.

See also ABLATION; DEEP BRAIN STIMULATION; MACROELECTRODE; MACROELECTRODE STIMULATION; THALAMOTOMY.

microelectrode recording A process for mapping the precise functional structure of a person's BASAL GANGLIA as a prelude to PALLIDOTOMY, THALAMOTOMY, or DEEP BRAIN STIMULATION (DBS) (SURGERY to reduce TREMORS, DYSKINESIAS, or BRADYKINESIA) in late stage Parkinson's disease. Following a path determined by functional imaging studies the neurosurgeon inserts a MICROELECTRODE (a probe that transmits electrical activity from individual neurons) through the brain toward the target (PALLIDUM, THALAMUS, or subthalamic nucleus [STN]). A computer controls the microelectrode's movements, advancing it literally one NEURON at a time. The microelectrode sends signals from each neuron it encounters back to the computer, which generates continually refreshed images of the microelectrode's location. This capacity allows the neurosurgeon to place precisely the ABLATION probe that will create a lesion (wound and scar), or the DBS electrode that electronically disrupts neuronal activity, to interrupt the chaotic messages the pallidus is sending, thereby calming motor symptoms. Microelectrode recording is tedious and time-consuming; it usually takes around two hours to locate one target, but depending on the target, the experience of the surgical team, and luck it may require several hours.

See also STEREOTAXIS; THALAMOTOMY.

micrographia The clinical term for the tiny, cramped style of handwriting that is characteristic of people who have Parkinson's disease. Micrographia, which literally means "tiny writing," is often one of the earliest symptoms of Parkinson's, although recognition occurs in retrospect. In the early to middle stages of Parkinson's, ANTI-PARKINSON'S MEDICATIONS relieve micrographia along with other symptoms. Handwriting continues to deteriorate as fine motor skills decline, however. Micrographia can be a simple yet an effective means of monitoring medication effectiveness (including FLUCTUATING PHENOMENON) and disease progression. Micrographia is a symptom of Parkinson's disease only when it is different from the person's usual handwriting and becomes progressively smaller and more cramped. Many people have small handwriting, which is not in itself a symptom of Parkinson's.

Although handwriting changes can reflect damage to specific areas of the brain, such as can occur with stroke, researchers believe micrographia in Parkinson's disease results from the same disruptions of neuron communication that cause other neuromuscular symptoms such as BRADYKINESIA (slowness of movement). Micrographia can make a person's signature difficult to read and to confirm, such as for identification purposes. If this becomes a problem, the person with Parkinson's can provide ON-STATE and OFF-STATE signature samples for key verifiers such as banks or for important documents.

See also ARCHIMEDES SPIRAL; DEXTERITY, PHYSICAL; MONEY MANAGEMENT, DAILY; READING.

midbrain See BRAIN.

mindfulness A method of MEDITATION that emphasizes nonjudgmental focus on the present. This increases awareness of events and circumstances to improve the ability to control the responses to them. Mindfulness has been reported to help reduce STRESS, improve sleep quality, relieve DEPRESSION and ANXIETY, and decrease many physical symptoms including PAIN. Many locations throughout the United States teach mindful meditation techniques; especially for the person who is new to meditation, taking a class is a good way to get started. For the person with Parkinson's, mindfulness might be considered as a method to help with issues of DENIAL AND ACCEPTANCE, loss of INDEPENDENCE, and the many frustrations that accompany a disease over which a person has no control and can help him or her feel more connected to body, mind, and spirit in ways that enhance self-understanding and personal insight. Mindful meditation is helpful for caregivers as well.

See also BREATH CONTROL; STRESS REDUCTION TECHNIQUES; YOGA.

Mini Mental Status Examination (MMSE) A simple method for assessing a person's basic COGNITIVE FUNCTION. Developed and introduced in 1975 by three psychiatrists at the Johns Hopkins Hospital (Marshal F. Folstein, M.D.; Susan E. Folstein, M.D.; and Paul R. McHugh, M.D.), the MMSE has become a standard clinical assessment tool. It consists of 11 items that a clinician administers in five to 20 minutes, although there is no time limit for completing the assessment. The items assess a person's orientation to time and place, memory, and abilities to maintain attention, follow verbal and written instructions, repeat sequences, write a sentence, and copy a drawing. Scoring accommodates the person's level of education and age.

Psychological Assessment Resources (PAR), Inc., produces and markets the MMSE in written and software versions. Only qualified health care professionals can purchase the MMSE. For further information contact

Psychological Assessment Resources (PAR), Inc.
16204 N. Florida Avenue
Lutz, FL 33549
(800) 331-8378 or (813) 968-3003
www.parinc.com

See also HOEHN AND YAHR STAGE SCALE; MEMORY; MEMORY IMPAIRMENT; MENTAL STATUS; PARKINSON'S IMPACT SCALE.

Mirapex See PRAMIPEXOLE.

mitochondrial complex I See COMPLEX I.

mitochondrial dysfunction Abnormal activity within a mitochondrion, an energy-producing structure within a cell. The word *mitochondria* is derived from Greek words meaning "threadlike cartilage" in reference to the appearance of these structures under the microscope when they were identified in the late 1890s. It was not until 100 years later, in the 1990s, that technological advances finally made it possible for scientists to recognize the full role and genetic influences of mitochondria, which have numerous shapes and sizes.

Mitochondria manufacture, or synthesize, the cell's primary energy source, adenosine triphosphate (ATP), which cells use to fuel their functions. A high-energy cell such as a brain cell (NEURON) or heart cell has hundreds of mitochondria. A lower-energy cell, such as a skin cell, has fewer. Mitochondria also synthesize a number of the proteins the cell requires to carry out its functions. Among these proteins are those that initiate APOPTOSIS, the natural sequence of events that causes a cell to die (often called programmed cell death), and those that play key roles in the efficiency of cellular metabolism, identified as complexes. COMPLEX I has received the most study because of its role in binding with FREE RADICALS, the molecular waste products of cellular metabolism, to prevent them from causing cellular damage.

Mitochondria are the only structures in the human body, other than cells, that have their own deoxyribonucleic acid (DNA). This mitochondrial DNA (mtDNA), as scientists designate it, is separate and distinct from the nuclear DNA of the cell in which the mitochondrion resides and provides the "map" for the mitochondrion's functions. Nuclear DNA has a spiral organization, which resembles a twisted ladder, that strengthens and helps to protect the genetic structures it contains. The organization of mtDNA, in contrast, is circular and spare. This structure makes mtDNA significantly more fragile than nuclear DNA and allows less space for the mtDNA's contents. To accommodate this, mtDNA draws on nuclear DNA to complete many of its activities including replication and repair. Mitochondria replicate far more rapidly than the cell that contains them; the life cycle of a cell encompasses numerous life cycles of mitochondria. These factors increase mtDNA's susceptibility to damage, or mutation. Although each mitochondrion contains several copies of its mtDNA, mutations can cause the copies to vary from each other.

The significance of these variations depends on the nature and prevalence of a particular mutation. Transient mtDNA mutations, which are slight changes or errors that occur during the process of replication, typically are random and do not themselves cause problems in the short term. In the long term, transient mtDNA mutations contribute to disease processes when enough of them are present to create widespread interference with the MITOCHONDRIAL ELECTRON TRANSPORT CHAIN, the process through which the mitochondrion carries the molecular particles that become ATP and cellular proteins. Some mtDNA mutations are inherited and may affect a few or many mitochondria. A person inherits all mitochondria, and hence mtDNA, from his or her mother as only the egg, and not the sperm, contribute mitochondria to the embryo. Diseases caused by inherited mtDNA mutations are passed along in a fashion called matrilineal inheritance: affected individuals inherit the mutation from their mothers. As well, nuclear DNA mutations affect mtDNA structure and function. Mutations in the ALPHA-SYNUCLEIN GENE and the PARKIN GENE in nuclear DNA that are linked to Parkinson's disease, for example, alter the proteins available for mitochondrial metabolism.

When a cell replicates, it carries its complement of mitochondria, mtDNA mutations and all, into the new cells that form. Over time mtDNA mutations can become prominent within numerous cells, causing widespread mitochondrial dysfunction. The results are reduced ATP synthesis, reduced complex I production, and increased production of proteins associated with apoptosis. Researchers believe this abnormal activity generates cumulative cell-level damage that results in disease and have now linked these to dozens of diseases from cancer and heart disease to NEURODEGENERATIVE conditions such as ALZHEIMER'S DISEASE and Parkinson's disease.

Mitochondrial dysfunction is emerging as a leading focus in the search for the causes of Parkinson's disease, as it represents an intersection between genetic and environmental factors. Many researchers believe science eventually will demonstrate that mitochondrial dysfunction plays a role in nearly all diseases. Preventing mitochondrial damage by controlling environmental influences appears the most effective means of minimizing mitochondrial dysfunction. Research involving COENZYME Q-10, an ANTIOXIDANT that increases complex I production, is showing promising, although not yet conclusive results.

See also CHROMOSOMES LINKED TO PARKINSON'S DISEASE; GENE MAPPING; GENE THERAPY; HUMAN GENOME PROJECT; LIPOPOLYSACCHARIDES; NEUROPROTECTIVE EFFECT; NEUROPROTECTIVE THERAPIES; OXIDATION; PARKINSON'S DISEASE, CAUSES OF; UBIQUITIN.

mitochondrial electron transport chain The process through which a mitochondrion, an energy-producing structure within a cell, carries the molecules it needs for its metabolic functions. The mitochondrial electron transport chain is significantly less active in the BRAIN cells (NEURONS) of people with Parkinson's disease, impairing mitochondrial metabolism and causing MITOCHONDRIAL DYSFUNCTION. This lack of activity shortchanges the cell of adenosine triphosphate (ATP), its primary fuel source, and proteins that it needs to carry out its functions, setting in motion a sequence of events that ultimately results in cumulative cell damage, which causes disease.

See also ALPHA-SYNUCLEIN GENE; CHROMOSOMES LINKED TO PARKINSON'S DISEASE; COENZYME Q-10; GENE MAPPING; GENE THERAPY; LIPOPOLYSACCHARIDES; NEUROPROTECTIVE EFFECT; NEUROPROTECTIVE THERAPIES; PARKIN GENE; PARKINSON'S DISEASE, CAUSES OF; UBIQUITIN.

mobility The ability to move. The neuromuscular symptoms of Parkinson's disease such as BRADYKINESIA and GAIT DISTURBANCES progressively impair MOVEMENT and mobility, with a significant and direct effect on independence. Mobility can be unassisted or assisted. SUPPORTIVE THERAPIES such as PHYSICAL THERAPY and OCCUPATIONAL THERAPY can help to maintain mobility for as long as possible through structured exercises and techniques that preserve BALANCE, COORDINA-

TION, and MUSCLE STRENGTH. These may include the following:

- Regular walking with intentional effort focused on aspects of GAIT such as body position, ARM SWING, and stride length.

- Gentle strength (resistance) exercises with light weights, to maintain muscle mass and strength. Resistance activities such as strength training and walking also help maintain bone density and strength, which are particularly important in women who are past menopause and in older men as well.

- Activities that practice movements to minimize gait freezing and other gait disturbances, such as concentrating on lifting each foot completely from the walking surface with each step. Other strategies to overcome freezing include marching, clapping out a cadence, or using a ribbon or other object for the person with Parkinson's to step over. Removing clutter and increasing open space often helps to reduce freezing in the home.

- Range of motion exercises to help to keep joints and the muscles that support them moving freely.

- Activities that practice HAND-TO-EYE COORDINATION, muscular coordination, and balance, such as catching and throwing a ball.

In the mid to late stages of Parkinson's, continued neuromuscular degeneration results in increased difficulty with motor skills and balance. As LEVODOPA and other ANTI-PARKINSON'S MEDICATIONS become less effective, symptoms become less predictable. MOBILITY AIDS such as walking sticks and walkers can provide stability, reducing the risk of FALLS. In late Parkinson's, mobility may require a wheelchair. ACTIVITIES OF DAILY LIVING (ADL) measures and assessment tools such as the PARKINSON'S IMPACT SCALE can help to determine a person's level of mobility.

Some aspects of mobility are psychosocial as much as they are physical. One of the toughest challenges for people with neurodegenerative diseases such as Parkinson's is the progressive loss of independence. For many people one of the first activities relinquished is driving; stopping driving significantly curtails independent mobility in ways that extend well beyond functional ability. Many communities have low-cost public transportation alternatives for seniors and people with mobility limitations that can accommodate mobility aids including wheelchairs. The AMERICANS WITH DISABILITIES ACT (ADA) has established widespread access to public facilities for people with mobility impairments. Although accepting the transition to assisted mobility can be emotionally difficult for the person with Parkinson's before a crisis such as a major fall demands it helps to extend independence. Innovation and creativity in dealing with mobility challenges are helpful, too, to adjustment to the changes that Parkinson's imposes.

See also ADAPTIVE EQUIPMENT AND ASSIST DEVICES; ADJUSTING TO LIVING WITH PARKINSON'S; POSTURAL INSTABILITY; QUALITY OF LIFE; RANGE OF MOTION.

mobility aids Devices that extend a person's ability to be mobile and independent. These include the following:

- Shoe ORTHOTICS for foot support and stability.
- Walking sticks.
- Canes, which are manufactured in various styles including ones with multiple points of contact for increased stability. It is important to have a cane that is the correct length. Some styles are adjustable.
- Walkers, which also are made in various styles. Some styles fold for easy storage and transport. Others look like modified carts, with baskets or shelves to hold objects such as books and packages. Models with wheels generally are easier to use, particularly for people with Parkinson's who have diminished muscle strength, balance, and coordination. Hand brakes and wheel size are important features for wheeled walkers. While most require a squeeze to apply the brakes, the models that require a squeeze to release the brakes are particularly helpful for people with Parkinson's, who have particular problems with falling backwards or forwards without being able to catch themselves. Handle

height is important. A seat is a useful feature as fatigue is often an issue.
- Wheelchairs are manual or battery-powered; there are various styles including powered scooters. Wheelchairs usually can be rented through suppliers that handle durable medical equipment (DME). A wheelchair should be sized to the person. It is also important to consider the home environment when choosing styles. Scooters require more space than wheelchairs for maneuvering and turning.

Some MEDICAL INSURANCE plans pay for certain mobility aids for home use as a DME benefit. MEDICARE and MEDICAID programs also pay for certain aids and devices.

See also GAIT; GAIT DISTURBANCE; OCCUPATIONAL THERAPY; PHYSICAL THERAPY.

modafinil A medication taken to improve alertness, most often prescribed to counteract the DAYTIME SLEEPINESS that is common with Parkinson's disease. Modafinil's use in people with Parkinson's is OFF-LABEL, hence some insurers are hesitant to cover it as it is fairly costly. However, there are several studies that confirm its usefulness in Parkinson's disease related drowsiness. Drowsiness and difficulty in staying alert during waking hours can result from taking LEVODOPA and other ANTIPARKINSON'S MEDICATIONS, disturbed sleep patterns that result in insufficient nighttime sleep, or from the disease itself. Although most people feel drowsy before falling asleep, some people with Parkinson's do not and sometimes fall asleep during activity. Modafinil (brand name Provigil) is a nonamphetamine stimulant. However, it has addictive potential similar to that of amphetamine. Possible side effects include NAUSEA, headache, dry mouth, DIZZINESS, and insomnia (inability to fall or stay asleep) if taken later in the day.

See also BEDROOM COMFORT; EPWORTH SLEEPINESS SCALE; FATIGUE; PARKINSON'S DISEASE SLEEP SCALE; SLEEP DISTURBANCES.

money management, daily The ability to handle personal financial matters, which becomes an increasing challenge for many people as Parkinson's disease progresses. There are several facets to this. One is the simple logistics of keeping up with financial tasks such as paying household bills, managing shopping expenses such as for groceries, and filing MEDICAL INSURANCE or MEDICARE claims. These tasks can be daunting enough without the limitations Parkinson's disease imposes, particularly for older people.

The motor symptoms of Parkinson's are another dimension, often making the physical actions of opening envelopes, writing checks, and preparing payments for mailing difficult. As well, ANTI-PARKINSON'S MEDICATIONS often impair alertness, and the disease process itself includes COGNITIVE IMPAIRMENT that can range from barely perceptible to significant. The person may write checks for more money than is in the account or for the wrong amount.

Daily money management is also an issue of independence. Most adults are accustomed to managing their personal affairs and do not recognize that health problems interfere with their abilities to continue doing so. Sometimes the focus on maintaining health is so intense that other aspects of daily living are shoved aside. It is beneficial for someone the person with Parkinson's disease trusts, such as a spouse or adult child, to help manage daily finances. This process can be collaborative, so the person with Parkinson's remains an active participant in daily affairs for as long as it is practical and does not feel "taken over."

For the person who receives regular payments such as those from a pension, retirement fund, or Social Security, banking services such as direct deposit and automatic bill payment can be efficient and effective ways to manage expenses that are consistent and predictable. Some banks do not charge for bill payment services when the account also has direct deposit; others charge a small fee. The person must still deal with unpredictable expenses such as medical costs and payment for groceries and such, but generally automatic deposit and payment programs cover the important basics. To make sure that there always is enough money in the account to cover automatic payments, it is a good idea to maintain a separate checking account for other uses. Some care management and senior services companies offer daily money management

assistance among the services they sell. For a fee, the company manages bank accounts and pays regular bills. It is essential to make certain such a company is appropriately licensed and bonded.

See also FINANCIAL PLANNING; PARENT/CHILD RELATIONSHIPS; RECORD KEEPING.

monoamine neurotransmitter A chemical formed from a single AMINO ACID group. The key monoamine neurotransmitters in the BRAIN are ACETYLCHOLINE, DOPAMINE, EPINEPHRINE, NOREPINEPHRINE, and SEROTONIN. These neurotransmitters facilitate NEURON communication related to MOOD, EMOTION, MEMORY, pleasure, and COGNITIVE FUNCTION. As well, dopamine and, to a lesser extent, acetylcholine have functions related to movement. Changes in the levels of these neurotransmitters are linked to various health conditions:

- Dopamine depletion in the BASAL GANGLIA is the hallmark of Parkinson's disease and causes impaired movement.
- Acetylcholine depletion in the basal forebrain is the hallmark of ALZHEIMER'S DISEASE and causes COGNITIVE IMPAIRMENT.
- Low levels of serotonin, norepinephrine, and cerebral dopamine contribute to DEPRESSION.
- Elevated levels of cerebral dopamine or hypersensitivity of dopamine receptors in the CEREBRUM contribute to PSYCHOSIS and SCHIZOPHRENIA.

As well, the proportions of these neurotransmitters to one another appear to be important to proper brain function; however, scientists do not entirely understand the intricacies of their relationships. Restoring them to normal levels to the extent that this is possible also restores their balance within the brain.

See also MONOAMINE OXIDASE; MONOAMINE OXIDASE GENE; MONOAMINE OXIDASE INHIBITOR (MAOI) MEDICATION; NEUROPROTECTIVE EFFECT; NEUROPROTECTIVE THERAPIES; NEUROPSYCHIATRY.

monoamine oxidase (MAO) An enzyme that metabolizes (breaks down) MONOAMINE NEUROTRANSMITTERS such as DOPAMINE, serotonin, epinephrine,

NOREPINEPHRINE, and ACETYLCHOLINE. Mitochondria, tiny structural units within a cell, produce MAO. Only NEURONS (nerve cells) contain MAO. There are two main forms of MAO, type A (MAO-A) and type B (MAO-B). MAO-A primarily acts on serotonin, epinephrine, and norepinephrine; MAO-B primarily acts on dopamine and acetylcholine. Through its metabolic actions, MAO affects many autonomic NERVOUS SYSTEM functions including regulation of heart rate and blood pressure (through its actions to metabolize epinephrine and norepinephrine) as well as functions related to MOOD, EMOTION, and behavior (through its actions on serotonin and cerebral dopamine).

The MONOAMINE OXIDASE (MAO) GENE regulates mitochondrial monoamine oxidase production. Mutations in the MAO gene appear in some people with Parkinson's, suggesting that flaws in MAO regulation may contribute to the disease's symptoms. MAO also plays a key role in depression, which is emerging as a significant symptom of Parkinson's disease. More than half of people with Parkinson's experience clinical depression at some point in the disease, and for many it is identified in retrospect as one of the earliest symptoms.

As DOPAMINERGIC NEURON loss continues in Parkinson's disease, the brain's supply of dopamine correspondingly diminishes. The supply of MAO, however, appears to remain normal, as it must for other brain functions to continue. As a result dopamine metabolism continues at a normal rate even though there is less dopamine than the brain requires. MONOAMINE OXIDASE INHIBITOR (MAOI) MEDICATIONS used to treat depression block the action of MAO nonselectively. Their use may have significant adverse consequences, including potentially life-threatening escalation of blood pressure. Using medications selectively to regulate the action of MAO-B shows great promise in treatment for Parkinson's disease, although at present only the drug SELEGILINE (Deprenyl) is used for this purpose; another drug, rasaligine, has already undergone trials in humans and may be approved by the U.S. Food and Drug Administration (FDA) soon. GENE THERAPY to address mutations in the MAO gene and other genes remains on the therapeutic horizon, with much research still necessary to determine

its effectiveness. As well, there is much scientists still do not know about the regulation, production, and role of MAO, including whether forms other than type A and type B exist.

See also 3-METHOXYTYRAMINE; 3-METHOXY-4-HYDROXYPHENYLACETIC ACID; 3,4-DIHYDROXYPHENYLACETIC ACID; CATECHOL-O-METHYLTRANSFERASE; LIPOPOLYSACCHARIDES; MITOCHONDRIAL DYSFUNCTION; NEUROPROTECTIVE EFFECT; NEUROPROTECTIVE THERAPIES.

monoamine oxidase (MAO) gene One of several GENES believed to have a causative role in Parkinson's disease. The MAO gene directs mitochondrial production of MONOAMINE OXIDASE (MAO), an ENZYME that metabolizes MONOAMINE NEUROTRANSMITTERS such as DOPAMINE. Researchers have found mutations of the MAO gene in some people with Parkinson's disease, often in conjunction with mutations of the ALPHA-SYNUCLEIN GENE and the PARKIN GENE that frequently appear in EARLY-ONSET PARKINSON'S DISEASE. Because MAO is just one of numerous substances involved in neurotransmitter metabolism, it is less likely to be a determinant cause of Parkinson's than a contributing factor. Some research has linked mutations in the MAO gene to disorders involving mood and emotion, other brain functions in which dopamine also plays a role.

See also ANTIDEPRESSANT MEDICATION; DEPRESSION; GENE MAPPING; GENE MUTATIONS; GENE THERAPY; GENETIC PREDISPOSITION; MONOAMINE OXIDASE INHIBITOR (MAOI) MEDICATION.

monoamine oxidase inhibitor (MAOI) medication A drug that blocks or interferes with the actions of MONOAMINE OXIDASE, an ENZYME that has a key role in the metabolism of the MONOAMINE neurotransmitters ACETYLCHOLINE, DOPAMINE, epinephrine, NOREPINEPHRINE, and serotonin. Scientists have known for decades that MAO activity is involved in functions of the brain related to MOOD, EMOTION, and behavior. An imbalance between MAO and neurotransmitters, through either a decrease in MAO production or an increase in neurotransmitter production, is linked to DEPRESSION.

MAOIs, which became available in the 1950s, were the first drugs available to treat depression and are still used for this purpose today. They work by blocking the action of MAO to extend neuro-transmitter presence and action. The earlier formu-lations of these drugs are nonselective for MAO type; they include phenelzine (Nardil), Isocarbox-azid (Marplan), and Tranylcypromine (Parnate), which block both MAO-A and MAO-B. However, these medications have significant side effects as well as extensive interactions with foods and other medications.

MAOIs to Treat Parkinson's Disease

Because conventional MAOIs do extend the avail-ability of dopamine, neurologists have tried using them to relieve symptoms of people with Parkin-son's disease. However, this effect also extends the

MONOAMINE OXIDASE INHIBITOR (MAOI) MEDICATION SIDE EFFECTS AND INTERACTIONS

Possible Side Effects	Medication Interactions	Food Interactions
Hypotension, orthostatic hypotension (low blood pressure)	Levodopa, dopamine agonists	Fava beans (broad beans, long beans)
Hypertension (high blood pressure)	Most antihypertensives (drugs that treat high blood pressure)	Caffeine (coffee, tea, cola)
Headache, drowsiness	Beta-blockers (propanolol, nadolol, metoprolol)	Chocolate, licorice
Hallucinations, disorientation, confusion, delirium, delusions, sleep disturbances	Thiazide diuretics	Aged cheese (cheddar, brie, camembert, emmenthaler, gruyère, mozzarella, parmesan, romano, bleu, roquefort)
Anxiety, psychosis	Tricyclic antidepressants (amitriptyline, nortriptyline)	Beer, red wine, sherry
Tremors, myoclonus, ataxia, sensory disturbances, blurred vision	Bupropion	Hard sausage (salami, pepperoni, Lebanon bologna), summer sausage
Dry mouth constipation	St.-John's-wort (hypericum), buspirone	Smoked meats and fish
Liver damage	Carbamazepine (Tegretol)	Pickled or kippered fish (herring), anchovies, caviar
Edema	SSRI antidepressants (fluoxetine, paroxetine, citalopram, sertraline)	Avocados, bananas, bean curd, figs, prunes, raisins, raspberries
Urinary retention, sexual dysfunction	Other MAOIs including selegiline	Liver (including chicken liver), liver pâté, liver sausage (braunschweiger)
	Oral antidiabetes medications	Sauerkraut, soy sauce, yeast
	Decongestants in cold medicines (ephedrine, pseudoephedrine, phenylephrine	
	Dextromethorphan cough suppressant	
	Methyldopa (Aldomet)	
	Sulfonamide antibiotics (oral, topical, ophthalmic)	
	Phenothiazine antipsychotics	
	Alcohol	
	Ginseng, 5-HTP supplement	

availability of norepinephrine and epinephrine, which can cause rapid heart rate, arrhythmias (irregularities in the heartbeat), and sudden and serious (sometimes fatal) escalations in blood pressure. As well, MAOIs interact with LEVODOPA, DOPAMINE AGONISTS, and many other ANTI-PARKINSON'S MEDICATIONS.

A new MAO, SELEGILINE (Deprenyl), blocks only MAO-B and extends the availability of dopamine without affecting MAO metabolism of other monoamine neurotransmitters. Doctors sometimes prescribe selegiline as one of the ADJUNCT THERAPIES with LEVODOPA, to allow a lower levodopa dose. Some people with DE NOVO PARKINSON'S (newly diagnosed and not yet treated) are able to forestall levodopa therapy by starting on MONOTHERAPY of selegiline. A five-year study conducted from 1987 to 1992, the DATATOP (Deprenyl and Tocopherol Antioxidative Therapy for Parkinson's Disease) study, found selegiline (as the brand name product Deprenyl) could delay the need for levodopa therapy by one to three years in de novo Parkinson's. Despite these findings, there remains considerable controversy within the medical community as to whether its use is therapeutically prudent when looking at the entire spectrum of anti-Parkinson's therapy. Most movement disorders specialists believe that because degeneration continues even with selegiline, symptoms are more severe and accordingly more difficult to control when more potent (levodopa or dopamine agonist) or possibly protective (dopamine agonist) therapy is delayed. Most neurologists believe that dopamine agonists are a better choice than selegiline in delaying the need for levodopa because selegiline is less potent, has similar side effect potential, and, at present, has no stronger (and, in the opinion of most experts, substantially weaker) evidence of a possible neuroprotective effect than dopamine agonists.

MAOIs and Tyramine

As well as blocking the action of MAO to metabolize monoamine neurotransmitters, MAOIs inhibit metabolism of the amino acid TYRAMINE. Tyramine, along with norepinephrine and epinephrine, helps to regulate blood pressure. When its levels rise, so does blood pressure. Many foods—especially those that are aged or smoked—contain tyramine. Eating such foods while taking a conventional MAOI causes sudden surges in tyramine levels, as the drug blocks the body's normal response mechanism (increasing MAO production). This can cause spikes in blood pressure that can result in severe headache as well as brain hemorrhage that causes stroke and death. For this reason, people taking conventional MAOIs have broad dietary restrictions.

The MAOI-B medication selegiline, because it selectively blocks MAO action to metabolize dopamine but not other MAO neurotransmitters, does not have the same effect with tyramine. Although it is prudent to avoid foods that are high in tyramine to minimize fluctuations in blood pressure, dietary restrictions are much less severe for people who use selegiline.

MAOIs and SSRIs

MAOIs, because they block the action of MAO on all brain MAO neurotransmitters, extend the availability of serotonin, a neurotransmitter that often is at lower than normal levels in people who have depression. This is one of the ways in which MAOIs exert an antidepressive effect. However, the newer antidepressants, SELECTIVE SEROTONIN REUPTAKE INHIBITOR (SSRI) MEDICATIONS, block the process by which neurons reabsorb serotonin after its release. This action also extends the availability of serotonin. If medications of each type are taken, the result is an excess of serotonin in the brain, which can cause a potentially fatal condition called serotonin syndrome, toxic serotonin syndrome, or serotonin toxicity. Symptoms include euphoria, drowsiness, abnormal movements of the foot, lack of coordination, restlessness, dizziness, sense of intoxication, tremors and twitching, muscle rigidity, elevated body temperature, confusion, diarrhea, and sometimes loss of consciousness and death. Serotonin syndrome requires emergency medical treatment. While much less likely to precipitate a serotonin syndrome than MAO-A inhibitors, taking selegiline or other MAO-B inhibitors with SSRIs is believed to carry some risk of causing this potentially life threatening condition.

See also ANTIDEPRESSANT MEDICATIONS; NEUROPROTECTIVE EFFECT; NEUROPROTECTIVE THERAPIES; SELECTIVE

SEROTONIN REUPTAKE INHIBITORS; TRICYCLIC ANTIDE-PRESSANT MEDICATIONS; NEUROPSYCHIATRY.

monotherapy   Use of a single ANTI-PARKINSON'S MEDICATION as primary treatment to control the symptoms of Parkinson's. A common monotherapy is the LEVODOPA, which the BRAIN metabolizes (converts) to DOPAMINE. This process provides a temporary replacement supply of dopamine to compensate for the depletion that occurs as a result of the death of DOPAMINERGIC NEURONS. As Parkinson's progresses and dopaminergic neurons continue to die higher dosages of levodopa are required to achieve symptom relief. As well, DOPAMINE RECEPTORS become less responsive (sensitized) and require higher amounts of dopamine for activation.

Sometimes other anti-Parkinson's medications are effective as monotherapy early in the course of the disease, particularly with DE NOVO PARKINSON'S (Parkinson's that is newly diagnosed and has never been treated). These include

- AMANTADINE. This antiviral medication was developed in the 1960s to shorten the course of influenza A. It also has central dopamine agonist action and can cross the BLOOD-BRAIN BARRIER. Although researchers do not know its precise mechanisms, amantadine either stimulates dopaminergic neurons to increase dopamine production or activates dopamine receptors in ways that simulate the action of dopamine. Amantadine monotherapy can delay the need for levodopa for up to two years; much longer delays are possible if dopamine agonists can be added first.

- DOPAMINE AGONISTS. These medications are chemically similar to dopamine and can bind with, or activate, dopamine receptors in the brain. They, like amantadine, are able to cross the blood-brain barrier. Because they do not have exactly the same molecular configuration as dopamine, dopamine agonists bind incompletely but enough to "bridge" neuron communication as a supplement to endogenous dopamine. The action is analogous to decoding word messages when the vowels are missing. As

dopamine levels continue to decline with the progression of Parkinson's, the limitations of this incomplete binding become more pronounced and the "bridge" carries less of the neuron messages—not enough gets through to deliver coherent communication. To extend the word messages analogy, consonants drop out as well as vowels, leaving inadequate clues for deciphering the words. Common dopamine agonists are BROMOCRIPTINE, PERGOLIDE, PRAMIPEXOLE, and ROPINIROLE. The latter two of these, which target specific dopamine receptors (D2, D3, D4), show promise of being as effective as levodopa in early Parkinson's and can postpone the need for levodopa for up to three to five years on average, with some people being able to be maintained on dopamine agonist monotherapy for over a decade.

- Monoamine oxidase inhibitor-type B (MAOI-B): MONOAMINE OXIDASE (MAO) is an enzyme that initiates metabolism of MONOAMINE NEURO-TRANSMITTERS. Monoamine oxidase type B (MAO-B) specifically targets dopamine. Inhibiting, or blocking, the action of MAO-B extends the availability of dopamine in the brain and thereby sometimes relieves the neuromuscular symptoms in early Parkinson's. The only MAO-B inhibitor medication available in the United States at present is selegiline (Deprenyl). It can postpone the need for levodopa for up to three years. Rasaligine, an MAO-B inhibitor that has undergone testing in people with Parkinson's, may be approved soon and has data that mainly supports its use as an adjunct therapy in people with moderate to severe Parkinson's.

There is debate among specialists who treat people with Parkinson's about how long to delay levodopa therapy by use of other anti-Parkinson's medications during the disease's early stages. Virtually all neurologists believe when symptom control is as effective, and side effects are not any higher, with another medication as monotherapy, delaying levodopa therapy is worthwhile. It is important to note that the listed alternative monotherapies to levodopa all pose a significantly greater risk of worsening cognition in elderly or cognitively impaired people than levodopa. What is more difficult to determine is when the less complete symptom control or more problematic side effects of other monotherapies reach the point that they unfavorably compare to the known risks of motor complications—and some possible theoretical risk of contributing to disease progression—which initiation of levodopa therapy engenders. Medications other than levodopa that are taken as monotherapy early in the course of Parkinson's typically remain effective later in the disease as ADJUNCT THERAPIES, when they are able to supplement and extend the effectiveness of levodopa.

See also ABLATION; FLUCTUATING PHENOMENON; PALLIDOTOMY; PHARMACOTHERAPY; SURGERY; THALAMOTOMY; THERAPEUTIC WINDOW; TREATMENT ALGORITHM.

mood swings   Sudden, extreme changes in emotion. Mood swings are common in Parkinson's disease and are often among the earliest symptoms, although this becomes clear retrospectively. Parkinson's disease develops when so many DOPAMINERGIC NEURONS die that there is no longer an adequate supply of DOPAMINE, the NEUROTRANSMITTER largely responsible for brain functions related to movement. Because dopamine is present in other parts of the brain that regulate MOOD, EMOTION, and COGNITIVE FUNCTION, many researchers believe there is also dopaminergic neuron loss in those areas as well, although not as pronounced as in the BASAL GANGLIA (the part of the brain that regulates movement). This, some researchers believe, accounts for mood swings in people with Parkinson's, as well as related symptoms such as DEPRESSION, MEMORY LOSS, and COGNITIVE DYSFUNCTION.

Many people with Parkinson's disease find that mood swings and related symptoms such as depression improve during an ON-STATE, when ANTI-PARKINSON'S MEDICATIONS are most effectively controlling neuromuscular symptoms or change when their medication regimens change, although CLINICAL RESEARCH TRIALS studying such correlations provide conflicting results. Mood swings are also symptoms of other conditions that may or may not be related to Parkinson's disease, such as ALZHEIMER'S DISEASE, or that occur as side effects of various anti-Parkinson's medications.

See also ANXIETY; DENIAL AND ACCEPTANCE; PARKINSON'S PERSONALITY; PSYCHOSOCIAL FACTORS.

Morris K. Udall Parkinson's Research Act of 1997
Significant legislation passed by the U.S. Congress in 1997 that increased federal funding for Parkinson's disease research from $34 million to $100 million a year. The act was named in honor of U.S. Representative Morris K. Udall (1922–98), a Democrat, who represented the state of Arizona in the U.S. House of Representatives from 1961 to 1991. Udall was diagnosed with Parkinson's disease in 1979 and died as a consequence of its symptoms in 1998.

The Morris K. Udall Parkinson's Research Act of 1997 was landmark legislation in that it marked the first extensive public push for funding for Parkinson's research. The former heavyweight boxing champion MUHAMMAD ALI, who was diagnosed with Parkinson's disease in 1982, testified in congressional hearings in support of the act. The act passed overwhelmingly and was signed into legislation by the then-president, Bill Clinton.

See also ALI, MUHAMMAD; FOX, MICHAEL J.; MICHAEL J. FOX FOUNDATION FOR PARKINSON'S RESEARCH; UDALL, MORRIS K.

Motilium   See DOMPERIDONE.

motor function   The integration among BRAIN, NERVOUS SYSTEM, and musculoskeletal functions that results in movement and speech. This integration is quite complex and encompasses physical structures as well as biomechanical and biochemical actions. Motor function is the essence of human movement.

See also BRAIN; MOBILITY; MOVEMENT; NERVOUS SYSTEM.

motor system disorders   A broad classification of dysfunctions and diseases that impair the body's ability to move, sometimes called motor function disorders or movement disorders. Many motor system disorders are progressive and DEGENERATIVE, such as Parkinson's disease, MULTIPLE SCLEROSIS, AMYOTROPHIC LATERAL SCLEROSIS (ALS), and MUSCULAR DYSTROPHY. These disorders often have genetic components. For such disorders, treatment typically targets symptom control. Other motor system disorders result from trauma or injury and remain stable or can improve with treatment, such as stroke and spinal cord injury.

See also CONDITIONS SIMILAR TO PARKINSON'S; DIAGNOSING PARKINSON'S; OCCUPATIONAL THERAPY; PARKINSON'S DISEASE, CAUSES OF; PHYSICAL THERAPY.

movement The actions that result in changing the body's position. Movement can be voluntary (under conscious control) or involuntary (beyond a person's ability to control). Voluntary movement allows MOBILITY and requires an integration of MOTOR FUNCTIONS involving the BRAIN, NERVOUS SYSTEM, and musculoskeletal system. Although basic movement such as WALKING or reaching for an object appears to be automatic, it is voluntary and intentional. The neuromuscular system "remembers" patterns of movement so the body seems to perform them without conscious effort. Involuntary movement may involve the same muscle groups as voluntary movement, but the person cannot direct or control it. The TREMORS, DYSKINESIA, and DYSTONIA (severe spasms) common in Parkinson's disease are involuntary movements.

See also BALANCE, GAIT; MUSCLE STRENGTH; MUSCLE TONE; POSTURAL RIGHTING REFLEX; RANGE OF MOTION.

movement disorder A widely inclusive term encompassing numerous health conditions that interfere with a person's ability to move. Neurologists who specialize in movement disorders tend to focus on degenerative diseases of the parts of the brain known as the basal ganglia and cerebellum, but many nervous system, muscular, or even skeletal conditions can present as abnormal alterations of one's ability to move. Parkinson's disease is a degenerative condition that affects the substantia nigra, structures that are considered part of the basal ganglia circuitry that controls the EXTRAPYRAMIDAL MOTOR SYSTEM, hence it is considered one of the MOTOR SYSTEM DISORDERS. A move-

ment disorder also can arise as a complication of surgery or nonmotor system disease, as a result of trauma such as from injury or stroke, or as a side effect of drugs such as ANTIPSYCHOTIC MEDICATIONS that can cause EXTRAPYRAMIDAL SYMPTOMS similar to those of Parkinson's. Movement disorders can involve localized disturbances such as tics (repetitious twitching movements that usually involve the face) and TREMOR, or generalized disturbances that affect the body unilaterally (on one side only) or bilaterally (both sides) such as BRADYKINESIA (slowed muscle response) and AKINESIA ("frozen" muscle response).

See also ATAXIA; CONDITIONS SIMILAR TO PARKINSON'S; GAIT DISTURBANCE; MOTOR FUNCTION; MULTIPLE SYSTEM ATROPHY; POSTURAL INSTABILITY; RESTLESS LEG SYNDROME.

MPTP, MPTP-induced parkinsonism See 1-METHYL-4-PHENYL-1,2,3,6-TETRAHYDROPYRIDINE.

multiple sclerosis A chronic NEURODEGENERATIVE disease characterized by random demyelination of motor and sensory NEURONS. Scar tissue forms where myelin is missing, creating LESIONS that block the neuron from transmitting electrical impulses. Cumulatively, this process results in hardening and stiffening of nerve structures where demyelination has taken place, giving rise to the name *sclerosis,* which means "hardening." The MYELIN SHEATH is a protective covering that surrounds the neuron's AXON, or tail, sheltering the nerve signals it transmits from interference. Researchers do not know what causes demyelination; it appears to be an interaction of genetic, autoimmune, and environmental factors. Multiple sclerosis is significantly more common in people with family members who have multiple sclerosis or who live in temperate parts of the United States and Europe. Multiple sclerosis most commonly emerges in early adulthood (between the late 20s and early 40s) but can appear at any age.

Impaired motor function sometimes can appear at first to be Parkinson's disease when multiple sclerosis is manifested in middle age, although symptoms do not fit the classic Parkinson's profile. It is rare for such confusion to persist after a careful neurologic evaluation. As in Parkinson's disease, there is no conclusive diagnostic test as yet for multiple sclerosis. Imaging studies such as MAGNETIC RESONANCE IMAGING (MRI) and COMPUTED TOMOGRAPHY (CT) SCAN certain studies of the cerebrospinal fluid (the fluid surrounding the brain), and some neurophysiologic studies such as visual evoked potentials often can detect the fingerprints of demyelination and the lesions that form there, helping to confirm the diagnosis of multiple sclerosis, and rule out other neurodegenerative diseases.

The symptoms and course of multiple sclerosis are unpredictable. Most people experience symptom-free periods (remission) that can last years, and others experience complete debilitation within a short period. Depending on the nerves that are involved, multiple sclerosis can impair motor skills and mobility, speech, vision, and sensory perceptions. Symptoms often are bilateral (affecting both sides of the body). Steroid medications that relieve inflammation relieve symptoms in some people. Motor function impairments do not respond to LEVODOPA or other ANTI-PARKINSON'S MEDICATIONS.

See also CONDITIONS SIMILAR TO PARKINSON'S; DIAGNOSING PARKINSON'S; NERVE CONDUCTION STUDIES; NERVOUS SYSTEM; POSITRON EMISSION TOMOGRAPHY; SINGLE PHOTON EMISSION COMPUTED TOMOGRAPHY.

Multiple Sleep Latency Test   (MSLT) A study of BRAIN activity during sleep, conducted to help determine the causes of SLEEP DISTURBANCES and DAYTIME SLEEPINESS. The MSLT, conducted in a sleep laboratory, consists of five 20-minute periods during which the person is in a darkened room and encouraged to fall asleep. For two hours between each sleep session the person must stay awake. An ELECTROENCEPHALOGRAM (EEG), for which electrodes attached to the scalp transmit electrical messages from the brain to a recording mechanism, captures changes that occur between waking and sleeping states.

The neurologist analyzes the electrical patterns to determine whether there are patterns that point to pathological causes of the sleep problems. Nar-colepsy (a neurological disorder in which the person suddenly and uncontrollably falls asleep), for example, has a particular pattern of electrical disturbance. The main reason for a person with Parkinson's to have an MSLT is to rule out pathological causes of sleep disturbances and daytime sleepiness. The neurologist might request an MSLT when adjustments to the ANTI-PARKINSON'S MEDICATION regimen do not alleviate the symptoms. Typically, Parkinson's disease does not cause discernible disturbances in the brain's electrical activity during waking or sleeping periods.

See also BEDROOM COMFORT; EPWORTH SLEEPINESS SCALE; FATIGUE; PARKINSON'S DISEASE SLEEP SCALE.

multiple system atrophy   (MSA) A triad of coexisting NEURODEGENERATIVE disorders that manifest collective symptoms of autonomic, ataxic (cerebellar), and extrapyramidal (parkinsonian) dysfunctions. The predominant set of symptoms determines the commonly assigned name for the disorder, although the overall syndrome is more appropriately designated as multiple system atrophy (MSA) type A (autonomic), type C (cerebellar), or type P (parkinsonian). Symptoms typically begin when a person is in the mid-40s to mid-50s; When PARKINSONISM is the predominant set of symptoms, it is not unusual for clinicians to misdiagnose the condition as Parkinson's disease; ataxic (cerebellar) and autonomic features may not become apparent until years later in some people. Some experts classify MSA as one of the PARKINSON'S PLUS SYNDROMES on the premise that its core element is Parkinson's disease with additional overlying dysfunctions.

Scientists estimate that about 10 percent of people who are incorrectly diagnosed with Parkinson's have MSA. However, only at autopsy after death can the diagnosis be certain for either MSA or Parkinson's. The main clue during the course of the disease that a person has MSA instead of Parkinson's is rapid and significant deterioration; typically MSA results in death within seven to 10 years of diagnosis. The causes of MSA are unknown but are likely as multiple and intertwined as its symptoms. There are few effective treatments after the early stage of MSA. MSA is a devastating diagnosis for the person who has the disorder as well as for loved ones.

Ataxic Dysfunction (MSA-C): Olivopontocerebellar Atrophy (OPCA)

Olivopontocerebellar atrophy (OPCA) is the progressive deterioration of key structures of the medulla called the olives (because they physically resemble olives); of the CEREBELLUM, the part of the BRAIN that coordinates muscle activity and movement; and of the pons, a structure of the BRAINSTEM. With the physical loss of cells and tissues there occurs a corresponding loss of function that is manifested as ATAXIA (lack of BALANCE and COORDINATION). Intentional or kinetic tremor (a tremor that is present during intentional actions such as reaching for an object) also often occurs. Other symptoms of cerebellar dysfunction are similar to the symptoms of Parkinson's, including DYSKINESIA (involuntary movements) and DYSTONIA (severe rigidity with muscles often "frozen" in awkward positions). DYSARTHRIA (difficulty in forming words) and choreic movements also are part of the OPCA component of MSA.

Autonomic Dysfunction (MSA-A): Shy–Drager Syndrome

Disturbances of involuntary functions are the hallmark of the Shy–Drager syndrome component of MSA. These include urinary INCONTINENCE or retention, intestinal problems such as diarrhea or CONSTIPATION, SEXUAL DYSFUNCTION (particularly ERECTILE DYSFUNCTION), changes in sensory perceptions, ORTHOSTATIC HYPOTENSION (drop in blood pressure on changing position), and irregularities in heartbeat. Medications appropriate for each of these dysfunctions often can relieve symptoms in the early stages of MSA but may not be very effective as the degeneration progresses.

Extrapyramidal Dysfunction (MSA-P): Striatonigral Degeneration

MSA's extrapyramidal symptoms are much the same as those of Parkinson's disease and often include Parkinson's four classic or CARDINAL SYMPTOMS: resting TREMOR, BRADYKINESIA (slowed movement), RIGIDITY (muscle stiffness and resistance to movement), and POSTURAL INSTABILITY. This similarity occurs because the same kind of damage develops in the STRIATUM, SUBSTANTIA NIGRA, and other structures of the BASAL GANGLIA that are key to movement. DOPAMINERGIC NEURONS in these parts of the BRAIN rapidly die and the brain's supply of DOPAMINE diminishes. Notably tremor is often less prominent in MSA-P than in Parkinson's, and postural instability both presents much earlier in the disease course and is more severe than in Parkinson's. The olivopontocerebellar atrophy aspect of MSA involves significant atrophy (shrinking) of the CEREBELLUM, another part of the brain that is important to motor functions, particularly COORDINATION. Often this atrophy appears in imaging studies such as MAGNETIC RESONANCE IMAGING (MRI) or COMPUTED TOMOGRAPHY (CT) SCAN, or in FUNCTIONAL IMAGING STUDIES such as POSITRON EMISSION TOMOGRAPHY (PET) and SINGLE PHOTON EMISSION COMPUTED TOMOGRAPHY (SPECT).

In MSA, neurons contain substances called inclusions, abnormal but indistinct deposits throughout the cell's cytoplasm that can be detected at autopsy. As are LEWY BODIES, the characteristic protein deposits that infiltrate brain neurons in Parkinson's disease, MSA inclusions are primarily ALPHA-SYNUCLEIN. However, these inclusions are distinct from Lewy bodies in structure and composition, microscopically and biochemically. As well, MSA inclusions also infiltrate brain cells called glial cells, whose function is to support and protect neurons. Inclusion infiltration is fairly widespread throughout the brain.

The neuromuscular symptoms of MSA progress more rapidly than in Parkinson's, often leading to debilitation within a few years of diagnosis when extrapyramidal dysfunction is the predominant cluster of symptoms. Bradykinesia, dyskinesia, dystonia, and AKINESIA (lack of movement) typically are more pronounced than TREMORS. When the person with MSA does have tremors, typically MYOCLONUS is also present. Cerebellar atrophy causes additional neuromuscular symptoms such as ATAXIA (lack of muscle coordination and balance), which affects postural stability, GAIT, and MOBILITY.

Differential Diagnosis and Treatment

Each of the conditions that MSA comprises has distinct anatomical characteristics that often can be visualized through imaging studies as well as distinct typical functional characteristics on functional imaging. These characteristics can help to differentiate MSA from Parkinson's disease. A test of LEVODOPA therapy also can provide clinical clues, as levodopa is not effective in about two thirds of people with MSA and is effective only for a short time in others.

There really are few therapeutic options for MSA at present. Making an accurate diagnosis nonetheless is important so people with either diagnosis can make informed and appropriate decisions. If the diagnosis is Parkinson's disease, immediate and aggressive treatment with ANTI-PARKINSON'S MEDICATIONS can improve quality of life and delay debilitation. In MSA's early stages, anti-Parkinson's medications sometimes control some motor symptoms, but not for long (generally no more than two or three years) because of MSA's swift progression, and not completely. Also because symptoms progress rapidly, relief through surgical therapies such as DEEP BRAIN STIMULATION (DBS) or PALLIDOTOMY is so minimal that the benefits of surgery do not outweigh the risks; surgery is seldom considered an option for MSA. When anti-Parkinson's medications fail, treatment for neuromuscular symptoms is primarily supportive. Other medications can provide relief for symptoms of the Shy–Drager syndrome component of the triad, such as orthostatic hypotension (fludrocortisone, minodrine) and urinary incontinence (tolterodine, oxybutynin).

See also COMPASSION; CONDITIONS SIMILAR TO PARKINSON'S; DIAGNOSING PARKINSON'S; EMPATHY; URINARY FREQUENCY AND URGENCY; URINARY RETENTION.

muscarinic   See CHOLINERGIC.

muscle strength   The ability of a muscle to perform work. Muscle strength correlates with muscle mass: The greater the muscle mass, or volume of muscle fibers, the greater the strength of the muscle. Strength training, also called resistance training and weight training, helps to build muscle mass by stimulating the growth of new muscle fibers. Muscle strength is important for movement; muscle groups must be able to support the body as it moves through the range of positions involved in activities such as walking.

Regular physical activity such as occurs in daily living—sitting, standing, walking, reaching—helps maintain a muscle group's strength. When the nature of that activity changes, so does its effectiveness in maintaining muscle strength. Common GAIT DISTURBANCES in Parkinson's disease are reduced ARM SWING and LEG STRIDE. The muscle groups that move the arms and legs gradually get less exercise as swing and stride shorten, and they have less strength. Muscle mass is reduced because the body has no need to carry the metabolic needs of tissues it does not use. Unused muscle fibers flatten and shorten, and fat cells infiltrate the spaces around them.

Suggestions for improving mobility and stability such as "Make a conscious effort to engage in a full arm swing and lift the foot completely up from the walking surface during each step" also help to maintain muscle strength by making muscles work to the full RANGE OF MOTION for the action. For most people, walking is one of the most effective strengthening activities. Gentle resistance exercises, such as lifting one-pound weights, also help to strengthen muscle groups.

See also BALANCE; EXERCISE AND ACTIVITY; GAIT; GAIT DISTURBANCE; MUSCLE TONE; OCCUPATIONAL THERAPY; PHYSICAL THERAPY.

muscle tone   The amount of resistance to movement that exists in a muscle. Muscle tone is increased in Parkinson's disease as a result of disruptions in the nerve signals from the BASAL GANGLIA, particularly the subthalamic nucleus (STN), and other areas of the brain involved with movement to the muscles. Delays and interruptions in these messages cause slowed or inappropriate response in the muscles.

The depletion of DOPAMINE that is the hallmark of Parkinson's disease allows a disproportion of ACETYLCHOLINE to exist in the brain. In addition to their separate functions related to brain activity, these two NEUROTRANSMITTERS seem to work as a "check and balance" system to regulate messages from brain neurons to muscle cells. In Parkinson's disease, the lack of dopamine prevents transmission of certain nerve signals, accounting for symptoms such as BRADYKINESIA (slowed movement). At the same time the excess of acetylcholine results in a chaotic jumble as other nerve signals are allowed through; other neuromuscular symptoms such as TREMORS, RIGIDITY, and COGWHEELING, classic symptoms of Parkinson's disease result.

The person with Parkinson's typically does not perceive that muscles are stiff or rigid. In the early and middle stages of the disease, many neuromuscular symptoms tend to disappear with voluntary movement. Regular physical activity helps the person with Parkinson's disease take advantage of this tendency, observing the common advice "Use it so you don't lose it." Walking and swimming are activities that exercise nearly all muscle groups in the body. As the disease progresses and damage to the PYRAMIDAL PATHWAYS becomes more extensive, however, this is less likely to occur. Doctors can assess muscle tone through clinical examination that involves passive movement of a muscle group. ELECTROPHYSIOLOGIC STUDIES such as ELECTROMYLOGRAM (EMG) can provide measures of the electrical activity within muscle groups, a more direct way to assess nerve function.

Muscle tone changes with ANTI-PARKINSON'S MEDICATIONS. It can be near-normal during ON-STATES when medication is at its most effective, and extremely heightened during an OFF-STATE, when medication levels in the body are lower than the levels necessary to control symptoms such as rigidity. Surgical treatments such as DEEP BRAIN STIMULATION (DBS), PALLIDOTOMY, and THALAMOTOMY can block chaotic neuron messages, helping to provide long-term control of symptoms related to muscle tone.

See also EXERCISE AND ACTIVITY; FLUCTUATING PHENOMENON; MUSCLE STRENGTH; OCCUPATIONAL THERAPY; PHYSICAL THERAPY; RANGE OF MOTION; RANGE OF MOTION EXERCISES.

muscular dystrophy   A group of neuromuscular disorders marked by progressive deterioration of motor function. The muscular dystrophies affect the pyramidal motor system and may involve the muscles, peripheral nerves, spinal cord, and brain stem primary motor neurons, or the pyramidal motor pathways in the brainstem and spinal cord. EXTRAPYRAMIDAL MOTOR SYSTEM diseases such as Parkinson's are not considered muscular dystrophies. Many forms of muscular dystrophy are genetic and hereditary; they result from GENE MUTATIONS or defects that are passed from parent to child. Some are autosomal dominant, requiring that the gene mutation be present in only one parent, and others are autosomal recessive, requiring that the gene mutation be present in both parents. Other forms of muscular dystrophy are autoimmune (the body's immune system attacks particular cellular structures) or idiopathic (a specific cause is not clear). There are as yet no cures for any of the identified forms of muscular dystrophy, and although some have fairly mild symptoms over a period of many years, treatment is limited to supportive care for many other forms.

Most forms of muscular dystrophy appear in childhood; a few do not produce symptoms until middle age. Symptoms are distinct from those of most other neurodegenerative diseases including Parkinson's. Researchers studying Parkinson's disease are interested in muscular dystrophy, particularly the forms that involve neuromuscular dysfunctions, because many gene mutations have been identified among this group of disorders.

See also AUTOSOMAL DOMINANT INHERITANCE; AUTOSOMAL RECESSIVE INHERITANCE; GENE MAPPING; GENE THERAPY.

myelin sheath   A protective covering that encases the AXON, or tail, of motor and sensory NEURONS in much the same way that plastic encloses an electrical wire. Myelin cells are made of lipids (fatty acids) and proteins. This composition gives the myelin sheath its characteristic whitish color. The myelin sheath insulates the axon, containing the electrical impulses the neuron carries. This insulation increases the speed with which the neuron transmits electrical signals as well as prevents interference from sources outside the neuron. Damage to the myelin sheath creates distortions of the neuron's signals that result in inappropriate or no muscle response and movement when motor neurons are involved or tingling and pain when sensory neurons are involved.

Many disease processes can cause myelin sheath damage in the peripheral nerves; among the most common is diabetes, in which such damage results in peripheral neuropathy (functional damage to the nerves serving the outer parts of the body such as the feet and hands). Kidney disease, liver disease, and certain vitamin deficiencies also cause myelin sheath damage and peripheral neuropathy. Demyelination, in which myelin sheath damage occurs in the central white matter tracts, is the hallmark of the NEURODEGENERATIVE disease MULTIPLE SCLEROSIS.

See also BRAIN; DENDRITE; NERVOUS SYSTEM.

myoclonus   A sudden, brief muscle contraction that gives the appearance of twitching or jerking. Myoclonus has several forms:

- Physiological myoclonus is an isolated myoclonic event that is not symptomatic of any disease, such as hiccups or the "sleep jump" (commonly of the head or limbs) that a person sometimes experiences when falling asleep.

- Symptomatic myoclonus is secondary and shows as a pattern of myoclonic movements consistent with neurological damage caused by a specific disease such as MULTIPLE SCLEROSIS, Parkinson's disease, multiple system atrophy (MSA), progressive supranuclear palsy, cortical basal ganglionic degeneration, ALZHEIMER'S DISEASE, CREUTZFELDT-JAKOB DISEASE (CJD), and some seizure disorders.

- Nocturnal or sleep myoclonus is spasmodic movement of the muscles during sleep at night.

- Essential myoclonus is repetitive, forceful myoclonic movement that is pathological in nature (the result of unknown damage to the neuromuscular system) and can be debilitating; it may be focal (restricted to a particular muscle group) or generalized (affecting multiple muscle groups).

- Epileptic myoclonus is myoclonic movement that occurs in some seizure disorders.

  Drugs (especially ANTIPSYCHOTIC MEDICATIONS and some illicit drugs), infection, hypoxia (lack of oxygen to the BRAIN), and trauma can cause temporary (reversible) or permanent damage to NERVOUS SYSTEM structures such as the BRAIN or SPINAL CORD that result in myoclonic episodes. Nocturnal myoclonus is common among people with middle to late stage Parkinson's, as medication schedules typically load dosages during daytime hours for maximal symptom control when it is needed most. Certain actions or events can trigger myoclonic episodes. most common are movements (such as taking a step to walk or reaching for an object), intense physical exercise, and ANXIETY.

It is important to establish the nature and likely cause of myoclonus in the person with Parkinson's disease. Some ANTI-PARKINSON'S MEDICATIONS can cause myoclonic episodes. As well, many medications prescribed to treat myoclonus, such as the antiseizure medication valproate, interact with anti-Parkinson's medications. the antispasmodic medications CLONAZEPAM and BACLOFEN often provide relief and do not interact with anti-Parkinson's medications.

See also DYSKINESIA; MOTOR FUNCTION; MOTOR SYSTEM DISORDERS; TREMORS.

N4A class The international therapeutic classification for ANTI-PARKINSON'S MEDICATIONS and other therapies for treating Parkinson's disease. CLINICAL PHARMACOLOGY TRIALS and CLINICAL RESEARCH STUDIES are sometimes listed according to their therapeutic classifications.

See also PHARMACOTHERAPY.

N-acetyl-transferase 2 gene One of a number of genes that influence the synthesis of *N*-acetyl-transferase, an enzyme that participates in many metabolic functions within the body. The *N*-acetyl-transferase 2 gene affects the relationship between *N*-acetyl-transferase and metabolism of the MONOAMINE NEUROTRANSMITTERS including DOPAMINE. Studies have been mixed as to whether mutations of the *N*-acetyl-transferase 2 gene are associated with an increased risk of Parkinson's disease in either familial or sporadic presentations. Some researchers believe it might prove to be one of the multiple factors that likely converge to cause Parkinson's to develop.

Scientists discovered the first *N*-acetyl-transferase gene in 1996 and by 2002 had identified nearly two dozen variants. Mutations in a number of these are linked to other diseases, most notably diabetes, bladder cancer, some kinds of breast cancer, colorectal cancer, systemic lupus erythematosus, and ALZHEIMER'S DISEASE. Collectively, scientists refer to the many variants of the *N*-acetyl-transferase gene as NATs.

See also ENVIRONMENTAL TRIGGERS; GENE MAPPING; GENE MUTATION; GENE THERAPY; HUMAN GENOME PROJECT; NEUROPROTECTIVE EFFECT; NEUROPROTECTIVE THERAPIES.

NADH See NICOTINAMIDE ADENINE DINUCLEOTIDE.

narcotic pain reliever See PAIN MANAGEMENT.

National Human Genome Research Institute (NHGRI) An institute of the U.S. NATIONAL INSTITUTES OF HEALTH (NIH) through which American researchers contribute to the international Human Genome Project and conduct other research that targets genetic causes of disease. The NHGRI provides funding and support for research projects related to human genetics and molecular medicine located at universities and research centers around the country and maintains extensive databases that catalog research findings. The NHGRI's website (www.nhgri.nih.gov or www.genome.gov) provides a vast array of information about sponsored research projects and gene research in general. The main contact for the NHGRI is

Communications and Public Liaison Branch
National Human Genome Research Institute
National Institutes of Health
Building 31, Room 4B09
31 Center Drive, MSC 2152
9000 Rockville Pike
Bethesda, MD 20892-2152
(301) 402-0911
http://www.genome.gov

See also GENE MAPPING; GENE MUTATIONS; GENE THERAPY; GENETIC PREDISPOSITION; MICHAEL J. FOX FOUNDATION FOR PARKINSON'S RESEARCH; PARKINSON STUDY GROUP.

National Institute of Neurological Disorders and Stroke (NINDS) An institute of the U.S. NATIONAL INSTITUTES OF HEALTH (NIH) that funds and supports biomedical research on diseases and disorders of the BRAIN and nervous system. The NINDS website (www.ninds.nih.gov) lists current clinical research trials doing neurological studies that are looking for participants and reports on research project status and findings. The main contact for the NINDS is

NIH Neurological Institute
P.O. Box 5801
Bethesda, MD 20824
(800) 352-9424 or (301) 496-5751
TTY (301) 468-5981
http://www.ninds.nih.gov

See also HUMAN GENOME PROJECT; MICHAEL J. FOX FOUNDATION FOR PARKINSON'S RESEARCH; NATIONAL HUMAN GENOME RESEARCH INSTITUTE; PARKINSON STUDY GROUP.

National Institutes of Health (NIH)   A collective of more than two dozen institutes and centers that sponsor, support, fund, coordinate, and oversee biomedical research in the United States. The NIH sets research guidelines and ethics standards, provides information and research findings for medical professionals and for the general public, and publishes extensive information about health topics. The NIH is part of the U.S. Department of Health and Human Services. The main contact for the NIH is

National Institutes of Health
Building 1
1 Center Drive
Bethesda, MD 20892
(301) 496-4000
http://www.nih.gov

Each institute and center of the NIH also has its own contact information. The NIH website (www.nih.gov) provides a directory of NIH institutes, centers, programs, and resources.
See also HUMAN GENOME PROJECT; NATIONAL HUMAN GENOME RESEARCH INSTITUTE; NATIONAL INSTITUTE OF NEUROLOGICAL DISORDERS AND STROKE.

National Parkinson Foundation   A private, not-for-profit organization founded in 1957 that is dedicated to finding the causes of and a cure for

Parkinson's disease. It sponsors a number of centers of excellence throughout the world that combine clinical care and research and basic science research, as well as providing publications and seminars aimed at educating people with Parkinson's. The National Parkinson Foundation's headquarters in Miami, Florida, houses research facilities as well as clinical services, in affiliation with the University of Miami School of Medicine, through which physicians and other health care practitioners provide care to people with Parkinson's disease. The main contact for the National Parkinson Foundation is

National Parkinson Foundation, Inc.
Bob Hope Parkinson Research Center
1501 N.W. 9th Avenue
Bob Hope Road
Miami, Fl 33136-1494
(800) 327-4545 or (305) 547-6666
http://www.parkinson.org

See also MICHAEL J. FOX FOUNDATION FOR PARKINSON'S RESEARCH; PARKINSON STUDY GROUP.

nausea   The unpleasant sensation of being about to vomit. Nausea is a common side effect of many DOPAMINERGIC MEDICATIONS, most notably LEVODOPA. Peripheral metabolism of these drugs is rapid after their absorption into the bloodstream; DOPAMINE is nearly immediately further metabolized to NOREPINEPHRINE and epinephrine. Whereas in the brain these substances function as neurotransmitters, in the body they are hormones that regulate heart rate, breathing rate, and blood pressure. The body responds to the sudden flush of epinephrine as an activation of its "fight or flight" mechanism, which affects numerous body chemicals and functions.
    The most effective way to minimize levodopa-induced nausea is to take sufficient amounts of DOPA DECARBOXYLASE INHIBITORS, such as CARBIDOPA (as in the medication Sinemet) or BENSERAZIDE (as in the medication Madopar); these drugs block the action of the enzyme that metabolizes levodopa, DOPA DECARBOXYLASE. This also slows the rate at which levodopa becomes converted to dopamine (and subsequently to norepinephrine and epineph-

rine) in the peripheral bloodstream. The therapeutic effect of this is to both permit a greater amount of levodopa to cross the BLOOD-BRAIN BARRIER so it can be converted to dopamine in the brain, and reduce the risk of side effects from the conversion of levodopa into dopamine in the bloodstream, which include levodopa-induced nausea.

Another strategy that often works in early to middle stages of the disease is to take the medication with food to slow the rate of levodopa's absorption into the bloodstream. This releases less levodopa at a time for peripheral metabolism, but this decreased absorption can also cause decreased control of Parkinson's symptoms in people with mid-stage to late-stage Parkinson's who are very dependent on getting very precise levels of levodopa to the brain. Taking levodopa with large amounts of protein is particularly risky. Some advanced patients even note worse symptoms after protein even when it is consumed well away from the time of their medications.

Other ANTI-PARKINSON'S MEDICATIONS sometimes can cause nausea as well, including tricyclic and SELECTIVE SEROTONIN REUPTAKE INHIBITOR (SSRI) MEDICATIONS taken for depression, some ANTICHOLINERGIC MEDICATIONS, and the MAOI-B inhibitor SELEGILINE. Nausea also can be a symptom of Parkinson's disease itself, as the altered balance of neurotransmitters in the brain affects many functions in the body including those related to digestion. Balance disturbances can cause a person to feel dizziness or "wooziness," of which nausea is often a component. Nausea that actually ends in vomiting can prevent medications from being fully digested and absorbed and should be brought to the doctor's attention. Mild and distracting activity such as walking sometimes reduces nausea.

See also ANTIDEPRESSANT MEDICATIONS; BIOAVAILABILITY; MEDICATION MANAGEMENT; MEDICATION SIDE EFFECTS.

nefazodone An atypical example of the ANTIDEPRESSANT MEDICATIONS generally taken when other antidepressants have unacceptable side effects, are not effective, or cannot be taken because of interactions with other medications. Nefazodone (Serzone) inhibits (blocks) serotonin reuptake to extend the availability of serotonin, a BRAIN NEUROTRANSMITTER that effects mood and emotion. Its biochemical actions differ from those of conventional SELECTIVE SEROTONIN REUPTAKE INHIBITOR (SSRI) MEDICATIONS, however, precluding some of the side effects of SSRIs that can be particularly troublesome for people with Parkinson's such as DAYTIME SLEEPINESS, ORTHOSTATIC HYPOTENSION, and nighttime SLEEP DISTURBANCES. Nefazodone does not interact with most ANTI-PARKINSON'S MEDICATIONS, although it can increase the risk of side effects if taken with the MAO-B inhibitor SELEGILINE. As with other antidepressants, nefazodone is not fully effective for four to six weeks, and the dosage should be tapered rather than suddenly stopped.

See also ANXIETY; FLUOXETINE; PAROXETINE; PSYCHOSOCIAL FACTORS; PSYCHOTHERAPY; SERTRALINE.

nerve cell See NEURON.

nerve conduction studies Diagnostic tests to determine the nature and extent of damage to peripheral nerve pathways. Nerve conduction studies often are performed in conjunction with an ELECTROMYOGRAM (EMG) to provide a comprehensive picture of the neuromuscular physiology in a certain group of muscles or part of the body. During a nerve conduction study, a technician applies recording electrodes to the skin over the muscle groups being tested and then uses a different set of electrodes to apply a very mild electrical current. The current travels through the nerves, which are the body's communication pathways, and the recording electrodes capture the electrical activity. The rate and consistency with which the nerves carry the electrical signals help to determine what, if any, nerve conduction problems are present.

A neurologist may request nerve conduction studies to evaluate weakness, numbness, gait and balance problems, and other neuromuscular symptoms. The findings are more significant for ruling out peripheral nerve injury and other diseases that have specific damage patterns and have no role in confirming a diagnosis of Parkinson's disease.

See also DIAGNOSING PARKINSON'S; ELECTROENCEPHALOGRAM; ELECTROPHYSIOLOGIC STUDIES; NEUROLOGICAL EXAMINATION.

nervous system The body network that regulates all bodily functions. The nervous system is complex and contains numerous structures and subsystems that are responsible for specific activities or processes. Billions of NEURONS, or nerve cells, compose these structures and their subsystems. There are three major divisions of the nervous system. Two are structural as well as functional: the central nervous system, which consists of the BRAIN and SPINAL CORD; and the peripheral nervous system, which consists of all other nerve structures. The autonomic nervous system is a functional division of the nervous system that includes peripheral and central components to control many of the bodies involuntary responses. Voluntary and involuntary actions require the concerted function of central and peripheral nervous system components. Parkinson's disease damages the structures of the central nervous system, thereby affecting voluntary and involuntary functions. In mid to late stages of the disease damage to the autonomic nervous system may become a significant source of disability.

Central Nervous System

The central nervous system consists of the brain and spinal cord and the functions of these structures that regulate the body's conscious (voluntary) and (involuntary) actions. It is the master control center of the entire nervous system from which other functional divisions emanate. Directly or indirectly, the central nervous system has a role in every body activity from breathing and movement to cognition and memory. Parkinson's disease affects the structures and functions of the central nervous system in numerous ways.

The BRAIN is the primary organ of the nervous system. It has three physically distinctive structures:

• The cerebrum, which controls conscious activity including intellect, thought, speech, emotions, and memory. The organizational units of the brain are its four paired lobes: frontal, temporal, parietal, and occipital. Voluntary movement begins in the cerebrum, with the conscious (although often unaware) decision to move. This initiates a complex and intricate sequence of nervous system functions. The DOPAMINE DEPLETION that is the hallmark of Parkinson's dis-

ease directly affects the structures and functions of the cerebrum.

• The cerebellum, which controls coordination of both voluntary and involuntary movement. A switching station of sorts, the cerebellum processes millions of messages that relay information between the cerebrum and the body's neuromuscular structures per second. Although the direct functions of the cerebellum remain intact in Parkinson's disease, the chaotic communication among brain neurons that results from dopamine depletion in the BASAL GANGLIA disrupts signals before and after they pass through the cerebellum.

• The brainstem, which is the conduit for communication between the brain and the body. Some of its direct functions, which control involuntary functions such as breathing and blood pressure, are part of the AUTONOMIC NERVOUS SYSTEM. Structures of the brainstem also control the function of smooth muscle, such as in the digestive tract, blood vessels, and heart. Some of these structures, most notably the midbrain, contain dopaminergic neurons that also die as Parkinson's progresses, impairing the functions of the midbrain and possibly other brainstem structures.

Nestled at the junction of these three structures are the basal ganglia, a cluster of specialized nerve structures that control voluntary movement. The death of DOPAMINERGIC NEURONS in the basal ganglia, primarily in the SUBSTANTIA NIGRA, initiates the changes that cause the neuromuscular dysfunctions such as TREMORS and BRADYKINESIA that characterize Parkinson's disease.

The spinal cord is a ropelike collection of nerve tissues and fibers that extends from the brain stem to immediately above the tail bone and is the "highway" through which nearly all nerves and nerve signals enter and leave the brain. In an adult, the spinal cord is about 18 inches long and the thickness of a thumb. The spinal cord carries motor signals from the brain and sensory signals to the brain. It also controls certain basic involuntary motor responses, for instances, reflexes such as the knee jerk. Its divisions are anatomical rather than functional, correlating to the sections of the body the spinal cord passes through: cervical (neck), thoracic (chest), lumbar (lower back), and sacral (tail bone). The spinal cord ends in a splay of nerve fibers, called the cauda equina ("horse's tail"), that extends downward along the final segments of the spine. Parkinson's disease does not affect the structure of functions of the spinal cord.

Peripheral Nervous System

The nerves that extend from the central nervous system to communicate with other structures of the body form the peripheral nervous system. This includes the cranial nerves, spinal nerve roots, nerve connection points (called ganglia), and peripheral nerves. Although the peripheral nervous system's structures remain intact in Parkinson's disease, the progressive degeneration of central nervous system structures and functions affects the functions of the peripheral nervous system. Distorted signals from the basal ganglia cause confused and chaotic responses in peripheral motor neurons, resulting in dysfunctional movement (TREMORS AND DYSKINESIAS) and impaired motor function.

Cranial nerves   The 12 paired cranial nerves originate in the brain. One pair, the olfactory, originate in the cerebrum, a second pair, the optic, originate in the thalamus; they have solely sensory functions. The remaining pairs originate in the structures of the brainstem and have mixed sensory and motor functions. The pair known collectively as the vagus nerve is a key structure of the autonomic nervous system that controls such functions as breathing and heart rate. Parkinson's disease affects some of the functions for which cranial nerves are responsible, for example, by creating disturbances of vision and smell, but scientists are not certain whether this effect involves damage to the cranial nerves or to the areas within the brain that interpret sensory signals. Parkinson's symptoms such as difficulty in moving the eyes or swallowing relate to neuromuscular disruptions that take place in the basal ganglia and affect neuron communication to the muscles, rather than to damage that involves the cranial nerves that also have functions related to the muscles that move the eyes, tongue, and face. The route of transit remains intact although the signals traveling it are distorted.

Spinal nerves   The spinal nerves branch from the spinal cord in 31 pairs named for their corresponding locations along the spine: eight cervical

		CRANIAL NERVES	
Nerve Pair	Nerve Name	Origin	Functions
1	Olfactory	Olfactory bulb in the cerebrum	Smell
2	Optic	Lateral geniculate nucleus of the thalamus	Vision
3	Oculomotor	Midbrain	Most eye movements (major eye muscles)
4	Trochlear	Midbrain	Eye movement (superior oblique muscle)
5	Trigeminal	Pons and medulla	Face sensations and jaw movement
6	Abducens	Pons	Eye movement (lateral rectus muscle)
7	Facial	Pons	Facial expressions and movements, taste, salivation
8	Vestibulocochlear	Pons and medulla	Balance and equilibrium (vestibular) hearing (cochlear)
9	Glossopharyngeal	Medulla	Palate sensation, sensory arm of autonomic reflexes controlling heart rate and blood pressure
10	Vagus	Medulla	Breathing, blood pressure, heart rate and rhythm, digestion
11	Spinal accessory	Medulla and spinal cord	Neck and shoulder movement
12	Hypoglossal	Medulla	Tongue movement

pairs, 12 thoracic pairs, five lumbar pairs, five sacral pairs, and one coccygeal pair. Each spinal nerve attaches to the spinal cord with two roots, a dorsal root containing afferent neurons that carry signals to thalamus and brainstem via the spinal cord and a ventral root containing the oxons (arms of the neuron that serve as communication cables) of efferent neurons that carry signals away from the spinal cord. The spinal nerves quickly branch as they leave the spinal cord, forming an extensive network of nerves that eventually reaches to all parts of the body. Parkinson's disease does not directly damage the spinal nerves, which continue carrying signals to and from the brain. However, there is no process within the spinal cord, spinal nerves, or other nerve pathways to decode or correct faulty nerve signals; signals from the brain that are incomplete or jumbled travel nerve pathways and reach their destinations just as incomplete or jumbled as when they left the brain.

Peripheral nerves   All of the nerve structures that branch from the cranial and spinal nerves are the peripheral, or outer, nerves. Nerves that serve organ systems are called visceral or enteric; nerves that serve the musculoskeletal system are called somatic. As with the cranial and spinal nerves, the peripheral nerves remain structurally and functionally sound in Parkinson's disease. The disruptions and dysfunctions that cause the neuromuscular symptoms of Parkinson's originate in the regions of the brain that control movement.

Autonomic Nervous System

The autonomic nervous system regulates the body's automatic functions such as heartbeat, blood pressure, breathing, digestion, excretion, temperature regulation, and actions of smooth muscle (such as in the heart, blood vessels, and intestinal tract). Its primary purpose is to sustain life; its structures and mechanisms are the nervous system's most primitive and most basic. The loss of DOPAMINERGIC NEURONS and corresponding DOPAMINE depletion that characterizes Parkinson's disease affects parts of the brainstem, particularly the subthalamic nucleus and the midbrain, the are involved in functions of the autonomic nervous system such as smooth muscle control.

The autonomic nervous system has two components that have counterbalancing functions, the sympathetic and parasympathetic nervous systems. Structurally these systems exit the central nervous system with certain cranial and spinal nerves. The sympathetic pathways then involve a connection with a neuron in a ganglia chain that parallels the spinal cord, this neuron then forms the connection with the end organ (usually the smooth muscle of viscera, the heart, or glands). Parasympathetic axons travel all the way to the wall of the target organ before connecting to the neuron that actually connects to the end organ. The sympathetic and parasympathetic nerve systems are important for sexual arousal and function, including erection and ejaculation in men. Many ANTI-PARKINSON'S MEDICATIONS, particularly anticholinergics and dopamine agonists, affect the functions of the autonomic nervous system.

Sympathetic nervous system   A nerve network that extends from the thoracic and upper two lumbar segments of the spinal cord constitutes the sympathetic nervous system. The main functions of this nerve network to maintain adequate heart rate, blood pressure, and breathing rate and to prepare the body for "fight or flight." The ganglia chains terminate in various organ systems; the adrenergic neurons at the ends of the chains release NOREPINEPHRINE, which causes neurotransmitters cause blood vessels to dilate, heart rate to increase, and blood pressure to rise. They also open airways in the lungs and accelerate breathing. At the same time, the sympathetic nervous system slows the function of smooth muscle in the digestive tract. The sympathetic nervous system is also important for ejaculation and sexual climax.

Parasympathetic nervous system   The nerve networks of the parasympathetic nervous system extend into the body from two points, the brainstem and the lower region of the spinal cord. The main functions of the parasympathetic nervous system are to relax the cardiorespiratory system (heart rate, blood pressure, breathing) and stimulate functions of digestion. The parasympathetic nervous system is also important for sexual arousal: erection in men, and probably vaginal lubrication, labial engorgement, and clitoral engorgement in women. The terminal neurons of the parasympathetic ganglia chains are cholinergic; when activated they release acetylcholine, which causes smooth muscle tissues to relax and dilates blood vessels, slows heart rate, and increases blood flow to organs such as the stomach and intestines.

See also CONDITIONS SIMILAR TO PARKINSON'S; EXTRAPYRAMIDAL SYSTEM; PYRAMIDAL PATHWAY.

neural graft Any of several procedures in which cells, usually dopaminergic, are transplanted to the brain of a person with Parkinson's disease. The intent is for these cells to take root and begin to reproduce, replacing the DOPAMINERGIC NEURONS that have died. At present, neural grafts are experimental and have produced inconsistent results. Graft sources include human fetal dopaminergic cells, fetal porcine brain cells, human stem cells, and AUTOGRAFT using adrenal medullary tissue.

See also ADRENAL MEDULLARY TRANSPLANT; BIOETHICS; BRAIN TISSUE TRANSPLANT; HOPE FOR A PARKINSON'S CURE; RETINAL CELL IMPLANT.

neurochemical brain imaging See FUNCTIONAL IMAGING STUDIES.

neurochemistry The balance and distribution of chemical messengers (neurotransmitters) of the BRAIN and NERVOUS SYSTEM. There is an intricate and complex interplay among them, making it virtually impossible to separate one from the other. Parkinson's is a disease of altered neurochemistry; the DOPAMINE DEPLETION that results from the death of DOPAMINERGIC NEURONS in the BASAL GANGLIA (brain structures that control movement) distorts and disrupts NEUROTRANSMITTER functions. Most ANTI-PARKINSON'S MEDICATIONS target the brain's neurochemistry by attempting to restore dopamine levels or to change the brain's neurochemical balance by inhibiting other neurotransmitters.

See also ACETYLCHOLINE; NEURON; NOREPINEPHRINE.

neurodegenerative A progressive loss of NERVOUS SYSTEM cells, structures, and functions. Some slow patterns of neurodegeneration occur as a function of normal aging. When neurodegeneration occurs in an abnormal pattern that affects function, it is deemed a neurodegenerative disease. The symptoms of neurodegenerative disease worsen as the disease progresses. GENE MUTATIONS are the sole cause of some neurodegenerative diseases, such as HUNTINGTON'S DISEASE, and are known to contribute to many others including ALZHEIMER'S DISEASE and Parkinson's disease. Infections (for example HIV, the AIDS virus, and some prion diseases such as Creutzfeldt-Jakob disease [CJD]) and toxic exposures also can lead to neurodegeneration. Scientists do not fully understand the mechanisms of most neurodegenerative diseases, from what causes them in development to how to slow or stop their progression.

See also BRAIN; NERVOUS SYSTEM; NEURON; NEUROPROTECTIVE EFFECT; NEUROPROTECTIVE THERAPIES; NEUROTRANSMITTER.

neurofibrillary tangles Deformities that develop within NEURONS that prevent them from functioning properly. The body of a neuron contains numerous tiny fibers, called neurofibrils, that conduct electrical impulses through the cell. Typically, neurofibrillary tangles form around abnormal protein deposits that collect in the cell's cytoplasm, such as the TAU deposits (amyloid plaques) that are characteristic of ALZHEIMER'S DISEASE and progressive supranuclear palsy (PSP), and the ALPHA-SYNUCLEIN deposits called LEWY BODIES that are characteristic of Parkinson's disease. Neurofibrillary tangles interfere with the neuron's ability to shuttle nutrients, raw materials, waste, and its end product neurotransmitters to the appropriate places and organelles within itself, greatly impairing the neuron's ability to function. This disrupts neuron communication in the nervous system. Scientists are not certain whether neurofibrillary tangles form as a consequence of other biochemical factors involved in the disease process or are themselves part of that process.

See also NERVOUS SYSTEM; NEUROPROTECTIVE EFFECT; NEUROPROTECTIVE THERAPIES.

neurological examination An assessment and evaluation of the structures and functions of the nervous system. Typically, a neurological examination covers COGNITIVE FUNCTION, MOTOR FUNCTION, and sensory function. Though all physicians have had some training in performing neurological examinations, neurologists are the most expert at performing them and interpreting their results. Often, the physician overlaps these areas during the examination to expedite the proceedings and also to help the person feel less self-conscious. The extent to which the examination probes these functions depends on whether the purpose is diagnostic or follow-up.

Cognitive Function

The neurologist assesses basic cognitive function by asking simple questions such as "What is today's date?" and "Who is the president?" These kinds of questions aim to establish whether the person is oriented to current time and events. The neurologist then may ask the person to repeat a sequence of letters, words, or numbers. These questions evaluate memory and recall, as well as attention span and concentration. The doctor may conduct a MINI MENTAL STATUS EXAMINATION (MMSE) or administer a more comprehensive cognitive assessment. This portion of the neurological examination also typically includes questions about sleeping and waking patterns, particularly SLEEP DISTURBANCES and DAYTIME SLEEPINESS. The doctor may ask the person to complete an EPWORTH SLEEPINESS SCALE (ESS) self-assessment. As well, the doctor should ask about his or her concerns or noticeable problems.

Motor Function

The motor function assessment begins before the person knows the examination is under way, when the doctor observes posture, BALANCE, and MOVEMENT. When extending a handshake for greeting, the doctor notices whether there is tremor or hesitation, full extension of the arm, and strength and firmness in the grip. More focused examination or motor function includes instructed movements such as walking down a corridor, which allow the doctor to evaluate GAIT and GAIT DISTURBANCES suggestive of Parkinson's disease such as reduced ARM SWING, slumping or stooped shoulders and upper posture, and short-

ened LEG STRIDE and step. Other kinds of gait disturbances, such as swinging one leg in an arclike pattern during forward stepping or dragging the heels, suggest neurological or neuromuscular disorders other than Parkinson's disease. A wide stumbling gait may suggest cerebellar problems rather than Parkinson's. Other gait and balance problems might suggest normal pressure hydrocephalus, neuropathy, or other disorders. The doctor watches for whether symptoms are asymmetrical (one-sided) or symmetrical (affect both sides); Parkinson's is nearly always asymmetrical until its later stages.

The doctor will instruct the person to squeeze his or her hand or fingers to determine whether strength is appropriate and even on both sides and to push and pull against the doctor's hands to test strength. The doctor puts the wrists, elbows, knees, and ankles through a series of passive movements to check for RIGIDITY, a classic sign of Parkinson's. During this part of the examination, the doctor also looks for other patterns of stiffness suggestive of disorders other than Parkinson's. The doctor checks the standard tendon tap reflexes, alteration of which may suggest a different or additional disorder in people suspected to have Parkinson's. Often the doctor tells the person to stand and push and pull the person at the shoulders to test balance and POSTURAL RIGHTING REFLEX. This is always done in such a way that the person cannot fall. It is normal to take a step forward or back to recover balance; a person with Parkinson's typically takes three or more steps before recovering.

Some motor function tests seem silly, such as wiggling the fingers and rapidly tapping heel–toe. But these activities challenge the brain's motor functions and draw out disturbances that might otherwise remain undetected. The doctor engages the person in conversation during the motor function examination and listens closely to the person's voice modulation and speech patterns. Soft, slow speech suggests Parkinson's disease and may be present without the person's awareness. The conversation additionally helps the doctor to assess cognitive function. During conversation the doctor observes the person's face for changes in facial expression, smiling, blinking, and eye movements. Reduced facial expression and slowed blinking are common early signs of Parkinson's.

Sensory Function

Sensory functions are those related to the five senses: vision, hearing, smell, taste, and touch. In most people with Parkinson's sensory perceptions are normal with the exception of smell. More than half of people with Parkinson's have an altered sense of smell or cannot detect smells. Parkinson's can cause visual disturbances when it affects the muscles that control eye movements; the doctor explores this function by asking the person to move the eyes to follow a moving object. There also seems to be some decrease in visual acuity from retinal changes in Parkinson's as well; the retina also needs dopamine (from dopaminergic cells on the retinal surface) to function properly. Disturbances of touch may suggest peripheral neuropathy (damage to the peripheral nerves); the doctor tests for this by touching the feet, legs, hands, arms, face, and sometimes back with a soft object such as a cotton swab and a hard object such as a tongue depressor or the stick end of the swab. Tests of sensory function help to establish whether the CRANIAL NERVES are functioning properly; sensory disturbances can suggest cranial nerve lesions or damage.

Symptom Assessment

Most people have a neurological examination because they have symptoms. The doctor should ask about these symptoms throughout the examination and may conduct focused tests to evaluate those that appear prominent or significant further. For example, the doctor may ask a person who is experiencing coordination and dexterity difficulties to perform a number of exercises such as touching the finger to the nose, rapidly tapping the fingers, reaching for a moving object, matching movements with the doctor, picking up small objects such as coins from a smooth surface, and writing a sentence or drawing (copying) a geometric figure. These kinds of exercises tell the doctor as much about the conditions the person does *not* have as about those he or she may have.

Further Testing

The physician may want the person to have MAGNETIC RESONANCE IMAGING (MRI) studies, laboratory testing of blood or other samples, FUNCTIONAL IMAGING STUDIES, ELECTROPHYSIOLOGIC STUDIES, or other tests to narrow the diagnosis further, assess the progression of the disease, or evaluate the effectiveness of a treatment regimen. As there are no conclusive diagnostic markers for Parkinson's disease, diagnostic testing is primarily used to rule out other causes of symptoms. LESIONS such as tumors or scars and injuries such as those from trauma or stroke that affect the BASAL GANGLIA or the BRAINSTEM can cause TREMORS and DYSKINESIAS, for example, and typically are detected on FUNCTIONAL IMAGING STUDIES such as COMPUTED TOMOGRAPHY (CT) SCAN or magnetic resonance imaging (MRI). None of these tests is necessary when the CARDINAL SYMPTOMS of Parkinson's—resting tremor, bradykinesia, postural instability, and rigidity—are present. The fewer of the cardinal symptoms that are present or younger the person is the more likely the doctor is to want additional diagnostic information.

See also ARCHIMEDES SPIRAL; COPING WITH ONGOING CARE OF PARKINSON'S; DIAGNOSING PARKINSON'S; MICROGRAPHIA; STAGING OF PARKINSON'S DISEASE.

neurology A specialty in the practice of medicine that focuses on caring for people with disorders, diseases, and injuries involving the BRAIN and NERVOUS SYSTEM. A physician who specializes in neurology is a neurologist. In the United States a physician must complete medical school, a comprehensive residency in neurology (usually four years of study), which focuses on the structures, functions, and dysfunctions of the nervous system, and then pass written and oral examinations conducted by the American Board of Psychiatry and Neurology. Some neurologists subspecialize in narrowly focused areas of neurology such as neuromuscular or movement disorders often undertaking additional training in the form of fellowships after residency. People with Parkinson's disease should receive care through a neurologist, either directly or through close collaboration with the PRIMARY CARE PHYSICIAN.

See also NEUROPSYCHIATRY; NEUROPSYCHOLOGY; NEUROSURGERY.

neuron The cell that is the basic unit of function of the NERVOUS SYSTEM. The nervous system contains billions of neurons. There are many kinds of neurons including sensory neurons, interneurons, and motor neurons. Interneurons are the most common. Some neurons within these basic types have specialized structures and functions. In general, neurons share the following common features:

- Cell body, which contains the nucleus bearing the cell's genetic instructions (deoxyribonucleic acid [DNA]), cytoplasm, neurofibrils, and mitochondria
- Dendrites, branchlike projections that receive incoming electrical signals
- Axon, a taillike structure that sends outgoing electrical signals; most axons are covered with a protective myelin sheath that insulates them

Neurons conduct electrical impulses that travel at speeds equivalent to several hundred miles an hour. Separating neurons from one another are corridors called synapses; NEUROTRANSMITTERS carry signals across the synapses from one neuron to another in an intricately timed sequence of events. A change in the neuron's electrical properties, called an action potential, heralds that start of an electrical transmission and causes the sending neuron, called the presynaptic neuron, to release its neurotransmitter. The neurotransmitters cross the synaptic gap and binds with receptors in the receiving, or postsynaptic, neuron's dendrites. This action alters the postsynaptic neuron's electrical properties, causing a signal to which the postsynaptic neuron responds. As soon as the transmission is complete the axon and other cells, including the non-neural glia, resorb the remaining neurotransmitters and their chemical remnants, and the neuron is ready to repeat the process. As complex as the sequence is, it takes place in less than a millisecond. A single neuron can "fire" many times a second and convey messages to multiple other neurons.

The sequence requires that the correct amount of neurotransmitter be present at the correct time and for the correct duration. In Parkinson's disease, there is a decreased number of dopaminergic neurons. This decrease causes DOPAMINE, the neurotransmitter essential for neuron communication in parts of the brain that control movement, to be in short supply. As a result, neurons cannot properly transmit signals, and neuron communication becomes disrupted and incomplete. Messages directing movement leave the brain jumbled and confused, resulting in dysfunctional muscle response in the body such as TREMORS, BRADYKINESIA, and other DYSKINESIAS that characterize Parkinson's disease.

A cluster or bundle of like neurons (neurons with similar structure and function) and their supporting structures is called a ganglion (plural, *ganglia*) if located outside the cortex where most neurons in the brain are found. Collections of neuron bodies form gray matter, and collections of axons (fibers) form white matter. The body does not generate new neurons or replace damaged or dead neurons. The neurons present at birth are the ones that remain throughout life; neurons gradually die as a result of damage or APOPTOSIS.

Sensory Neurons

Sensory neurons are afferent (from the Latin meaning "carry toward"); they respond to external sensory stimuli such as touch and carry signals to the brain. A sensory neuron typically has a tightly focused, somewhat bulbous dendrite structure and a long (up to several feet), myelinated axon with multiple axon terminals (branches). Sensory neurons are concentrated in structures that receive sensory messages, such as the dorsal root ganglion, which conveys signals from touch receptor organs in the skin to the spinal cord and then to thalamic neurons, which complete the transmission of the sensory signals to the sensory cortex, and the retina, which conveys visual signals to neurons in the lateral geniculate nucleus of the thalamus, which in turn sends axons to the primary visual cortex.

Motor Neurons

Motor neurons are efferent (from the Latin meaning "carry from"); they convey signals from the brain to the muscles. A motor neuron typically has a widely branched dendrite structure and a long (up to several feet), myelinated axon ending in a small cluster of axon terminals.

- Upper motor neurons originate in the brain; their axons extend from the brain and into the spinal cord. They send signals to lower motor neurons.

- Lower motor neurons originate in the anterior horn of the spinal cord; their axons extend from the spinal cord to the skeletal (striated) muscles. They send signals to muscle cells.

Parkinson's disease disrupts upper motor neuron function. Lower motor neurons function normally but convey jumbled messages because the signals sent from the brain via the upper motor neurons are confused and incomplete.

Interneurons

Interneurons are the most abundant neurons in the nervous system. They are associative: They convey messages among neurons, rather than from neurons to the cells of body structures, to expedite the communication process. An interneuron typically has a short axon (no longer than a few centimeters), often unmyelinated, and sparsely placed dendrites. Interneurons are found throughout the nervous system.

See also AGING; CONDITIONS SIMILAR TO PARKINSON'S; MOTOR FUNCTION; NEUROPROTECTIVE EFFECT; NEUROPROTECTIVE THERAPIES.

neuroprotective effect The result of biochemical actions that help to shield NEURONS from damage by slowing FREE RADICAL activity and OXIDATION. Natural substances such as vitamins and other nutrients contain ANTIOXIDANTS. Antioxidants bind with free radicals, the waste by-products of metabolism, to prevent them from forming unstable molecular structures that cause cumulative damage to neurons and other cells. Some medications, such as MONOAMINE OXIDASE INHIBITOR (MAOI) MEDICATIONS, also have neuroprotective effects by limiting the formation of free radicals.

See also ANTI-PARKINSON'S MEDICATIONS; NEUROPROTECTIVE THERAPIES; SELEGILINE.

neuroprotective therapies Treatment approaches and medications that attempt to prevent damage to neurons. In people with Parkinson's disease, such therapies target preservation of the function of remaining dopaminergic neurons. Practical application of neuroprotective therapies for Parkinson's disease is fairly limited at present. None of the ANTIOXIDANTS tested so far (tocopherol, selegiline, vitamin C, glutathione) demonstrate any clear proof of neuroprotection when given to humans with Parkinson's, though a recent report on the use of COENZYME Q-10 is encouraging. Most Parkinson's experts recommend nutritional supplementation only to meet the body's nutritional needs when diet alone cannot do so. CLINICAL RESEARCH TRIALS are exploring other neuroprotective therapies such as genetic interventions whose purpose is to correct GENE MUTATIONS and MITOCHONDRIAL DYSFUNCTION.

Neuroprotection is an important factor in Parkinson's disease not only because it slows or prevents further loss of dopaminergic neurons but also because the cornerstone of medication therapy, LEVODOPA, has been found in some cell culture studies to possibly contribute to neuron damage through increased oxidation. It is important to note that animal studies have not been very suggestive of this problem, and all human studies to date fail to demonstrate any increase in cell death from the use of levodopa. In fact, the human data clearly suggest that levodopa provides a survival benefit versus no treatment and is the most potent medication for relieving the symptoms of Parkinson's. A recent large study suggests that it may have a mild protective effect against progression of off-medication symptoms.

See also ANTI-PARKINSON'S MEDICATIONS; GENE THERAPY; MONOAMINE OXIDASE; NEUROTROPHIC FACTORS; TREATMENT ALGORITHM.

neuropsychiatry A specialty in the practice of medicine that focuses on the relationships between neurological diseases and damage and psychiatric symptoms such as PSYCHOSIS, executive dysfunction, language disorders, and DEMENTIA. It is sometimes erroneously used interchangeably with NEUROPSYCHOLOGY, a complementary field, which, though very similar, is based in the profession of psychology and, hence, has less of a focus on neurochemistry and pharmacology. Practitioners of neuropsychiatry are physicians who have completed a residency in neurology or psychiatry and, usually, additional training in the form of a fellowship. Symptoms often accompany NEURODEGENERATIVE diseases and will significantly affect about a third of people who have Parkinson's disease. The physical deterioration that takes place in the brain with Parkinson's disease causes changes in many brain functions such as cognition and MEMORY. Providing treatment to relieve these symptoms requires understanding and addressing the underlying changes as well as the symptoms themselves. Many ANTIPSYCHOTIC MEDICATIONS taken to treat psychiatric symptoms can cause the neuromuscular symptoms of Parkinson's disease to worsen.

See also NEUROLOGY; NEUROSURGERY; NEUROPSYCHOLOGY.

neuropsychology   A specialty of psychology that addresses many of the same conditions as NEUROPSYCHIATRY but with a focus on evaluative testing and nonpharmacologic interventions and therapies to assist patients in coping with their neuropsychiatric symptoms. A clinical neuropsychologist has completed at least a master's degree in psychology, with most having completed a doctoral degree, and usually additional clinical education.

neurosurgery   A specialty in the practice of medicine that focuses on surgical treatments for diseases and disorders of the BRAIN and other structures of the NERVOUS SYSTEM. For most people with Parkinson's disease, surgery becomes a viable treatment option only when ANTI-PARKINSON'S MEDICATIONS and other medical treatments do not control symptoms. Surgical therapies to treat the symptoms of Parkinson's disease include PALLIDOTOMY and THALAMOTOMY, in which the neurosurgeon uses ABLATION to create lesions, or scar tissue, in brain structures that control movement. DEEP BRAIN STIMULATION of either the THALAMUS, subthalamic nucleus, or PALLIDUM is currently a more popular procedure because it lacks the irreversibility of ablation, can be titrated to provide benefit and avoid side effects, and has much less risk of side effects when a bilateral procedure is necessary. Because brain function and the course of Parkinson's disease are unique to each individual, surgical therapies have variable success. And because Parkinson's is progressive, symptoms may eventually return. Many people who have surgical treatment for Parkinson's experience long-term relief of symptoms such as TREMORS, BRADYKINESIA (slowed movement), AKINESIA (inability to move), and other DYSKINESIAS (abnormal, involuntary movements).

See also MEDICAL MANAGEMENT; NEUROLOGY; NEUROPSYCHIATRY; SURGERY; TREATMENT ALGORITHM.

neurotoxin   A substance that damages or destroys NEURONS (nerve and brain cells). Neurotoxins can originate outside the body, such as through exposure to chemicals such as polychlorinated biphenyls (PCBs) and to certain heavy metals, pesticides, and herbicides. Some medications also can have neurotoxic effects, even when taken at recommended dosages. Neuro toxins also can arise within the body, such as from bacteria (ENDOTOXINS and EXOTOXINS) and OXIDANTS. There are thousands of known neurotoxins that cause various symptoms. Those that have been linked to Parkinson's disease or Parkinson's-like symptoms include PCBs, the pesticide rotenone, MPTP the inadvertent contaminant of illicit attempts to synthesize narcotics and metals introduced through industrial or pollutant exposure such as mercury or manganese, and metals such as copper or iron that may accumulate due to genetic defects. Some neurotoxic damage reverses when the neurotoxin exposure ends, but much of it is permanent.

See also ACERULOPLASMINEMIA; ANTIOXIDANT; ANTIPSYCHOTIC MEDICATION; FREE RADICAL; HALLERVORDEN–SPATZ SYNDROME; NEUROPROTECTIVE EFFECT; NEUROPROTECTIVE THERAPIES; WILSON'S DISEASE.

neurotransmitter   A biochemical substance that facilitates communication among NEURONS. There are dozens of neurotransmitters. Those that are the most active in the brain are ACETYLCHOLINE, DOPAMINE, EPINEPHRINE, GLUTAMATE, NOREPINEPHRINE, GAMMA-AMINOBUTYRIC ACID (GABA), and SEROTONIN. Although neurons are very close together, they do not touch; corridors called synapses separate them. When a neurotransmitter binds with a receptor, it usually causes an ion channel (electrified pathway) to open: Either the receptor itself is a channel that changes its conformation to open up when the neurotransmitter binds or it triggers a cascade of activity in the cell that either results in ion channels opening or the release of calcium stores within the cell. This results in a change in the cell's membrane potential that causes it to fire, propagating the electrical signal (action potential) from the presynaptic cell. Neurotransmitters bridge the synapses, conducting action potentials from one neuron to those of another.

The neuron's AXON terminals synthesize, or manufacture, the neurotransmitter the neuron needs and packages it into a unit called a synaptic vesicle. The axon stores synaptic vesicles until it needs to use them. When an action potential arises in the neuron, the axon releases a synaptic vesicle that transports the needed neurotransmitter to the synaptic cleft. Here it travels to activate receptors on the post synaptic neuron's DENDRITE terminal. Neuron communication always moves in one direction: the dendrites receiving and the axon sending. This intricately synchronized sequence of events takes place in less than a millisecond each time it occurs, giving neurons the capacity to "fire" multiple times a second. Neurotransmitters allow neurons to communicate simultaneously with multiple other neurons.

Although most neurons are specific for a particular neurotransmitter according to their functions—such as DOPAMINERGIC NEURONS, which produce and bind with DOPAMINE, or adrenergic neurons, which produce and bind with epinephrine—some neurons can synthesize and bind with more than one kind of neurotransmitter. Once the neurotransmitter is "used," it rapidly leaves the synapse through one of three mechanisms:

- The neuron reabsorbs, or reuptakes, it (most common).

- It diffuses or drifts out of the synapse.

- Enzymes dismantle it into molecular components that are then reused by the neuron to synthesize additional neurotransmitters.

A neurotransmitter's effect at a receptor is either excitatory (stimulates the post-synaptic neuron's activity) or inhibitory (blocks the post-synaptic neuron's activity). Some neurotransmitters such as dopamine and serotonin may have either an excitatory or inhibitory effect depending on the receptor. Acetylcholine and glutamate are excitatory neurotransmitters; lycine and gamma-aminobutyric acid (GABA) are inhibitory neurotransmitters. Scientists believe the balance among these neurotransmitters in the brain has important effects on their overall functions. Even though the amount of acetylcholine remains the same in the brain as Parkinson's progresses, for example, it exerts more of an effect as dopamine amounts diminish. This process results in symptoms such as TREMORS.

See also CATECHOLAMINE; DOPAMINE AGONIST MEDICATION; DOPAMINE DEGRADATION; DOPAMINE RECEPTOR; DOPAMINE TRANSPORTER; MONOAMINE OXIDASE.

neurotrophic factors Naturally occurring proteins, also called neurotrophic proteins, that stimulate the growth or repair of NEURONS. BRAIN-DERIVED NEUROTROPHIC FACTORS (BDNF) stimulate the growth of new neurons; found primarily in the fetal brain, they are the critical substances in FETAL DOPAMINERGIC CELL TRANSPLANT, an experimental therapy still in the early stages of research. GLIAL DERIVED NEUROTROPHIC FACTOR (GDNF) is found in the hippocampus of the adult brain and helps to repair damaged neurons. Its use is also experimental. In research studies involving animal models, GDNF injected directly into the BRAIN has had some success in limiting the loss of DOPAMINERGIC NEURONS. Very limited clinical research studies are investigating the effectiveness of GDNF in people with Parkinson's disease; these studies are ongoing but initial reports of infusing GDNF directly into the putamen in a few people with Parkinson's have been encouraging.

See also BASAL GANGLIA; NEUROPROTECTIVE EFFECT; NEUROPROTECTIVE THERAPIES.

nicotinamide adenine dinucleotide (NADH)   An energy source that mitochondria generate within a cell. NADH stimulates DOPAMINE production, through mechanisms scientists do not fully understand. NADH also is the COENZYME structure of vitamin B$_3$ that is sometimes taken as an ANTIOXIDANT to help protect cells throughout the body from OXIDATIVE STRESS and damage, and specifically to protect them against the loss of DOPAMINERGIC NEURONS in Parkinson's disease. NADH became popular among people with Parkinson's disease as a nutritional supplement in the 1990s, when several uncontrolled studies reported anecdotal improvement of symptoms and the reduction of LEVODOPA dosages among people with Parkinson's who added NADH supplement to their medication regimens. As a nutritional supplement, NADH is the COENZYME of vitamin B$_3$.

Research continues to explore NADH's role in neuroprotection and ability, if any, to reduce the symptoms of Parkinson's or slow the progression of the disease. At this time, most medical professionals do not recommend NADH supplementation as one of the ADJUNCT THERAPIES or ALTERNATIVE THERAPIES for Parkinson's disease. The only people known to have deficiency of vitamin B$_3$ are those who have chronic alcoholism. Because NADH is also an energy source for cells, its use as a supplement can cause feelings of jitteriness and agitation similar to those produced by high caffeine intake. For people who want to take NADH supplement, nutritional experts recommend starting with a low dosage and gradually increasing to the therapeutic dosage.

See also ALPHA-SYNUCLEIN GENE; COENZYME Q-10; LIPOPOLYSACCHARIDES; MITOCHONDRIAL DYSFUNCTION; MITOCHONDRIAL ELECTRON TRANSPORT CHAIN; OXIDATION; UBIQUITIN.

nicotine   An addictive chemical stimulant that occurs naturally in tobacco. For nearly a century doctors have noticed that people with Parkinson's disease who use tobacco (primarily by cigarette smoking) report that their symptoms seem to improve shortly after tobacco use. Researchers also noticed that Parkinson's disease is less likely to develop in people who smoke. This finding has given rise to the theory that cigarette smoking can protect against Parkinson's disease.

Nicotine, the key active ingredient that enters the body with tobacco use, appears to have several actions in the brain. One is that it blocks certain cholinergic receptors, called nicotinic acetylcholine receptors, preventing them from binding with ACETYLCHOLINE, a NEUROTRANSMITTER important to motor function. Acetylcholine is one of the monoamine neurotransmitters that, in health, exist in balance in the brain. DOPAMINE is also a MONOAMINE NEUROTRANSMITTER. When dopamine levels drop in Parkinson's disease, the ratio of dopamine to other monoamine neurotransmitters such as acetylcholine changes. Acetylcholine becomes more active, overstimulating cholinergic receptors. Nicotine's mild anticholinergic effect helps to slow cholinergic transmissions to the muscles, easing symptoms such as TREMORS (although in some people with Parkinson's disease, nicotine has the opposite effect and causes tremors to worsen).

Nicotine also blocks MONOAMINE OXIDASE B (MAO-B), an enzyme that aids the metabolism of dopamine. This effect extends the availability of dopamine in the BASAL GANGLIA and other areas of the brain involved with motor function. For the person with Parkinson's, this effect helps to mitigate neuromuscular symptoms such as BRADYKINESIA (slowed movements). This MAO-B blocking effect also extends the availability of dopamine in the cerebrum, where it affects brain centers related to mood and pleasure. Researchers believe this effect of nicotine accounts for its addictive qualities, as dopamine stimulates those centers. Nicotine also activates receptors in areas of COGNITIVE FUNCTION, improving focus, concentration, and MEMORY.

Although research shows that nicotine administration, such as through the common "stop smoking" patches and gums, can relieve some of the symptoms of Parkinson's disease, there is not yet adequate evidence to support its use as a therapeutic approach. The health risks and consequences of cigarette smoking and other forms of tobacco use are too high to offset any potential benefit from nicotine. The cardiac and vascular complications of smoking (for example heart attack, stroke, and hypertension) appear to be due to the effects of nicotine itself, hence nicotine patches are hardly any safer for long-term use than smoking.

See also ALCOHOL; MONOAMINE OXIDASE; NEURO-PROTECTIVE EFFECT; NEUROPROTECTIVE THERAPIES.

nightmares See SLEEP DISTURBANCES.

nighttime wakefulness See SLEEP DISTURBANCES.

nigral pigment The dark coloration of the cells in the SUBSTANTIA NIGRA (literally "black substance"), the structure in the BRAIN that regulates motor function. A chemical called melanin, the same substance responsible for skin color, causes the coloration. However, there is no correlation between skin color and the amount of melanin in the substantia nigra. Scientists do not know why these cells deep within the brain contain melanin; there does not seem to be a functional purpose. Melanin in the skin helps to protect the skin from ultraviolet radiation damage that results from Sun exposure; it is what causes light-colored skin to "tan." There does not appear to be any connection between melanin and Parkinson's disease.

See also APOPTOSIS; BASAL GANGLIA; PARKINSON'S DISEASE, CAUSES OF.

nigrostriatal fibers Filaments from the DOPAMIN-ERGIC NEURONS in the SUBSTANTIA NIGRA that transport DOPAMINE into the STRIATUM and other structures of the BASAL GANGLIA that require dopamine. In Parkinson's disease the numbers of these fibers decrease as the numbers of dopaminergic neurons diminish, further restricting the supply of dopamine available to facilitate neuromotor communication. This loss can only be detected at autopsy after death. Scientists consider it one of the defining pathological conditions of Parkinson's disease. In other neurodegenerative diseases that produce Parkinson's-like symptoms have normal numbers or nigrostriatal fibers (such as drug induced parkinsonism) or more wide-

spread neuronal loss in the basal ganglia in addition to nigrostriatal fiber loss (such as progressive supranuclear palsy [PSP] and multiple system atrophy [MSA]).

There are also filaments from dopaminergic neurons that originate in and transport dopamine from the striatum, called striatonigral fibers as the striatum is their point of origin, toward the substantia nigra and other structures of the basal ganglia. The numbers and apparent function of these fibers remain normal in Parkinson's disease. However, the striatum does not produce enough dopamine to meet the brain's needs, and so the normal functioning of striatonigral fibers cannot offset the loss of nigrostriatal fibers. The loss of striatonigral fibers is a characteristic of the Parkinson's-like disease striatonigral degeneration (SND), which is a component of the MULTIPLE SYSTEM ATRO-PHY (MSA) disease complex.

Differentiating between these fibers and their roles in dopamine transport has no therapeutic consequence at present. However, understanding of their functions provides additional insights into the mechanisms of Parkinson's disease.

See also BRAIN; CONDITIONS SIMILAR TO PARKIN-SON'S; DIAGNOSING PARKINSON'S; NEURON; NEURO-TRANSMITTER.

nocturia The frequent need to urinate at night. Nocturia tends to become a problem with aging as the structures of the urinary tract become less resilient, as well as being a consequence of Parkinson's disease. If often is the first manifested of a triad of symptoms related to bladder function; urinary urgency (feeling of the need to urinate even when the volume of urine in the bladder is low) and URINARY FREQUENCY typically develop as well.

The frontal lobes of the cerebrum regulate most voluntary physiological functions related to urination. However, the reticular formation within the brainstem also plays a role. The dopamine depletion that results as Parkinson's disease progresses affects the function of this structure and can cause a symptom called detrusor hyperactivity—increased stimulation of the detrusor, the layer of smooth muscle that lines the bladder. This stimulation causes the sensation of bladder fullness, generating the urge to urinate.

For many people, reducing fluids for the four hours or so before bedtime and urinating immediately before going to bed are effective measures for reducing or eliminating nocturia. It is important to make sure that this nocturnal fluid restriction does not lead to dehydration, which is particularly problematic for people with Parkinson's because dehydration can contribute to both constipation and ORTHOSTATIC HYPOTENSION (lightheadedness from a fall in blood pressure when one stands up). ANTICHOLINERGIC MEDICATIONS that act primarily on the smooth muscle of the urinary tract such as oxybutynin (Ditropan) or tolterodine (Detrol) often helps. Propantheline (Pro-Banthine), which often is taken to reduce excess sweating, can also be considered, but it has a slightly higher risk of side effects. Nocturia can interfere with restful sleep. There is also an increased risk of falling when getting up at night, particularly when the person is drowsy and ANTIPARKINSON'S MEDICATIONS typically are at their lowest levels in the body. These circumstances make coordination of movement more difficult.

See also ADJUSTING TO LIVING WITH PARKINSON'S; BATHING AND BATHROOM ORGANIZATION; BEDROOM COMFORT; COPING WITH THE ONGOING CARE OF PARKINSON'S; SLEEP DISTURBANCES.

nocturnal myoclonus   See MYOCLONUS.

nonfluctuating response   A state of therapeutic stability in which anti-Parkinson's medication predictably and consistently control the symptoms of Parkinson's. Typically, this is the expected response in the early and mid stages of the disease and can continue for years and sometimes decades, depending on the rate of progression and severity of symptoms. During this time, many people with Parkinson's who have no other medical conditions feel and function as though they are in full health and are able to participate in work and family activities with few limitations. Good NUTRITION AND DIET, regular EXERCISE AND ACTIVITY, and stress management practices such as meditation help to maintain lifestyle stability and overall health and well-being as well.

See also ADJUNCT THERAPIES; ADJUSTING TO LIVING WITH PARKINSON'S; ANTI-PARKINSON'S MEDICATIONS; CARE MANAGEMENT AND PLANNING; FLUCTUATING PHENONEMON; MEDICATION MANAGEMENT; OFF-STATE; ON-STATE; TAI CHI; WALKING; YOGA.

norepinephrine   A naturally occurring chemical in the body that functions as a HORMONE or a NEUROTRANSMITTER. Norepinephrine is a CATECHOLAMINE that is present centrally (in the BRAIN) and peripherally (in the body). One of its key functions is to regulate blood pressure by stimulating blood vessels to constrict (narrow and stiffen) when the blood pressure drops below a certain level. The noradrenergic neurons of the sympathetic nervous system produce, and the adrenal medulla produces and stores, norepinephrine. Chemically, norepinephrine is closely related to the other catecholamines, DOPAMINE and epinephrine. Peripheral dopamine becomes metabolized to norepinephrine and to epinephrine; norepinephrine also can become metabolized to epinephrine.

Scientists do not fully understand norepinephrine's role in Parkinson's disease. Research in the late 1990s discovered that people with Parkinson's disease appear to have decreased numbers of peripheral noradrenergic receptors in the heart, suggesting some relationship between dopamine and norepinephrine. It is not clear whether the relationship is related to brain depletion of dopaminergic neurons and dopamine or to peripheral metabolism of LEVODOPA. In the brain, there do not seem to be many overlaps in the functions of norepinephrine and dopamine. Norepinephrine, along with the other catecholamines, cannot cross the BLOOD-BRAIN BARRIER; therefore, central and peripheral norepinephrine levels remain separate.

See also ADRENAL MEDULLARY AUTOGRAFT; CAROTID BODY CELL GRAFT; MONOAMINE OXIDASE; MONOAMINE NEUROTRANSMITTER; NERVOUS SYSTEM; NEUROTRANSMITTER.

nortriptyline   A tricyclic ANTIDEPRESSANT MEDICATION taken to relieve depression and improve mood and sometimes to relieve chronic neurogenic (nerve-based) pain. Common brand names are Pamelor and Aventyl. As do other tricyclic antidepressants, nortriptyline extends the brain's NEUROTRANSMITTER action by blocking neurotransmitter reuptake. It primarily acts on NOREPINEPHRINE and SEROTONIN. A significant side effect of use of nortriptyline is ORTHOSTATIC HYPOTENSION, or a drop in blood pressure that occurs when one changes position from lying down to sitting or sitting to standing. As many ANTI-PARKINSON'S MEDICATIONS can have a similar side effect, adding nortriptyline to the mix can compound the problem.

Nortriptyline has been reportedly associated with EXTRAPYRAMIDAL SYMPTOMS such as DYSKINESIA (especially TARDIVE DYSKINESIA) in a few case reports and can rarely worsen existing symptoms of Parkinson's disease. Generally, a person who has Parkinson's should first consider other medications for depression, such as SELECTIVE SEROTONIN REUPTAKE INHIBITOR (SSRI) MEDICATIONS, before taking nortriptyline or any of the other tricyclic antidepressants. Nortriptyline cannot be taken when other antidepressants are also taken.

See also AMITRIPTYLINE; ANXIETY; DESIPRAMINE; IMIPRAMINE; MEDICATION MANAGEMENT; MEDICATION SIDE EFFECTS; MONOAMINE OXIDASE INHIBITOR (MAOI) MEDICATIONS; PSYCHOTHERAPY; SELEGILINE.

nursing home   See LONG-TERM CARE FACILITY.

nutrition and diet   Eating properly is essential, but sometimes a challenge, for the person with Parkinson's. There is no specific "diet" for people with Parkinson's disease. Good nutrition helps to support the body's ability to remain as healthy as possible and to provide enough energy to meet the body's needs. In the early to middle stages of Parkinson's, most people can continue EATING favorite foods with few changes (except to healthier choices, if appropriate). As Parkinson's progresses to affect the muscles of the face, mouth, and throat, the mechanics of eating become more challenging. Chewing foods such as meats and fresh, raw vegetables can become difficult. Cutting these foods into small pieces and cooking them until they are tender make them easier to manage and less of a choking hazard.

In the later stages of Parkinson's disease the timing of medications and meals becomes essential. Dietary PROTEIN interferes with the absorption of LEVODOPA, the primary ANTI-PARKINSON'S MEDICATION. In the early stages of levodopa therapy it is possible to take a larger dosage than the brain needs, knowing that some will be lost, so the levodopa can be taken with food to mitigate the nausea that is a common side effect of its use. As the loss of DOPAMINERGIC NEURONS in the SUBSTANTIA NIGRA continues, the BRAIN needs greater amounts of levodopa to replace the diminishing levels of DOPAMINE.

The dosage soon reaches the maximal tolerable dosage of levodopa; at that time it becomes important to make the best possible use of that dosage. No longer is there the luxury to "waste" any part of the dosage by cushioning its side effects with food. It becomes necessary to adjust meals and medications to take levodopa doses on an empty stomach (or with just a light, protein-free snack such as crackers if nausea is a problem) and to limit the amount of protein in meals. Protein is necessary for tissue health and many body functions as it supplies the amino acids the body needs for cell activity and repair. It is important to eat enough protein to meet the body's requirement, which for a typical adult is about 40 to 60 grams a day.

Many people who are experiencing FLUCTUATING PHENOMENON in response to levodopa therapy shift nearly the full amount of their daily protein needs to the evening meal, when their levodopa dosage is the smallest; most people take higher dosages during the day to relieve symptoms during the times they prefer to be active. This method helps to meet nutritional needs and to obtain the maximal benefit from levodopa therapy. Maintaining adequate nutrition in the late stages of Parkinson's disease becomes difficult as the challenges of eating increase. A NUTRITIONIST can help plan meals that meet nutritional needs that the person can consume.

See also ADJUSTING TO LIVING WITH PARKINSON'S; COOKING; COPING WITH ONGOING CARE OF PARKINSON'S; DYSPHAGIA; FEEDING TUBE; FOOD PREPARATION; FOODS TO AVOID; FOODS TO EAT; PARENTERAL NUTRITION; PROTEIN RESTRICTIONS, DIETARY; SWALLOWING.

nutritional supplements Products that help to supply the body's nutritional needs along with diet. The range of products available is vast, and most are unnecessary for the person with Parkinson's. Many doctors recommend a general multivitamin/multimineral product, particularly for people who are having problems in eating nutrient-dense foods such as fresh vegetables and fruits. Many people choose to take ANTIOXIDANTS such as COENZYME Q-10 for their neuroprotective effects. The person with Parkinson's disease should consult a nutritionist for advice on meal planning and food preparation to accommodate the challenges of Parkinson's as well as to meet nutritional needs.

See also ALTERNATIVE THERAPIES; VITAMINS.

occupational therapy A specialty of health care that focuses on improving a person's ability to function in the ACTIVITIES OF DAILY LIVING (ADLs) (formerly referred to as "occupations") and other life tasks. Occupational therapy considers a person's abilities, limitations, physical environment (home, work, and social) and their effects on typical or necessary tasks. An occupational therapist can help the person develop methods and techniques to accomplish needed tasks. For the person with Parkinson's disease, there is a particular focus on preserving abilities for as long as possible but with an eye toward adapting to changing circumstances. This may include integration with PHYSICAL THERAPY to maintain physical skills, functions, and environmental and behavioral approaches to combat gait freezing; activities to support COGNITIVE FUNCTION; assessment of visual function and strategies to improve performance in vision-based skills such as driving; and help in learning to use ADAPTIVE EQUIPMENT AND ASSIST DEVICES to extend INDEPENDENCE.

In the United States, there are two levels of occupational therapy practitioners, the certified occupational therapy assistant (COTA) and the registered occupational therapist (OTR). The COTA is a technical practitioner who completes an accredited two-year program and passes a national certification examination. An occupational therapist completes an accredited four-year undergraduate program and passes a national certification examination to earn the professional designation of occupational therapist, registered. There are also postgraduate programs in occupational therapy that award master's or doctoral degrees for additional study. All states require both levels of practitioner to be licensed and to complete continuing education courses to remain current in practice standards.

Occupational therapy services require a physician's referral or prescription that specifies the kinds of services the person needs. The occupational therapist completes an assessment of the person's status and can make other recommendations, which must be approved by the physician. Occupational therapy can be provided on an inpatient basis for people who are hospitalized but is most often an outpatient service. Private MEDICAL INSURANCE, MEDICARE, and MEDICAID programs typically provide benefits for occupational therapy services.

See also ADJUSTING TO LIVING WITH PARKINSON'S; BATHING AND BATHROOM ORGANIZATION; BEDROOM COMFORT; CARE MANAGEMENT AND PLANNING; COOKING; COPING WITH ONGOING CARE OF PARKINSON'S; INSTRUMENTAL ACTIVITIES OF DAILY LIVING; KITCHEN EFFICIENCY; MOBILITY AIDS; SHOPPING.

off-label drug A medication taken for purposes other than those for which it is approved by the U.S. Food and Drug Administration (FDA). Off-label use of medications is a very common and accepted practice throughout medicine. It is particularly common in neurologic diseases because they tend to be less common, and, therefore, drug companies are unlikely to invest the enormous resources required to obtain FDA approval for another on-label use of a drug they can already sell on the market. The effectiveness and safety of common off-label uses are typically well supported by clinical studies in the scientific literature. Some off label uses are so commonplace that many physicians don't even think of them as off-label unless they happen to review the insert on a medication.

Quite a number of medications taken to control various symptoms of Parkinson's disease have

OFF-LABEL DRUG USES IN PARKINSON'S DISEASE

Medication	Approved Use	Off-Label Uses in Parkinson's
Acetylcholinesterase inhibitor medications (donepezil, galantamine, rivastigmine, tacrine)	Reduction of dementia and improve cognitive function in people with Alzheimer's disease	Reduce dementia and improve cognitive function
Baclofen, intracathal baclofen therapy	Relieve muscle spasms in multiple sclerosis, cerebral palsy, and spinal cord injury	Relieve dystonia and severe tremors
Dopamine agonists (cabergoline, bromocriptine, pergolide, pramipexole, ropinirole)	Adjunct therapies in Parkinson's disease	Monotherapy in Parkinson's disease relieve restlessly syndrome; relieve dystonia
Atypical antipsychotic medications (clozapine, olanzapine, quetiapine, reserpine)	Schizophrenia, psychosis	Reduce dementia; improve tremors that do not respond to other treatment
Modafinil	Increase alertness and wakefulness in narcolepsy	Overcome daytime sleepiness related to Parkinson's and anti-Parkinson's medications
Anticholinergic medications (trihexyphenidyl, benztropine, procyclidine, biperiden	Adjunct therapies in Parkinson's disease	Monotherapy in de novo Parkinson's and early-onset Parkinson's to treat stiffness and tremor
Beta-antagonist medications (propanolol, nadolol, metoprolol)	Control tremors in essential tremor disorder, reduce elevated blood pressure	Control tremors in Parkinson's that do not respond to other medications

off-label uses. It is important that the person taking an off-label drug fully understand the expected benefits and possible side effects of the drug. Typically off-label drug use involves trying the medication to treat similar symptoms in a different condition, such as using ACETYLCHOLINESTERASE INHIBITOR MEDICATIONS approved for use to improve COGNITIVE FUNCTION in people with ALZHEIMER'S DISEASE as a therapy to improve cognitive function of people with Parkinson's disease. Although the symptoms of COGNITIVE IMPAIRMENT appear similar in these two conditions, they arise from different pathological conditions (physiological and neurochemical causes). Other off-label uses may involve using dosages that are different from those approved or in combination with other medications.

Often off-label medication use evolves through anecdotal reports of its effectiveness. As a result, the off-label use may become an approved use, as occurred with AMANTADINE, which started its pharmaceutical life as an antiviral medication to prevent or shorten the course of influenza A and is

now an approved and effective DOPAMINERGIC MEDICATION used as MONOTHERAPY in DE NOVO PARKINSON'S and EARLY-ONSET PARKINSON'S and as one of the ADJUNCT THERAPIES in middle-to-late stage Parkinson's to alleviate dyskinesias. Influenza is a particular health risk among older people, who also are more likely to have NEURODEGENERATIVE diseases such as Parkinson's. Doctors noticed that their older patients who had Parkinson's disease and took amantadine to head off influenza also experienced dramatic improvement in their Parkinson's symptoms. Open-label use of amantadine to control the symptoms of Parkinson's spread, eventually leading to CLINICAL RESEARCH TRIALS that confirmed the drug's effectiveness as an anti-Parkinson's medication.

See also INVESTIGATIONAL NEW DRUG; INVESTIGATIONAL TREATMENTS; MEDICATION MANAGEMENT; PHARMACOTHERAPY; TREATMENT ALGORITHM.

off-state (off-time)   The period in the middle to late stages of Parkinson's disease when dosages of

ANTI-PARKINSON'S MEDICATIONS are on the downward side of peak effectiveness or can no longer fully suppress symptoms and symptoms "break through." Most people with Parkinson's disease structure their medication dosages to provide the most substantial relief during waking hours (ON-STATE). Medication coverage is lowest in the early morning, when symptoms such as TREMORS and BRADYKINESIA (slowed movement) are likely to be prominent. Early-morning off-state dystonia, in which the person with Parkinson's awakens to find a foot, most commonly, "frozen" in an awkward and sometimes painfully contorted position, is particularly distressing. Sometimes a muscle relaxant medication such as BACLOFEN can help relieve this off-state symptom, but it has a high risk of causing sedation and thinking problems. Other DYSKINESIAS and DYSTONIA (intense muscle rigidity) are common during off-state episodes as well, and COGNITIVE IMPAIRMENT, particularly DEMENTIA and MEMORY LOSS, can become more pronounced.

As Parkinson's disease progresses and DOPAMINE DEPLETION in the brain becomes more severe, current anti-Parkinson's medications are no longer able to compensate for the changes in the brain's NEUROCHEMISTRY. Medication dosages reach the threshold at which the adverse effects of the drug outweigh the benefits; the medications begin to cause symptoms, such as dystonia, chorea (involuntary fidgeting movements often described as dancelike) and ATHETOSIS (involuntary slow, writhing, repetitive movements), that are as debilitating as the symptoms of Parkinson's. As well, remaining DOPAMINE RECEPTORS in the brain become sensitized to activation by the exogenous (from a source outside the body) dopamine the brain metabolizes from LEVODOPA or the exogenous dopaminergic activity from dopamine agonists.

Altering ADJUNCT THERAPIES—adjusting the kinds and combinations of medications, dosages, and timings—often provides short-term improvements in the balance between on-state and off-state when off-state episodes begin. In the late stages of Parkinson's, this approach becomes less effective. MEDICATION MANAGEMENT becomes strategic, as the person takes dosages for maximal benefit during times when he or she desires the greatest relief from symptoms and plans activities around peak on-states. PATIENCE, EMPATHY, and HUMOR are helpful in coping with off-state episodes, which often are frustrating and can be frightening for the person with Parkinson's as well as for loved ones.

See also CARE MANAGEMENT AND PLANNING; COMPASSION; COPING WITH ONGOING CARE OF PARKINSON'S; FLUCTUATING PHENOMENON; HOPE FOR A PARKINSON'S CURE; RESCUE DRUG; TREATMENT ALGORITHM.

oily skin   See DERMATITIS, SEBACEOUS.

olanzapine   One of the ANTIPSYCHOTIC MEDICATIONS taken to treat symptoms of PSYCHOSIS such as HALLUCINATIONS, CONFUSION, DELUSIONS, PARANOIA, and DEMENTIA. About one third of people in the late stages of Parkinson's disease have symptoms of psychosis. These symptoms can arise as a consequence of Parkinson's disease, be present because of coexisting ALZHEIMER'S DISEASE, or develop as undesired side effects of ANTI-PARKINSON'S MEDICATIONS, particularly LEVODOPA and DOPAMINE AGONIST MEDICATIONS.

Though olanzapine (Zyprexa) is classified as an atypical antipsychotic because it affects the brain's neurochemical processes in different ways than conventional antipsychotics do, making it less likely to worsen Parkinson's symptoms than antipsychotic medications are necessary, olanzapine still causes extrapyramidal motor side effects in about 30 percent of people with Parkinson's disease who take it. As do other antipsychotic medications, olanzapine has some action as a DOPAMINE ANTAGONIST (it blocks dopamine activity) on selective DOPAMINE RECEPTORS, primarily D1, whereas conventional antipsychotic medications act nonselectively. The dopamine receptors primarily involved with motor function are D1, D2, D3, and D4. Quetiapine (Seroquel) and clozapine (clozaril) are better choices for people with Parkinson's balance between enough focused dopamine antagonist activity to suppress the symptoms of psychosis but not so much that it carries over to motor disturbances.

The first therapeutic approach for psychotic symptoms in a person with Parkinson's should be to evaluate the medication regimen, as often making adjustments to medications and dosages can reduce or alleviate such symptoms. Antipsychotic medications often exacerbate motor and COGNITIVE IMPAIRMENTS in people diagnosed with Parkinson's disease and should be used only when other therapeutic approaches are ineffective and the psychotic symptoms are severe enough to mandate MEDICAL MANAGEMENT. Atypical antipsychotic medications are commonly used to treat symptoms of psychosis in people with Alzheimer's disease, and when such extrapyramidal side effects occur can create a confusing clinical picture as Parkinson's and Alzheimer's frequently coexist. It can be difficult to determine whether Parkinson's-like symptoms are in fact a manifestation of Parkinson's disease or side effects of the antipsychotic medication. Doctors generally presume the former when symptoms persist after stopping of the antipsychotic medication and respond to anti-Parkinson's medications such as levodopa.

See also CARE MANAGEMENT AND PLANNING; MEDICATION MANAGEMENT; NEUROCHEMISTRY; NEUROPSYCHIATRY; QUETIAPINE; RISPERIDONE; SCHIZOPHRENIA.

olivopontocerebellar atrophy See MULTIPLE SYSTEM ATROPHY.

on–off state (on–off effect) See FLUCTUATING PHENOMENON.

on-state (on-time) The time in the mid to late stages of Parkinson's disease when ANTI-PARKINSON'S MEDICATIONS are at peak effectiveness and are keeping the symptoms of Parkinson's disease under control. In the early to mid stages of Parkinson's when LEVODOPA is most effective, most people do not experience a differentiation between on-state and OFF-STATE because anti-Parkinson's medications can maintain a fairly constant level of symptom control during which symptoms are barely, if at all, perceptible.

As DOPAMINERGIC NEURONS (dopamine-producing brain cells) continue to die and the brain's supply of endogenous DOPAMINE (dopamine that the brain's dopamine-producing neurons manufacture) diminishes, so does the capacity of anti-Parkinson's medications to maintain adequate NEUROTRANSMITTER function. Higher dosages of

medications begin to cause more severe side effects, such as DYSKINESIAS (involuntary movements) and DYSTONIA (severe muscle rigidity), that are as debilitating as the symptoms of Parkinson's.

Strategic manipulation of medications and dosages can help to extend on-state times or to structure them to occur when they are needed or desired, such as during times of activity. OFF-STATE episodes are most pronounced in the early morning, when medication levels are at their lowest. On-state time becomes both shorter per episode and less frequent as the disease advances, however, and eventually anti-Parkinson's medications have limited effect in mitigating symptoms. Nonpharmacotherapeutic methods such as PHYSICAL THERAPY and OCCUPATIONAL THERAPY can help to maintain MUSCLE TONE, MUSCLE STRENGTH, and MOTOR FUNCTION for as long as possible. Planning activities to take place during on-state times as much as this is predictable eases frustration. During on-state times, the person with Parkinson's can appear fairly normal in motor function, MOVEMENT, and COGNITIVE FUNCTION even in later stages of the disease.

See also CARE MANAGEMENT AND PLANNING; COMPASSION; COPING WITH ONGOING CARE OF PARKINSON'S; FLUCTUATING PHENOMENON; HOPE FOR A PARKINSON'S CURE; RESCUE DRUG; TREATMENT ALGORITHM.

1-methyl-4-phenyl-1,2,3,6-tetrahydropyridine (MPTP) A chemical derivative of the illicit narcotic known as MPPP, pethidine or MPP+ (chemically, 1-methyl-4-phenyl-4-propionoxypiperidine). When this synthetic heroin breaks down in the body, one of the substances it forms is the toxin 1-methyl-4-phenyl-1,2,3,6-tetrahydropyridine, known as MPTP, which interferes with the action of mitochondrial enzyme COMPLEX I. This interference causes cells to die. In the 1980s MPPP became briefly popular as a "designer drug" to enhance or substitute for heroin among addicts, until its dangers became clear. Many who used it experienced rapid and severe onset of Parkinson's symptoms, which researchers finally were able to conclude were the result of exposure to MPTP as accidental by-product of attempting to synthesize MPPP. Researchers exploring the connection discovered, by injecting MPTP into laboratory monkeys, that

MPTP creates lesions in the SUBSTANTIA NIGRA that prevent DOPAMINE production in a replication of the pathological course of Parkinson's disease. This was the first time that scientists were able to reproduce Parkinson's disease in laboratory animals, opening the door to new directions in research.

Because MPTP is a common ingredient in many pesticides currently used for outdoor application throughout the United States, speculation about a possible correlation between IDIOPATHIC Parkinson's disease and long-term, low-level exposure to such chemicals in the environment has led to research studies about their potential association. Although initial findings appeared promising, extended studies have not been conclusive. Exposure to environmental toxins remains one of several theorized causes of Parkinson's disease. Researchers continue to study MPTP-induced parkinsonism to explore new treatments as well as to gain better understanding of the on–off state and WEARING-OFF STATE that are typical of the mainstay of drug treatment for Parkinson's disease, LEVODOPA.

Although MPTP-induced Parkinson's disease in the laboratory offers scientists the best understanding yet of the mechanisms and pathological process of Parkinson's disease, MPTP-induced parkinsonism differs in several key ways from the idiopathic form of the disease that most commonly afflicts humans. MPTP-induced parkinsonism symptoms appear rapidly and severely, sometimes within just a few days, in addicts injecting MPTP-contaminated drugs. Damage occurs only in the substantia nigra, and LEWY BODIES are not present. Also, unlike most other drug-induced parkinsonisms, MPTP-induced parkinsonism is permanent and often quickly fatal.

See also DRUG-INDUCED PARKINSON'S; ENVIRONMENTAL TOXINS; PARKINSONISM; PARKINSON'S DISEASE, CAUSES OF.

open-label drug study   A study of the effects of a drug in a group of patients in which both the patient and the person evaluating the effectiveness of the therapy know exactly what drug and dose of drug is being taken. Typically a drug of interest is compared to either an existing standard (control) treatment, or no treatment if there is not an established effective therapy. Though much easier to perform than double-blind clinical trials, the reliability and applicability of the results of open label drug studies are less clear since both patients and the evaluators might have a bias towards wanting the study drug to work better than the control treatment.

optimism   The ability to find the positive in situations and events. Focusing on the challenges Parkinson's disease presents, whether actual or potential, is a natural tendency. The person who has Parkinson's should look ahead and to plan for the future but do so with the sense that the future will include joys and pleasures as well as challenges. Most people who have Parkinson's find that day-to-day life does not change much for quite some time after diagnosis. There is every reason for most people with Parkinson's disease to enjoy years and even decades doing what makes them happy and sharing their life with friends and family as they always have.

Optimism is looking at the reality of a situation and choosing to feel and act in ways that make the best of it. It is acknowledging that there are challenges and finding ways to meet them. Most importantly, optimism is living each day for the joy of the day itself as well as expecting that tomorrow will have its own joys. Health care professionals know that the people with chronic illness who do best are those who can find the positive in less than ideal circumstances. There is no one, regardless of health status, who can afford to waste today worrying about tomorrow, and the person with Parkinson's is no exception.

There is more HOPE FOR A PARKINSON'S CURE today than there has been at any other time since James Parkinson identified the disease that bears his name, and people with Parkinson's have good reason to believe they can manage the course of their disease to an extent to which its interference with everyday life is minimal. New and exciting research that is taking place is rapidly expanding what scientists know and understand about Parkinson's disease, leading to different ways of looking at treatment options and to new treatments. When the people who are today being diagnosed with

Parkinson's were born, there was no effective treatment for the disease. Today there are so many options that physicians use a TREATMENT ALGORITHM—a chart of symptoms and approaches for managing them—to help them decide what treatments are likely to be most effective. Barely a generation ago there was a single treatment for Parkinson's disease—LEVODOPA. Although levodopa remains the cornerstone of Parkinson's treatment today, there are numerous other medications to fine-tune symptom control and others in various stages of clinical research trials.

See also COMPASSION; COPING WITH DIAGNOSIS OF PARKINSON'S; COPING WITH ONGOING CARE OF PARKINSON'S; DENIAL AND ACCEPTANCE; EMPATHY; QUALITY OF LIFE.

orofacial chorea   See CHOREA.

orthotics   Appliances or devices used to stabilize and support weakened muscles and joints. The word's Greek origin means "to straighten." For many MOTOR SYSTEM DISORDERS, splints and braces improve mobility. Upper extremity splints sometimes are helpful for people who have intentional TREMORS (tremors that occur with purposeful action but not at rest), and ankle braces can help keep the foot and leg in proper alignment for walking. Only rarely are these methods useful for the person with Parkinson's. However, most orthotics can become impediments to movement because they create additional interference with movement or because the person focuses attention on them.

Occasionally the person with Parkinson's disease experiences bruxism, an involuntary clenching of the jaw and grinding of the teeth that are consequences of symptoms such as RIGIDITY that affect the muscles of the jaw and face. A person with Parkinson's who is able to swallow normally and has no concerns about choking may want to wear a dental splint that protects the teeth from damage. However, bruxism tends to be a problem in later Parkinson's, as are swallowing difficulties.

Shoe orthotics also can be helpful for the person with Parkinson's. Inserts that fit inside the shoes help to hold the foot in a particular position during walking and can sometimes improve stability, balance, and GAIT in the person with Parkinson's.

See also GAIT DISTURBANCE; MOBILITY; MOBILITY AIDS; WALKING.

oxidation   Technically chemical process that involves the transfer of electrons, the atomic subparticles that orbit around the nucleus of an atom. In biochemistry, it is best typified by the biochemical processes within a cell that utilize oxygen to produce energy. Oxidation breaks down a molecule such as glucose into its atomic components. Electrons from oxygen then bond or transfer to the chemical energy sources, primarily adenosine triphosphate (ATP), that fuel a cell's functions. The remainder of atomic components re-form into other molecular structures, some of which are waste by-products called FREE RADICALS. A free radical is an unstable molecule that binds with the first available molecular structure it encounters. Such binding forms a structure, called an oxidant, that has no purpose. These oxidants mill about within cells, and as they accumulate they begin to damage the components of the cell, and may lead to the cell's death. OXIDATIVE STRESS, as scientists call this interference, eventually develops the potential to cause disease.

Oxidation is normal and necessary for cells to carry out the functions that support life. There is much about oxidation and oxidative stress that scientists as yet do not understand. Both exist in health as well as disease; it seems to be the balance between them that determines which circumstance, health or disease, prevails. Naturally occurring enzymes called antioxidants help to regulate this balance by dismantling free radicals into harmless structures that the body can discharge as waste. This process has led to the presumption that increasing consumption of antioxidants, which are abundant in fruits, vegetables, and whole grains, reduces free radical presence.

However, most controlled studies to date have not conclusively supported this premise. One large study conducted over five years, the DATATOP (DEPRENYL AND TOCOPHEROL ANTIOXIDATIVE THERAPY FOR PARKINSON'S DISEASE) STUDY, examined the antioxidant effect of vitamin E (in its active form, tocopherol) and found no effect on oxidative stress and oxidative damage in people with EARLY-ONSET PARKINSON'S. Evidence for the monoamine oxidase-

B inhibitor medication SELEGILINE did initially suggest possible slowing of the progress of Parkinson's, but longer follow-up of the same patients has led to the belief that selegiline only has mild effects on treating Parkinson's symptoms and that it has no effect on the progression of the brain damage that the disease causes.

See also ANTIOXIDANT THERAPY; APOPTOSIS; COMPLEX I; LIPOPOLYSACCHARIDES; MITOCHONDRIAL DYSFUNCTION; MITOCHONDRIAL ELECTRON TRANSPORT CHAIN; PARKINSON'S DISEASE, CAUSES OF.

oxidative stress Molecular changes within cells that occur over time with repeated exposure to FREE RADICALS, the waste by-products of OXIDATION. Scientists believe that oxidative stress exposes cells to cumulative damage that results in diseases such as cancer, diabetes, heart disease, ALZHEIMER'S DISEASE, and Parkinson's disease, among many others. In response to the presence of free radicals, cells manufacture ANTIOXIDANTS—enzymes whose job it is to bind with free radicals to render them harmless.

Unbound free radicals do not stay unattached for long; their molecular structures are such that they can bind with nearly any other molecule. When they do so, they create a molecular structure that prevents the original molecule from fulfilling its intended purpose. Because the newly formed free radical struc-

ture has no purpose of its own, cells have no use for it. Over time these useless structures, called oxidants, accumulate, much as dust might accumulate within the workings of a precision timepiece, and interrupt normal functions. Such interruptions may cause various kinds of damage, sending cell replication awry or causing breaks in genetic codes. This damage eventually can result in disease.

Many people eat foods or take nutritional supplements that are high in antioxidants such as vitamin C and vitamin E as a means of minimizing the formation of oxidants. Although in moderation this practice likely presents no health risks, there is as yet no conclusive scientific evidence that it produces health benefits. Scientists suspect antioxidants are valuable for fighting disease development but are still searching for empirical evidence that they are. Numerous research studies continue to explore how the body manages oxidation and oxidative stress in health, as well as how these events come into play in illness. Many scientists believe oxidative stress is a key factor in allowing Parkinson's disease to develop.

See also ALTERNATIVE THERAPIES; ANTIOXIDANT THERAPY; APOPTOSIS; CHEMICAL TOXINS; COENZYME Q-10; COMPLEX I; LIPOPOLYSACCHARIDES; MITOCHONDRIAL DYSFUNCTION; MITOCHONDRIAL ELECTRON TRANSPORT CHAIN; NEURODEGENERATIVE; PARKINSON'S DISEASE, CAUSES OF.

pain A common secondary symptom in Parkinson's disease. Although Parkinson's disease itself does not seem to affect sensory pathways responsible for conveying pain messages to the BRAIN, its neuromuscular symptoms can create awkward postures and limb positions that become uncomfortable. BRADYKINESIA, in which movement and motor response are slow, causes people with Parkinson's to feel as though they are working against great resistance for every move. This effect causes muscles to tire and ache, in the same way as they might with vigorous exercise in a healthy person. DYSTONIA, in which a muscle group becomes so rigid as to be immobilized, can cause painful distortions, spasms, and cramps. Early morning and off-time dystonia, which emerges when ANTI-PARKINSON'S MEDICATIONS are at their lowest levels in the body, commonly affects the feet in later stages of Parkinson's and can cause considerable pain. RESTLESS LEG SYNDROME (RLS), in which painful spasms cause the muscles in the legs to twitch and jerk when lying in bed awake at night (or sometimes while sitting quietly during the day), also emerges when anti-Parkinson's medication levels are low. In addition to being uncomfortable, RLS causes SLEEP DISTURBANCES.

Other conditions not related to Parkinson's disease also can cause pain. One of the most common is osteoarthritis, which causes irritation, inflammation, and swelling in the tissues surrounding the joints. The awkward movements and positions that sometimes result from the neuromuscular symptoms of Parkinson's can exacerbate osteoarthritis. IDIOPATHIC pain syndromes occur in people with Parkinson's as well and seem to be more common in EARLY-ONSET PARKINSON'S. These conditions tend to attract less attention, from the person with Parkinson's as well as from doctors, because the primary therapeutic focus is on relieving the symptoms of Parkinson's disease. The person with Parkinson's may not recognize that some pains and discomforts are unrelated to Parkinson's disease.

Pain often is worse at night, as a result of several factors. Among the factors are the hormonal cycles of the body, which influence the release of chemicals in the body that affect pain perception such as endorphins, enkephalins, and prostaglandins. The levels of these substances are lowest during sleep, when the body's physical and mental functions are slowed. As well, the levels of anti-Parkinson's medications are at their lowest during sleep, when they are needed least. This state can allow symptoms to emerge.

Most people with Parkinson's disease can take common over-the-counter PAIN RELIEF MEDICATIONS such as nonsteroidal antiinflammatory drugs (NSAIDs) to relieve intermittent discomforts, aches, and pains. It is a good idea to check with the doctor or pharmacist about possible interactions between the pain reliever and the anti-Parkinson's medications. Always discuss persistent or sudden pain with the doctor before self-treating. Pain is a message from the body that something is not right, and determining whether that message is an alert to a serious problem is important. Pain that begins suddenly is called acute; pain that is ongoing is called chronic.

See also ALTERNATIVE THERAPIES; CONSTIPATION; EXERCISE AND ACTIVITY; PAIN MANAGEMENT.

pain management A therapeutic method of reducing, relieving, and preventing pain. There are numerous methods of pain management, including nonmedication techniques and PAIN RELIEF MEDICATIONS. Most people who have regular or chronic pain benefit from a combination of methods tailored to address their individual needs and circumstances. Keeping the neuromuscular symptoms of Parkinson's disease in check and treating depression and anxiety aggressively are the most important factors in minimizing discomfort. Taking ANTI-PARKINSON'S MEDICATIONS as prescribed and scheduled and striving to maintain as much function as possible are the most effective ways to do this.

Nonmedication techniques can be as effective as medication for some causes and kinds of pain. PHYSICAL THERAPY modalities such as diathermy (heat therapy), general stretching exercises, and specific exercises to strengthen muscle groups according to individual need improve stability and function. Therapeutic massage relaxes stiffened muscles, and the structured movements of TAI CHI and YOGA improve flexibility and RANGE OF MOTION. These methods target the causes of muscle and joint pain. MEDITATION and BIOFEEDBACK, approaches that integrate the body and the mind, often are effective for reducing chronic discomfort and pain. Regular physical activity and exercise such as walking and swimming help sustain balance, coordination, and mobility. These methods have the added benefit of improving overall well-being and reducing stress.

Many common pain relief medications are effective for pain management in a person who has Parkinson's disease, although possible interactions with anti-Parkinson's medications must be considered. Generally, over-the-counter medications such as nonsteroidal antiinflammatory drugs (NSAIDs) and acetaminophen do not cause interactions. Narcotics (such as codeine, hydrocodone, and oxycodone) are a less desirable option for people with Parkinson's as they can worsen daytime somnolence and constipation, which is already a likely problem as a result of the disease's disruption of smooth muscle function in the digestive tract or as a side effect of medications such as anticholinergics. Muscle relaxants and tricyclic antidepressants also sometimes relieve pain. Pain medications taken for chronic pain work best when they are

taken regularly rather than after pain becomes noticeable.

See also ALTERNATIVE THERAPIES.

pain relief medications Drugs taken to relieve discomfort and pain. Over-the-counter pain medications, called analgesics, are available without a doctor's prescription. They include aspirin, acetaminophen (Tylenol), and nonsteroidal antiinflammatory drugs (NSAIDs) such as ibuprofen (Advil, Motrin IB) and naproxen (Naprosyn). These medications are effective for relieving mild to moderate pain such as that of headache, backache, and muscle discomfort. Aspirin and NSAIDs have mild anticoagulation effects (reduce blood clotting) and can irritate the stomach. People who are taking prescription anticoagulants (blood thinners) or prescription medications for osteoarthritis or who have gastroesophageal reflux disorder (GERD) should not use aspirin or over-the-counter NSAIDs.

Prescription medications to treat pain include strong NSAIDs such as oxaprozin (Daypro) and nabumetone (Relafen), often taken for osteoarthritis and other chronic inflammatory conditions. These drugs act by inhibiting the release of prostaglandins, hormones that the body produces as part of the inflammatory response. Another class of prescription NSAIDs, the selective COX-2 inhibitors like rofecoxib (Vioxx), seem to have less risk of gastritis, and recent animal studies and some retrospective studies of groups of humans suggest that they might have a protective effect against developing Parkinson's disease. Narcotic pain relievers such as hydrocodone (Vicodin) and oxycodone (Percodan, Percocet) tend to cause or worsen constipation; mild narcotics such as propoxyphene (Darvon, Darvocet) and acetaminophen with codeine (Tylenol No. 3) are less likely to have this side effect. It is important to drink plenty of fluids when taking any narcotic pain reliever, to minimize the risk for constipation. Narcotics affect the ways in which the brain receives and interprets pain messages from the peripheral nerves.

Muscle relaxants such as CLONAZEPAM (Klonopin) and BACLOFEN (Lioresal) often alleviate discomfort and pain related to muscle spasms, RIGIDITY, and DYSTONIA. They act by slowing nerve stimulation of the muscles, allowing them to relax, return to normal positions, and ease the tension on joints. Tricyclic ANTIDEPRESSANT MEDICATIONS such as AMITRIPTYLINE (Elavil, Endep) and NORTRIPTYLINE (Pamelor) often relieve chronic pain due to IDIOPATHIC pain syndromes such as fibromyalgia, although doctors do not know exactly why these drugs are effective for pain relief. Narcotic pain relievers, muscle relaxants, and tricyclic antidepressants commonly cause drowsiness and dullness of thinking, affect balance and coordination. Muscle relaxants and tricyclic antidepressants interact with numerous other medications including ANTI-PARKINSON'S MEDICATIONS.

See also DEPRESSION; DOPAMINE AGONIST MEDICATIONS; LEVODOPA; MEDICATION MANAGEMENT; MEDICATION SIDE EFFECTS; QUALITY OF LIFE.

COMMON PAIN RELIEF MEDICATIONS

Type	Examples	Taken to Relieve	Interactions with Anti-Parkinson's Medications
OVER-THE-COUNTER (OTC)			
Analgesics	Aspirin acetaminophen (Tylenol)	Minor aches and discomforts, headache, backache, muscle ache, toothache	No
Nonsteroidal anti-inflammatory drugs (NSAIDs)	Ibuprofen (Advil, Motrin IB, Nuprin) Naproxen (Naprosyn, Aleve) Ketoprofen (Orudis KT)	Mild to moderate pain, headache, back pain, muscle pain, tooth pain Inflammation and swelling Osteoarthritis, injury	No
PRESCRIPTION			
Nonsteroidal anti-inflammatory drugs (NSAIDs)		Moderate pain Osteoarthritis Rheumatoid arthritis	No
Muscle relaxants	Baclofen (Lioresal) orphenadrine (Norflex) cyclobenzaprine (Flexeril) tizanidine (Zanaflex) alprazolam (Xanax), clonazepam, (Klonopin), diazepam (Valium)	Pain due to muscle spasms, rigidity, dystonia	MAOI antidepressants, selegine, sleep medications
Tricyclic antidepressants	Amitriptyline (Elavil, Endep), nortriptyline (Pamelor)	Chronic pain Fibromyalgia, chronic pain syndromes	MAOI antidepressants, selegine, SSRI antidepressants, levodopa, dopamine agonists, anticholinergics
Non-narcotic analgesics	Tramadol (Ultram)	Moderate to significant pain Postsurgical pain	MAOI antidepressants, muscle relaxants, sleep medications
Narcotic analgesics	Codeine, propoxyphene (Darvon, Darvocet), hydrocodone (Vicodin), oxycodone (Percodan, Percocet)	Moderate to significant pain Postsurgical pain Pain that other medications do not relieve	Antidepressants, muscle relaxants, sleep medications

palliative care   Supportive care that focuses on relieving symptoms as much as possible and making a person comfortable when a medical condition and health status will not improve. End of life care and HOSPICE care are forms of palliative care given to sustain comfort when death is imminent. The point at which it is appropriate to shift from treatment to palliative care is indistinct in Parkinson's disease and often relates more to other problems and resulting decline than to the Parkinson's.

As Parkinson's is a progressive disease, however, it is helpful for the person with Parkinson's and loved ones to have frank and honest discussions early in the course of the disease about what the person wants with regard to nutritional support, medication, and other interventions so that when the situation arises the decisions have already been made. Such decisions may also include the most appropriate location to meet the person's care needs. Most people want to remain at home, but this choice is not always practical when the person has become totally dependent. ADVANCE DIRECTIVES can formalize these choices.

Typically, the physician and family members make the determination that palliative care has become appropriate, on the basis of the person's medical condition and expectations for further decline. Family members often need emotional support and reassurance that they are making the right choices for their loved one's best interests.

See also ADVANCE DIRECTIVES; CARE MANAGEMENT AND PLANNING; END OF LIFE CARE AND DECISIONS; FEEDING TUBE; RESPITE CARE.

pallidotomy   A surgical treatment for Parkinson's disease in which targeted areas of neurons in the PALLIDUM, one of the BRAIN structures that control movement, are destroyed. This process interrupts the flow of nerve signals the globus pallidus sends to the motor cortex, which in turn controls the muscles, reducing many of the symptoms of Parkinson's such as TREMORS, BRADYKINESIA, DYSTONIA, and other DYSKINESIA. It also can decrease or end ON–OFF STATE fluctuations and decrease the amount of LEVODOPA, the standard medical therapy, necessary to control symptoms. Because the risks of surgical treatments are greater than the risks of nonsurgical treatments

and can be significant (such as infection and permanent cognitive and functional disabilities), pallidotomy generally becomes an option only when ANTI-PARKINSON'S MEDICATIONS can no longer control symptoms.

Radiosurgical techniques such as gamma knife provide a way to perform ablative procedures such as pallidotomy without many of the surgical risks, but because they depend upon cells dying over the ensuing months, their effectiveness or side effects often evolve over months. Many movement disorders specialists are of the opinion that the evidence for radiosurgical ablative techniques does not support its widespread use.

Although the effects of pallidotomy are permanent, they do not cure Parkinson's disease or prevent its progression. It is necessary to continue taking anti-Parkinson's medications, although usually the person can significantly reduce the dosages. Symptoms eventually return as DOPAMINERGIC NEURONS continue to die and brain DOPAMINE levels correspondingly decline. However, 70 to 85 percent of people who have pallidotomy experience years of significant improvement.

The pallidotomy procedure takes several hours. The neurosurgeon first attaches to the person's skull a stereotactic frame, a device that keeps the head motionless during the surgery. MAGNETIC RESONANCE IMAGING (MRI) is performed with the frame in place to allow surgeons to plan the surgical path to take to the globus pallidus. Computerized equipment attached to the stereotactic frame also assures that the electrical probes advance properly into the brain. The person remains awake although sedated during the surgery, as it is necessary for his or her responses to inform the neurosurgeon whether the probe is on target. The functional regions of the brain are not visually distinctive from one another and vary among individuals. The pallidus is very close to optic tract, the nerve structure that conveys visual signals from the optic nerve to the CEREBRUM. The neurosurgeon makes sure to avoid this tract by asking the person to report any visual perceptions such as "seeing" lights or stars during the surgery.

The neurosurgeon uses a local anesthetic to numb the surface tissues of the skull, which is the only location there are nerve endings capable of sensing pain, and drills a small hole through the skull through which the probe is inserted. MICRO-ELECTRODE RECORDING and MACROELECTRODE STIMU-LATION help to guide the probe into position within an interior portion of the pallidus called the GLOBUS PALLIDUS internus (GPi). Microelectrode recording, which allows the neurosurgeon to hear the changing spontaneous firing frequencies of neurons as the probe encounters them, further refines the probe's placement; electrical activity produces a different frequency in each type of neuron. Macro-electrode stimulation serves as a test of both the probable effectiveness and side effects of lesioning the apparent target area before any tissue is actually destroyed.

Once the probe is in place, the neurosurgeon sends a small electrical current through it to ablate or "burn" a very small number of the surrounding neurons. ABLATION interrupts the flow of electrical signals enough to reduce the activity of the pallidus to more normal levels, thereby quelling much of the overstimulation that causes neuromuscular symptoms such as BRADYKINESIA. Because the person is conscious and can respond to questions and directions, the neurosurgeon knows the results immediately. The person can usually notice the change as well.

Most pallidotomies are unilateral, performed on the side of the pallidus opposite the side of the body with the more severe symptoms as the functions of the brain are contralateral (the right side of the brain controls functions on the left side of the body and the left side of the brain controls functions on the right side of the body). This technique reduces the likelihood that any side effects from the surgery would be debilitating, because they, too, would affect only one side of the body. Bilateral pallidotomies carry a significant risk of affecting speech, swallowing, problems with eyelid opening, and neuropsychological side effects such as depression, extreme passivity, and obsessive behavior. Though the probe is very thin, it must pass through brain cells on its way to its destination and can inadvertently cause damage. It also is possible for ablation to leave a larger scar than anticipated, creating some movement difficulties or vision problems. The computerized stereotactic systems that neuro-surgeons use allow the probe to target specific cells, with a precision that minimizes the risk of such problems.

See also DEEP BRAIN STIMULATION; STEREOTAXIS; THALAMOTOMY.

pallidum A functional division of the BASAL GAN-GLIA, the cluster of neurons responsible for voluntary movement that is also called the globus pallidus. As other brain structures, the pallidum is a paired formation; the right structure controls movements on the left side of the body and the left structure controls movements on the right side of the body.

Each pallidum has two parts, the GLOBUS PAL-LIDUS externus (designated as the GPe) and the globus pallidus internus (GPi). Both receive nerve signals from the putamen, and the GPi also receives inputs from the subthalamic nucleus (STN) other structures of the basal ganglia. The GPi then sends out nerve signals to the THALAMUS, which channels them to sections of the cerebrum that direct voluntary movement, and to the brainstem, which regulates coordination of movement and sends nerve signals to the muscles. GPi nerve signals are inhibitory to these structures; that is, they slow their actions. In a healthy brain, DOPAMINE helps to regulate the activity of neurons throughout the basal ganglia. It acts as an inhibitory NEUROTRANS-MITTER among the neurons in the GPi, where it functions to keep their activity in check. Dopamine affects the GPi via direct and indirect pathways from the putamen, which receive dopamine via the NIGROSTRIATAL FIBERS from the SUBSTANTIA NIGRA that produces it.

In Parkinson's disease, the GPi malfunctions. As dopaminergic neurons continue to die, as is the hallmark of Parkinson's disease, the number of nigrostriatal fibers also decreases. There is less dopamine in the brain, and there are fewer fibers to carry it where it needs to go. Without dopamine to curtail them the neurons in the GPi intensify their activity, sending increased inhibitory signals to the thalamus. The resulting decrease in thalamic stimulation to the cerebral motor cortex results in BRADYKINESIA (slowed movements), AKINESIA (lack of movement or "freezing"), DYSTONIA (extreme RIGIDITY), and other DYSKINESIAS (abnormal movements) of Parkinson's.

ANTI-PARKINSON'S MEDICATIONS that restore dopamine levels reestablish temporary control over neuron activity in the GPi, easing these symptoms. Levodopa and other medications become less effective as Parkinson's progresses, however, and GPi activity again intensifies. SURGERY called PALLIDO-TOMY that interferes with the GPi's neuron communication can produce long-term relief of neuromuscular symptoms for some people with late stage Parkinson's disease.

See also ABLATION; ADJUNCT THERAPIES; DEEP BRAIN STIMULATION; MEDICATION MANAGEMENT; TREATMENT ALGORITHM.

palsy An antiquated term for temporary or permanent paralysis or inability to move. Parkinson's disease was once called the SHAKING PALSY in reference to its more prominent symptoms of TREMOR, BRADYKINESIA, and FREEZING OF GAIT.

See also ADJUSTING TO LIVING WITH PARKINSON'S; CARDINAL SYMPTOMS; CONDITIONS SIMILAR TO PARKINSON'S; GAIT DISTURBANCE.

paralysis agitans An antiquated term for Parkinson's disease that describes the blend of TREMORS, BRADYKINESIA, and freezing of gait, that characterize the disease. It is the Latin form of the term "SHAKING PALSY."

See also MULTIPLE SYSTEM ATROPHY; PARKINSON, JAMES; PARKINSONISM; PARKINSON'S PLUS SYNDROMES.

paranoia A psychiatric disorder of DELUSION: Any set of false beliefs in which the person holding them structures perception of random events and circumstances to support them. Paranoia is the delusion that others are out to cause one harm. Paranoia can develop as an aspect of psychiatric illnesses such as PSYCHOSIS or SCHIZOPHRENIA, as a consequence of organic degeneration of the brain, or as an element of drug-induced psychosis (as a side effect). In the person with Parkinson's, paranoia is a common element of cognitive impairment. It can be present as the consequence of another pathological process such as dementia (as in ALZHEIMER'S DISEASE,) which often coexists with Parkinson's disease, or as the result of degenerative changes in the brain due to the Parkinson's.

As ANTI-PARKINSON'S MEDICATIONS can cause cognitive changes and symptoms such as delusions and hallucinations, it is important first to determine whether they are the source of the paranoia by lowering dosage or changing to a different medication. Anti-Parkinson's medications most likely to cause psychotic symptoms including paranoia are ANTICHOLINERGIC MEDICATIONS such as BENZTROPINE (Cogentin) and trihexyphenidyl (Artane) and DOPAMINE AGONIST MEDICATIONS such as ROPINIROLE (Requip), PRAMIPEXOLE (Mirapex), PERGOLIDE (Permax), and BROMOCRIPTINE (Parlodel). Switching to a different drug within a particular classification often eliminates the side effects yet maintains the benefits of the medication type. ANTIPSYCHOTIC MEDICATIONS taken to treat dementia and psychosis also can ameliorate symptoms such as paranoia, people with Parkinson's disease should avoid taking these drugs because they may exacerbate EXTRAPYRAMIDAL SYMPTOMS although some of the newer (atypical) antipsychotic agents such as quetiapine (Seroquel) and clozapine (Clozaril) are safer choices to avoid these side effects.

When paranoia is severe enough to interfere with everyday activities, trying antipsychotic medications and being especially alert for side effects may be necessary. Paranoia in which the person has a fear of being poisoned may cause him or her to refuse to take medications or eat, for example, in that case intervention is essential.

See also ANXIETY; ANTIANXIETY MEDICATIONS; ANTIDEPRESSANT MEDICATIONS; DEPRESSION; MEDICATION MANAGEMENT; MEDICATION SIDE EFFECTS; MENTAL STATUS.

parasympathetic nervous system See NERVOUS SYSTEM.

parent/child relationships Many changes take place in the relationships between adult children and their parents when the parent has a degenerative disease such as Parkinson's. In many respects the child becomes the parent figure, taking on responsibility for the parent's care and overall well-being. Some adult children may already be in such a role as a result of changes in the parent due to aging. It can be a challenging balance for the adult child and the parent to maintain, and either or both may be resistant to changing roles. It is difficult to relinquish independence at any age, regardless of the reason, and the person doing so often focuses his or her resentment on the person who is stepping in to pick up caregiving responsibilities. Compassion and empathy help each to see the other's perspective, and to treat the other with appropriate respect. The relationship can become particularly strained if the adult child and the parent have not been close and the parent's condition now forces them to become so.

When there is more than one adult child, there are sometimes disagreements about how to divide responsibilities. It is important for families to talk through these issues and to involve the parent with Parkinson's in discussions to the extent that this is reasonable. Sometimes the parent's cognitive impairment becomes a significant factor, and he or she cannot participate in dialogue and decisions regarding his or her care and circumstances. When families are not able to have such conversations before it becomes necessary to take action, resentment and uncertainty about doing the right things often result. When the diagnosis of Parkinson's is made early enough and before other health problems become factors, family members including the person with Parkinson's can plan for future needs.

The challenges of a chronic, degenerative disease such as Parkinson's can bring out the best or the worst in families and in parent/child relationships. Strained relationships can but do not necessarily improve because the parent's situation has changed; it often requires concerted effort particularly by the adult child to reconcile past differences to focus on present and future needs. The adult child may resent the changing roles as much as the parent; it is an intense emotional transition for most people. Strong family relationships, however, tend to become even stronger as family members draw together to support one another. Candor, humor, and kindness help to maintain open lines of communication.

See also ADJUSTING TO LIVING WITH PARKINSON'S; ADVANCE DIRECTIVES; COPING WITH ONGOING CARE OF PARKINSON'S; MARRIAGE RELATIONSHIP; PLANNING FOR THE FUTURE.

parenteral nutrition   Meeting of the body's nutritional needs through means other than eating, sometimes called artificial feeding. The word *parenteral* means "around the intestine." Parenteral nutrition becomes a consideration when the person with Parkinson's is not able to obtain adequate nourishment by eating. This may be the result of swallowing difficulties (DYSPHAGIA), significant COGNITIVE IMPAIRMENT, neuromuscular impairments that ANTI-PARKINSON'S MEDICATIONS cannot control, or factors related to other health problems.

Parenteral nutrition involves infusing specially prepared and formulated nutrient-dense intravenous (IV) solutions through a catheter inserted into a large vein, going directly into the bloodstream, and bypassing the digestive system. This method, called central line infusion, can sustain a person's nutritional needs for quite a long time, but it is typically only utilized as a short-term solution when the gastrointestinal tract is temporarily unavailable (usually from abdominal surgery or disease). Risks of its use include infection and blood clots (thromboembolisms), infection, and inflammation of the pancreas.

Though not parenteral, enteral feeding via a FEEDING TUBE through which liquid supplements are channeled directly to the stomach or intestine often is a better choice for short-term and long-term nutrition in patients with an intact digestive system but who cannot be safely fed by mouth.

The decision about whether to implement enteral or parenteral nutrition is often a struggle for family members. Ideally the person with Parkinson's and family members discuss this option well before it is necessary to consider it and formalize preferences through ADVANCE DIRECTIVES. Many people are loath simply to prolong living when the resulting quality of life is questionable or undesirable, given that the Parkinson's will continue to progress.

See also CARE MANAGEMENT AND PLANNING; COPING WITH ONGOING CARE OF PARKINSON'S; END OF LIFE CARE AND DECISIONS.

parkin gene A gene located on chromosome 6 that is mutated in some people who have Parkinson's disease, particularly EARLY-ONSET PARKINSON'S. Researchers in Japan first isolated and identified the parkin gene and some of its mutations in the late 1990s when studying a rare form of early-onset Parkinson's called autosomal recessive juvenile parkinsonism (AR-JP). Because people with AR-JP do not have the classic LEWY BODY structures (protein deposits within BRAIN neurons) that characterize IDIOPATHIC Parkinson's disease, whether AR-JP is a true form of Parkinson's disease or produces similar symptoms but has a different pathological origin is controversial.

For the parkin gene to clearly cause disease, the person must have identical mutations from both mother and father. Because the number of possible mutations is significant, the conditions necessary for the disease to be manifested happen only in siblings from the same nuclear family and then only in approximately one-quarter of the siblings. However, researchers believe parkin gene mutations of any kind, even just a single mutation from one parent, may increase a person's vulnerability to Parkinson's, creating an interaction with environmental factors that causes development of the disease. Scientists have since found numerous defects in structures of the parkin gene called exons, primarily in people with early-onset Parkinson's, throughout the world. As the technology to identify gene mutations is just becoming available, researchers will be able to examine a wider sample of people, both with and without diagnosed Parkinson's disease, to attempt to determine how widespread these mutations are.

As does the ALPHA-SYNUCLEIN GENE mutation, another known gene mutation associated with Parkinson's disease, the parkin gene mutation alters the way in which neurons handle protein. This alteration, scientists believe, allows toxic levels of oxidative stress to accumulate, leading to premature cell death. Incorrectly oxidized proteins become toxic OXIDANTS, or FREE RADICALS, which are capable of causing significant cell and tissue damage over time. Some chromosomal defects also appear linked to whether LEVODOPA therapy is effective. Further research in this area could pro-vide new insights into how and why levodopa functions in the brain and perhaps establish more effective TREATMENT ALGORITHMS.

See also CHROMOSOMES LINKED TO PARKINSON'S DISEASE; GENE MAPPING; GENE THERAPY; GENETIC PREDISPOSITION; HUMAN GENOME PROJECT.

Parkinson, James The 18th-century British physician (1755–1824) who first described the symptoms and progression of the disease that now bears his name. Parkinson's father, John, also was a physician, and James Parkinson eventually took over his practice. In 1817 Parkinson published a medical paper, "Essay on the Shaking Palsy," in which he discussed the collection of symptoms he had observed in numerous patients through his years of practice. The shaking palsy, he wrote, was marked by

> involuntary tremulous motion, with lessened muscular power, in parts not in action and even when supported with a propensity to bend the trunk forwards and to pass from a walking to a running pace: the senses and intellects being uninjured.

The medical community paid little attention, however, until the French neuropathologist Jean Martin Charcot rediscovered Parkinson's paper some 40 years after its publication and added his observations about the disease to Parkinson's. Not until the 20th century did the medical community begin to refer to the shaking palsy as Parkinson's disease.

During his lifetime Parkinson was better known as an amateur paleontologist than as a physician. He traveled extensively to collect fossils and published a three-volume series about his efforts to identify them, *Organic Remains of the Former World.* The three books were published in 1804, 1808, and 1811. He published a follow-up volume, *Elements of Oryctology: An Introduction to the Study of Fossil Organic Remains,* in 1822. These writings remain highly regarded in Great Britain today for their work in laying the foundation of fossil identification and study for the region.

See also CONDITIONS SIMILAR TO PARKINSON'S; PALSY; PARALYSIS AGITANS.

Parkinson Study Group A not-for-profit organization of medical and research centers throughout the United States and Canada that coordinates CLINICAL RESEARCH STUDIES and whose research findings provide information regarding improved treatment options for people with Parkinson's disease. The Parkinson Study Group funds and supports numerous research studies and partners with various experts such as pharmaceutical companies to introduce new treatments. The group's website, www.parkinson-study-group.org, maintains a listing of active clinical research studies, including those that are recruiting participants. It also reports on the findings of completed studies. Because the Parkinson Study Group is a network of providers and facilities, its central address is that of its current chairperson. Access to the group and the information it provides is obtained through the website.

See also HOPE FOR A PARKINSON'S CURE; MICHAEL J. FOX FOUNDATION FOR PARKINSON'S RESEARCH; MORRIS K. UDALL PARKINSON'S RESEARCH ACT; NATIONAL INSTITUTE OF NEUROLOGICAL DISORDERS AND STROKE; NATIONAL PARKINSON'S DISEASE FOUNDATION.

Parkinsonian An adjective used to describe symptoms and physical exam findings that suggest an extra pyramidal disorder such as Parkinson's disease.

See also PWP.

parkinsonism A noun that describes a constellation of EXTRAPYRAMIDAL SYMPTOMS that resemble those of Parkinson's disease but may result from other causes or conditions. These generally result from either Parkinson's or damage to the same areas of the BRAIN Parkinson's disease affects. The distinction becomes important from a treatment perspective, as sometimes Parkinson's-like symptoms that are not true Parkinson's disease do not respond to LEVODOPA therapy and other ANTI-PARKINSON'S MEDICATIONS. Because there are no clear pathological biomarkers that definitively differentiate Parkinson's disease from conditions that generate similar damage and symptoms, doctors must rely on a careful and comprehensive clinical examination and medical history. Several distinct parkinsonisms are known; as with Parkinson's disease, diagnosis can be confirmed only at autopsy after death.

Postencephalitic Parkinsonism

Postencephalitic parkinsonism develops as a result of damage to the brain after infection with a viral form of encephalitis called encephalitis lethargica. The causative virus has never been identified. Although sporadic cases of this encephalitis occur throughout the world today, it became of medical significance in the years after World War I (1916–27) when it infected millions of people. The classic symptom of extended sleep, sleep attacks, and extreme alteration of normal sleep-wake cycles earned the infection the nickname "sleepy sickness." About a third of those who contracted it died, and about half of those who survived suffered permanent brain damage with symptoms very similar to those of Parkinson's disease as well as significant cognitive impairment that left them in a state of reduced consciousness. Some who recovered were seemingly normal and then experienced sudden neuromuscular and cognitive symptoms years later. At the time there were neither treatments for Parkinson's disease nor antibiotics, and those who experienced severe neuromuscular dysfunction quickly succumbed to other infections such as pneumonia.

The American psychiatrist Oliver Sacks drew attention to postencephalitic parkinsonism in the 1970s in his book *Awakenings*. Intrigued by the similarities of neuromuscular impairment in the few survivors of the post–World War I epidemic of encephalitis lethargica and aware of research using the then-new drug LEVODOPA to treat Parkinson's disease, Sacks administered levodopa for some of his patients' symptoms. This dramatically "awakened" the patients, many of whom had not been capable of voluntary movement for the decades since the virus struck them.

Postencephalitic parkinsonism is rarely reported today, but when it does occur, it often responds at least partially to levodopa therapy and other anti-Parkinson's medications that extend the availability of DOPAMINE. The damage to the brain appears to be permanent but not progressive. The most prominent symptoms are AKINESIA and AKATHISIA, which cause the person to become nearly motionless. At autopsy after death the brain shows a dramatic loss of DOPAMINERGIC NEURONS in the SUBSTANTIA NIGRA, as is characteristic of Parkinson's disease, but no NIGROSTRIATAL FIBER loss or LEWY BODY formation.

Arteriosclerotic Parkinsonism

Arteriosclerotic parkinsonism occurs when there is damage to blood vessels in the brain, typically small strokes, that affects the blood supply to the substantia nigra and other structures of the BASAL GANGLIA. The neuromuscular symptoms that result are similar to those Parkinson's disease because the brain's dopamine-induced activity patterns in the basal ganglia diminish. However, other brain functions are affected as well, and anti-Parkinson's medications such as levodopa and dopamine agonists have little effect on symptoms as the putamenal neurons that dopamine modulates are often damaged. This parkinsonism is sometimes called pseudoparkinsonism.

Secondary Parkinsonism

Neuromuscular symptoms similar to those of Parkinson's disease such as TREMORS and DYSKINESIA sometimes accompany posttraumatic encephalopathy (changes in brain function that follow brain injury) and other NEURODEGENERATIVE diseases such as HUNTINGTON'S DISEASE and CREUTZFELDT-JAKOB DISEASE. These parkinsonisms do not respond to levodopa or other anti-Parkinson's medications.

Toxin-Induced Parkinsonism

Certain environmental toxins produce damage in the brain that causes Parkinson's-like symptoms. The most common are pesticides such as rotenone, manganese poisoning (through industrial exposure to manganese dust), mercury poisoning (through industrial or other exposure to mercury-based pollutants), carbon monoxide, carbon disulfide (an industrial pollutant), polychlorinated biphenyls (PCBs), and the illicit drug MPTP, an inadvertent contaminant from botched attempts to illicitly synthesize a narcotic. The damage that exposure to these toxins produces is usually permanent, and symptoms do not respond to levodopa and other anti-Parkinson's medications. Since environmental standards and regulations have been enacted over the past several decades to protect people from dangerous levels of these chemicals, poisonings and parkinsonisms related to them are rare but still do occur.

Drug-Induced Parkinsonism

Some medications can cause extrapyramidal symptoms that resemble Parkinson's disease. Those most noted for doing so are older antipsychotic medications such as HALOPERIDOL (Haldol) and chlorpromazine (Thorazine), the antihypertensive (high blood pressure) medication RESERPINE, antinausea medications such as promethazine (Phenergan) and prochlorperazine (Compazine) and metoclopramide (Reglan) taken for gastroesophageal reflux disorder (GERD). People who have Parkinson's disease or Parkinson's-like symptoms should not use any of these medications; there are alternatives available that produce similar therapeutic results without the risk of extrapyramidal side effects. When these drugs cause extrapyramidal symptoms as side effects, reducing the dosage or stopping the drug usually ends the symptoms. Rarely symptoms can permanently persist as parkinsonism or in forms such as TARDIVE DYSKINESIA.

See also 1-METHYL-4-PHENYL-1,2,3,6,-TETRAHYDROPYRIDINE; CHEMICAL TOXINS; CONDITIONS SIMILAR TO PARKINSON'S; EXTRAPYRAMIDAL SYSTEM; HALLERVORDEN–SPATZ SYNDROME; MULTIPLE SYSTEM ATROPHY; PARKINSON'S PLUS SYNDROMES; PROGRESSIVE SUPRANUCLEAR PALSY; SACKS, OLIVER.

Parkinson's Awareness Month Parkinson's disease organizations worldwide have designated April as Parkinson's Awareness Month. Each year during the month of April, these organizations sponsor special fund-raising and educational events to increase public awareness of Parkinson's disease and support for research to find a cure.

Parkinson's crisis An exaggeration of Parkinson's symptoms caused by sudden stopping of an ANTIPARKINSON'S MEDICATION, especially a DOPAMINE AGONIST, and sometimes by extreme ANXIETY. Some people experience episodes of Parkinson's crisis in the late stages of the disease when FLUCTUATING RESPONSE becomes a problem. During a Parkinson's crisis the person's body seems to freeze and the person is unable to move. This is very frightening, even when the person knows what it is, and creates anxiety that can further intensify the situation. The most effective treatment is injection of a RESCUE DRUG, usually APOMORPHINE, as this dopamine agonist acts within minutes. Rarely, a crisis may be more severe and take the form of involuntary rolling of the eyes (occulogyric crisis) which is a portent of a withdrawal syndrome of labile blood pressure, extreme fever, extreme rigidity, and alterations of consciousness that mimics the neuroleptic malignant syndrome that antipsychotic medications can cause. Any signs of this more severe withdrawal syndrome would indicate the need for immediate medical care and treatment.

See also DRUG "HOLIDAY"; PENJET SYSTEM; STAGING OF PARKINSON'S DISEASE; TREATMENT ALGORITHM.

Parkinson's disease   An incurable NEURODEGENERATIVE disorder affecting the parts of the BRAIN that direct voluntary movement. Researchers believe most Parkinson's disease is caused by a combination of genetic and environmental factors. Some people with Parkinson's have a clear family history of the disease; in those cases GENE MUTATIONS likely are a stronger influence than in people without such a family history. There do not appear to be any forms of Parkinson's that are exclusively genetic, unlike in other neurodegenerative diseases such as HUNTINGTON'S DISEASE, the disease will develop in a person who has the gene mutation.

Most people with Parkinson's have what doctors call IDIOPATHIC Parkinson's disease, to indicate that the reason for its development is unknown. Though Parkinson's disease has been diagnosed in only about 0.3 percent of the U.S. population, reports of its presence in the elderly is much higher. One report found that 50 percent of community-dwelling people over age 85 met criteria for parkinsonism; another study found parkinsonism in 10 percent of general medicine clinic patients order than age 60. Parkinson's disease that develops in a person before age 50 is considered EARLY-ONSET PARKINSON'S. Somewhat more men than women have Parkinson's disease. Although Parkinson's is incurable and progressive, it is seldom fatal and does not shorten life expectancy for most people who have it. It is possible to live with Parkinson's disease for several decades. The disease's progression and symptoms are unpredictable and inconsistent, however, and those who have it respond differently to treatment.

Pathological Features and Symptoms
An excessive loss of DOPAMINERGIC NEURONS (dopamine-producing neurons) in the SUBSTANTIA NIGRA region of the BRAINSTEM in the BRAIN is the hallmark pathological condition of Parkinson's disease. The substantia nigra is closely connected to structures of the basal ganglia, which regulate voluntary movement in the body. DOPAMINE is the brain NEUROTRANSMITTER essential to this regulation. When the number of dopaminergic neurons declines to about 20 percent of normal, the level of dopamine they produce is no longer adequate. This mechanism establishes a situation of dopamine depletion. The results are manifested by various motor symptoms, the most characteristic of which are

- Resting TREMOR
- BRADYKINESIA
- POSTURAL INSTABILITY
- RIGIDITY

These four primary or CARDINAL SYMPTOMS are asymmetrical (predominantly affect one side of the body) until the disease is fairly advanced. The presence of one or two of these symptoms is somewhat inconclusive, with the triad of tremor, bradykinesia, and rigidity being most indicative of Parkinson's disease. The presence within the first three years of symptoms of postural instability strongly argues against Parkinson's. The presence of abnormalities on exam that suggest other motor system abnormalities, other than signs that are typical of the extrapyramidal tract, or early dysfunction of the autonomic nervous system, are also suggestive of a diagnosis other than Parkinson's disease; three or four of them is considered conclusive of the diagnosis. There is no specific diagnostic test or BIOMARKER that identifies Parkinson's. As a result misdiagnosis, particularly in early stage disease, is common; as many as 25 percent of people receive an incorrect diagnosis. Other symptoms that may accompany the cardinal symptoms include

- DEPRESSION
- Soft voice and difficulty in speaking
- GAIT DISTURBANCES
- AKINESIA (lack of movement) typically in a single body part such as a finger

The other conclusive pathological feature of Parkinson's disease is the presence of Lewy bodies, protein-based inclusions that develop within the neurons in the substantia nigra. These distinctive structures are made mostly of a protein called ALPHA-SYNUCLEIN and are detectable only at autopsy after death. Lewy bodies are always present in Parkinson's disease, but there are a handful of other diseases that also are characterized by the presence of Lewy bodies. Some, but not all, people who have Parkinson's have mutations of the ALPHA-SYNUCLEIN GENE, which controls how the body handles alpha-synuclein. Researchers do not fully understand what causes Lewy bodies to form or how they affect neuron function; the deposits appear to "clog" the cell and interfere with its metabolic activities.

Causes

The causes of Parkinson's disease remain unknown. Most researchers believe a complex interplay of various genetic and environmental factors sets in motion the events that result in the disease's development. Some scientists believe this interplay accelerates APOPTOSIS (natural cell death); others believe damage to neurons, such as through exposure to NEUROTOXINS or MITOCHONDRIAL DYSFUNCTION, causes them to die. Although there are families in whom Parkinson's disease is prevalent and those in whom it develops have specific GENE MUTATIONS, there is no evidence to date that specific gene mutations unequivocally cause Parkinson's disease or that there is a solely genetic cause of Parkinson's disease. Some chemicals are known to cause Parkinson's disease irrespective of genetic factors. These include the illicit narcotic contaminant MPTP. However, researchers do not know the mechanisms through which these chemicals act on the brain or why they selectively affect dopaminergic neurons. Most of the time doctors do not know what causes the development of Parkinson's disease.

Risk Factors

Although most Parkinson's disease is IDIOPATHIC, there are four key risk factors that make it more likely a person will develop the disease. The more of these factors that are present, the higher the risk. They are

- Age
- Cumulative exposure to environmental toxins
- Genetic mutations
- Alzheimer's disease

The leading risk factor for Parkinson's disease is age. Eighty-five percent of people with Parkinson's disease are older than age 60; the percentage of people who have Parkinson's disease increases with each decade of life after age 60. Some scientists speculate that in every person who lives long enough Parkinson's disease will in fact develop, as APOPTOSIS (regular, programmed cell death) among dopaminergic neurons would eventually drop the neurons' level below that capable of meeting the brain's dopamine needs. Genetic risk factors include mutations of the alpha-synuclein gene and the PARKIN GENE, as well as numerous mutations in certain areas on more than a half-dozen chromosomes. Environmental risk factors include cumulative exposure to chemical toxins such as pesticides and herbicides and to industrial pollutants such as mercury and polychlorinated biphenyls (PCBs). Medications such as the potent antipsychotic HALOPERIDOL also cause damage to the brain that manifests in the form of Parkinson's disease.

Diagnosis

The diagnosis of Parkinson's is clinical, based on an assessment of symptoms; there are no conclusive biomarkers or tests for the disease. About 25 percent of people are misdiagnosed, particularly in the early stages, when symptoms can suggest a number of neurodegenerative CONDITIONS SIMILAR TO

PARKINSON'S that also lack definitive tests. The most conclusive diagnostic evidence includes

- The presence of three or all four of the CARDINAL SYMPTOMS
- Asymmetrical (predominantly one-sided) symptoms
- Positive response to a trial of LEVODOPA therapy

Functional imaging studies such as COMPUTED TOMOGRAPHY (CT) SCAN or MAGNETIC RESONANCE IMAGING (MRI) are most useful for ruling out other causes such as stroke or lesions in the basal ganglia or BRAINSTEM. If symptoms are markedly relieved by levodopa, the diagnosis is almost certainly Parkinson's. One exception is the Parkinson's-like complex of disorders known collectively as MULTIPLE SYSTEM ATROPHY (MSA), which is characterized by a similar loss of dopaminergic neurons and dopamine depletion. About a third of people with MSA also respond favorably to initial levodopa therapy.

Treatment

The DOPAMINE PRECURSOR levodopa remains the cornerstone of treatment for advanced Parkinson's disease. Although the dopamine molecule is too large to cross the BLOOD-BRAIN BARRIER, the levodopa molecule is small enough for such passage. Once levodopa is in the brain it must enter a surviving substantia nigra neuron where DOPA DECARBOXYLASE metabolizes it to dopamine and it is stored as a neurotransmitter. The substantia nigra neuron eventually releases the stored dopamine into the synapse where its effect is temporary, as once in the synapse it is in turn metabolized into another element. Early in Parkinson's a levodopa dose might provide benefit for many hours, as there are many surviving substantia nigra neurons and, hence, both lots of storage capacity for dopamine and little significant dopaminergic deficit; late in the disease, the symptomatic effects of a levodopa dose can last less than an hour. The loss of dopamine storage capacity and increasing dopamine deficit in the brain is complicated by poorer digestive system absorption of levodopa making it necessary to take dosages that are signif-

icantly higher than the amount of the drug that will reach the brain.

Peripheral levodopa metabolism causes a number of unpleasant side effects including nausea, lightheadedness, and palpitations. For this reason most people take levodopa in combination with CARBIDOPA (Sinemet) or BENSERAZIDE (Madopar). These drugs are DOPA DECARBOXYLASE INHIBITORS that slow peripheral metabolism of levodopa to allow more of it to reach the brain. The occurrence of the above side effects with initiation of Sinemet therapy usually resolves with the addition of more carbidopa (Lodosyn). For this reason, Sinemet 10/100 tablets are usually a poor choice for initiation of therapy and should be reserved for people with advanced disease who are taking more than 800 mg of levodopa per day. Though motor complications commonly occur after a few years on levodopa, and the underlying disease progresses, levodopa remains an effective treatment for motor symptoms throughout the course of the disease, supplying significant relief from symptoms for decades in many people. Most people with advanced Parkinson's remain on it until intolerable side effects develop.

Other anti-Parkinson's medications have a role as monotherapy in early or moderate disease and may supplement levodopa in advanced disease. They include

- Amantadine, which has a mild dopamine agonist effect and reduces levodopa-induced dyskinesias
- Anticholinergics, which inhibit acetylcholine to control tremors
- COMT inhibitors, which increase the duration and effectiveness of levodopa
- Dopamine agonists, which activate dopamine receptors in the brain to simulate dopamine
- Muscle relaxants, which act on the muscles to relieve rigidity

Course of Disease and Prognosis

Although the progression of Parkinson's disease is inevitable, the rate of degeneration and the kinds and severity of symptoms vary widely among individuals. Some people have virtually no symptoms and go for many years on dopamine agonists or very low dose with levodopa therapy and others are significantly debilitated within a few years despite trying multiple medications and attempting to maximize levodopa. Most people have a course between the extremes, with periods when symptoms are repressed and other periods when they are not. There is no way to predict how a person will respond to treatment, whether Parkinson's will become debilitating, or which symptoms will be prominent.

Most people who have Parkinson's disease when they die do not die of the disease. Parkinson's disease is seldom a cause of death, although it can establish the circumstances that allow life-threatening infections such as pneumonia to develop. Other diseases that coexist with Parkinson's, such as diabetes or heart disease, are likely to have a far greater effect on QUALITY OF LIFE and longevity than is Parkinson's disease.

Outlook for a Cure

Hundreds of research studies are under way in the quest for a cure for Parkinson's. Some of the most promising results are those from the field of genetics, as scientists continue to decode the human genome and gain further insights into the effects of genes on health. Other research explores new drugs that can specifically and precisely target certain cells and functions in the brain. Still other studies are looking at ways to protect neurons, which the body does not replace when they die, from OXIDATIVE STRESS and other factors known to cause cell damage and death.

See also ADJUSTING TO LIVING WITH PARKINSON'S; COPING WITH DIAGNOSIS OF PARKINSON'S; COPING WITH ONGOING CARE OF PARKINSON'S; HUMAN GENOME PROJECT; LEWY BODY; MEDICAL MANAGEMENT; 1-METHYL-4-PHENYL-1,2,3,6-TETRAHYDROPYRIDINE; PARKINSON'S DISEASE, CAUSES OF; SURGERY; THERAPEUTIC WINDOW; TREATMENT ALGORITHM.

Parkinson's disease, causes of   There are a number of theories about the causes of Parkinson's disease, most of which are related to a combination of genetic and environmental factors that interact to result in disease. At present, however, there is no clearly identified cause of Parkinson's disease. Researchers understand the symptoms of Parkinson's disease to be the result of dopamine depletion in the brain that prevents brain NEURONS from communicating properly with one another, disrupting the flow of signals from the brain to the muscles of movement in the body. They know that the death of DOPAMINERGIC NEURONS in the SUBSTANTIA NIGRA, causes the dopamine depletion. But there is no clear understanding of how or why this degeneration develops, or why it progresses.

Aging

Eighty-five percent of people with Parkinson's disease are older than age 50; Parkinson's disease is estimated to affect as much as 1 percent of the American population older than age 50 and a third of those older than age 75. Researchers believe that dopaminergic neurons in the substantia nigra begin to die, as a natural function of aging, after about age 40 at the rate of 10 percent a decade. Parkinson's symptoms begin to manifest when the level of surviving dopaminergic neurons falls below roughly 20 percent. Although age clearly is correlated as the older a person is the more likely he or she is to have Parkinson's, it is not the only factor. Projecting the normal course of dopaminergic neuron death, a person would reach age 100 or 110 before the loss would be significant enough to produce symptoms. When Parkinson's disease develops, other factors accelerate the loss.

Chromosome Defects and Gene Mutations

Scientists have identified defects in areas on numerous chromosomes as well as mutations of the ALPHA-SYNUCLEIN GENE and the PARKIN GENE in some people with Parkinson's disease who have participated in research studies. However, not all people with Parkinson's who have been tested have these defects. And the extent to which these defects and mutations exist in people who do not have Parkinson's is unknown. So far, there is no "absolute" genetic defect that results in Parkinson's disease, unlike in HUNTINGTON'S DISEASE, a NEURODEGENERATIVE disorder in which disease eventually develops in every person who has the defective gene (unless death occurs prematurely of other causes). Rather, it appears that certain defects and mutations predispose a person to development of Parkinson's. Other factors then converge with this predisposition, allowing Parkinson's to emerge as a disease.

Some families have drawn the attention of researchers because of the high rate of Parkinson's among relatives across generations. Even in these families, the presence of chromosome defects and gene mutations is inconsistent. However, scientists hope that by studying these families they can learn more about how Parkinson's gets its start.

Environmental Toxins

Various chemicals are known to cause Parkinson's-like symptoms, which are sometimes permanent. There is also a higher rate of Parkinson's disease among people with long-term exposure to certain chemicals than among the general population, leading scientists to suspect environmental toxins play a role in why and how Parkinson's disease develops. CHEMICAL TOXINS under suspicion include industrial pollutants such as mercury, carbon disulfide, and polychlorinated biphenyls (PCBs). PCBs were once common in thousands of chemicals from household cleaning products to industrial solvents, and although banned in the United States in the 1970s they remain pervasive contaminants in the soil and in water supplies. Numerous common pesticides and herbicides still in use also are suspect, although the connections between them and Parkinson's are not conclusive. Scientists believe exposure to these substances affects the body's ability to manage FREE RADICALS, particles of metabolic waste that, when they accumulate, interfere with normal cell function.

Mitochondrial Dysfunction

Mitochondria are tiny structures within the cell that generate the energy that the cell needs to fuel its functions. Although scientists have known of the existence of mitochondria for more than a century, recent technological advances are just now making it possible for them to understand how mitochondria function. Mitochondria are the only structures in the body other than cells that have

deoxyribonucleic acid (DNA). They manufacture not only the cell's energy source but also contain substances that enable the cell to clean up its metabolic waste, proteins that can bind with free radicals to render them harmless. Scientists know that people with Parkinson's disease have fewer of these proteins than people without Parkinson's disease. Mitochondria also contain proteins that initiate APOPTOSIS, the natural sequence of events in which cells die. A number of the genetic defects linked to Parkinson's disease relate to functions of these proteins (such as ALPHA-SYNUCLEIN). Mitochondrial dysfunction has been associated with numerous diseases.

See also AGING; ANTIOXIDANTS; CHROMOSOMES LINKED TO PARKINSON'S DISEASE; ENDOTOXIN; EXOTOXIN; GENE MAPPING; GENE THERAPY; LIPOPOLYSACCHARIDES; OXIDATIVE STRESS.

Parkinson's Disease Foundation, Inc. (PDF) A not-for-profit organization whose mission is to provide education and information about Parkinson's disease for medical professionals, people with Parkinson's disease and their family members, and the media. The PDF also provides referral and resource contacts to clinical practice groups throughout the United States that specialize in treating people with Parkinson's disease and similar movement disorders. The PDF initiated and continues to support the Brain Bank at Columbia-Presbyterian Medical Center, which collects and provides to scientists brain tissue samples from people with Parkinson's who died, supporting research efforts to find the causes of and a cure for Parkinson's. The main contact for the Parkinson's Disease Foundation is

Parkinson's Disease Foundation
William Black Medical Building
Columbia-Presbyterian Medical Center
710 West 168th Street
New York, NY 10032-9982
(800) 457-6676 or (212) 923-4700
http://www.pdf.org

See also MICHAEL J. FOX FOUNDATION FOR PARKINSON'S RESEARCH; NATIONAL PARKINSON'S DISEASE FOUNDATION; PARKINSON STUDY GROUP.

Parkinson's Disease Quality of Life Questionnaire (PDQL)

A proprietary assessment tool to measure the effect of Parkinson's disease on the person's quality of life. Designed by Dutch researchers, the PDQL consists of 37 questions that a clinician asks the person with Parkinson's disease. Questions relate to symptoms, interference of Parkinson's disease with daily activities, emotional factors, and social factors. Scoring rates the responses and gives an assessment of quality of life perceptions in key areas as well as overall. The PDQL is often used in clinical research studies to provide comparative assessments among individuals as well as within different treatment approaches.

See also BECK DEPRESSION INVENTORY; HAMILTON DEPRESSION RATING SCALE; INSTRUMENTAL ACTIVITIES OF DAILY LIVING; MINI MENTAL STATUS EXAMINATION; PARKINSON'S DISEASE QUESTIONNAIRE; SICKNESS IMPACT PROFILE; UNIFIED PARKINSON'S DISEASE RATING SCALE.

Parkinson's Disease Questionnaire (PDQ-39)

A proprietary quality of life assessment consisting of 39 health-related questions that a clinician asks of the person with Parkinson's. The PDQ-39 can also be completed as a self-assessment and scored by the clinician. Researchers commonly use the PDQ-39 as one of the assessment tools to measure changes in quality of life perceptions with medical or surgical treatments that are in CLINICAL RESEARCH TRIALS. The PDQ-39 is not commonly used in clinical practice.

See also BECK DEPRESSION INVENTORY; HAMILTON DEPRESSION RATING SCALE; INSTRUMENTAL ACTIVITIES OF DAILY LIVING; MINI MENTAL STATUS EXAMINATION; PARKINSON'S DISEASE QUALITY OF LIFE QUESTIONNAIRE; SICKNESS IMPACT PROFILE; UNIFIED PARKINSON'S DISEASE RATING SCALE.

Parkinson's Disease Sleep Scale (PDSS)

A fairly simple self-assessment of the quality of sleep. The PDSS consists of 15 questions that the person with Parkinson's rates by marking along a line that represents a continuum from worst (0) to best (10). The clinician or scorer then measures the marks and assigns values to them. The PDSS asks about movement during the night, awkward positions or difficulty in changing positions, NOCTURIA (the need to get up at night to urinate), nightmares, and other factors that interrupt sleep. It is primarily useful for physicians in trying to assess the need for nighttime ANTI-PARKINSON'S MEDICATIONS. Many people try to stagger their medications to provide the highest dosages and greatest relief of symptoms during daytime hours, but this schedule often results in an increase in symptoms at night. As well, some anti-Parkinson's medications can cause side effects such as HALLUCINATIONS that interfere with sleep. SLEEP DISTURBANCES are common in Parkinson's disease and contribute to problems such as DAYTIME SLEEPINESS as well as irritability from lack of restful sleep.

See also BEDROOM COMFORT; EPWORTH SLEEPINESS SCALE; INAPPROPRIATE SLEEP COMPOSITE SCORE (ISCS) QUESTIONNAIRE; MULTIPLE SLEEP LATENCY TEST; RESTLESS LEG SYNDROME.

Parkinson's Impact Scale (PIMS)

An assessment questionnaire to measure the effect of Parkinson's disease on QUALITY OF LIFE. The Parkinson Foundation Canada developed the PIMS in cooperation with several clinical and research centers across Canada. The questionnaire asks the person with Parkinson's to rate the effect of the disease on 10 central aspects of life on a five-point scale (0 to 4). The aspects are

- Self—positive (optimism, happiness)
- Self—negative (anxiety, depression)
- Family relationships
- Community relationships
- Work (job or home tasks)
- Travel (ability to get to desired locations)
- Leisure (activities for pleasure)
- Personal safety (ability to participate in tasks and functions without injury)
- Financial security (ability to pay bills and meet financial obligations)
- Sexuality/sexual relationship

Assessments such as the PIMS are helpful in evaluating how well treatment mitigates the limitations Parkinson's disease can impose on a person's lifestyle and enjoyment of life. The PIMS does not address physical symptoms or the direct effectiveness of the treatment regimen.

See also ACTIVITIES OF DAILY LIVING; BECK DEPRESSION INVENTORY; HAMILTON DEPRESSION RATING SCALE; INSTRUMENTAL ACTIVITIES OF DAILY LIVING; MINI MENTAL STATUS EXAMINATION; PARKINSON'S DISEASE QUALITY OF LIFE QUESTIONNAIRE; PARKINSON'S DISEASE QUESTIONNAIRE; SICKNESS IMPACT PROFILE; UNIFIED PARKINSON'S DISEASE RATING SCALE.

Parkinson's personality   The perception that the person with Parkinson's disease is lethargic, uninterested, and depressed. The term is really inaccurate, as it identifies a perception of personality based on limited outward expression, especially the lack of facial expression that often develops early in the disease and the slowed movement that appears from the outside observer's perspective to be intentional and methodical. These limitations result from the effects of Parkinson's on muscle control and movement, however, and have relation to the person's real feelings. Unless and until the Parkinson's causes COGNITIVE IMPAIRMENT, the genuine personality of the person with Parkinson's remains unchanged.

People do change their behavior and attitudes in response to major life changes, and learning that they have Parkinson's disease is certainly one of those changes. Many people who are diagnosed with Parkinson's when they are in their 50s and 60s find themselves reevaluating their priorities and interests and make changes in their lives as a result. When a person's personality seems to change dramatically, it is important to look for a reason. A change in personality is a key symptom of DEPRESSION, which affects nearly half of those who have Parkinson's at some point in the course of the disease. It also can suggest medication side effects or interactions, which should be considered if the change in personality can be linked to a change in medication.

Cognitive impairment, which occurs in about a third of people in the later stages of Parkinson's disease, does cause personality changes. The person may become volatile, with outbursts of anger or crying. Often there is DEMENTIA with HALLUCINATIONS, DELUSIONS, AGITATION, ANXIETY, PARANOIA, and even frank PSYCHOSIS. These changes typically evolve over time and correlate with worsening motor symptoms, however. MOOD SWINGS are common in mid to late stages of Parkinson's, likely as the effect of a combination of progressive degeneration in the brain and increased number and dosages of medications.

Before doctors understood the pathological mechanisms of Parkinson's disease, there was a widespread belief that people who were by nature cautious, slow, and methodical were more likely to have Parkinson's disease than people who were outgoing and risk taking; the former were said to have the "Parkinson's personality." This idea can be compared to the similarly faulty association that being outside in cold, inclement weather and "catching a chill" lead to development of pneumonia. Neither is accurate.

See also AKINESIA; BRADYKINESIA; HYPOMIMIA; NEUROPSYCHIATRY; PROGRESSIVE SUPRANUCLEAR PALSY; PSYCHOSIS; PSYCHOSOCIAL FACTORS.

Parkinson's plus syndromes   A collective designation for conditions that include Parkinson's disease or Parkinson's-like symptoms but have additional features that alter their pathological presentation and therapeutic potential. The Parkinson's plus syndromes account for the majority of misdiagnosies of Parkinson's disease, particularly in early stages of disease development when symptoms are similar. Nearly always, one of the key markers that the condition is not Parkinson's disease is the lack of symptom response to LEVODOPA therapy. The Parkinson's plus syndromes include

- CORTICOBASAL DEGENERATION (CBD), a rare disorder in which there is extensive loss of NEURONS and GLIAL CELLS in the cerebral cortex and BASAL GANGLIA, as well as widespread NEUROFIBRILLARY TANGLES. There are significant speech and articulation problems, and neuromuscular dysfunction fairly rapidly progresses to an inability to walk.

- MULTIPLE SYSTEM ATROPHY (MSA), a disorder characterized   by   progressive   motor   system (extrapyramidal, cerebellar, and pyramidal), autonomic, and cognitive dysfunctions. Neuron loss is widespread throughout the brain. Generally one of the three prototypical coexisting disorders—Shy–Drager syndrome (MSA-A, so named for the prominent autonomic nervous system dysfunction), striatonigral degeneration (MSA-P for the prominent parkinsonism), and olivopontocerebellar atrophy (MSA-C, so named for the prominent signs of cerebellar dys-

Parkinson's Plus Syndrome	Difference from Parkinson's Disease		
	SYMPTOMS	PATHOLOGY	TREATMENT
Corticobasal degeneration (CBD)	Older than age 50 First unilateral and remain markedly asymmetric Significant dysarthria and motor control problems of face Early inability to walk Myoclonus Focal rigidity and dystonia "Alien limb" in which arm or leg appears to move of its own volition Early speech alterations	Extensive loss of neurons and glial cells in cerebral cortex as well as basal ganglia Widespread tau-based neurofibrillary tangles Enlargement of surviving neurons	No response to levodopa; primarily palliative treatment
Multiple system atrophy (MSA)	Age 35 to 75 Men more than women Significant autonomic dysfunction (blood pressure, intestinal immobility, sexual dysfunction, urinary system dysfunction) Significant cerebellar ataxia Significant cognitive impairment, dementia, memory loss Progressive (most are wheelchair bound by 5 years and die by 10 years)	Widespread loss of neurons White matter demyelinization Glial inclusions Cerebellar atrophy	Response of motor symptoms to levodopa for a limited time, followed by palliative treatment
Progressive supranuclear palsy (PSP)	Impaired eye movements, vision, swallowing, breathing Personality changes Cognitive impairment	Subcortical neuron loss and atrophy Loss of neurons and glial cells in areas of brainstem Tau-based neurofibrillary tangles	No response to levodopa; primarily palliative treatment
Lewy body disease	Variable cognitive impairment Visual hallucinations Sudden onset of neuromuscular symptoms	Presence of Lewy bodies throughout brain	Frequent response of motor symptoms to levodopa but no improvement of cognitive impairment

function)—is prominent at the onset. Most frequently this is striatonigral degeneration.

- PROGRESSIVE SUPRANUCLEAR PALSY (PSP), in which symptoms first resemble those of Parkinson's disease but quickly include significant problems with eye movements, swallowing, and breathing. Neuron loss affects the structures of the cerebral subcortex including the SUBTHALAMIC NUCLEUS (STN), PALLIDUS, and SUBSTANTIA NIGRA, as well as of the BRAINSTEM including the pons and thalamus. Glial cells have a characteristic "tufted" appearance.

- LEWY BODY DISEASE, which has degeneration and symptoms that appear to be a blend of Parkinson's disease and ALZHEIMER'S DISEASE. The presence of Lewy bodies in the structures of the basal ganglia is a characteristic of Parkinson's disease; in Lewy body disease they infiltrate other parts of the brain as well, causing significant COGNITIVE IMPAIRMENT and DEMENTIA. Visual hallucinations and personality changes are earlier and more prominent symptoms in Lewy body disease as compared to Alzheimer's disease.

For a good percentage of people with Parkinson's plus syndromes, diagnosis becomes conclusive only after death, at autopsy. The Parkinson's plus syndromes are particularly frustrating for people who have them as well as physicians who try to treat them, because they are not always distinguishable from Parkinson's disease and often respond briefly or incompletely to treatment with ANTI-PARKINSON'S MEDICATIONS. As finding the right mix of medications to treat Parkinson's disease can take time, determining whether lack of response is a result of the TREATMENT ALGORITHM (determination of which medications to use and in what combinations) or of misdiagnosis becomes challenging.

See also MEDICATION MANAGEMENT; PARKINSONISM; PARKINSON'S DISEASE, CAUSES OF.

Parlodel   See BROMOCRIPTINE.

paroxetine   A medication taken to relieve symptoms of DEPRESSION, which affects nearly half of those who have Parkinson's. Paroxetine (Paxil) belongs to the class of drugs called SELECTIVE SEROTONIN REUPTAKE INHIBITOR (SSRI) MEDICATIONS. It extends the availability of SEROTONIN, a NEUROTRANSMITTER important to brain functions related to mood and emotion. Paroxetine requires about four weeks to become fully effective. Paroxetine generally does not interact with ANTI-PARKINSON'S MEDICATIONS, although it, like other SSRIs, cannot be taken simultaneously with MONOAMINE OXIDASE INHIBITOR (MAOI) OR tricyclic antidepressant medications. Caution should be used when it is taken with SELEGILINE, a selective monoamine oxidase-B inhibitor that some people with Parkinson's disease take for its NEUROPROTECTIVE EFFECTS, as there is some theoretical risk of side effects from an excess of serotonin. Common side effects include headache and TREMORS, which often end at lower dosages or over time. SEXUAL DYSFUNCTION is also common (typically decreased libido or delayed ejaculation) and may persist even with lower dose. Switching to a different drug within the SSRI classification often eliminates side effects.

See also ANXIETY; MONOAMINE OXIDASE INHIBITOR (MAOI) MEDICATIONS; MOOD SWINGS; PSYCHOTHERAPY.

patience   Parkinson's disease is frustrating for the person who has it as well as for loved ones. Everything, it seems, takes more time, which people to whom time has become precious do not want to waste. Yet it is essential to allow enough time, extended time, for what were once ordinary activities. No amount of frustration or pushing makes the situation any better for the person with Parkinson's, whether self-imposed or by others, and in fact it often makes symptoms worse. ANXIETY further disrupts the concentration and effort that motor functions, particularly fine motor movements, require as Parkinson's progresses. When the world around them is running in fast-forward, many people with Parkinson's feel that despite their best efforts, it is all they can do to stand still. Parkinson's disease changes the pace of life, yet outwardly the person with Parkinson's appears no different from the person who was once the master of multitasking.

Maintaining a realistic sense of the time required to accomplish functions such as bathing, dressing, and eating and allowing half again as much time for them are helpful. They allow the person who has Parkinson's disease to complete activities without feeling the need to rush. As much as possible, avoid imposing any sense of time limitation around activities. The person with Parkinson's cannot move any faster even when he or she desires to do so; this is the nature of the disease and the block it places between "want to do" and "can do," and it is a block that no amount of urging, pushing, or frustration can dislodge.

Flexibility, planning, and HUMOR are key when there are time factors to accommodate, as when having a doctor appointment. It is nearly impossible to start preparations too far in advance for most such events; allowing what might seem an endless amount of time is seldom a mistake. Although the INDEPENDENCE that the person with Parkinson's insists on may at times appear to be stubbornness, independence is essential to the person's ability to maintain as much function as possible. Completing a task quickly is much less important than simply completing it. Loved ones and caregivers often can be most helpful by "running interference" to protect the person with Parkinson's from distractions and interruptions, establishing a cooperative and collaborative process.

See also ACTIVITIES OF DAILY LIVING; ADAPTIVE EQUIPMENT AND ASSIST DEVICES; ADJUSTING TO LIVING WITH PARKINSON'S; CAREGIVER WELL-BEING; COMPASSION; EMOTIONS; EMPATHY; TASK SIMPLIFICATION.

patterned movement Movement that has the appearance of a sequence of individual events but that the brain processes as a single but collective event. Clusters of NEURONS receive simultaneous signals from the BASAL GANGLIA, which they then pass on to clusters of neurons in the motor cortex. Because patterns are faster and easier to learn and to repeat than individual events, the brain can initiate and control movement with great efficiency. Patterned movements make use of the EXTRAPYRAMIDAL SYSTEM, which includes brain structures such as the basal ganglia and area of the BRAINSTEM and nerve pathways that control movement. Any damage to the extrapyramidal system affects the body's ability to carry out patterned movements. The cerebellum, the brain's coordination center, also is critical for patterned movements. Most movements of the lower extremities, such as walking, are patterned movements.

Scientists believe that the brain "maps" certain neuron clusters for specific patterns. These same clusters always handle the same patterns. When the brain learns new patterns, such as when a person takes up a new physical activity, the brain shifts its mapping to include additional clusters to handle related patterns. People who use muscle groups in specialized and refined ways such as athletes, musicians, and dancers refer to this as "muscle memory"—the muscle groups involved function as though they automatically engage in the movements of, for example, a diving position or a complex musical scale. The movements remain voluntary, of course, but occur with such efficiency that they appear to require no conscious thought.

The brain appears to have a broad ability to learn new patterned movements and a more limited context for reassigning previously learned ones. Relearning typically becomes necessary when areas of the brain become damaged. Part of the neuron cluster may remain functional but cannot handle the entire task, or there are not enough healthy specialized neurons, such as those that direct movement, available to accept large patterns (like walking). In Parkinson's disease, the damage is dynamic, ever extending as the disease process progresses. Patterned movements such as those of walking are incredibly complex despite the efficiency of clustering their multitude of sequential and simultaneous actions and reactions. All neurons in the cluster must carry out their assignments to allow the pattern to be executed properly. As neurons within pattern zones die, pieces of the pattern fall out. Signals become chaotic and confused, movements disrupted.

Understanding of patterned movements has led to successful rehabilitative strategies for brain dysfunction in which the damage is fixed, such as after injury due to trauma or stroke, or in conditions such as cerebral palsy. The extent to which disturbance of patterned movements matters in Parkinson's disease is unclear, however, as the more significant factor is the progressive loss of DOPAMIN-ERGIC NEURONS. The loss thwarts any attempts the brain may make to remap neuron clusters.

See also GAIT; GAIT DISTURBANCE; POSTURAL INSTABILITY; PROPRIOCEPTION; PYRAMIDAL PATHWAY.

penjet system   A needleless method for injecting APOMORPHINE, a potent DOPAMINE AGONIST MEDICATION used as a RESCUE DRUG for PARKINSON'S CRISIS. The penjet system delivers a premeasured amount of medication, which is injected into the subcutaneous tissue in the abdomen, thigh, or upper arm, where the body rapidly absorbs it. The penjet contains a small cylinder of pressurized nitrogen, an inert gas that, when released, propels the drug through the skin and into the subcutaneous tissue. This delivery allows the caregiver to administer the rescue drug. The penjet with apomorphine requires a doctor's prescription.

See also ANTI-PARKINSON'S MEDICATIONS.

pergolide   A DOPAMINE AGONIST MEDICATION that binds selectively with D1 and D2 DOPAMINE RECEPTORS in the SUBSTANTIA NIGRA and the NIGROSTRIATAL FIBERS (areas of the brain integral to movement) to simulate DOPAMINE action. Pergolide is commonly taken as either one of the ADJUNCT THERAPIES employed to enhance the effectiveness of LEVOPODA; or as MONOTHERAPY in early Parkinson's disease when symptoms are minor to moderate. Because it is an ERGOT-DERIVED MEDICATION, it has an effect on blood vessels as well. Although the most common consequence of its use is ORTHOSTATIC HYPOTENSION (a drop in blood pressure with a change in position), a sudden surge in blood pressure also can occur. Other side effects include daytime somnolence, hallucinations, headache, nausea, and changes in personality or mood. Unlike other agonists, pergolide's ergot derivation also puts it at risk of causing scarring (fibrosis) of the lungs, the covering of the heart, or the so-called retroperitoneal tissues and organs in the back of the abdomen. Pergolide usually is titrated to a therapeutic dosage to minimize side effects, and the person takes increasingly larger dosages over several weeks. It should be discontinued in similar fashion, in decreasing dosages over several

weeks. Women who are pregnant or trying to become pregnant should not take pergolide or other ergot alkaloids, as ergot affects reproductive hormones.

See also ANTI-PARKINSON'S MEDICATIONS; MEDICATION MANAGEMENT; MEDICATION SIDE EFFECTS; PREGNANCY; TREATMENT ALGORITHM.

peripheral neuropathy   Injury or damage to the nerves that supply body organs and structures including the muscles that results in tingling, numbness, pain, or loss of sensory perception and sometimes motor function. Peripheral neuropathy can occur in people with Parkinson's disease, but it is not a symptom of, or caused by, the Parkinson's, which affects the body's neuromotor system within the brain rather than the peripheral sensory motor nerves.

One of the most common forms of peripheral neuropathy is carpal tunnel syndrome, in which the nerves that serve the hand become compressed in the structures of the wrist. Peripheral neuropathy involving the toes and feet in particular, and sometimes the fingers and hands, is common with diabetes, a disease of metabolism in which fluctuations in blood sugar levels damage the tiny blood vessels that supply peripheral nerves. Pain as well as circulatory problems result.

Neurodegenerative diseases in which damage to central neuronal pathways that is similar to the peripheral nerve damage that occurs in peripheral neuropathy, leading to sometimes similar symptoms, include AMYOTROPHIC LATERAL SCLEROSIS (ALS) and MULTIPLE SCLEROSIS (MS), conditions in which the protective myelin sheathing that surrounds the AXONS of NEURONS is destroyed. This destruction causes neuromuscular dysfunctions as well as pain. Pain present with what appear to be symptoms of Parkinson's disease, is usually an indication that the condition is one other than Parkinson's.

See also CONDITIONS SIMILAR TO PARKINSON'S; NERVOUS SYSTEM; PAIN MANAGEMENT.

peristalsis   The rhythmic or wavelike contractions of the smooth muscle tissues in the digestive system. Peristalsis begins in the esophagus as food is swallowed and continues through the intestinal tract, culminating in defecation (bowel movement). Peristaltic movements differ in the various parts of the digestive system. In the esophagus they are strong, frequent waves that forcefully push food into the stomach. Esophageal peristalsis is so forceful, in fact, that it can push food into the stomach against the force of gravity. The walls of the stomach contract in different directions simultaneously to provide a churning action that mixes food with the stomach acids that begin the digestive process.

In the small intestine, peristalsis changes to more of a back-and-forth agitation, somewhat like the motion of a washing machine, that further "mashes" food with digestive enzymes and also moves the mixture, called a bolus, through the 20 to 22 feet of small intestine where the majority of digestion takes place. Contractions occur every few seconds to minutes, depending on the intestinal contents. When the bolus reaches the large intestine it has become compact, and there is less of it to move. Peristalsis slows to a contraction every 20 to 30 minutes, inching the bolus through the six or so feet of large intestine to the rectum, where, when the rectum fills, a final strong contraction expels the fecal matter through the anus.

Parkinson's disease slows peristalsis somewhat, as the involvement of motor function structures in the brain has an effect on certain smooth muscle action. ANTI-PARKINSON'S MEDICATIONS, particularly anticholinergic medications taken to relieve TREMORS, further slow peristalsis. These medications act on smooth muscle fibers in the digestive and urinary systems, slowing them significantly. A number of medical conditions, including diabetes, also adversely affect peristalsis. Slowed peristalsis has several adverse effects for the person with Parkinson's:

- It slows GASTRIC MOTILITY, the rate at which food leaves the stomach. This slowing influences the effectiveness of LEVODOPA, which must be absorbed through the small intestine. The longer the levodopa remains in the stomach, the less of it is available for absorption. This is particularly a concern later in the course of the disease when levodopa EFFICACY becomes critical.

- It decreases appetite, as food remains in the digestive system longer. This causes the person to eat less or to eat less frequently; nutritional deficiencies may result.

- It interferes with digestion and the absorption of nutrients, further contributing to nutritional deficiencies.

- It causes CONSTIPATION, an accumulation of unexpelled fecal matter, which is uncomfortable at the least and can result in intestinal blockages that require medical intervention.

Eating enough foods that are high in fiber (fresh fruits and vegetables, whole grains and whole grain products) and drinking plenty of water are the two most effective ways to maintain optimal intestinal function. Sometimes it is necessary to adjust medication dosages, particularly of anticholinergics that directly affect intestinal function. Regular physical activity, especially walking, also helps to keep the digestive tract as active as possible. Many of the medications to combat slowed peristalsis, including metoclopramide (Reglan) and cisapride (Propulsid), are apt to worsen the motor symptoms of Parkinson's.

See also ADJUSTING TO LIVING WITH PARKINSON'S; EATING; EXERCISE AND ACTIVITY; FOODS TO AVOID; FOODS TO EAT; NUTRITION AND DIET.

Permax   See PERGOLIDE.

perphenazine   A medication prescribed to treat either PSYCHOSIS or NAUSEA. Perphenazine (Trilafon) is a DOPAMINE ANTAGONIST. It nonselectively blocks DOPAMINE RECEPTORS throughout the BRAIN including the BASAL GANGLIA, where this effect counteracts LEVODOPA and dopamine agonists in people who are taking it for Parkinson's disease and can cause a PARKINSON'S CRISIS (sudden and severe worsening of motor symptoms). It also has strong anticholinergic actions, which give it its effectiveness in mitigating nausea. Perphenazine is an old drug, on the market since the late 1950s. There are many newer medications to treat either PSYCHOSIS or NAUSEA that do so without the high risk of extrapyramidal consequences. The person with Parkinson's disease should not use perphenazine. Perphenazine cannot be taken with LEVODOPA or DOPAMINE AGONIST MEDICATIONS such as BROMOCRIPTINE, PRAMIPEXOLE, ROPINEROLE, OR PERGOLIDE.

See also ALTERNATIVE THERAPIES; ANTICHOLINERGIC MEDICATIONS; ANTI-PARKINSON'S MEDICATIONS; ANTIPSYCHOTIC MEDICATIONS; GINGER AS A TREATMENT FOR NAUSEA; MEDICATION MANAGEMENT; MEDICATION SIDE EFFECTS; TREATMENT ALGORITHM.

personal care assistance   Help with tasks and activities related to personal care such as bathing, dressing, and feeding. Under certain circumstances, MEDICARE (on a temporary basis only) and some MEDICAID programs pay for a personal care assistant in the home. Such an assistant should be affiliated with an organization that provides personal care and other services, such as HOME HEALTH CARE or HOSPICE. Some states require that such service providers be certified or registered; many do not. It is important to obtain and verify references and other relevant credentials when hiring a personal assistance agency or individual. Personal care assistance can help the person with Parkinson's retain INDEPENDENCE and can provide relief for caregivers.

See also ADJUSTING TO LIVING WITH PARKINSON'S; BATHING AND BATHROOM ORGANIZATION; COPING WITH ONGOING CARE OF PARKINSON'S; LONG-TERM CARE; QUALITY OF LIFE.

pesticides and herbicides   Numerous research studies in the late 1990s established a connection between a higher rate of Parkinson's disease and long-term exposure to common poisons used to kill pests (pesticides) and weeds (herbicides). Key support for this connection includes an unusually high rate of Parkinson's disease among people who live in farm communities where pesticide and herbicide use is frequent. People who often use home pesticides and herbicides, such as for gardening and lawn care, also have higher rates of Parkinson's disease. As well, autopsy evidence consistently demonstrates that people who have Parkinson's when they die have higher levels of chemicals found in pesticides and herbicides in their brain than people who do not have Parkinson's.

What this connection means as far as proving that they might cause Parkinson's remains uncertain. Researchers know that there are close chemical similarities between many pesticides and herbicides and the illicit narcotic contaminant (from amateurish attempts to synthesize the synthetic narcotic pethidine) 1-METHYL-4-PHENYL-1,2,3,6-TETRAHYDROPYRIDINE (MPTP) that is used in the laboratory to create a Parkinson's model in research animals. Yet far more people who live in farming communities with ostensibly the same exposure to pesticides and herbicides do not have Parkinson's than do. Limiting exposure to these substances is prudent, regardless of the connection to Parkinson's disease, as they are known NEUROTOXINS that can produce a wide range of damage to the brain and nervous system.

See also CHEMICAL TOXINS; ENDOTOXIN; ENVIRONMENTAL TRIGGERS; EXOTOXIN; PARKINSON'S DISEASE, CAUSES OF.

pharmacotherapy   The use of medications to treat the symptoms of disease. The primary therapeutic approach for Parkinson's disease is pharmacotherapy, with LEVODOPA and dopamine agonists as its mainstays. Pharmacotherapy involves managing multiple medications to relieve specific symptoms, as well as monitoring drug interactions, side effects, and complications. MEDICATION MANAGEMENT of the person with Parkinson's can become complex as the disease progresses, as many of the ANTI-PARKINSON'S MEDICATIONS interact with each other or with other medications the person may be taking, for example, to treat hypertension, diabetes, heart disease, and other health conditions common in the age group in which Parkinson's is most prevalent.

See also ADRENERGIC MEDICATIONS; ANTIANXIETY MEDICATIONS; ANTICHOLINERGIC MEDICATIONS; ANTIDEPRESSANT MEDICATIONS; ANTIHISTAMINE MEDICATIONS; CATECHOL-*O*-METHYLTRANSFERASE (COMT) INHIBITOR MEDICATIONS; DOPAMINE AGONIST MEDICATIONS; DOPAMINE PRECURSOR MEDICATIONS; ERGOT-DERIVED MEDICATIONS; MEDICATION SIDE EFFECTS; PAIN RELIEF MEDICATIONS; SLEEP MEDICATIONS; TREATMENT ALGORITHM.

phonation See SPEECH.

physical therapy A specialty of health care that focuses on improving and restoring physical function after injury or disease. Physical therapy employs various modalities; those that seem to be most effective for people with Parkinson's are prescribed exercises and activities to maintain muscle tone and strength, joint flexibility and range of motion, and functions of mobility such as balance, posture, and walking. Physical therapy often integrates with OCCUPATIONAL THERAPY, which focuses on improving ability for ACTIVITIES OF DAILY LIVING (ADLs) environmental safety issues, and adapting to the slowing of movements, visual processing, and thinking processes that often accompanies Parkinson's.

In the United States, there are two levels of physical therapy practitioners, the certified physical therapy assistant (CPTA) and the registered physical therapist (PTR). The CPTA is a technical practitioner who completes an accredited two-year program and passes a national certification examination. A physical therapist completes an accredited four-year undergraduate program and passes a national certification examination to earn the professional designation of physical therapist, registered. There are also postgraduate programs in physical therapy that award master's or doctorate degrees following additional study. All states require both levels of practitioner to be licensed and to complete continuing education courses to remain current in practice standards.

Physical therapy services require a physician's referral or prescription that specifies the kinds of services the person needs. The physical therapist completes an assessment of the person's status and can make other recommendations, which the physician must approve. Physical therapy is often provided on an inpatient basis for people who are hospitalized, but is more often an outpatient service. Private MEDICAL INSURANCE, MEDICARE, and MEDICAID programs typically provide benefits for physical therapy services.

See also ALTERNATIVE THERAPIES; GAIT; GAIT DISTURBANCE; MUSCLE STRENGTH; MUSCLE TONE; PATTERNED MOVEMENTS.

pills See MEDICATION MANAGEMENT.

pill-rolling movements The manifestation of resting TREMORS characteristic of PARKINSON'S DISEASE in which the fingers (usually forefinger and thumb) rub together as though rolling a pill between them, with an accompanying slight wrist flexion and extension (up and down movement). Often this is one of the earliest symptoms of Parkinson's and the person is unaware that it is present. The movements (at least in the early stages) often stop when the person notices them or takes another action such as reaching for an object. When measured with an ELECTROMYOGRAM (EMG) or an accelerometer (a device that measures the changes in speed and direction of movement), the tremor has a slow cycle of four to six hertz. This helps to differentiate it from ESSENTIAL TREMOR, which is more rapid and usually does not involve the pill-rolling movements so much as rhythmic trembling sorts of movement, although at this stage differential diagnosis can be difficult. Pill-rolling movements can be the only symptom of Parkinson's disease for quite some time, up to years. When this is the case, the person usually does not need ANTI-PARKINSON'S MEDICATIONS or can control the tremor, if desired, with drugs such as ANTICHOLINERGIC MEDICATIONS.

See also DIAGNOSING PARKINSON'S; MEDICAL MANAGEMENT; MEDICATION MANAGEMENT; TREATMENT ALGORITHM.

placebo A therapeutically inert substance given to see whether it results in changes in symptoms. Placebo use is most common in CLINICAL RESEARCH STUDIES, most often those testing INVESTIGATIONAL NEW DRUGS. Placebo controls, as this approach is called, allow researchers to measure and quantify responses and present them as comparable comparisons when objective measurement is difficult. If, for example, 5 percent of those who take an investigational new drug report that muscle aches diminish but 5 percent of those who take the placebo make the same report, the effectiveness of the investigational new drug is questionable. If, however, 30 percent of those taking the drug being tested make such a report compared to 5 percent taking the placebo, and the investigational group has been well designed (for example, is large enough), the difference is statistically significant and becomes a factor supporting the investigational new drug's effectiveness.

The ethical issue for researchers, and a critical health issue for research study participants, in PLACEBO-controlled research studies is to make sure that administration of the placebo does not jeopardize the person's health or well-being because in general it is unethical to withhold treatment with an effective substance for a significant amount of time. A person considering participation in a clinical research trial should make sure to understand fully whether placebo controls are being used and what this means in terms of other possible treatment options.

Some controversial trials of surgical methods have involved placebo surgery in which the surgeon makes a small incision in the skin and gives the appearance of conducting surgery but does not. The ethical issue here is that the placebo surgery is nonetheless invasive even though it has no therapeutic effect and exposes the person to the risk, however slight, of infection, bleeding, and other complications.

There is a phenomenon called the placebo effect in which the person's belief that a substance is providing relief causes him or her to perceive that relief occurs. Even the symptoms of Parkinson's disease are at least in the short term somewhat amenable to this effect as they are often susceptible to subconscious control.

See also BIOETHICS; CLINICAL PHARMACOLOGY TRIALS; INFORMED CONSENT.

planning for the future　The first reaction many people have when they learn they have Parkinson's disease is the feeling that their future has been taken away. Indeed, the future has been altered. But most people will enjoy years and even decades of near-normal function and activities. Honest and candid discussions and assessments of plans and life circumstances can help make those years as pleasant as possible.

On a pragmatic level, it is essential to evaluate financial circumstances and stability early after diagnosis, because as Parkinson's progresses they will become increasingly important. The person who is employed at the time of diagnosis should consider factors such as MEDICAL INSURANCE, life insurance, disability insurance, long-term care insurance, and pension or retirement funds. The person who is retired should consider the limitations of his or her fixed income in the context of increasing medical expenses and begin planning to accommodate these shifts. Planning may necessitate consulting an attorney who specializes in elder law to assess matters such as MEDICAID spend down. Even though this may seem a long way off, the course of Parkinson's is unpredictable and can veer drastically without warning. Only careful strategic planning can protect financial resources.

On the medical front, it is important to consider the kinds of treatments the person may desire, and where he or she wants to draw the line. The mainstay of treatment is currently LEVODOPA therapy, with ADJUNCT THERAPIES incorporating other medications as necessary. But there is much research under way, and there are many opportunities to participate in clinical testing for new drugs and methods. Surgical options such as DEEP BRAIN STIMULATION (DBS) and experimental cell replacement techniques are also gaining renewed interest as technology allows greater refinement of results. Although the person with Parkinson's cannot fully evaluate these options until they become viable for his or her circumstances, it is important to learn as much as possible about Parkinson's disease, current treatments, potential treatments, and ongoing research and to remain informed.

Planning for the future also should include an evaluation of what is important to the person with Parkinson's and to his or her loved ones. Many people reevaluate plans such as retirement and travel and engage in those activities sooner rather than later. Other people prefer not to make fundamental changes in such plans, especially those who are close to fulfilling them, but to continue working toward them with the resolve to follow them through. Factors such as other health problems affecting the person with Parkinson's or a spouse or partner may further shape choices and decisions.

See also ADJUSTING TO LIVING WITH PARKINSON'S; ADVANCE DIRECTIVES; ESTATE PLANNING; FINANCIAL

PLANNING; MEDICAL MANAGEMENT; MEDICATION MANAGEMENT; TREATMENT ALGORITHM.

pneumonia Irritation and inflammation of the lungs. There are many causes of pneumonia; the most common and the most dangerous is infection. The cause of the infection can be bacterial or viral. Antibiotics can treat bacterial pneumonia, but the only treatments for viral pneumonia are preventive (vaccination) and supportive to relieve symptoms such as tissue swelling and fluid accumulation. Pneumonia is a leading cause of hospitalization, debilitation, and death of people older than age 65 and is a frequent complication of viral influenza infections. In combination, influenza/ pneumonia is the seventh leading cause of death in the United States.

People with limited mobility are at particular risk for pneumonia, as allows shallow physical inactivity breathing and enables infective agents (bacterial or viral) to collect in the airways. In the person with Parkinson's aspiration pneumonia is a significant risk as well; it can be damaging itself as well as set the stage for bacterial infection. Aspiration pneumonia develops when swallowing difficulties allow food or fluids to enter the trachea instead of continuing down the esophagus. This process allows bacteria that are normally present in the mouth to enter the lungs, causing an infection.

Health experts recommend influenza vaccinations (flu shots) and pneumonia vaccinations for people such as those with Parkinson's disease who are at high risk for these infections. A medication taken to prevent or minimize the course of influenza A, AMANTADINE, also has dopamine agonist actions. People who are taking amantadine receive some protection against influenza A but should still receive annual vaccinations for both influenza and pneumonia unless there are medical reasons for them not to have them.

In Parkinson's, the actions of the chest muscles and diaphragm become limited, as do those of other voluntary muscles. Shallow breathing that does not fully expand the lungs results. Regular physical activity such as walking, and even just sitting upright in a chair as opposed to lying in bed, helps the lungs to clear debris and mucus to keep infection at bay. Breathing exercises further help to expand the lungs. When late stage Parkinson's disease immobilizes a person, frequent position changes, including sitting if possible, help to prevent infective agents from settling in the lungs, but the risk of pneumonia is very high at this stage.

See also BREATH CONTROL; HEIMLICH MANEUVER.

position changes Frequent moving to minimize the pressure a position imposes on body structures. Position changes are especially important for people whose symptoms confine them to wheelchairs or to bed. At a minimum, a person should change position every two hours during waking hours and should not remain in the same position more than four hours even at night. Most people even when sleeping change position frequently; position changes become challenging for the person with Parkinson's, who may fidget and have trouble falling asleep and then remain in the same relative position much of the night. Skin that is in contact, under pressure, with a surface for a prolonged period is vulnerable to tissue tenderness and breakdown.

People with Parkinson's tend to maintain one position for extended periods often because moving requires too much effort or they cannot move independently. Standing to stretch, or at least stretching out the arms and legs, for a few minutes every hour during waking hours is good for the muscles; relieves pressure, even if slightly, on contact points; and helps maintain alertness. Engaging in movement such as walking is even better. When changing positions becomes a problem because of Parkinson's disease's physical limitations, creativity is often required to create the support the person needs.

See also ACTIVITIES OF DAILY LIVING; BEDSORES.

positive outlook The ability to see the good aspects of a situation and to look to the future with hope and OPTIMISM. Countless studies demonstrate that people who have a positive outlook do better and enjoy a better QUALITY OF LIFE when dealing with chronic or serious illness. There are many aspects of Parkinson's disease that are beyond control, but there are equally numerous opportunities to make the best of matters. Many people live with Parkinson's for decades, and to allow its limitations to shape life is to allow the disease to take control.

- Stay active and engaged in life. Busy people do not have time to worry or dwell on the "what ifs" and other uncertainties of Parkinson's.
- Enjoy favorite events for as long as possible. Go to the movies or the theater, work in the garden, take grandchildren to the park.
- Learn as much as possible about Parkinson's disease. Find a good physician who understands the disease's subtleties and takes interest in personalizing treatment approaches to meet individual needs.
- Allow the challenges of Parkinson's to draw family members and friends closer rather than to push them away. People who care want to help—let them.
- Maintain the best health possible. Eat nutritiously, exercise regularly, meditate.

See also ADJUSTING TO LIVING WITH PARKINSON'S; DENIAL AND ACCEPTANCE; FRIENDSHIPS; HOPE FOR A PARKINSON'S CURE; JOY.

positron emission tomography   (PET) A sophisticated functional imaging study that uses radioactive "tags" in combination with COMPUTED TOMOGRAPHY to create three-dimensional pictures of internal organs and structures. For a PET scan, the person receives an injection of a solution containing radioactive isotopes—small particles that the tissues to be studied will "uptake" or absorb more than the surrounding tissues will. In most studies in people with Parkinson's, a radioactively labeled form of dopamine, called fluorodopa, is used. They highlight the tissues that absorb them, making those tissues detectable by radiation detectors. An array of detectors provides data that a computer assembles into two- or three-dimensional pictures.

PET allows doctors to visualize structures deep inside the BRAIN such as the BASAL GANGLIA and BRAINSTEM and provides as much information about what it does not show as about what it does. Problems such as lesions (tumors) or damage due to stroke show up on a PET scan. This capacity helps to diagnose conditions other than Parkinson's. The absence of cells and tissue that should be present also becomes apparent with PET scanning. Doctors often can identify areas of atrophy (tissue loss) in the SUBSTANTIA NIGRA where DOPAMINERGIC NEURONS have died, for example, in middle to late stages of Parkinson's. Although this does not constitute a conclusive diagnosis of Parkinson's, it can help doctors mark the progression of the disease and make some treatment choices. Atrophy is also apparent in other NEURODEGENERATIVE conditions such as CREUTZFELDT-JAKOB DISEASE (CJD).

The equipment necessary to conduct PET scanning is very sophisticated and very expensive, including a device called a cyclotron to prepare the radioactive isotopes, which typically must be used within minutes of their creation. Typically only major research centers have the necessary equipment and personnel to do PET scans. Some large hospitals have the less costly SINGLE PHOTON EMISSION COMPUTED TOMOGRAPHY (SPECT), which provides somewhat less precise but similar imaging.

See also COMPUTED TOMOGRAPHY (CT) SCAN; MAGNETIC RESONANCE IMAGING.

postencephalitic parkinsonism (PEP)   See PARKINSONISM.

postural instability An inability to make adjustments in body position to maintain BALANCE, EQUILIBRIUM, and appropriate momentum during MOVEMENT. Postural instability develops in Parkinson's disease as a convergence of several factors: progressively degenerative motor function that inhibits appropriate response, disruption of the body's POSTURAL RIGHTING REFLEXES, disturbances of the body's PROPRIOCEPTION (orientation to spatial location) mechanisms, and postural changes such as stooping, reduced ARM SWING, and shortened LEG STRIDE. Postural instability generates numerous GAIT DISTURBANCES as the body attempts to use other means to return itself to stability.

A common test for postural instability is to push the person when he or she is standing (with due caution for the person's safety to prevent falling). The person with Parkinson's often takes several steps in the direction in which he or she is pushed before being able to recover. Stepping forward is called PULSION; stepping backward is RETROPULSION. A person with normal extrapyramidal function may take one short step in the direction of the push. Making turns by taking multiple small steps rather than pivoting on the ball of the foot is a mechanism of attempted compensation for postural instability. Postural instability usually improves with ANTI-PARKINSON'S MEDICATIONS, especially levodopa, but it can be very resistant to treatment in Parkinson's disease, accounting for a significant number of falls.

See also EXTRAPYRAMIDAL SYSTEM; MUSCLE STRENGTH; MUSCLE TONE; POSTURE, STOOPING; WALKING.

postural righting reflex The body's automatic responses to adjust BALANCE and maintain EQUILIBRIUM. This reflex depends upon inputs from the vestibular system (inner ears), cerebellum, sensory system (proprioception), and even vision. It is fundamental to the ability to sit, stand, and walk or engage in any movement of mobility. In Parkinson's disease, failure of the postural righting reflex results from the loss of DOPAMINERGIC NEURONS and NIGROSTRIATAL FIBERS that reduces the availability of DOPAMINE. Motor areas of the brain can no longer function, creating breaches in the reflex pathways. It is possible to train other parts of the brain to take over the functions of the postural righting reflex, and during the early and mid stages of Parkinson's the person often can overcome postural righting reflex inadequacies through conscious reaction and response. However, the progressive deterioration of Parkinson's makes this a difficult and ultimately unsuccessful challenge by the disease's later stages.

See also BODY SCHEME; GAIT; GAIT DISTURBANCE; POSTURAL INSTABILITY; PROPRIOCEPTION; WALKING.

posture, stooping A characteristic symptom of Parkinson's disease marked by forward-sloping shoulders and limited upper body movement during walking. Stooped posture is one of the earliest symptoms of Parkinson's but often is not linked with Parkinson's until other symptoms begin to emerge. In older people stooping sometimes is dismissed as a postural change reflecting aging. As Parkinson's progresses the forward inclination of the upper body advances. It develops as a consequence of RIGIDITY, or changes in MUSCLE TONE that cause the muscle fibers to shorten and the muscles to resist movement. This rigidity holds the muscles in tense, somewhat contracted postures. It can cause discomfort, interferes with BALANCE and the POSTURAL RIGHTING REFLEX, and restricts breathing as it limits movement of the chest muscles and diaphragm. The same process causes the arms to bend and the hands to adopt clawlike positioning. Although stretching exercises can help to relieve some of the rigidity, it and the postures it causes are involuntary. ANTI-PARKINSON'S MEDICATIONS relieve stooped posture as they relieve other motor symptoms.

One easy exercise nearly everyone with Parkinson's disease can do is to stand with hands on the hips. This position inherently straightens the spine, stretching the muscles of the back and the chest. Raising the hands simultaneously and extending them upward over the head also help to stretch muscles. This action relieves discomforts that often arise from the unnatural positions the body tends to take, and it maintains flexibility and RANGE OF MOTION.

See also DYSKINESIA; DYSTONIA; EXERCISE AND ACTIVITY; GAIT; GAIT DISTURBANCES; MICROGRAPHIA; OCCUPATIONAL THERAPY; PHYSICAL THERAPY.

power of attorney See ADVANCE DIRECTIVES.

pramipexole A DOPAMINE AGONIST MEDICATION taken as MONOTHERAPY in early Parkinson's or as one of the ADJUNCT THERAPIES in middle to late stages of the disease. Pramipexole (Mirapex) has shown promise in postponing the need to start LEVODOPA therapy when symptoms are mild, thus, some neurologists believe, extending the therapeutic options available to people with Parkinson's. A nonergot dopamine agonist, pramipexole is selective for D2 and D3 DOPAMINE RECEPTORS and causes fewer significant side effects, such as DYSTONIA, than ERGOT-DERIVED MEDICATIONS such as BROMOCRIPTINE (Parlodel) or pergolide (Permax) that bind unselectively. Pramipexole does carry a dose-related risk of daytime somnolence, and sudden sleep attacks that come without warning have been reported in some people who take the medication. Pramipexole is a bit longer lived in the bloodstream than ropinerole, though still shorter lived than pergolide, and it joins ropinerole in having some evidence that it may be neuroprotective, delaying the progression of dopaminergic neuronal loss in Parkinson's. Pramipexole can cause NAUSEA, DIZZINESS, and HALLUCINATIONS, but these side effects occur infrequently.

See also ANTI-PARKINSON'S MEDICATIONS; DOPAMINE PRECURSOR; PERGOLIDE; ROPINEROLE.

preclinical Parkinson's disease   The start of the process of an accelerated or excessive loss of DOPAMINERGIC NEURONS from the SUBSTANTIA NIGRA that does not yet manifest symptoms of Parkinson's disease. Advanced functional imaging studies such as POSITRON EMISSION TOMOGRAPHY (PET) and SINGLE PHOTON EMISSION COMPUTED TOMOGRAPHY (SPECT), used primarily in research settings at the present time, can detect radioactive markers that allow neurologists to view such degenerative processes in the BRAIN before they become severe enough to cause symptoms. As there are as yet no NEUROPROTECTIVE THERAPIES or other therapeutic interventions that can slow or stop the dopaminergic neuron loss, interest in diagnosing preclinical Parkinson's disease also remains primarily academic. For the person with preclinical Parkinson's, currently there is little value in knowing of the disease's imminent manifestation.

For researchers, knowing when the degeneration begins and when symptoms start may provide valuable insights into the way the disease develops. This is important in understanding its causes and working toward more effective treatments, including prevention. Monitoring changes in the brain over time can help scientists to calculate the rate of deterioration and determine whether it is linear or variable. However, at present such monitoring relies on retrospective analysis as to date scientists have not been able to pinpoint the precise start of the deterioration; it must already be under way for the imaging techniques to detect it. As well, there are so many variations in the clinical progression of Parkinson's disease after symptoms are manifested

that the course of the disease cannot be predicted from one individual to the next.

See also CLINICAL RESEARCH STUDIES; DIAGNOSING PARKINSON'S; NEUROPROTECTIVE EFFECT; NEUROTROPHIC FACTORS; PARKINSON'S DISEASE, CAUSES OF.

precursor   A substance that, via chemical reactions, develops into a different substance. LEVODOPA is a precursor for DOPAMINE; ENZYMES facilitate a series of metabolic reactions that create the new chemical structure that is molecularly close to the precursor's molecular structure. Similarly dopamine is a precursor for another NEUROTRANSMITTER, NOREPINEPHRINE, which is a precursor for EPINEPHRINE. All such conversions require interaction with other substances, however, which often are enzymes (protein-based structures), as this conversion is a key role of enzymes in the body.

A precursor also can be a circumstance or condition that subsequently becomes a disease. Insulin resistance from obesity is a precursor for type 2 diabetes, for example. A genetic defect such as a mutation in the ALPHA-SYNUCLEIN GENE may be a precursor for Parkinson's disease, if there are events that occur to activate the gene's defective functions and cause development of Parkinson's.

See also ANTI-PARKINSON'S MEDICATIONS; DOPAMINE PRECURSOR; DOPAMINE RECEPTOR; GENE MUTATION.

pregnancy   There is very little data available on pregnancy in people with Parkinson's disease. Women with EARLY-ONSET PARKINSON'S who are of childbearing age do appear to have some risk of their Parkinson's symptoms worsening during pregnancy, but they require no special care or precautions, and there do not appear to be any particular risks for the fetus. The safety of ANTI-PARKINSON'S MEDICATIONS in pregnancy is largely unknown: there are case reports (totaling 15 pregnancies in 12 patients) of uniformly no adverse effects on the unborn baby of SINEMET, but there have been no reports of pregnancy's on the nonergot-derived agonists. Amantadine might be associated with first-trimester obstetric complications including spontaneous abortion. A woman who is pregnant or attempting to become pregnant should not take ERGOT-DERIVED MEDICATIONS such as the dopamine agonists BROMOCRIPTINE (Parlodel) and PERGOLIDE (Permax), as these drugs influence the body's production of prolactin, a HORMONE related to fertility and lactation, though the only report of a pregnancy on bromocriptine in the literature had no maternal or fetal complications. It is recommended that women who have Parkinson's disease forgo breast-feeding, partly because some anti-Parkinson's medications are expressed in breast milk and partly because the added fatigue factor tends to exacerbate Parkinson's symptoms. Nonergot dopamine agonists have less effect on prolactin but still influence its production and thereby can cause reduced milk production.

See also MEDICATION MANAGEMENT; MEDICATION SIDE EFFECTS.

prescription assistance programs   Programs that drug manufacturers sponsor to provide low-cost or free prescription medications to people who cannot afford to buy the medications they need. Most of these programs target seniors (people older than age 60 or 65), who often have only MEDICARE or MEDICAID to cover the expenses of medical care. They require the person to complete an application form and submit it along with a statement from the person's physician that attests to the person's need for the medication. Doctors know of the various programs that are available and usually offer them to people they know are in need. Doctors also typically have samples of medications that they often give to people who are trying a new drug. No one should be without medication needed to treat Parkinson's disease; assistance with drug costs is usually available in some form.

Many state health programs also have prescription assistance programs that are available to people whose income falls within a certain relation to the federal poverty level, such as 120 percent (the person is allowed to earn 120 percent of the federal poverty level and still qualify for the program). As of 2004, Medicare did not cover prescription medications and most state Medicaid programs at best offered coverage for those drugs on their formularies (lists of drugs for which Medicaid will pay).

ANTI-PARKINSON'S MEDICATIONS may cost several thousand dollars a year—a significant expense for most people.

The National Council on the Aging (NCOA) sponsors an Internet-based program called BenefitsCheckUpRx, at the website www.BenefitsCheckUp.org, that is designed to help people find low-cost or free prescription drugs. Prescription assistance programs usually provide limited medications; programs have different requirements and services.

See also MEDICAL INSURANCE; MEDICATION MANAGEMENT.

primary care physician   A doctor who provides general medical care for adults. Most primary care physicians in the United States are M.D.'s (doctor of medicine) or D.O.'s (doctor of osteopathic medicine) with specialty designation in family medicine (family practice physician) or internal medicine (internist). In many health care systems, the primary care physician functions as the "gatekeeper" for health care services and oversees all care that a person receives. Most specialists such as neurologists require a referral from a primary care physician.

Either a primary care physician or a neurologist can diagnose and treat Parkinson's disease. Most people including physicians are more comfortable when a neurologist makes or confirms the diagnosis, as there is a high rate of misdiagnosis particularly in the early stages of the disease. Due to the recent proliferation of treatments for Parkinson's disease, a neurologist's input is often very useful even in the early to mid stages of Parkinson's disease. Because primary care physicians provide the majority of care for the elderly (some specialize in geriatrics, the branch of medicine that focuses on such care), they sometimes are experienced in diagnosis and treatment of classic Parkinson's and many provide good oversight and medical management during the disease's early and middle stages. Late stage Parkinson's usually requires the expertise of a neurologist, at least in consultation.

See also CARE MANAGEMENT AND PLANNING; DOCTOR VISITS; NEUROLOGICAL EXAMINATION; NEUROLOGY; NEUROPSYCHIATRY; NEUROSURGERY.

prognosis   A projection of a condition's clinical course and outcome. The prognosis for Parkinson's disease is both certain and highly variable. Parkinson's disease is chronic and progressive, so what is certain is that its symptoms will worsen over time. But the course of disease that is manifested in each individual is highly variable, as there is no predictable pattern to the progression and severity of symptoms. As well, many factors influence Parkinson's course, including lifestyle, other health conditions, attitude, expectations, and outlook. This variation is both a drawback and an advantage; the person can live life as usual yet knows that circumstances can suddenly and unexpectedly change.

Diagnosis—determining that a disease or condition exists—and prognosis are the cornerstones of medical assessment. In many medical conditions, each is well defined. Laboratory tests establish positive evidence of infections; X rays and imaging studies such as COMPUTED TOMOGRAPHY (CT) SCAN show fractures. There are parameters for the effectiveness of treatment that make prognosis fairly certain. Strep throat typically clears up after two weeks on antibiotics; a broken wrist or arm heals after six weeks in a cast. Although even under the best of circumstances prognosis is a process of educated guessing predicated on the statistics of what happens with most people most of the time, it is far more precise in situations such as these. In complex, and particularly chronic, conditions, prognosis becomes a great challenge. Most people want definitive answers about such matters, but for Parkinson's those answers are in short supply. Parkinson's disease is a continuum with no obvious beginning, no clear path, and no foreseeable finish.

For the person with Parkinson's, prognosis is a balance between taking each day as it comes and anticipating future care needs. ANTI-PARKINSON'S MEDICATIONS hold symptoms at bay for many years in most people, allowing near-normal function. Yet the inevitable deterioration that continues in the BRAIN establishes the reality that the disease demands careful planning and management for optimal QUALITY OF LIFE.

See also ADJUSTING TO LIVING WITH PARKINSON'S; CARE MANAGEMENT AND PLANNING; CONDITIONS SIMILAR TO PARKINSON'S; COPING WITH ONGOING CARE OF PARKINSON'S; DIAGNOSING PARKINSON'S; END OF LIFE CARE AND DECISIONS; LIFESTYLE FACTORS; MEDICATION MANAGEMENT; PLANNING FOR THE FUTURE.

progressive supranuclear palsy (PSP)   A rare neurodegenerative disease with symptoms that are similar to those of Parkinson's disease. However, PSP has enough distinctive features that misdiagnosis is uncommon or short-lived. Early in the onset of PSP, symptoms such as TREMORS, BRADYKINESIA (slowed movement), POSTURAL INSTABILITY (balance and equilibrium problems), and GAIT DISTURBANCES (difficulty in starting, stopping, and changing direction when walking) often are prominent; postural instability is rarely a prominent sign in the first few years of Parkinson's disease. Another distinctive sign of PSP is difficulty with vertical eye movements, especially looking down. People with PSP also have more severe and earlier problems with swallowing and speaking than is typical for Parkinson's. Personality changes, sleep disturbances, and cognitive problems are also usually earlier and more severe in PSP compared to Parkinson's. As PSP almost always develops in people older than age 50, the combination of age and slowness with which neurologic symptoms develop frequently leads to an inaccurate diagnosis of Parkinson's disease. Because many symptoms and a portion of the disease process are Parkinson-like, PSP is considered one of the PARKINSON'S PLUS SYNDROMES (conditions that have Parkinson's symptoms as well as other distinctive symptoms).

Though it is a more aggressive disease than Parkinson's, PSP is still fairly slowly progressive, with patients surviving years, often well over a decade. Although pneumonia, often from aspirating food or liquids due the swallowing difficulties, is the most common causes of death in PSP, people with PSP often do not die from their PSP and eventually succumb to unrelated causes. The loss of other brain cells causes PSP's other symptoms, which include visual disturbances such as double vision or blurred vision, difficulty in breathing, personality changes, and DEMENTIA.

PSP is sometimes misdiagnosed as CREUTZFELDT-JAKOB DISEASE (CJD), an even more rare neurodegenerative disease in which there is widespread tissue loss in the brain. Such misdiagnosis is most likely when the primary symptoms of PSP are dementia and personality changes, which are hallmarks of CJD. Differential diagnosis often does not occur until autopsy after death. Because there is no adequate treatment for either disease (though some experimental treatments for CJD hold some promise), misdiagnosis has little or no therapeutic consequence.

AMYOTROPHIC LATERAL SCLEROSIS (ALS), also widely known as Lou Gehrig's disease, is also a potential misdiagnosis in people with PSP, due to the fact that problems with swallowing, keeping the airway open (so called stridor from involuntary closure of the vocal cords), and producing speech can be fairly early and prominent in both diseases. As with CJD, the consequences of such a misdiagnosis are small because ALS lacks an effective treatment as well.

Pathology of PSP

PSP primarily affects the structures of the BRAINSTEM that regulate COORDINATION, in particular the PONS and THALAMUS, and the subcortical nuclei that regulate voluntary movement, in particular the subthalamic nucleus (STN), PALLIDUM, and SUBSTANTIA NIGRA. Scientists do not know how the deterioration that leads to PSP starts. Although this deterioration causes symptoms similar to those of Parkinson's widespread death of both subcortical NEURONS and GLIAL CELLS (specialized brain cells that support and protect neurons) occurs throughout the subcortex. Glial cells acquire a characteristic "tufted" appearance that results from the accumulation of TAU-based NEUROFIBRILLARY TANGLES similar to those found in Alzheimer's disease.

These are distinguishing factors apparent only at autopsy after death, although FUNCTIONAL IMAGING STUDIES SUCH AS POSITRON EMISSION TOMOGRAPHY (PET) and SINGLE PHOTON EMISSION COMPUTED TOMOGRAPHY (SPECT) often can detect atrophy (loss of tissue) in the subcortical nuclei in the mid to late stages of the disease. The MRI often develops characteristic abnormalities by the mid to late stages as well. The neurologist may order one of these studies if questions remain about diagnosis as the disease progresses; although the findings are not conclusive, they help to distinguish PSP from

Parkinson's because such atrophy does not occur with Parkinson's.

Differential Diagnosis

Diagnosis of PSP is primarily clinical as there are no definitive tests. Differentiating PSP from Parkinson's disease and other neurodegenerative conditions often is a matter of time. The most significant differentiating factor is that Parkinson's disease responds to treatment with LEVODOPA or DOPAMINE AGONIST MEDICATIONS and PSP does not. However, TREMORS in both conditions respond to treatment with ANTICHOLINERGIC MEDICATIONS. This common response can perpetuate an incorrect diagnosis when tremor is the predominant symptom until symptoms worsen. As establishing a medication regimen that effectively relieves the symptoms of Parkinson's disease requires up to several months, the lack of response of motor symptoms to treatment with anti-Parkinson's medications may not be immediately apparent. Indeed, it is not uncommon for fine-tuning a medication regimen to take as long as a year. However, there is usually a noticeable improvement even if incomplete, and improvement this does not occur, the Parkinson's diagnosis is questionable.

Visual disturbances often are overlooked or misunderstood in early PSP yet provide distinctive diagnostic clues. Vision problems in older people are fairly common, and blurred vision can occur in both PSP and Parkinson's. However, the person with PSP often has significant difficulty in controlling eye movements and aiming the eyes. This is a consequence of cell loss in areas of the BRAINSTEM that coordinate vision and probably reflects damage to the optic tract and possibly the third, fourth, and sixth cranial nerves, which originate in the midbrain and the PONS (structures of the BRAINSTEM). The person with Parkinson's who has visual symptoms may have a problem in moving the eyes downward but has control over other eye movements. This problem is a consequence of the loss of dopaminergic neurons in the areas of the BASAL GANGLIA that regulate voluntary movement.

Treatment Options

Unfortunately, there are few effective treatments for PSP. Anti-Parkinson's medications sometimes help to control tremors or, other motor symptoms, but usually only incompletely and temporarily; as symptoms progress past the mild stages, usual Parkinson's treatments are rarely effective. Treatment is primarily palliative, aiming to maintain comfort as much as possible. PSP does not cause pain, although its DYSKINESIAS and DYSTONIA can cause uncomfortable postures and positions. Muscle relaxants sometimes relieve these discomforts. Medications used to improve COGNITIVE FUNCTION in people who have ALZHEIMER'S DISEASE are largely ineffective in those who have PSP, although many physicians would try them in people with PSP and cognitive decline.

Why PSP Interests Parkinson's Researchers

PSP interests Parkinson's researchers because part of the disease process is the same in PSP and Parkinson's—the loss of dopaminergic neurons. Yet the motor symptoms of PSP do not respond to dopamine replacement strategies as they do in Parkinson's disease. As well, there are intriguing differences, such as the loss of nigrostriatal fibers that occurs in Parkinson's disease but not in PSP, that raise questions about how the disease processes evolve. PSP's cognitive and personality changes support the premise that functions in the brain are linked in ways that researchers do not yet understand; unraveling these connections will provide greater insights into brain function as well as dysfunction.

See also AMYOTROPHIC LATERAL SCLEROSIS; CORTICOBASAL DEGENERATION; LEWY BODY DISEASE; MULTIPLE SCLEROSIS; MULTIPLE SYSTEM ATROPHY.

prooxidant   A substance that increases metabolic actions that result in OXIDATION, the biochemical pathway through which cells generate energy. Oxidation causes the production of FREE RADICALS, unstable molecules that many scientists believe are the cumulative cause of numerous diseases. When the body's health is in balance, cells produce sufficient amounts of substances that function as ANTIOXIDANTS to neutralize free radicals. Through normal degenerative processes, aging, and exposure to various toxins, this balance becomes altered and free radical production exceeds the body's ability to control it. Common prooxidants include minerals such as iron. OXIDATIVE STRESS (damage to cells over time that results from oxidation) is one of the factors scientists are exploring as a possible cause of Parkinson's disease.

See also ACERULOPLASMINEMIA; ANTIOXIDANT THERAPY; HALLERVORDEN–SPATZ SYNDROME.

proprioception   The body's ability accurate perception of its spatial relationship to its surroundings. It represents automatic communication between peripheral nerves and the brain and determines the body's ability to respond with appropriate force during activities such as lifting, pushing, or WALKING. Proprioception is an essential component of BALANCE, EQUILIBRIUM, and MOVEMENT. Proprioception mechanisms integrate closely with POSTURAL RIGHTING REFLEXES. Proprioceptive receptors are distributed widely throughout the musculoskeletal system as well as the inner ear structures related to balance.

Disturbances of the neuromuscular system can interfere with the body's proprioception mechanisms by inhibiting or distorting muscle response. Some scientists believe that treatment with DOPAMINERGIC MEDICATIONS such as LEVODOPA suppresses proprioception, contributing to dyskinesias.

See also BODY SCHEME; GAIT; MOBILITY; MOTOR FUNCTION.

protein   Chemical structure consisting of oxygen, hydrogen, and nitrogen. The body requires a continuous supply of protein to meet its functional and energy needs. Proteins compose numerous substances in the body including ENZYMES, HORMONES, cell structures, and deoxyribonucleic acid (DNA). Scientists have identified a number of proteins and corresponding GENE MUTATIONS that direct their functions that have roles in Parkinson's disease. Proteins are constructed of hundreds to thousands of amino acids, the smallest units of organic structure. Although there are only about 20 amino acids, the ways in which they combine allow them to form countless proteins. DNA, a cell's genetic code, determines how each cell synthesizes (makes) and uses proteins. The more complex the protein, the greater the likelihood of errors in its synthesis.

In the 1990s scientists identified mutations in the ALPHA-SYNUCLEIN GENE and the PARKIN GENE in significant numbers of people with Parkinson's disease. These genes regulate the synthesis of ALPHA-SYNUCLEIN, a complex protein that facilitates synaptic communication among brain NEURONS, and a number of other proteins that scientists know are present in the BRAIN but do not fully understand. Alpha-synuclein has been one of the most extensively studied brain protein to date. Researchers also know that the neurons often contain structures called inclusions. In the brain of people with Parkinson's disease, these inclusions are characteristic structures called LEWY BODIES, which are composed primarily of alpha synuclein. The correlation between these protein-based inclusions, the role of alpha-synuclein in synaptic communication, and the neurodegeneration that occurs in Parkinson's disease remains unclear.

ALZHEIMER'S DISEASE was the first neurodegenerative disease for which scientists discovered a conclusive protein connection, that of the TAU protein, which forms the characteristic deposits and NEUROFIBRILLARY TANGLES that are the pathological hallmark of Alzheimer's. As with Parkinson's, there are gene mutations that correspond with the apparent malfunction of tau protein synthesis. And also as with Parkinson's, the correlation of tau, the deposits, and the disease process in Alzheimer's is not fully understood. Both proteins—alpha-synuclein and tau—are present in healthy brains, but not as deposits. People who have one of these diseases, Parkinson's or Alzheimer's, also have a much higher risk than other people their age of having the other, raising intriguing questions about connections between the two disease processes and the role of protein synthesis in health and in disease. Researchers are optimistic that unraveling these connections will provide crucial understanding of the causes of and possible cures for both, as well as related diseases.

See also CONDITIONS SIMILAR TO PARKINSON'S; GENE MAPPING; GENE THERAPY; LEWY BODY DISEASE; PARKINSON'S DISEASE, CAUSES OF.

protein restrictions, dietary Dietary protein and orally administered LEVODOPA, the primary ANTI-PARKINSON'S MEDICATION, can compete for absorption into the bloodstream. Levodopa is a large-molecule amino acid structure that, to be absorbed into the bloodstream, requires attachment to a carrier molecule. The availability of these carriers is limited during each digestive "transport," and they accept large molecule amino acids from other dietary sources as well. Once these carrier molecules are all attached, any remaining large molecule amino acids are passed on through the digestive system and eventually become waste.

In the early stages of Parkinson's disease it is not a problem for most people that only small amounts of dopamine need to eventually get to the brain. Even small doses contain much more than their brain requires, so that lost in the gut is of no consequence. As the Parkinson's progresses and symptom management requires higher dosages of levodopa, it becomes necessary to manage its absorption better. The most effective way to do this is to separate dietary protein from levodopa dosages.

- During waking hours when levodopa doses are highest, eat primarily fruits, vegetables, whole grains, and whole grain products. Avoid dairy products, meats, nuts, and legumes (dried beans), all of which are high in protein.

- Eat five or six small meals spread throughout the day to help to counter feelings of hunger and to increase the nutritional value of the day's food intake.

- Incorporate the day's protein into the evening meal, or other meals that follow at least one hour after the last and at least two hours before the next dose of levodopa. An adult should consume two or three servings of protein (50 to 60 grams) daily.

Taking levodopa doses with meals that do not contain protein allows the food to neutralize the nausea that levodopa can cause but does not provide competition for absorption.

See also COOKING; FOOD PREPARATION; FOODS TO AVOID; NUTRITION AND DIET.

Provigil See MODAFINIL.

psychosis A condition of mental dysfunction in which a person loses contact with reality. DELUSIONS, HALLUCINATIONS, CONFUSION, DISORIENTATION, and PARANOIA are common in psychosis. In the person with Parkinson's disease, psychosis can develop as a separate disease entity, as a manifestation of the brain deterioration taking place as a result of the Parkinson's, or as a side effect of ANTIPARKINSON'S MEDICATIONS. The primary treatment for psychosis employs ANTIPSYCHOTIC MEDICATIONS, but a person with Parkinson's disease should exercise great caution in taking these. Many of them, particularly HALOPERIDOL (Haldol) and PERPHENAZINE (Thorazine), are dopamine agonists that can cause the symptoms of Parkinson's to worsen dramatically. Safer antipsychotic choices for people with Parkinson's include low dose quetiapine (Seroquel) and clozapine (Clozaril).

The symptoms of dementia are similar to those of psychosis, and the two conditions can coexist. Treatment decisions should consider how disruptive the person is and whether there is a threat of injury to self or others. If medication is determined to be necessary to treat psychosis of a person with Parkinson's, it is important to watch Parkinson's symptoms very carefully. Psychotherapy and other interventions generally are not helpful with psychosis because the person does not perceive reality. Psychosis is a biochemical disorder, the result of imbalances among the neurotransmitters in the brain.

See also DEMENTIA; SCHIZOPHRENIA.

psychosocial factors The numerous psychological and social aspects of life that influence a person's ability to manage daily functions. Psychosocial factors include family, friends, and perceptions about health and illness. Often these factors are significant in defining how well a person copes with the needs of a chronic, NEURODEGENERATIVE disease such as Parkinson's. People with strong support networks are better able to handle such demands.

Although Parkinson's disease clearly arises from physical changes in the structures of the brain, a person's attitudes, fears, worries, level of self-confidence, and sense of self-worth influence the severity of symptoms. Older people who have Parkinson's disease may remember knowing people when they were growing up who had Parkinson's and progressed to significant impairment quickly—just 40 years ago, there were no effective treatments for Parkinson's disease. Younger people who are diagnosed with Parkinson's disease may have no frame of reference for a chronic health condition and may have developed no mechanisms for coping with significant stress.

SUPPORT GROUPS are extremely helpful to people who have Parkinson's disease. They provide information gained from experience and a network of understanding. It is important for the person with Parkinson's as well as family members and friends to learn as much as possible about Parkinson's disease, to equip themselves with the knowledge that helps in coping. Family support is crucial, yet family members often do not know what to do or how to help. Support groups, as well as health care providers, can offer suggestions and guidance.

See also ADJUSTING TO LIVING WITH PARKINSON'S; COMPASSION; COPING WITH ONGOING CARE FOR PARKINSON'S; EMPATHY; PATIENCE; QUALITY OF LIFE; SELF-ESTEEM.

psychotherapy Professional assistance from a mental health specialist to deal with emotional issues. Social workers, therapists, psychologists, and psychiatrists are among the professionals who may provide psychotherapy. Generally, a psychiatrist, who is a medical doctor, becomes involved only when there is a need to prescribe medications. People who are experiencing ANXIETY or DEPRESSION often benefit from a combination of medication and psychotherapy. Psychotherapy can help a person or family understand fears and worries that contribute to anxiety and depression and to develop positive coping mechanisms.

See also ANTIANXIETY MEDICATIONS; ANTIDEPRESSANT MEDICATIONS; PSYCHOSOCIAL FACTORS; STRESS REDUCTION TECHNIQUES.

pulsion See GAIT DISTURBANCE.

putamen See BASAL GANGLIA.

PWP Acronym for *person with Parkinson's*. See also PARKINSONIAN.

pyramidal pathway A large mass of nerve fibers that originate in the motor control areas of the cerebral cortex in an area called the primary motor cortex and travel through the cerebral hemispheres (including the posterior internal capsule, which lies between the thalamus and globus pallidus), the brainstem (crossing at the bottom of the medulla), and the lateral part of the spinal cord before synapsing on the motor neurons that exit the spinal cord as nerve roots, eventually joining nerves to innervate individual muscles. It also is called the pyramidal tract or the corticospinal tract. The pyramidal pathway is so named because its course over the surface of the brainstem's medulla resembles a pyramid in shape. Pyramidal nerves control gross voluntary and reflexive muscle function; the EXTRAPYRAMIDAL SYSTEM refines this control to regulate fine motor movements. The extrapyramidal system often uses the same nerve structures to conduct its signals. The pyramidal pathway is not damaged in Parkinson's disease, but the extrapyramidal system is, affecting the functions of both. A common representation of the relationship between the two is that of the relationship between musical instrument and musician. The pyramidal pathway is the instrument; the extrapyramidal system, the musician.

See also BASAL GANGLIA; BRAIN; NERVOUS SYSTEM.

quality of life   The perceptions of a person of the well-being and satisfaction of his or her daily living experiences. Many factors influence quality of life for people with Parkinson's disease, from physical symptoms and the limitations they impose to problems such as depression, anxiety, urinary disturbances, constipation, SLEEP DISTURBANCES, MEDICATION SIDE EFFECTS that impair MEMORY and COGNITIVE FUNCTION, and SEXUAL DYSFUNCTION. Quality of life is of course a subjective measure and perceptions of what is acceptable vary widely. The variable course of Parkinson's, the range of symptoms, and a person's lifestyle before diagnosis are all important factors. A person's expectations, before and after the diagnosis of Parkinson's, also have a great effect on his or her perception of quality of life. Reduced independence is the leading quality of life issue for many people with Parkinson's.

Small changes can make big differences in quality of life. Actions as simple as removing throw rugs and rearranging furniture can make walking through the house appreciably easier for the person with Parkinson's. Adaptive equipment such as raised toilet seats and bathroom grab bars, and assist devices such as a "sock aid" or zipper pulls that make it easier to dress and undress improve independence. Sleep medications often can improve the amount and quality of sleep a person gets, in turn improving his or her ability to function in many areas of life.

Adjustments in the ANTI-PARKINSON'S MEDICATION regimen can provide more complete symptom relief during times when the person desires such relief, which may not necessarily be according to the standard schedule. The person with Parkinson's who is more of a "swing shift" person by nature may prefer symptom relief well into the evening, whereas the "morning person" wants to swing out of bed ready to plunge into the day's activities. It is important to accommodate, as much as is practical, the person's individual needs and preferences. Often doing so requires surprisingly little extra effort.

Although quality of life is highly subjective, a number of assessment tools attempt to measure it in quantifiable terms, include:

- PARKINSON'S DISEASE QUESTIONNAIRE (PDQ-39): A 39-item proprietary assessment survey used mainly in research studies that can be a self-assessment (the person with Parkinson's completes the questionnaire) or be administered by a clinician (usually a researcher or research assistant, who asks the questions and fills out the form). Questions are related to general health, specific Parkinson's symptoms, and perceptions of whether medical or surgical treatments improve quality of life.

- PARKINSON'S DISEASE QUALITY OF LIFE QUESTIONNAIRE (PDQL): A 37-item assessment survey usually given by a clinician. This proprietary survey is available for clinicians to purchase through the French company Mapi Research Institute, Inc., which specializes in quality of life assessment tools for health care.

- PARKINSON'S IMPACT SCALE (PIMS): A five-point assessment scale that measures the effect of Parkinson's disease in 10 core areas of life including self-image and relationships with partners, family members, and friends. The Parkinson Foundation Canada developed the PIMS.

Other commonly used survey tools such as ACTIVITIES OF DAILY LIVING (ADLS) assessments and the HOEHN AND YAHR STAGE SCALE measure the progression of symptoms and the level of disability that results, but not their direct effect on a person's quality of life.

Often perceptions about what matters in daily life shift as Parkinson's disease exerts a greater influence on daily living decisions, with a corresponding adjustment in satisfaction with life circumstances. Priorities change. Most people with Parkinson's find that they want to simplify their lives so they have the energy and the time to engage in activities they truly enjoy and have less tolerance for events that detract from them. A person who spent every walking minute before Parkinson's working may find it is now more important to spend time with children or grandchildren and find life more satisfying after making this shift even when physical symptoms limit mobility and independence. Quality of life becomes a process of adjustment and, to some extent, compromise. Not everything will be possible, but with ingenuity and persistence, the important things often can be put within reach.

Suffering in silence—not telling family members and doctors about problems or concerns—diminishes quality of life. Some people do not want to burden others and so keep their discomforts to themselves. As well, this can be a symptom of DEPRESSION, which itself interferes with the person's ability to experience JOY in everyday living. Regardless of the reason, keeping quiet about symptoms or fears can mean missing treatments that could reduce or end the problem. It also often creates frustration for family members, who may sense that the person with Parkinson's is holding back and fear the worst. On the flip side, some people dwell on the difficulties that Parkinson's creates in their life. This preoccupation makes it difficult to see the positives in situations and can cause family members to become resentful or to withdraw. Open and honest communication gives the person with Parkinson's and loved ones the opportunity to work together to find solutions and ways to deal with problems.

See also ADAPTIVE EQUIPMENT AND ASSIST DEVICES; ADJUSTING TO LIVING WITH PARKINSON'S; COPING WITH ONGOING CARE OF PARKINSON'S; FAMILY RELATIONSHIPS; FRUSTRATION; SUPPORT GROUPS.

quetiapine   One of the ANTIPSYCHOTIC MEDICATIONS taken to relieve symptoms of PSYCHOSIS, DELUSIONS, AND HALLUCINATIONS in people with Parkinson's disease. Often these symptoms are the side effects of ANTI-PARKINSON'S MEDICATIONS, particularly ANTICHOLINERGIC MEDICATIONS that block the action of ACETYLCHOLINE, a NEUROTRANSMITTER with a key role in neuron communication related to thought processes and memory. At present this is an open-label use of the drug, which is U.S. Food and Drug Administration–(FDA)-approved for SCHIZOPHRENIA and psychosis.

A significant drawback of most antipsychotic medications is that although they may relieve symptoms of psychosis or DEMENTIA, they do so through a strong DOPAMINE ANTAGONIST action. They block the action of dopamine in the brain, an effect that alters neuron activity related to cognitive functions but at the same time inhibits the action of LEVODOPA and the binding of DOPAMINE AGONIST MEDICATIONS such as BROMOCRIPTINE (Parlodel) and PRAMIPEXOLE (Mirapex). This effect dramatically worsens the neuromuscular symptoms of Parkinson's. Even in a person without Parkinson's, these drugs can cause Parkinson's-like symptoms or a sometimes permanent form of neuromuscular dysfunction called TARDIVE DYSKINESIA.

Quetiapine (Seroquel) is most physicians' antipsychotic of first choice in people with Parkinson's. It is an atypical antipsychotic that has less action on DOPAMINE RECEPTORS, particularly the D2 receptors that function to direct movement, than other antipsychotic medications. Quetiapine is much less likely to exacerbate Parkinson's symptoms than even other atypical antipsychotics such as olanzapine (Zyprexa), risperidone (Risperidal). Clozapine (Clozaril) is the only choice that clearly has less risk of worsening Parkinson's symptoms, but it can cause a deleterious decrease in white blood production and, hence, is rarely used. The new atypical antipsychotic (Abilify) might be even safer than quetiapine in theory, but it does not have much data or experience to support its safety in people with Parkinson's. Common side effects in addition to worsening of neuromuscular symptoms include headache, dizziness, drowsiness, and ORTHOSTATIC HYPOTENSION.

See also MENTAL STATUS; NEUROPSYCHIATRY; OFF-LABEL DRUG; OPEN-LABEL DRUG STUDY.

randomized double-blind study A prospective study of an intervention via a CLINICAL RESEARCH STUDY or CLINICAL PHARMACOLOGY TRIAL. In this type of trial neither the researchers nor the participants know who receives what agent or treatment, and participants are randomly assigned to a group without any qualifying factors. A pharmacist may prepare medication dosages (typically in forms that appear identical), which are dispensed to, or a clinician administers to, participants. Cross-referenced records are created to document all procedures; researchers compile the records when the trial is completed. The randomized double-blind study is considered to be one of the most objective models for conducting research because it prevents bias and expectations of either participants or researchers from influencing observations and outcomes or findings as neither knows which participants are in which group until the study is finished.

Typically a randomized double-blind study compares one agent or treatment with another, and participants in each group receive some form of treatment. There may be two or more groups, depending on the topic researchers are investigating. This is a common method for evaluating an INVESTIGATIONAL NEW DRUG (IND), for example, or for determining which of two or more commonly used treatments is more effective.

When there is also a group that does not receive any treatment, the trial is also called a controlled trial—those who do not receive treatment are the control group, a representation of a general population against which researchers can compare the outcome or findings of the agent or treatment being evaluated. A placebo-controlled study uses a control group that receives a PLACEBO (inert substance or agent) instead of medication. Control groups are not used as commonly in trials involving treatments for Parkinson's disease because people with Parkinson's must have treatment and there usually is little value in comparisons to people who do not have Parkinson's. Studies involving lifestyle factors or nutritional supplements may be among the exceptions.

Randomized double-blind studies generally produce the most reliable results; findings are compared against statistical standards for perspective. A randomized double-blind study is not always possible, as when a treatment is invasive (surgery). Anyone considering participation in any clinical research trial should make sure to understand fully what agent or treatment is being evaluated, what the expected results are, what the potential risks are, and what signs and symptoms are indications of possible adverse reactions.

See also BIOETHICS; INFORMED CONSENT.

range of motion The normal extent to which a joint flexes and extends. Range of motion is a crucial element of mobility; limited range of motion restricts mobility. The neuromuscular deterioration of Parkinson's disease affects range of motion physiologically as well as mechanically. RANGE OF MOTION EXERCISES keep joints as flexible as possible. Regular movement, such as walking, and focusing on full motion of a joint during movement (such as consciously swinging the arms and fully extending the legs with each stride), is also important. A device called a GONIOMETER measures the degree of motion. Range of motion can be passive (no resistance) or active (against resistance).

Joint	Full Range of Motion
Knee	140° Flexion (bending) 0° Extension (straightening)
Hip	125° Flexion (pulling leg forward) 25° Extension (pulling leg back) 45° Abduction (pulling leg outward from the body's median) 25° Adduction (pulling leg inward from the body's median) 60° Rotation outward (external) 40° Rotation inward (interior)
Ankle	20° Dorsiflexion (toes upward) 45° Plantar flexion (toes downward)
Shoulder	180° Flexion (above head) 180° Adduction (straight out from side)
Elbow	145° Flexion (bending) 0° Extension (straightening)
Wrist	70° Extension (back of hand up) 80° Flexion (palm down) 20° Radial deviation (thumb side toward body) 45° Ulnar deviation (pinky side away from body)
Neck	50° Flexion (chin toward chest) 60° Extension (head tipped back) 45° Flexion to left (tilt ear toward left shoulder) 80° Rotation to left (turn head toward left shoulder) 45° Flexion to right (tilt ear toward right shoulder) 80° Rotation to right (turn head toward right shoulder)
Back	60° Flexion (bend forward at waist) 25° Extension (bend backward at waist) 25° Lateral flexion left (bend at waist to left side) 25° Lateral flexion right (bend at waist to right side)

The motor symptom of Parkinson's that most directly affects range of motion is RIGIDITY, in which the endless barrage of nerve signals from the BRAIN to the muscle fibers keep them in a constant state of contraction. Over time the muscle fibers change physiologically, shortening and stiffening and becoming less responsive to nerve signals. This process causes greater resistance at the joint, and the natural inclination of the person who has Parkinson's disease is to accept the boundaries of

this resistance. Range of motion exercises that gently but consistently stretch muscle groups around joints help to keep the muscle fibers more resilient and lessen the extent of shortening.

Restricted range of motion in the person with Parkinson's is most obvious in the GAIT DISTURBANCES characteristic of the disease, particularly minimal ARM SWING and short, shuffling steps. The lack of upper body movement reflects rigidity affecting the muscles in the neck and spine (contributing to the stooped posture), shoulders, elbows, and wrists. The shuffling GAIT reflects rigidity affecting the hips and pelvic joints, knees, and ankles. Factors not related to Parkinson's disease, such as osteoarthritis and previous injuries involving shoulders and knees, affect range of motion, too, and can contribute to further restrictions.

"Use it or lose it" is an apt adage that applies to range of motion. Although the physiological changes that Parkinson's causes are unpreventable, regular movement of the joints can slow their development. Once these changes take place, offsetting their effects on the mechanics of movement becomes increasingly difficult. As Parkinson's progresses other motor symptoms such as BRADYKINESIA (slowed muscle response) and AKINESIA (freezing) limit MOBILITY in other ways, also affecting range of motion. The extent of restriction of range of motion is one of the factors doctors consider when STAGING PARKINSON'S DISEASE (determining the level of severity of symptoms and the degree to which they impair the ACTIVITIES OF DAILY LIVING).

See also CARDINAL SYMPTOMS; COGWHEELING; DIAGNOSING PARKINSON'S; LEAD PIPE RESISTANCE; LEG STRIDE; OCCUPATIONAL THERAPY; PHYSICAL THERAPY; TAI CHI; YOGA.

range of motion exercises Structured movements that help to stretch and flex the muscle groups around the joints to keep the joints supple and unrestricted. A physical therapist can teach range of motion exercises specific for each joint that take into consideration any existing injuries or limitations. In general, range of motion exercises gently extend, flex, bend, or rotate the joint through all of the positions it can accommodate.

All movements should be slow and steady. YOGA and TAI CHI are excellent structured activities that improve range of motion as well as FLEXIBILITY, BALANCE, and strength. Walking, swimming, and other activities that get the body in motion are also good. Whatever the activity, it should attempt to use each joint to its fullest.

See also EXERCISE AND ACTIVITY; MOVEMENT; MUSCLE STRENGTH; MUSCLE TONE.

rapid speech   See SPEECH.

reading   Although Parkinson's disease does not directly affect the optic nerve or the physical mechanisms of vision, the disease often affects the muscles that control the eyelids. This effect can result in reduced BLINK RATE (one of the earliest symptoms of Parkinson's disease), BLEPHAROSPASMS (involuntary and sometimes protracted closure resulting from intense, extended muscle contractions), excessive tearing that causes BLURRY VISION, and RIGIDITY of the lower eyelid. BRADYKINESIA and DYSKINESIA that affect other muscles, such as freezing, also can affect EYE MOVEMENTS and the ability to focus or to distinguish among objects. Although the optic tracts remain intact, neuromuscular impairments interfere with the mechanics of eye function.

ANTICHOLINERGIC MEDICATIONS taken to treat TREMORS can cause dryness of the eyes and either constricted or dilated pupils (both of which affect depth perception and the eye's ability to focus). Anticholinergics and LEVODOPA can cause increased pressure within the eye (intraocular pressure), causing rapid-onset glaucoma in rare individuals who are susceptible to closed angle glaucoma. By the time there are vision-related symptoms, it may be too late to prevent significant visual impairment or blindness. Glaucoma typically manifests no symptoms until the disease is fairly advanced. Anyone who is taking ANTIPARKINSON'S MEDICATIONS should have regular eye examinations that include checks for glaucoma. Most people with glaucoma have the open angle variety, and can usually take SINEMET or anticholinergics without ill effect, but they require close supervision by an ophthalmologist (a physi-

cian who specializes in the medical and surgical treatment of eye disease).

Other problems with reading arise as Parkinson's progresses and the person has increased difficulty with fine motor control in the hands and fingers, and it becomes more challenging to hold a book or magazine or to turn its pages. Tremors can cause constant movement, making seeing or focusing on words difficult. Large-print books can overcome this problem to some extent. Assist devices that provide hands-free support help hold books and other materials flat and steady; there are page-turning aids as well.

Audiobooks (books on tape) allow an avid reader to continue enjoying books. Many titles available in print are also available on audiotape. Reading aloud to a loved one who has Parkinson's disease provides a good opportunity to share an activity together. Some public libraries, senior centers, and organizations that assist the visually impaired have "read aloud" programs in which volunteers read to groups and individuals. Some people with Parkinson's disease may enjoy plays, movies, and other nonreading forms of entertainment as alternatives to reading.

Eye problems that cause reading difficulties can interfere with a person's ability to perform job functions, read directions on medication labels, and drive a motor vehicle. Adjusting medication dosages or trying different drugs sometimes improves control over the muscles of the eyelids and eye itself, and using lubricating eye drops can help to mitigate eye dryness and irritation.

See also ADAPTIVE EQUIPMENT AND ASSIST DEVICES; ADJUSTING TO LIVING WITH PARKINSON'S; GLAUCOMA, TREATMENT WITH PARKINSON'S; MEDICATION MANAGEMENT; MEDICATION SIDE EFFECTS.

receptor   A molecular structure on a cell that allows binding with a biochemical such as a NEUROTRANSMITTER or a HORMONE. Most receptors are "open" to just one such substance; some can bind with multiple substances. Some receptors in the brain can bind with either NOREPINEPHRINE or DOPAMINE, for example. Generally multiple bindings involve substances in the same chemical family; norepinephrine is a DOPAMINE PRECURSOR (the body can convert it into dopamine). Binding either activates or inhibits a function within the cell. Many ANTI-PARKINSON'S MEDICATIONS either block binding, as do ANTICHOLINERGIC MEDICATIONS, or mimic the natural biochemical and bind in its place, as do DOPAMINE AGONIST MEDICATIONS.

See also ALPHA-ADENOSINE RECEPTOR; DOPAMINE RECEPTOR.

record keeping Maintaining copies and files of important records, including medical, legal, financial, tax, and insurance paperwork and documents. This is important for PLANNING FOR THE FUTURE as well as preparing for sudden and unexpected changes in the condition of the person with Parkinson's. Most people have systems of some sort for keeping track of bills, payments, tax documents, and related records. Key family members or friends should know where records and documents are located and have access to them should the need arise. This is especially critical when the person who has Parkinson's is the one who has been responsible for maintaining records. Among many couples, one person handles finances and related records and the other person knows little about them. As difficult as it can be to share or give up this responsibility, it often creates unnecessary hardship when no one else knows where records are or how they are managed.

Medical Records

Get copies of all medical records from each doctor seen and each hospital or clinic that performs procedures or tests. Some providers charge a fee for making copies; many make one copy available at no charge. Individuals are entitled to copies of their medical records. When consulting new doctors, take copies of the records but do not give up the only copy. It is a good idea to keep lifelong medical records. As the medical environment continually changes as new treatment options become available, knowing what treatments have been tried and whether they were successful is important. A person with Parkinson's who participates in a CLINICAL RESEARCH TRIAL should also obtain and keep records related to the study, such as the drugs or procedures that were tested, their effect on symp-

toms, and any complications that resulted from participation in the study.

Financial and Tax Records

Keep all financial records and tax documents for at least seven to 10 years. These records will be essential for MEDICAID, if that becomes a necessity. Medicaid requires precise documentation of expenses for the previous three years to determine eligibility; as few people know exactly when they may need Medicare, it is prudent to keep this documentation as complete as possible. The burden of proof is on the person with Parkinson's to demonstrate that he or she meets Medicaid requirements for income as well as spend down. Keep receipts for pharmacy and medical expenses. An accountant or attorney who specializes in estate planning or elder law can provide specific advice about what to keep and how long.

Insurance Records

Insurance records should include medical, dental, life, and disability declaration pages; full contracts whenever possible; and documentation related to claims paid and claims rejected. It is also a good idea to keep copies of records related to auto insurance, if the person with Parkinson's owns a car and still drives, as well as property insurance (homeowner's or renter's insurance).

Other Important Documents

Deeds, pension records, bank statements, wills, living trusts, prepaid funeral trusts, and powers of attorney documentation are among the miscellaneous records that should be kept. Wills and records related to funeral plans in particular should be stored in a safe place at home or with a relative, not in a bank safe deposit box. In some states the law requires banks to seal safe deposit boxes until after probate, generally long after the need for these records arises.

See also ADVANCE DIRECTIVES; ESTATE PLANNING; FINANCIAL PLANNING.

relaxation techniques See STRESS REDUCTION TECHNIQUES.

REM sleep behavior disorder (RBD) See SLEEP DISTURBANCES.

remacemide An antiseizure medication sometimes taken as an OPEN-LABEL DRUG for the NEUROPROTECTIVE EFFECTS of its GLUTAMATE ANTAGONIST actions. GLUTAMATE is an AMINO ACID that functions as a brain NEUROTRANSMITTER; normally DOPAMINE counterbalances glutamate and keeps its actions in check. When dopamine levels decline in Parkinson's disease, this inhibitory effect is lost and glutamate overstimulates receptive neurons. Scientists believe this effect leads to their premature death. Clinical research trials so far have produced inconclusive findings about remacemide's effectiveness in slowing the progression of Parkinson's disease.

The drug has also been explored for open-label use in HUNTINGTON'S DISEASE, another neurodegenerative disorder, so far with similarly inconclusive results. At this point remacemide remains of questionable value in Parkinson's disease. AMANTADINE, sometimes taken as MONOTHERAPY in early Parkinson's, is believed to have some glutamate antagonist action; its effectiveness in postponing the need for LEVODOPA therapy raises hopes that other glutamate antagonists can have similar effects.

See also AMANTADINE; ANTIOXIDANT; ANTIOXIDANT THERAPY; COENZYME Q-10; OXIDATIVE STRESS.

Reno, Janet The 78th attorney general of the United States, who was diagnosed with Parkinson's disease in late 1995 at age 57, two years into her appointment. Reno was the first woman to serve as U.S. attorney general and held the office during the two presidential terms of Bill Clinton, from 1993 to 2000. She spoke openly and candidly about her diagnosis and her symptoms, which included noticeable TREMORS of her left hand, and completed her term as attorney general. Reno ran for governor of her home state, Florida, in 2002 but did not make it past the primary. Her bid drew considerable attention to Parkinson's disease and particularly to the potential development of DEMENTIA (deterioration of cognitive function), which Reno's doctors said was not one of her symptoms.

See also ALI, MUHAMMAD; FOX, MICHAEL J.; MORRIS K. UDALL PARKINSON'S RESEARCH ACT; UDALL, MORRIS K.; WHITE, MAURICE.

replacement therapy See LEVODOPA.

Requip See ROPINIROLE.

rescue drug An ANTI-PARKINSON'S MEDICATION taken to provide immediate relief from motor symptoms such as severe bradykinesia, rigidity, or freezing when the regular medication regimen cannot control them. Such OFF-STATE episodes can occur in the disease's later stages when conventional anti-Parkinson's medications are no longer effective in meeting the brain's DOPAMINE needs.

Extra oral doses of regular release LEVODOPA, as levodopa/carbidopa (Sinemet) or levodopa/benserazide (Madopar), often can act as rescue drugs, although they can take 45 minutes to an hour to become effective. Extended release formulas such as Sinemet CR, which many people with Parkinson's take because the effect lasts longer between doses, do not work well as rescue drugs because they are designed to enter the bloodstream slowly over a controlled period.

For extreme symptoms, subcutaneous injection of the drug APOMORPHINE, a potent DOPAMINE AGONIST medication chemically similar to morphine that is not a narcotic and acts on different receptors in the BRAIN, can provide relief within five to 15 minutes. Other dopamine agonists, because of their receptor activations, tend to be less effective than apomorphine when taken as rescue drugs. The primary drawback of apomorphine is that at present it is available only in injectable form and it almost invariably causes moderate to severe nausea and vomiting in most people. For this reason, rescue drug doses are almost always taken with an antiemetic medication such as trimethobenzamide (Tigan). Also the risk of undesired side effects, particularly dyskinesia (fidgety movements) DYSTONIA (extreme muscle rigidity) is quite high when rescue drugs are added to one's usual dose of medications. It can be a fine balance between relieving one set of symptoms and causing another.

See also BENSERAZIDE; CARBIDOPA; DOPAMINE DEGRADATION; MEDICATION MANAGEMENT; TREATMENT ALGORITHM.

reserpine A medication taken to lower high blood pressure (antihypertensive) that can cause Parkinson's-like symptoms. The risk for experiencing those symptoms is high enough, and there are so many alternative antihypertensive medications, that people with Parkinson's disease generally should not use reserpine. Doctors sometimes prescribed reserpine to take advantage of this side effect, in fact, to reduce DYSKINESIAS in NEURODE-GENERATIVE conditions such as Huntington's disease or in tardive dyskinesia before other medications became available. And this side effect made it possible to create the first laboratory model of Parkinson's, a crucial step in understanding the disease's pathological process and developing effective treatments.

Reserpine became available in 1952 as one of the first drugs to treat hypertension after it was isolated as the active ingredient in a botanical remedy, rauwolfia (snakeroot), that had long been used in herbal medicine to treat high blood pressure. Rauwolfia also was known to have a powerful sedative effect and was given to calm people who had severe psychiatric disorders. This effect intrigued the Swedish neuroscientist Arvid Carlsson, who began investigating the relationship between reserpine and serotonin and NOREPINEPHRINE, brain NEU-ROTRANSMITTERS related to emotion and mood.

During his research, Carlsson serendipitously discovered that high dosages of reserpine administered to laboratory animals caused the development of TREMORS and BRADYKINESIA (slowed muscle response), the hallmark symptoms of Parkinson's disease. Following this trail led Carlsson to recognize that dopamine is an independent neurotransmitter; previously scientists had believed it to be solely a NOREPINEPHRINE precursor. From Carlsson's work evolved the current understanding of Parkinson's disease as the consequence of DOPAMINERGIC NEURON death and DOPAMINE DEPLETION in the brain and of current treatment regimens based on dopamine replacement with LEVODOPA. Carlsson shared the 2000 Nobel Prize in medicine or physiology for his groundbreaking work that started with reserpine.

As a plant alkaloid, reserpine has numerous side effects in addition to its tendency to cause Parkinson's-like symptoms, including potentially serious cardiac arrhythmias (irregular heartbeat) and depression. It also interacts with numerous medications, in particular levodopa. Reserpine cannot be taken with the ANTIDEPRESSANT MEDICA-TION class MONOAMINE OXIDASE INHIBITORS (MAOIs) and the selective MAO-B inhibitor SELEGILINE, which some people with Parkinson's take for its neuroprotective effect, or with tricyclic antidepressants and SELECTIVE SEROTONIN REUPTAKE INHIBITOR (SSRI) antidepressants.

Reserpine is available in numerous products, some of which combine it with a diuretic such as hydrochlorothiazide. Common brand name products include Ser-Ap-Es, Regroton, Hydropres and Salutensin.

See also 1-METHYL-4-PHENYL-1,2,3,6-TETRAHY-DROPYRIDINE; DRUG-INDUCED PARKINSON'S; HEART DISEASE AND PARKINSON'S; HORNYKIEWICZ, OLEH; PARKINSONISM.

residential care Live-in care in a group facility. Residential care becomes an option to be considered or a necessity when the person who has Parkinson's disease can no longer live independently or becomes debilitated beyond the capability of family members to manage. Because care must include medical attention such as medications, most often residential care involves an ASSISTED LIVING FACILITY or a LONG-TERM CARE FACILITY where there are qualified medical staff on duty 24 hours a day.

Some facilities feature progressive services, in which the facility adjusts the level of care and the corresponding cost as the needs of the person with Parkinson's become more extensive. Often these are complexes on a single campus with separate facilities for independent living which can range from "senior apartments" with no care services to minimal care services (perhaps food preparation, housekeeping, and transportation services), assisted living (mostly independent with moderate care needs), and living in a nursing facility (fully dependent with extensive care needs). Small, often family-run group homes are at the other end of the spectrum. Some people prefer their more homelike setting; it is crucial to make sure such a home has properly trained and credentialed staff. There are also residential care facilities that specialize in NEU-RODEGENERATIVE disorders such as Parkinson's disease, HUNTINGTON'S DISEASE, AMYOTROPHIC LATERAL SCLEROSIS (ALS), and MULTIPLE SCLEROSIS. As about one in four people with Parkinson's disease also has dementia, it is often worthwhile to determine what services the facility offers to meet the unique needs of people who have both physical and cognitive deterioration.

The determination that residential care is necessary can be difficult for family members when there has been little discussion of the possibility before the need becomes apparent. Because many people with Parkinson's enjoy a relatively normal life, as ANTI-PARKINSON'S MEDICATIONS keep their symptoms in control for many years and even decades, they and their families can be lulled into complacency about the disease's inevitable progression. This decline is as unpredictable as it is progressive and can proceed gradually over time or take a sudden and dramatic turn for the worse. The latter in particular catches families unprepared.

It is good for loved ones and the person with Parkinson's to discuss the possibility of residential care and their preferences and to agree on the criteria that will establish the need for such care, for example, when the person is unable to bathe and dress unassisted or can no longer walk. There are no set criteria for families; determining factors are unique to each person's circumstances. Certain kinds of care facilities do have admission criteria that often use scoring systems such as the HOEHN AND YAHR STAGE SCALE, THE UNIFIED PARKINSON'S DISEASE RATING SCALE (UPDRS), or a basic ACTIVITIES OF DAILY LIVING (ADLs) assessment. If MEDICAID will be necessary to cover the expenses of the residential living facility, matters such as eligibility and spend down that must be considered long before the need arises, as well as potential residential care options that are Medicaid-approved. MEDICARE does not pay for residential care unless it is medically necessary (usually requiring a preceding acute hospitalization of several days), is of limited duration (there is no coverage for care beyond 100 days), and falls within the criteria for SKILLED NURSING FACILITY (SNF) services.

See also ADVANTAGE DIRECTIVES; CARE MANAGEMENT AND PLANNING; COPING WITH ONGOING CARE OF PARKINSON'S; ESTATE PLANNING; FINANCIAL PLANNING; RESPITE CARE.

resonation   See SPEECH.

respite care   Short-term care for the person with Parkinson's, either in a group setting or in the home, to allow the primary caregiver to a break from caregiving responsibilities. Most respite care is provided for a few hours. Out-of-home respite programs allow the person with Parkinson's a change of scenery and opportunity to socialize at the same time they give caregivers much-needed time for themselves. When the person with Parkinson's is too debilitated to leave home easily or is reluctant to do so, or there are complicating factors such as coexisting ALZHEIMER'S DISEASE or DEMENTIA, in-home respite care may be the better option. Often respite care providers send two people for in-home respite care, to assure that the person with Parkinson's is never left alone and that activities such as ASSISTED TRANSFER can be performed safely.

Whether respite care occurs in the home or in a group setting away from home, it is prudent to provide written instructions about essential information such as medications, dosages, and schedules; particular problems such as loss of balance during a change from a sitting to a standing position; food preferences; and other details that will make it easier for the respite staff to provide good care. Many but not all states regulate respite care services; it is essential to verify credentials and references, particularly for in-home respite care. Some MEDICAID programs pay for respite care services; MEDICARE and most private MEDICAL INSURANCE plans do not. Senior centers, churches, and hospitals sometimes offer volunteer, low-cost, or donation-funded respite care programs and services.

Caregivers sometimes feel guilty about leaving the person with Parkinson's in the care of strangers, even for just a few hours. It is important for caregivers to take care of themselves, and taking a short break now and again helps them to recharge and revitalize their own energy. When circumstances become such that the person with Parkinson's requires fairly constant attention and care, it is a treat for the caregiver to sit quietly and read a book, go to a movie, or just wander around a mall. Some caregivers use respite care to allow them to take care of extended chores such as servicing the car or going to the dentist. However, caregivers should try to use some of their respite time entirely for themselves. Circumstances permitting, it is good to schedule respite care on a regular basis. This pattern lets the caregiver plan activities and gives the person with Parkinson's the opportunity to get to know the respite staff or program.

See also CAREGIVER WELL-BEING; CAREGIVING; COPING WITH ONGOING CARE OF PARKINSON'S; FAMILY RELATIONSHIPS.

restless leg syndrome (RLS) A condition in which the legs twitch involuntarily usually when sitting or lying quietly at rest. It may be mild, with occasional tingling and small areas of twitching, or severe enough that the legs appear to be walking or running of their own volition. Most people also experience "crawling" or "pins and needles" sensations, feelings of hot or cold liquid running through their muscles, muscle cramps, muscle spasms, and sometimes outright pain that affects both legs equally as aspects of RLS. These sensory symptoms and their symmetrical (bilateral) nature help to distinguish RLS from Parkinson's symptoms. Restless leg syndrome is not confined to people with Parkinson's and can occur in people who do not have any other medical problem; doctors consider it an independent movement disorder rather than a symptom of Parkinson's disease, although RLS is common in people who have or later develop Parkinson's. RLS can significantly interfere with sleep, although it is not itself considered a SLEEP DISORDER.

DOPAMINE AGONIST MEDICATIONS such as PRAMIPEXOL (Mirapex), ROPINEROLE (Requip), or PERGOLIDE (Permax) are typically the first line agents used for this disorder. Other agents used include levodopa (Sinemet), muscle relaxants such as CLONAZEPAM (Klonopin) or TEMAZEPAM (Restoril), GABAPENTIN (Neurontin), clonidine, or opiates. Adjusting the ANTI-PARKINSON'S MEDICATIONS regimen is usually enough to end, or at least significantly reduce, the symptoms. In most peo-

ple who have restless leg syndrome, whether or not they have Parkinson's, symptoms tend to appear gradually over many years. Doctors do not know what causes RLS or why, even in people who do not have Parkinson's, it responds to treatment with dopaminergic medications (including, in people who do not have Parkinson's disease, LEVODOPA).

Restoril See TEMAZEPAM.

restraint A device, substance, or procedure that restricts a person's ability to move as desired. Restraints can be physical, such as LAP BUDDIES, geri-belts, posey jackets, and other items that fasten to a chair or bed to prevent the person from rising. Restraints also can be chemical, such as sedatives and ANTIPSYCHOTIC MEDICATIONS that reduce a person's interest in or capacity for movement. Generally, safety features such as bedrails are not considered restraints.

The use of restraints is controversial. No one likes the idea of a loved one's being "tied up" or otherwise restricted from movement. Restraints are most frequently used when a person has COGNITIVE IMPAIRMENT significant enough to interfere with judgment combined with physical limitations, and unsupervised mobility is likely to result in falls and injuries. State and federal regulations and guidelines strictly define appropriate use of restraints in hospitals and residential care settings such as LONG-TERM CARE FACILITIES and SKILLED NURSING FACILITIES (SNFs), and some states outlaw their use altogether.

Many facilities have internal policies and procedures for the use of restraints that are more explicit than state and federal laws and often provide examples as well as explanations for proper application of restraints. When considering a residential facility for a person with Parkinson's, ask about restraints and ask to see the facility's written policy documents. Also check whether residents appear to be restrained. Most facilities allow families to request that loved ones not be restrained. An open and frank discussion with the doctor and the facility's director can help family members to decide whether restraints are necessary to protect a loved one.

retinal cell implant An experimental procedure in which retinal pigment epithelial (RPE) cells, which produce DOPAMINE, are surgically implanted into the PUTAMEN, a structure of the BASAL GANGLIA. Once there, they "root" and begin producing dopamine in the BRAIN, helping to replace dopamine lost with the death of DOPAMINERGIC NEURONS that characterizes Parkinson's disease. The RPE cells are collected from donor eye tissue and then cultivated in the laboratory. Each implantation procedure requires about 350,000 RPE cells. In the very limited open-label studies done to date, people with Parkinson's who received the RPE implant had better motor function both on and after withholding medications and were able to reduce the amount of ANTI-PARKINSON'S MEDICATIONS necessary to control symptoms significantly though they still required LEVODOPA therapy. Much research remains necessary to determine whether retinal cell implant is a viable treatment option for Parkinson's disease.

See also ADRENAL MEDULLARY TRANSPLANT; FETAL DOPAMINERGIC CELL TRANSPLANT; FETAL PORCINE BRAIN CELL TRANSPLANT.

retirement Ending employment after meeting specified time-in-service and other requirements. There is no set retirement age, which varies among industries and employers. Some people retire with pensions and other benefits; others either are too young to qualify though they meet the organization's retirement criteria or have only SOCIAL SECURITY. Disability retirement follows different criteria and is generally health-related; people with Parkinson's who are otherwise not qualified to retire (too young or not employed long enough) often meet disability retirement qualifications when symptoms interfere with their ability to perform job tasks. However, in most situations federal and state laws prohibit employers from forcing a person to take disability retirement.

Early Retirement

People who have EARLY-ONSET PARKINSON'S often opt for early retirement, whereby they forfeit certain benefits but may collect other benefits. It is essential to know whether this forfeiture is temporary or permanent. A pension program that pays a reduced benefit for retirement before age 53, for example, when the age for full retirement is 58, may provide full benefits at age 58 or maintain them at the level in effect when the person retired at age 53. It often is best to consult a financial specialist to determine the true costs and value of these decisions.

Another key factor to consider with early retirement is medical insurance. A few pension programs award medical insurance coverage as part of the retirement benefit package, but most do not. Some allow the person to maintain medical insurance by paying the monthly premiums, which can be hefty. Most retirement programs do not offer medical insurance. Because MEDICARE qualification does not begin until age 65, early retirement can have serious implications for the person with Parkinson's disease whose health care needs will continue to grow.

Emotional Issues of Retirement

People who have worked all of their adult lives often have emotional attachments to their jobs, careers, and companies. They identify themselves with their work, and retirement ends this sense of self defined by career. Some people find it emotionally challenging to make this separation and may become depressed after retirement. If disability retirement or early retirement has been due to Parkinson's disease, the emotional challenges are intensified as the person may feel resentful about being "forced" into the decision. Having other activities to fill in the time—favorite hobbies, travel (if practical), all those chores and tasks put off until there was enough time to do them—can offset this reaction. It is important for family members to be understanding and supportive.

Financial Issues of Retirement

Few people who retire retain the same income level that they had when they were working. Pension programs may pay from 20 percent to 80 percent of the working salary, depending on the benefit structure. By retirement age most people have fewer financial responsibilities and have been anticipating retirement long enough to plan for the reduction in income. When a condition such as Parkinson's disease forces a change in plans, it is easy to minimize or ignore the potential financial challenges. The consequences can be devastating, however. FINANCIAL PLANNING is crucial.

See also AMERICANS WITH DISABILITIES ACT; ESTATE PLANNING; MEDICAL INSURANCE MEDICAID; MEDICARE.

retirement community A residential setting for people older than a certain age, usually age 50. Retirement communities have many different configurations. Some are homes converted to accommodate a small number of residents, some are large apartment buildings, some are smaller units such as fourplexes or duplexes, some are gated or secured communities of single-family houses, and some are large campuses that feature a combination of housing arrangements. Some such campuses include ASSISTED LIVING FACILITIES, SKILLED NURSING FACILITIES, and LONG-TERM CARE FACILITIES on the same property to provide what the industry refers to as a continuum of care.

Many retirement communities require that residents be fully independent: that is, capable of meeting their own personal care needs including transportation and functions such as shopping just as they would be if they were living alone anywhere else. Generally there is a higher level of security, and there are staff available to perform necessary maintenance and upkeep tasks, and sometimes to provide extra services such as grocery shopping. Some retirement communities, particularly those that are like apartment buildings, provide amenities such as community dining rooms that serve at least one meal a day, recreational facilities, computer rooms, and planned events ranging from day outings to vacation cruises. Full-service retirement communities may also provide meals, laundry services, and housekeeping services. The cost of living in a retirement community varies widely but generally is correlated with the level of services provided.

For the person with Parkinson's, moving to a retirement community often is an interim step between totally independent living and assisted living. The person feels more secure and comfortable in a more protected environment, and family members are reassured to know that there are people to check

on their loved one to make sure all is well. Spouses may live together, and in many retirement communities so too may unmarried partners. For all intents and purposes, there is little difference in many settings between the retirement community and independent living, aside from the age requirement.

Retirement communities that belong to an umbrella of residential services are becoming increasingly popular as the American population ages. Although the person must move from one facility to another when care needs change, the facilities are usually on the same campus and the person can maintain friendships and contacts as well as a sense of continuity of procedures. The advantage of these arrangements is that once a person moves into the retirement community, he or she is assured of availability in any of the other facilities should the need arise. As Parkinson's disease can shift course suddenly, this is a significant advantage for the person with Parkinson's as well as for family members.

It is important to take a full tour of the community before making any decisions or paying any fees and to visit several times unannounced. Such visits give a feel for the overall environment and the consistency of staff and procedures. Determine the community's accreditations, certifications, licensure, and other credentials and check with the local Better Business Bureau and other resources to see whether there is an unusual number of complaints about the community. Know exactly which services are included in the regular fees and charges and which services cost extra. As with other planning related to Parkinson's disease, considering retirement communities several years before anticipating a move is prudent. Many retirement communities have waiting lists.

See also ADJUSTING TO LIVING WITH PARKINSON'S; CARE MANAGEMENT AND PLANNING; COPING WITH ONGOING CARE OF PARKINSON'S; ESTATE PLANNING; INDEPENDENCE; PLANNING FOR THE FUTURE.

retropulsion See GAIT DISTURBANCE.

righting reflex See POSTURAL RIGHTING REFLEX.

rigidity An increase in muscle tone that causes resistance to passive movement. Rigidity is a cardinal sign of Parkinson's disease, typically manifested first as COGWHEELING or LEAD PIPE RESISTANCE. These manifestations are apparent to the physician during passive manipulation of the structures around a joint, most notably the wrists and ankles. In cogwheeling the foot or hand moves as though along a notched wheel, with hesitation and then sudden release. In lead pipe resistance, the rigidity is constant rather than intermittent. Most neurologists recognize cogwheeling as really just a sign of tremor, but lead pipe rigidity is recognized as a separate cardinal sign of parkinsonism. Rigidity is distinct from spasticity (a "clasp-knife" like catch on rapid passive movements) that is the form of stiffness associated with most strokes or other injuries to the brain or spinal cord that affect motor function. Rigidity expands to involve more muscle groups as Parkinson's progresses and can reach a point at which it prevents use of the muscles, such as in the leg or arm. The person with Parkinson's disease perceives rigidity as stiffness, and it causes the same kind of aching and discomfort as would holding an arm or leg in a contracted position. Rigidity results from a shortening of the muscle fibers in response to the continuous signals from the brain that cause them to stay contracted.

ANTI-PARKINSON'S MEDICATIONS that restore neuron communication in the structures of the BRAIN that regulate movement help to ease rigidity by slowing nerve signals for contraction and allowing nerve signals that instruct the muscles to relax to pass. For the duration of the medication's effectiveness, motor function can be near-normal in the early to middle stages of Parkinson's. In later stages anti-Parkinson's medications have difficulty in fully restoring neuron communication so rigidity tends to persist at a low to moderate level. This condition contributes to the stooped, closed posture that characterizes Parkinson's disease. As medications become less effective, rigidity causes episodes of AKINESIA or freezing, in which muscles remain so tightly contracted that they do not respond for movement. This contraction can cause abnormal and uncomfortable positions, such as "clawing" of a hand, that become permanent deformities. Rigidity accounts for one of Parkinson's more distressing symptoms, the lack of facial expression (HYPOMIMIA).

Surgical treatments such as DEEP BRAIN STIMULATION (DBS) or PALLIDOTOMY sometimes provide relief when anti-Parkinson's medications no longer do so. Because of their invasive nature these treatments have significant risks including infection and neurologic and neuropsychiatric side effects from disruption of the target and nearby structures. THALAMOTOMY, another surgical procedure, is effective in reducing TREMORS but not rigidity.

See also ABLATION; DYSTONIA; LESION; TREATMENT ALGORITHM.

risk factors for Parkinson's   Circumstances or events that influence a person's probability of development of Parkinson's disease. Researchers believe that numerous and varied factors interact to cause Parkinson's and that there are not a few key identifiable factors. Risk factors are either fixed or mutable. Fixed risk factors, such as age and genetic characteristics, cannot be changed. Mutable risk factors, such as exposure to environmental toxins, can be modified.

RISK FACTORS FOR PARKINSON'S DISEASE	
Fixed Risk Factors (Unchangeable)	**Mutable Risk Factors (Changeable)**
Age	Exposure to chemical toxins (pesticides herbicides, cleaning solutions)
Genetic mutations	Exposure to drugs that cause Parkinson's-like mutations damage and symptoms (MPTP, antipsychotic medications, illicit hallucinogens)
Family history	
Alzheimer's disease	Excessive oxidation (poor nutrition)

Fixed Risk Factors

The most significant risk factor for Parkinson's is age; more than 80 percent of people who have Parkinson's are older than age 60, which scientists attribute to possible dysfunction involving APOPTOSIS, the normal process by which cells in the body die. Research has established that the healthy adult BRAIN loses about 10 percent of its DOPAMINERGIC NEURONS through apoptosis each decade of life, beginning at age 40. Symptoms of Parkinson's disease become apparent when 80 percent of these neurons have died, indicating that under normal aging circumstances, few people would live long enough to experience Parkinson's disease solely as a process of aging.

Genetic research has isolated a number of chromosomes that are linked to Parkinson's, as well as several specific GENES. Genetic damage can be spontaneous, implicating interaction with environmental factors, or familial, reflecting hereditary mutations (mutations passed through family lines). Family history is a suspected risk factor when more than two close relatives (grandparents, aunts, uncles) have Parkinson's. EARLY-ONSET PARKINSON'S is more likely to have genetic components, although it is not clear whether the damage is spontaneous or hereditary.

Mutable Risk Factors

Also implicated as risk factors are exposure to environmental toxins that damage NEURONS in the BRAIN and the deleterious effects of normal cell metabolism. People who live and work where pesticide and herbicide use is high, as in farming communities, are more likely to develop Parkinson's than people who live in areas where these toxins are uncommon. People who are avid hobbyist gardeners also have an increased risk for Parkinson's, which scientists attribute to insecticide and herbicide exposure as well.

Illicit hallucinogenic drugs such as Ecstasy may be linked to Parkinson's, as is the illicit narcotic 1-METHYL-4-PHENYL-1,2,3,6-TETRAHYDROPYRIDINE (MPTP), a synthetic form of heroin that was popular in the 1980s and occasionally surfaces today among drug users. Legal drugs such as antipsychotics, some antiemetics, and the antihypertensive medication reserpine also can cause Parkinson's-like symptoms and DRUG-INDUCED PARKINSON'S disease. Stopping the drug sometimes allows the brain to recover with minimal residual damage; however, often the damage is permanent, as is almost always the case with MPTP. Eliminating exposure to the causative factor can prevent further damage, although scientists are uncertain at what point damage to neurons sets in motion an irreversible sequence of events that results in Parkinson's disease.

Scientific attention has recently been focused on metabolic damage to DOPAMINERGIC NEURONS by OXIDATION. A normal aspect of cell metabolism is waste production; when the body is healthy, it also produces substances (ANTIOXIDANTS) to "clean up" such waste to prevent it from accumulating to damaging levels. When antioxidant activity is inadequate, the free radicals that form during oxidation (molecules that have no specific function and attract themselves to other molecules at random) can interfere with normal cell functions and ultimately cause cell damage and death. Although many people believe taking antioxidant supplements helps to offset this process, current research supports a beneficial antioxidant effect primarily from natural antioxidants such as occur in fruits, vegetables, and whole grains. Most researchers consider appropriate nutrition is more effective in reducing oxidation damage.

Reducing Risk Factors

The multiplicity and intertwining nature of the causes of Parkinson's make it difficult to eliminate risk altogether. The most prudent approach is to eliminate or reduce those risks that are within control, such as exposure to chemicals. Good nutrition and maintenance of overall good health, including regular physical activity, help the body to accommodate oxidation. These efforts are particularly important when fixed risk factors such as family history are present. Most people do not know whether they have gene mutations that place them at increased risk for Parkinson's; at present gene testing is both costly and of uncertain value as researchers do not fully understand the correlation between genetic damage and Parkinson's disease.

See also CHROMOSOMES LINKED TO PARKINSON'S; GENE MAPPING; GENE MUTATIONS; GENETIC PREDISPOSITION; PARKINSON'S DISEASE, CAUSES OF.

rivastigmine An ACETYLCHOLINESTERASE INHIBITOR MEDICATION (brand name Exelon) that prevents the action of the enzyme ACETYLCHOLINESTERASE from metabolizing ACETYLCHOLINE, a NEUROTRANSMITTER in the BRAIN that is key to COGNITIVE FUNCTION. This drug is approved in the United States for treating the DEMENTIA of ALZHEIMER'S DISEASE. Doctors sometimes prescribe it to treat dementia in Parkinson's disease as well, and there are randomized controlled studies that support its usefulness for dementia in Parkinson's disease, including its safety in not worsening motor symptoms. Rivastigmine is the acetylcholinesterase inhibitor of first choice for most Parkinson's experts. Not all people with dementia who take rivastigmine experience improved cognitive function, and so far there is no way to assess who is likely to benefit. Side effects are uncommon, but when they occur they can include nausea, diarrhea, headache, DIZZINESS, and SLEEP DISTURBANCES.

See also COGNITIVE IMPAIRMENT; DONEPEZIL; GALANTAMINE; NEUROCHEMISTRY; OPEN-LABEL DRUGS; TACRINE.

rocking Intentional side-to-side movement that sometimes helps a person with Parkinson's break free of akinetic (freezing) episodes during walking and other movements such as when changing from sitting to standing or getting out of bed. Freezing occurs in the middle to late stages of Parkinson's as BRAIN DOPAMINE levels become significantly depleted and nerve signals to the muscles become increasingly erratic. The movement of side-to-side rocking stimulates different muscle fibers from those involved in forward movement, activating different nerve signals that can at least get the muscles moving. Once this happens, it seems to free the blockage of signals and movement resumes. Rocking also gives the person a different conscious focus, which helps to relieve anxiety about freezing.

Scientists believe there are connections between neuromuscular symptoms such as AKINESIA (freezing) and BRADYKINESIA (slowed muscle response) and PROPRIOCEPTION, the body's system for maintaining its spatial orientation. Proprioception relies on intricate interplays among visual cues, balance signals, muscle actions and reactions, and brain patterning of movement sequences. Researchers believe that a combination of dopamine depletion and a function of Parkinson's disease causes disruptions such as freezing and start hesitation. Rocking and other rhythmic movements alter the patterns and sequence of interplays, helping to restore more normal neurocommunication pathways.

In akinetic episodes that occur during walking, shifting the body's weight from one leg to the other initiates the rocking movement. During sitting or getting out of bed, moving the knees from side to side accomplishes the same effect.

See also GAIT; GAIT DISTURBANCE.

ropinirole A DOPAMINE AGONIST MEDICATION that binds with DOPAMINE RECEPTORS in the BRAIN, simulating the NEUROTRANSMITTER actions of DOPAMINE. Because ropinirole (Requip) is selective for D2 receptors, its use minimizes some of the undesired side effects such as nausea that occur with ergot-derived dopamine agonists such as BROMOCRIPTINE (Parlodel) or pergolide (Permax) that bind unselectively. It is even slightly more selective than pramipexole (Mirapex) and may carry a bit lower risk of daytime somnolence. Ropinerole is less potent and shorter lived in the bloodstream than the other two commonly used agonists in the United States (pergolide and pramipexole), but it joins pramipexole in showing some evidence that it may be neuroprotective, delaying the progression of dopaminergic neuronal loss in Parkinson's disease. Ropinirole is sometimes effective as MONOTHERAPY in early Parkinson's and can postpone the need for LEVODOPA therapy for up to three years. Ropinirole is one of the ADJUNCT THERAPIES used in late Parkinson's disease, when it extends the availability of dopamine and can allow the levodopa dosage to be reduced.

Ropinirole also is sometimes taken as an OPEN-LABEL DRUG to relieve RESTLESS LEG SYNDROME (RLS), a condition in which the legs feel as if they must move. RLS is a common cause of SLEEP DISTURBANCES in people with Parkinson's but also afflicts people who do not have the disease. Headache, DIZZINESS, and drowsiness are ropinirole's primary potential side effects.

See also ERGOT-DERIVED MEDICATIONS.

Sacks, Oliver A neurologist who attracted public attention through his book *Awakenings,* which told of a group of people, patients at Beth Abraham Hospital in New York City in the mid-1960s, who "awakened" from decades-long inability to move after Sacks gave them LEVODOPA. When Sacks examined these patients, he discovered they had all contracted a form of encephalitis, commonly called sleepy sickness, that swept through North America and Europe in the 1920s. Because of his experience as a neurologist treating people with Parkinson's disease, Sacks believed these patients, too, were suffering from a form of Parkinson's as a complication of the encephalitis.

The drug levodopa had just become available, and Sacks administered it to these patients, who immediately responded, giving the impression of "awakening" from the immobility that had contained them. The experience prompted medical recognition of postencephalitic PARKINSONISM, which Sacks wrote about in articles published in medical journals before publishing the book *Awakenings* in 1973. When in 1990, the book was made into a fictionalized account in the movie of the same title, starring Robin Williams and Robert De Niro, it drew widespread public attention to Parkinson's disease.

schizophrenia A form of PSYCHOSIS, a psychiatric illness, in which the person experiences DELUSIONS and HALLUCINATIONS, usually auditory (hearing voices), severe enough to interfere with everyday living. Disturbance of thought patterns and other COGNITIVE IMPAIRMENT also occur. The so-called negative symptoms of social withdrawal are sometimes the most debilitating. Schizophrenia, as do other psychotic disorders, occurs when there is an imbalance of brain NEUROTRANSMIT-TERS. Scientists speculate that an excess of DOPAMINE or a heightened sensitivity to dopamine, and perhaps other neurotransmitters, occurs in some areas of the brain.

ANTIPSYCHOTIC MEDICATIONS such as HALOPERIDOL (Haldol), CHLORPROMAZINE (Thorazine), and PERPHENAZINE (Trilafon) are dopamine antagonists; they suppress the symptoms of schizophrenia by blocking the action of dopamine. Newer drugs such as risperidone (Risperdal) have less dopamine antagonist action but also block the action of SEROTONIN, a brain neurotransmitter associated with MOOD, DEPRESSION, and ANXIETY. Symptoms generally improve with medication, although treatment often is long-term. PARANOIA (misperceptions that others want to hurt the person in some way) is common in schizophrenia and often causes people to refuse to take medications.

The dopamine antagonist action of antipsychotic medications often causes Parkinson's-like symptoms such as BRADYKINESIA (slowed muscle response and movement), rigidity, tremor, and AKINESIA ("freezing" episodes). These symptoms can be quite severe and occasionally are permanent, although often they cease when the person stops taking the antipsychotic medication. Quetiapine (Seroquel), clozapine (Clozaril), and aripiprazole (Abilify) have a more partial dopamine agonist activity, making them safer choices to avoid these Parkinson's-like side effects. Neurologists sometimes use antipsychotic medications to produce such side effects in NEURODEGENERATIVE diseases that cause hyperactive muscle activity, such as HUNTINGTON'S DISEASE. Among the first questions a doctor should ask when evaluating a person for possible Parkinson's disease is whether he or she is taking, or has taken, antipsychotic medications.

Doctors also prescribe antipsychotics to treat the aberrant behaviors of people with DEMENTIA such as can occur with ALZHEIMER'S DISEASE. However, even when symptoms of dementia are present, people who have Parkinson's disease should only take those atypical antipsychotics least likely to exacerbate the Parkinson's symptoms, although even they have some risk of worsening motor function. Psychotic behavior develops in about 20 to 25 percent of people who have Parkinson's disease, likely as a consequence of disturbances in the sensitivity of brain NEURONS to dopamine.

See also NEUROPSYCHIATRY; PSYCHOTHERAPY.

Schwab and England scale of capacity for daily living   See ACTIVITIES OF DAILY LIVING.

sebaceous dermatitis   See DERMATITIS, SEBACEOUS.

second opinion   A neurological examination by a second physician or by a movement disorder specialist obtained to confirm the findings and diagnosis of the original examination. Seeking a second opinion is a good idea when there is any question about the diagnosis, as in EARLY-ONSET PARKINSON'S or when symptoms are atypical. Most MEDICAL INSURANCE plans pay for second opinion consultations. People sometimes worry that the original physician will be offended by their seeking a second opinion, but this is a very common practice and most doctors are supportive if not encouraging of second opinions and may in fact themselves suggest them. DIAGNOSING PARKINSON'S can be a challenge as there are no definitive BIOMARKERS to assure that the diagnosis is correct. About 20 percent to 25 percent of people receive an incorrect initial diagnosis, which can delay appropriate treatment.

For a second opinion consultation, the physician should be a specialist, preferably a NEUROLOGIST specializing either in Parkinson's disease or in MOVEMENT DISORDERS. Take copies of all test and diagnostic procedures to the appointment for the second physician to review and evaluate. It is not usually necessary to repeat diagnostic tests unless the findings are questionable or inconsistent, although the second physician may want additional tests especially if clinical evidence to support

a diagnosis is scant. The second physician should perform a comprehensive NEUROLOGICAL EXAMINATION just as the first physician did, rather than relying on medical records and the first physician's assessment, although it is reasonable for the second physician to conduct this exam differently as often there are various methods for obtaining the same assessments.

If the two physicians differ sharply in their respective diagnoses it may be necessary to obtain additional opinions. This does not happen often but it does occur, especially when the symptoms are uncharacteristic, the person is younger than is typical in Parkinson's disease (younger than age 50), or another condition such as ALZHEIMER'S DISEASE also is present. Denial is a significant factor in any chronic, degenerative disease. Consultation of doctor after doctor, particularly when findings are similar, may be an indication of denial. Most medical insurance companies refuse to pay for multiple consultations unless the physician can present evidence that such consultations are medically necessary: that is, that each doctor is providing a unique aspect of care for the person.

See also CONDITIONS SIMILAR TO PARKINSON'S; COPING WITH DIAGNOSIS OF PARKINSON'S; DENIAL AND ACCEPTANCE; DOCTOR VISITS; MEDICAL MANAGEMENT.

secondary symptoms   Problems and symptoms that develop as consequences of the primary, or cardinal, symptoms of PARKINSON'S DISEASE. MICROGRAPHIA (small, cramped handwriting), for example, develops as a consequence of damage to fine motor control in the hands. Vision problems develop because Parkinson's symptoms affect the muscles controlling movements of the eyes. CONSTIPATION develops as a consequence of slowed muscle response in the gastrointestinal tract. Strictly speaking, all symptoms beyond the four CARDINAL SYMPTOMS—resting tremor, BRADYKINESIA, RIGIDITY, and POSTURAL INSTABILITY—are considered secondary.

This does not mean they are less significant; in fact, secondary symptoms often are more frustrating to people with Parkinson's because they are the symptoms that interfere with the small details of everyday living. Treating Parkinson's disease's cardinal symptoms also reduces or eliminates secondary symptoms, but treating secondary symptoms has little, if any, effect on cardinal symptoms. As Parkinson's progresses, it becomes necessary to use ADJUNCT THERAPIES to treat secondary symptoms, mainly because ANTI-PARKINSON'S MEDICATIONS are no longer able to keep cardinal symptoms in check.

See also BRADYPHRENIA; DAILY LIVING CHALLENGES; DIAGNOSING PARKINSON'S; DYSPHAGIA; GASTRIC MOTILITY; TREATMENT ALGORITHM.

selective serotonin reuptake inhibitor (SSRI) medications A classification of ANTIDEPRESSANT MEDICATIONS that work by delaying the reuptake, or reabsorption, of serotonin, a BRAIN NEUROTRANSMITTER essential to MOOD. These drugs are considered "selective" because they block only the reabsorption of serotonin, extending its presence and activity without directly altering the functions of other brain neurotransmitters. Because of this, SSRIs typically are the drugs of first choice prescribed to relieve DEPRESSION in people with Parkinson's as other antidepressants such as tricyclics (amitriptyline, imipramine) and MONOAMINE OXIDASE INHIBITORS (MAOIs) affect the actions of other brain neurotransmitters including DOPAMINE.

Depression is common in people with Parkinson's, affecting as many as four in 10 who have the disease (many clinicians believe the number to be much higher, as many as seven in 10). The reasons for this are not entirely clear. Depression has multiple biochemical, emotional, and psychosocial components and is a common companion of many degenerative, progressive, and incurable diseases. Some researchers believe depression is an early sign of Parkinson's, which develops in response to the fluctuating brain DOPAMINE levels that occur in the earliest stages of Parkinson's and in some people even before other symptoms are apparent. In the SUBSTANTIA NIGRA and other structures of the BASAL GANGLIA, dopamine conducts nerve signals related to voluntary muscle control and movement. In the CEREBRUM and parts of the BRAIN other than those involved in movement, dopamine facilitates neuron communication related to mood, emotion, and pleasure (and is believed a key player

in addiction). Researchers suspect the diminishing dopamine levels characteristic of Parkinson's affect function and activity throughout the brain, though the primary consequences are focused in the substantia nigra and the basal ganglia. As well, the declining dopamine levels affect the overall balance of neurotransmitters in the brain, thus altering the way each of them functions.

SSRIs became available in the 1980s; the first to debut was fluoxetine, better known by its trade name Prozac. For most people SSRIs cause fewer side effects than other antidepressants such as tricyclics and MAOIs and they are usually the antidepressants of choice for people with Parkinson's as they have fewer interactions with ANTI-PARKINSON'S MEDICATIONS. Commonly prescribed SSRIs include:

- Fluoxetine (Prozac)
- Paroxetine (Paxil)
- Fluvoxamine (Luvox)
- Sertraline (Zoloft)
- Citalopram (Celexa)

Although the SSRIs generally are considered therapeutically equivalent to one another, each medication has a different chemical formulation and method of action within the body and brain. For this reason, people respond differently to the SSRIs. If one SSRI does not relieve depression, another may. Side effects of SSRIs, which are generally mild, include NAUSEA, CONSTIPATION, weight loss, ANXIETY, and SEXUAL DYSFUNCTION. Often these side effects end after the medication is taken for six to eight weeks; if they do not, another SSRI may be equally effective and not produce the side effects. As many people who have Parkinson's have these symptoms as a function of the disease process, determining their causes can be difficult.

Because SSRIs have relatively long half-lives, they remain at high enough levels in the blood to exert a serotonin reuptake inhibitory effect for as long as several days after a dose. A rare but serious complication of SSRIs is serotonin syndrome, in which an excess of serotonin accumulates in the brain. This occurs most often in people who are taking other antidepressants (including over-the-counter products such as St.-John's-wort) that also extend the activity of serotonin. Symptoms of serotonin syndrome include CONFUSION, DISORIENTATION, MYOCLONUS (involuntary muscle contractions), TREMORS, RIGIDITY, rapid heartbeat, excessive sweating (diaphoresis), and high fever. These symptoms require immediate medical evaluation.

It is important to stop taking any other antidepressant at least 14 days before starting an SSRI. It also is important to tape the dose gradually (over two weeks) when stopping an SSRI at the high end of its therapeutic range, to give the brain's biochemistry opportunity to adjust to the drug's withdrawal. Although SSRIs are the least likely of the antidepressants to interact with anti-Parkinson's medications, they can intensify the effects of LEVODOPA, the cornerstone of PHARMACOTHERAPY for Parkinson's disease, causing symptoms such as DYSTONIA (extreme rigidity) and CHOREIOFORM DYSKINESIA (involuntary, dancelike movements). The SSRI that seems most likely to do this is fluoxetine. Because these side effects can appear even after the SSRI has been taken for some time, associating their occurrence with the SSRI sometimes is difficult.

See also COPING WITH ONGOING CARE OF PARKINSON'S; ELECTROCONVULSIVE THERAPY; MEDICATION MANAGEMENT; MEDICATION SIDE EFFECTS; NEUROPSYCHIATRY; TRICYCLIC ANTIDEPRESSANTS.

selegiline A selective monoamine oxidase-B inhibitor (MAOI-B) medication prescribed for people with Parkinson's disease to extend the activity and presence of DOPAMINE in the BRAIN. Selegiline is called selective because it specifically blocks the action of MONOAMINE OXIDASE-B, an ENZYME that participates in metabolism of the MONOAMINE NEUROTRANSMITTERS ACETYLCHOLINE and DOPAMINE. Other MONOAMINE OXIDASE INHIBITORS (MAOIs), taken primarily as antidepressants, nonselectively block metabolism of the other monoamine neurotransmitters epinephrine, NOREPINEPHRINE, and SEROTONIN as well; this action produces their antidepressant effects but also their potentially serious side effects. Nonselective MAOIs can allow dangerously high levels of epinephrine and the amino acid TYRAMINE to

accumulate, causing jumps in blood pressure and irregularities in heart rhythm.

Selegiline, as the then-new brand name drug Deprenyl, drew attention within the Parkinson's community in the 1980s when doctors noticed that it seemed to improve the symptoms of Parkinson's disease without creating many of the adverse effects (such as extensive food interactions and the risk of dangerous spikes in blood pressure) typical of nonselective MAOIs. A major study conducted from 1987 to 1992 called the DATATOP (Deprenyl and Tocopherol Antioxidative Therapy for Parkinson's Disease) study showed that selegiline could postpone the need for LEVODOPA therapy in DE NOVO PARKINSON'S DISEASE (disease in people who had not yet received treatment) for up to three years, raising interest in its potential for NEUROPROTECTIVE THERAPY. However, clinical use in the more than a decade since the study ended has not borne out this idea conclusively, and neurologists remain divided on the existence of selegiline's NEUROPROTECTIVE EFFECTS. The current consensus is that selegiline is of mild benefit in reducing the symptoms of Parkinson's, but it does not have any clear evidence of a neuroprotective effect.

Although selegiline is effective as MONOTHERAPY for some people who have early Parkinson's, the drug does not appear to delay the disease's progression. Rather, it seems to have a mild to moderate dopamine agonist action, binding with DOPAMINE RECEPTORS in brain NEURONS. This action, combined with its capacity to inhibit monoamine oxidase-B and delay metabolism of dopamine, allows selegiline to relieve Parkinson's motor symptoms while dopamine depletion in the brain is still mild. In later stages of Parkinson's, selegiline sometimes is effective as one of the ADJUNCT THERAPIES used to boost the effectiveness of levodopa.

The list of medications that potentially interact with selegiline, as with other MAOIs, is extensive. It includes any other antidepressant medications such as tricyclics (amitriptyline, imipramine), SSRIs (fluoxetine, paroxetine), and other MAOIs (phenelzine, isocarboxazid, tranylcypromine). Mild to moderate side effects are common: nausea, constipation, dry mouth (anticholinergic effects), DIZZINESS, headache, vivid dreams, and HALLUCINATIONS, among many others.

Because of its action on both acetylcholine and dopamine, selegiline occasionally worsens, rather than improves, the motor symptoms of Parkinson's, especially TREMORS and BRADYKINESIA (slowed muscle response and movement). It also can cause DYSTONIA (extreme rigidity). In a person who has Parkinson's, determining whether these symptoms are side effects of the selegiline or indicate progression of the disease can be difficult, particularly as side effects of selegiline do not always occur immediately. Because selegiline has negligible action on norepinephrine, epinephrine, and tyrosine, there are no restrictions on medications containing tyrosine when taking selegiline as there are when taking nonselective MAOIs.

There have been serious and some fatal interactions between selegiline and the narcotic pain relief medication meperidine (Demerol), and both drugs carry warnings not to use them at the same time. Doctors commonly administer meperidine by injection for moderate to severe pain after surgery or serious injuries such as fractures. The greatest risk for unintentionally combining selegiline and meperidine occurs during emergency treatment for injuries. The person who has Parkinson's should carry a list of the medications he or she is currently taking, as many ANTI-PARKINSON'S MEDICATIONS interact with other drugs as well.

See also MEDICATION MANAGEMENT; MEDICATION SIDE EFFECTS; MONOAMINE OXIDASE; MONOAMINE OXIDASE GENE.

self-care techniques Nonclinical methods to maintain or improve overall health and well-being to moderate the effects of the symptoms of PARKINSON'S DISEASE, and to retain as much INDEPENDENCE as possible. Self-care techniques include good NUTRITION AND DIET, regular physical EXERCISE AND ACTIVITY, regular RANGE OF MOTION EXERCISES, participation in functions and events that give them JOY and a sense of satisfaction about living, and centering and relaxation methods such as MEDITATION and YOGA. People with Parkinson's who engage in self-care techniques generally feel that they are more in control of their lives and consequently enjoy their lives more.

See also ADJUSTING TO LIVING WITH PARKINSON'S; DENIAL AND ACCEPTANCE; MINDFULNESS; OPTIMISM; QUALITY OF LIFE; STRESS REDUCTION TECHNIQUES.

self-esteem A person's perception of his or her value, capabilities, and contributions in life. Self-esteem can suffer when a person has a NEURODE-GENERATIVE disease such as Parkinson's. The physical changes the disease causes lead to altered appearance, reduced mobility, diminished physical dexterity, and decreased independence. Other people react to these changes in ways that are not always consistent with what the changes actually signify and without understanding that the person with Parkinson's remains who he or she has always been despite outward appearances. The person with Parkinson's often must become recentered in his or her sense of self to accommodate these reactions—not just once, but numerous times during the course of the disease as symptoms progress and cause other lifestyle changes. This recentering is particularly necessary for people who are younger than most people who have the disease at the time of diagnosis and may still be employed. Much of an individual's sense of identity is derived through job and occupation; loss of that connection can threaten self-esteem.

As well, partnerships with spouses or significant others shift, changing the dynamic of such relationships. This change can cause confusion and disorientation for all involved as roles and responsibilities become rearranged. Although actions such as taking over tasks such as driving, SHOPPING, and managing the finances seem matters of practicality to other family members, to the person with Parkinson's these moves represent losses that affect his or her value in the household and the family.

Family and friends can help and support the person with Parkinson's by focusing on each day's positives and by looking for innovative ways to nurture and encourage independence. Strong self-esteem is important in giving the person with Parkinson's the ability to draw from inner reserves to cope with the challenges of the disease. Maintaining self-esteem can be one of the more difficult aspects of coping with the continually changing landscape of Parkinson's as symptoms progress.

Staying active and engaged in daily living, participating in chores and household functions, and maintaining FRIENDSHIPS and FAMILY RELATIONSHIPS (such as outings and visits with children and grandchildren) are ways to foster a sense of self-value.

See also ADJUSTING TO LIVING WITH PARKINSON'S; BODY IMAGE; COMPASSION; COPING WITH ONGOING CARE OF PARKINSON'S; EMPATHY; MARRIAGE RELATIONSHIP; QUALITY OF LIFE.

sertraline   An ANTIDEPRESSANT MEDICATION that is a SELECTIVE SEROTONIN REUPTAKE INHIBITOR (SSRI). Although, as do other SSRIs, sertraline (Zoloft) has a unique chemical formulation, it acts in the brain to extend the availability of SEROTONIN by preventing its reuptake (reabsorption) after it is released. Sertraline has minimal effect on other brain NEUROTRANSMITTERS. Sertraline is more likely than other SSRIs to cause SEXUAL DYSFUNCTION (delayed ejaculation in men and reduced libido, or interest in sex, in both men and women) as a side effect. Other common side effects include NAUSEA, diarrhea, DIZZINESS, and headache. These problems, when they do occur, generally go away within eight weeks after starting treatment with sertraline.

People with Parkinson's who are taking SELEGILINE, a selective MONOAMINE OXIDASE-B INHIBITOR (MAOI-B), should not take sertraline or any other SSRI at the same time, as serious interactions can occur between these two kinds of drugs. People who are taking MONOAMINE OXIDASE INHIBITOR (MAOI) antidepressants also should not take sertraline or other SSRIs; people who have Parkinson's disease seldom take MAOI antidepressants as there are significant interactions between them and ANTI-PARKINSON'S MEDICATIONS.

See also ANXIETY; DEPRESSION; ELECTROCONVULSIVE THERAPY; PSYCHOTHERAPY; TRICYCLIC ANTIDEPRESSANTS.

sexual dysfunction   Difficulty in enjoying a satisfying sexual relationship that develops as a result of Parkinson's disease or the medications taken to treat symptoms. The physical symptoms of Parkinson's such as TREMORS and BRADYKINESIA make movement and coordination difficult during sexual activity just as during walking. Many of the

ANTI-PARKINSON'S MEDICATIONS affect smooth muscle function, which in turn affects sexual response in both men and women. Levodopa can induce dyskinesias that make the coordinated movements of sexual activity difficult. As well, emotional factors related to sexuality can result in sexual dysfunction.

Disruptions of nerve signals to smooth muscle tissue affect the ability of the penis to become erect, causing ERECTILE DYSFUNCTION and delayed ejaculation in men. As well, factors of aging contribute to erectile difficulties. High blood pressure and diabetes, two medical conditions that become more common as people become older, can damage the tiny blood vessels, slowing the response of nerves in the penis and the flow of blood that creates an erection. Medications, such as some ANTI-PARKINSON'S MEDICATIONS and ANTIDEPRESSANT MEDICATIONS, can further contribute to erectile dysfunction by slowing the physiological processes that result in a man's sexual arousal. These same kinds of problems—impaired circulation and nerve function, and medication side effects—can cause difficulty with sexual response in women as well, interfering with the physiological processes of arousal and orgasm.

Certain dopamine receptors in the brain, most notably D1 receptors, play a role in perception of pleasure and in sexual desire. As DOPAMINE levels in the brain decline, there is less dopamine present to bind with dopamine receptors. Although the most significant effect occurs on the D2 and D3 receptors that facilitate neuron communication related to movement, all dopamine receptors feel the effect. Ergot-derived DOPAMINE AGONIST MEDICATIONS, such as BROMOCRIPTINE (Parlodel) and PERGOLIDE (Permax), taken to provide dopamine-like stimulation in the brain sometimes produce a mild to moderate increase in libido in both men and women by increasing the activation of D1 receptors as well as suppressing the pituitary gland's production of prolactin, a hormone associated with lactation in women and sex drive in both men and women. Lowering the body's prolactin level increases sex drive.

Sexual dysfunction affects perhaps 60 percent or more of people who have Parkinson's, men and women alike. Many are reluctant to discuss this problem with their doctors, either because they feel embarrassed or because they consider it unimportant as a medical disorder. Improving sexual response and function could be as simple as changing the anti-Parkinson medication regimen, however, or adjusting dosages of other medications that are known to contribute to sexual dysfunction such as antidepressants and antihypertensive drugs taken for high blood pressure. As well, the medication SILDENAFIL, better known as Viagra, can significantly improve a man's ability to have and maintain erections.

See also BODY IMAGE; INTIMACY; MARRIAGE RELATIONSHIP; QUALITY OF LIFE; SEXUALITY.

sexuality   Sexuality is an important aspect of human existence and of intimacy in adult relationships. Its importance does not change with a diagnosis of Parkinson's disease, although the ways in which a couple deals with their needs for INTIMACY often do. Changes in body appearance that take place as Parkinson's disease progresses sometimes cause people to feel embarrassed and insecure about whether they remain sexually attractive to their partner. Sometimes the healthy partner is reluctant to initiate sexual encounters or to discuss matters of sexuality; such reluctance can create even greater self-doubt in the partner who has Parkinson's. Partners need to be reassuring and loving to each other and to enjoy physical closeness in ways they are capable of and feel comfortable with using. It is important for partners to maintain open and honest dialogue about concerns that are fundamental to their relationship.

Issues related to interest in sex, such as diminished libido, often have both physical and emotional components. Neuromuscular symptoms such as TREMORS and BRADYKINESIA can make the physical act of sexual intercourse more difficult. The disease takes a toll on the stamina and energy level of the person with Parkinson's, and by bedtime when couples typically engage in sexual activity, he or she is physically exhausted and cannot participate. Just as the body often does not cooperate when a person is walking across the kitchen or navigating through the living room, it can balk during the physical activity of lovemaking. Partners

may find that the "right time" is any time that happens to be right for both of them, which is not necessarily related to the clock or to previous habits. PATIENCE, HUMOR, and innovation are key to a continuing, mutually satisfying sexual relationship between partners.

See also BODY IMAGE; MARRIAGE RELATIONSHIP; SELF-ESTEEM; SEXUAL DYSFUNCTION.

shaking palsy   The name physician James Parkinson, who was the first to identify the disease that now bears his name, gave to the symptoms he described in his 1817 paper "Essay on the Shaking Palsy," which presented the first published case studies of Parkinson's disease. *Shaking* refers to the TREMORS that characterize Parkinson's disease. *Palsy* is an archaic term for paralysis, a reference to the BRADYKINESIA (slowed muscle response and movement) and AKINESIA (lack of muscle response and movement) that are hallmark symptoms of Parkinson's disease. At the time Parkinson published his observations, there were no treatments for the disease so its course was rapidly debilitating and inevitably fatal.

See also PARALYSIS AGITANS; PARKINSON, JAMES.

shoes   Without a conscious focus on lifting the feet, the person who has Parkinson's disease tends to shuffle his or her feet along the floor or walking surface. Shoes with a sticky type of sole, such as crepe, become tripping hazards as they grip the surface and then release suddenly. Jogging shoes and other shoes that have rugged tread designs present a similar hazard. The best shoe for the person with Parkinson's is one that has a low heel and a smooth but not slick or stiff sole, such as a comfort walking shoe with a sole that slides without sticking or snagging but that does not cause slipping. People are reluctant to give up their favorite shoes, but because there are many styles available today, an acceptable compromise between fashion and function usually is possible.

Shoes that tie, buckle, or have narrow or tall (more than one-half inch) heels are difficult to put on and take off when fine motor skills are impaired. Laces and buckles require greater dexterity than the person with Parkinson's is likely to have. In frustration the person is likely to leave the shoes unfastened, thus creating a tripping hazard. Better options are shoes that slip on or have hook-and-loop fasteners (such as Velcro). Long-handled shoehorns and other devices can help the person with Parkinson's to pull on shoes without bending down to reach them.

Shoes provide the person's connection with solid ground and should themselves feel and fit snugly. There should be little side-to-side movement in the heel cup, and the person's heel should stay firmly within the shoe during walking. The heel supports the person's sense of balance and orientation to the walking surface, both of which are essential for proper GAIT. Slip-on shoes, although easy to put on and take off, may feel too loose across the top, increasing the tendency to slide the feet when walking. As walking is one of the best forms of exercise and mobility, finding shoes that fit properly and are easy to manage is worth the extra effort.

See also ADAPTIVE EQUIPMENT AND ASSIST DEVICES; CLOTHING; DAILY LIVING CHALLENGES; DEXTERITY, PHYSICAL; DRESSING.

shopping Going out to shop is both a functional task and a social outing. For the person with Parkinson's, it can be both a pleasure and an ordeal. When Parkinson's symptoms are mild and well controlled through ANTI-PARKINSON'S MEDICATIONS, shopping and other social ventures do not change much after the Parkinson's diagnosis, particularly if the person is still driving and can go out independently. Often in the early stages of Parkinson's, the person notices no differences in mobility or stamina.

As symptoms begin to involve more of the body, this condition changes. People with BRADYKINESIA (slowed muscle response and movement) sometimes describe it as walking through mud: Every movement, every muscle response, takes extraordinary effort and concentration for less than ordinary results. Short shopping trips such as to the grocery store to pick up a few items become exhausting, and longer trips such as to a mall to shop for a variety of items become impossible.

By the mid stages of Parkinson's, there are many facets to planning to go shopping. Key points include:

- Plan shopping trips to take place during peak medication coverage. Always carry a 24-hour supply of medication so extra doses are available if needed.

- Know where bathroom facilities are located in stores and shopping malls.

- Plan twice as much time as anticipated to allow plenty of opportunity to rest.

- Make a list of items to buy, in any kind of shopping, not just grocery shopping.

- If the store or mall is more than 15 or 20 minutes from home, have a bag in the car with a complete change of clothing to accommodate spills and accidents.

- Discuss in advance how the person with Parkinson's wants to handle situations such as freezing to minimize awkwardness and embarrassment should they occur.

- Be flexible. Shop for essential or important items first. If the person with Parkinson's tires more quickly than usual, end the shopping trip and go back another day.

It is important, though sometimes difficult, for family members and friends to have PATIENCE on outings with the person who has Parkinson's. The tendency is to rush to the store, find needed items, and rush out. This rushing creates a lot of stress for the person with Parkinson's, who can no longer move at that pace. If physical stability when walking is a problem, pushing a shopping cart is often an easy solution. The handle is usually at about the right height for the person to grip or even lean on, and full-size shopping carts are relatively stable, particularly as they begin to fill with groceries or other items. Shopping malls usually have wheelchairs available; if the person does not want to ride in one, pushing one provides additional support and an available chair if needed.

Some people with Parkinson's become frustrated or embarrassed about their symptoms and prefer, by the middle stages of the disease, to stay home rather than go out to shop. Catalogs and the Internet can allow the person to do his or her own shopping without leaving home. In many locations grocery stores make arrangements to deliver groceries, usually for just a nominal fee. The person can select items online over the Internet or telephone in a grocery list. Another alternative is for a caregiver, friend, or family member to shop for the person.

See also ADJUSTING TO LIVING WITH PARKINSON'S; GAIT; GAIT DISTURBANCE; MOBILITY AIDS; SOCIAL INTERACTION.

short form 36 (SF-36) A general health status questionnaire designed to measure the well-being and everyday function of people who have chronic disease. Although it is not specific for Parkinson's disease, clinicians and researchers sometimes use the SF-36 to get a broad perspective of the person's perception of Parkinson's disease's overall effect on his or her daily activities. The SF-36 contains 36 questions, rated from 0 to 100. The higher the score, the greater the person's satisfaction with his or her ability to function on a daily basis. The SF-36 is a proprietary assessment tool.

See also ACTIVITIES OF DAILY LIVING; PARKINSON'S DISEASE QUALITY OF LIFE QUESTIONNAIRE; PARKINSON'S DISEASE QUESTIONNAIRE; PARKINSON'S IMPACT SCALE; QUALITY OF LIFE; SICKNESS IMPACT SCALE.

short stay services Some LONG-TERM CARE FACILITIES offer full care for short visits, from a few days to three weeks, for people who cannot live independently to give caregivers an extended break. Sometimes a short stay is a welcome break for the person with Parkinson's as well, as facilities offer many activities. Some facilities have secured units and specialized staff for people with ALZHEIMER'S DISEASE.

The facility should charge a standard rate for such short stay services; this fee usually is not covered by any insurance. Services include nursing and attendant care just as if the person were a resident at the facility. When considering short stay services, evaluate the facility and its staff as if it were a long-term care option. Go on a tour, meet with the facility's manager and director of nursing, and talk with staff if possible. Visit several times, at different times of the day on weekdays and on at least one weekend day, before arranging for a loved one to stay there.

See also CAREGIVER WELL-BEING; RESPITE CARE.

shuffling gait See GAIT DISTURBANCE.

Shy–Drager syndrome See MULTIPLE SYSTEM ATROPHY.

sialorrhea See DROOLING.

sickness impact profile (SIP) A quality of life assessment designed to measure the effect of a chronic health condition on the everyday living experience of the person who has it. Although not specific for Parkinson's disease, the SIP covers a broad range of topics that address quality of life concerns relevant to people with Parkinson's. A clinician may use the SIP to monitor the extent to which ANTI-PARKINSON'S MEDICATIONS allow a person to experience what he or she perceives as a "normal" life. Researchers and some disability insurance companies also use the SIP, which is a proprietary assessment tool.

See also ACTIVITIES OF DAILY LIVING; PARKINSON'S DISEASE QUALITY OF LIFE QUESTIONNAIRE; PARKINSON'S DISEASE QUESTIONNAIRE; PARKINSON'S IMPACT SCALE; QUALITY OF LIFE; SHORT FORM 36.

sildenafil A medication taken to treat ERECTILE DYSFUNCTION in men, better known by its trade name, Viagra. Sildenafil is a nitric oxide compound that enhances the sequence of biochemical events that increases blood flow to the penis and relaxes smooth muscle tissue, allowing an erection to develop in response to sexual stimulation. Generally a man should take a dose of sildenafil 30 minutes to an hour before intended sexual intercourse, although the drug can produce its effects for as long as four hours. If there is no sexual stimulation, erection does not occur. Sildenafil often is effective in men with Parkinson's disease as it acts directly on smooth muscle tissue rather than through neuromuscular communication from the BRAIN. It also is effective when erectile dysfunction is related to age or is a side effect of medications such as antidepressants and adrenergic antagonists.

Men who are taking nitrate-based medications for heart conditions such as ischemic heart disease, angina, arrhythmias, or congestive heart failure cannot use sildenafil; the combination of nitrates can cause fatal heart attacks. Sildenafil does not interact with DOPAMINERGIC MEDICATIONS (such as LEVODOPA) or DOPAMINE AGONIST MEDICATIONS (such as BROMOCRIPTINE and ROPINIROLE); therefore, it is generally safe for men with Parkinson's as long as they are not taking other medications that can interact with it. Although there has been OPEN-LABEL USE of sildenafil for treatment of sexual dysfunction (difficulty with physical arousal and orgasm) in women, at present this use is not U.S. Food and Drug Administration–(FDA)-approved, and evidence of its effectiveness is inconclusive.

Sildenafil's common side effects include flushing, headache, sweating, hypotension (low blood pressure), and the perception of looking through a blue filter (which affects blue–green color differentiation). This color misperception occurs because an enzyme in the retina, phosphodiesterase type 6 (PDE6), is chemically similar to the enzyme in the erection sequence, phosphodiesterase type 5 (PDE5), that sildenafil suppresses. The coincidental suppression of PDE6 reduces the retina's ability to perceive green, allowing blue to become dominant. This is a short-term effect that has no health consequences, but men who experience it sometimes find it disconcerting. A rare but serious side effect is priapism, a persistent erection that lasts longer than four hours. This is often painful and can require medical attention to prevent permanent damage to the penis.

See also INTIMACY; MARRIAGE RELATIONSHIP; SEXUAL DYSFUNCTION; SEXUALITY.

Sinemet The brand name formulation of the anti-Parkinson's medication most commonly used in the United States, a combination of LEVODOPA and CARBIDOPA that is manufactured by Du Pont. About 80 percent of people with Parkinson's disease use this drug or one of its generic counterparts. In the early stages of Parkinson's, Sinemet typically is so effective that symptoms entirely disappear. As the disease progresses, however, Sinemet's effectiveness diminishes. Although increasing the drug's dosage can prolong its effectiveness, it also increases its side effects, which can include NAUSEA, DYSKINESIAS, and DYSTONIA (extreme muscle rigidity).

Sinemet, or levodopa/carbidopa, is generally preferred to levodopa alone because the carbidopa helps to mitigate the more distressing side effects of levodopa (primarily nausea and a sense of queasiness). The dosage must introduce enough levodopa into the body to produce a level sufficient to pass the BLOOD-BRAIN BARRIER, enters the BRAIN, and there supply enough dopamine to meet the brain's needs. After being absorbed into the bloodstream, levodopa is subject to rapid peripheral metabolism through the actions of the enzyme DOPA DECARBOXYLASE (DDC). The high levels of peripheral dopamine cause moderate to severe nausea, lightheadedness, and other side effects.

Carbidopa is a DOPA DECARBOXYLASE INHIBITOR (DDCI), which slows peripheral levodopa metabolism. Taking the proper amount of carbidopa (usually 50 mg to 75 mg per day is sufficient for most people) both avoids the side effects of nausea and lightheadedness and increases the amount of levodopa that reaches the brain where brain DDC helps metabolize the levodopa to DOPAMINE for use by brain neurons. As the BLOOD-BRAIN BARRIER prevents dopamine in the BRAIN from passing back into peripheral circulation, high levels of dopamine in the brain have no effect on functions elsewhere in the body. As levodopa depends on active transport from the gut, taking it with protein, which competes for the same transporters, significantly limits the amount of levodopa that can be absorbed. For this reason, most physicians recommend taking levodopa on an empty stomach (at least an hour before or two hours after eating) to avoid dietary protein causing variations in the amount of levodopa absorbed. This is particularly important in people with more advanced Parkinson's disease who have clear motor fluctuations (frequent medication wearing off or dyskinesias). Many people with advanced disease note sensitivity to dietary protein even when they have taken steps to take Sinemet only well away from meal times.

Sinemet is available in tablets of varying strengths, with the 10/100 tablets seldom being used, except in patients taking eight or more tablets per day, due to the risk of their containing insufficient carbidopa to prevent the peripheral conversion of levodopa and the attendant side effects. CONTROLLED RELEASE (Sinemet CR) tablets are formulated to dissolve slowly in the digestive system and enter the bloodstream in a controlled fashion over time; ideally this provides more prolonged and smoother levels of levodopa, but in practice the long digestion makes absorption of the levodopa in Sinemet CR very variable and unreliable. Regular release Sinemet also can function as a RESCUE DRUG, since it often reaches therapeutic levels in about a half hour; Sinemet CR commonly takes well over an hour to kick in. A formulation that combines carbidopa, levodopa, and entacapone in one pill should be on the market by late 2003, which provides the reliability and fast onset of regular release Sinemet with an extended duration of effect.

Generic formulations produced by other manufacturers include the brand names Atamet and Laradopa. Some people with Parkinson's report that generic products are not as effective as the Sinemet brand name product. This is likely because formulation and manufacturing processes can affect how rapidly and completely the drugs dissolve and absorb into the bloodstream, and switching from one brand to another can change the level of levodopa that reaches the brain. Generally, clinicians recommend staying with the same brand, whether Sinemet or generic.

Although most people experience relief of most symptoms with the first dose, it can take several weeks to get the dosage to the desired therapeutic level. Dosing depends on symptoms and response, and it changes as the Parkinson's progresses. The typical starting point is to take the prescribed dose of the regular release formula three or four times a day or take Sinemet CR, the extended release formula, twice daily. However, doctors may recommend taking the drug less or more frequently, depending on symptoms. As the course of Parkinson's disease is highly variable among individuals, each person must work closely with the doctor to achieve balance between therapeutic benefit and undesired side effects. The potential drug interactions with levodopa, Sinemet's therapeutic ingredient, are extensive; they are discussed in the LEVODOPA entry.

See also ADJUNCT THERAPIES; ANTI-PARKINSON'S MEDICATIONS; BENSERAZIDE; DOPAMINE AGONIST MEDICATIONS; MEDICATION MANAGEMENT; MEDICATION SIDE EFFECTS; MONOTHERAPY; THERAPEUTIC WINDOW.

single photon emission computed tomography (SPECT)

A functional imaging procedure developed in the 1960s that uses radionuclides (radioactive substances injected into the body that specific cells and tissues absorb) to create perceptions of internal body structures that are then constructed and projected through computerized imaging techniques. SPECT can provide insights into the functioning of internal brain structures such as the BASAL GANGLIA and it constitutes a basic method of monitoring the loss of dopaminergic neurons of a person who has Parkinson's disease, if this is desired. The primary value of this application is to research, although some neurologists use SPECT to help determine whether dopaminergic medications are improving dopamine presence and action in the brain.

In SPECT, the person receives an injection of the radionuclide and lies on a table that moves inside a large donut-shaped device. There is no discomfort beyond the placement of the IV for the initial injection, although some people feel claustrophobic while inside the device. Special detectors within this device collect the signals that the radionuclides emit and send the signals to the computer. Using complex mathematical formulas and physiological models, the computer creates multidimensional images of the body structures and representations of their functioning.

SPECT is less precise than radionuclide imaging technology such as POSITRON EMISSION TOMOGRAPHY (PET), which uses a dual collection procedure that allows greatly refined images. However, PET requires sophisticated and expensive equipment and highly trained specialists to operate it, and its cost is about three times higher than the cost of SPECT. For most clinical applications in Parkinson's disease, SPECT provides adequate information and is more readily available. There are no adverse effects of having SPECT.

See also COMPUTED TOMOGRAPHY (CT) SCAN; FUNCTIONAL IMAGING STUDIES; MAGNETIC RESONANCE IMAGING.

skilled nursing facility (SNF) A health care facility that has the staff and equipment to provide nursing care for people who need intravenous (IV) lines, wound care, mechanical ventilation, high intensity acute rehabilitation therapy, and other medical treatments but who do not require the more intensive attention of a hospital setting. Some SNFs are affiliated with hospitals and others with LONG-TERM CARE FACILITIES. Some long-term care facilities have SNF and long-term care floors or units and provide both levels of care within the same physical facility. The person with Parkinson's is likely to need an SNF for further recovery after an injury such as a fracture from a fall, an illness such as pneumonia, or another medical condition. Parkinson's disease itself seldom meets the criteria for admission to an SNF.

An SNF must have a certain number and percentage of registered nurses (RNs) on staff and on duty at all times to perform skilled nursing functions within the scope of their licensure and direct the functions of other staff such as licensed practical nurses (LPNs) and certified nursing assistants (CNAs) in performing supportive functions. SNFs also have registered physical therapists, certified occupational therapists, speech pathologists, and other allied health practitioners who contract with the facility or who are on staff.

Generally a person enters an SNF after HOSPITALIZATION and stays no longer than about three months, with an expectation of measurable improvement over that time. After this period the person's care needs typically are for maintenance rather than treatment, even when the necessity for medication and total personal care remains. MEDICARE requires three consecutive days of hospitalization before it will pay for SNF services and covers 100 days of care per episode of illness (along with other criteria). Most private insurance plans, medical or long-term care, that cover SNF services follow the same guidelines.

Many areas have several SNFs. When this is the case, visit at least two or three to get a sense of how they differ. Unlike in hospitalization, admission to an SNF requires planning to arrange for a bed and to confirm that the SNF can meet the person's specific needs and that the appropriate payment arrangements (Medicare, private insurance, private payment) can be made. For SNFs that are of interest, it is important to verify the following:

- The facility's licensing and Medicare certification: This is important whether or not the person is covered under Medicare. Medicare inspects certified facilities and requires them to maintain certain standards of care. A facility that does not meet these standards typically cannot provide adequate skilled nursing care. All states have licensing procedures for SNFs. The state's department of health generally oversees this process. As well, look for an SNF that is accredited by the Joint Commission on Accreditation of Healthcare Organizations (JCAHO); this certification assures that the SNF meets health care industry standards of care.

- The physical setting: Take a tour, making sure to see several patient rooms as well as common areas. Pay attention to smells, sights, sounds, and perceptions of whether the facility "feels" right. Is it clean? Are the hallways clear of clutter? Talk with staff and talk with people who are visiting their loved ones, if possible, to find out what they think of the facility. Visit again, at a different time of the day and unannounced. If possible, visit in the early evening if your tour occurred during the day and in the early morning if your tour was in the late afternoon. And make a short visit on a weekend, if possible.

- The financial details: Know exactly what services are included in the basic charges and what services are billed extra. Also know what services are paid for by Medicare, MEDICAL INSURANCE, LONG-TERM CARE INSURANCE, and MEDICAID, whichever of these payers is applicable.

Most hospitals have discharge planners who help make arrangements for transfer to an SNF when this is necessary, although the final decision always rests either with the person or with the family. As the person with Parkinson's who is admitted to an SNF will enter it for health reasons other than the Parkinson's, the person's primary care physician or neurologist must know of the admission and oversee matters such as MEDICATION MANAGEMENT.

See also CARE PLANNING AND MANAGEMENT.

sleep disturbances Problems in falling or staying asleep are common in people with Parkinson's disease. Symptoms such as RIGIDITY (muscle resistance to movement) and BRADYKINESIA (slowed muscle response and movement) make turning over in bed and finding comfortable positions difficult. Sometimes these symptoms cause aching and even pain as muscles held in the same position too long become cramped and exhausted. An uncomfortable feeling in the legs as one lies in bed trying to fall asleep that is at least partially relieved with movement. It is known as RESTLESS LEG SYNDROME and is common in those with Parkinson's and is often a precursor to actual Parkinson's in some cases. Once asleep, the person often thrashes around. Many people with Parkinson's have extraordinarily vivid dreams and nightmares. The reasons for these disturbances seem to be a combination of factors related to the disease process of Parkinson's, the effects of ANTI-PARKINSON'S MEDICATIONS, and normal changes in sleep patterns that take place with increasing age.

Consequences of Inadequate Sleep

Although researchers do not fully understand what happens during sleep or why sleep is essential, they do know that the consequences of sleep deprivation can be severe and may include physical as well as cognitive and psychological impairment. Studies of extended sleep deprivation in healthy volunteers reveal significant disruptions of concentration, ability to think, and reason, and even seizures, which suggest strong connections between physical and cognitive functioning in the brain.

Sleep is the body's time to slow its functions, allowing cells the opportunity to repair and recover from the stresses of daily activity. When the rest the body receives is inadequate, cells (and accordingly tissues and structures) must continue functioning at full activity, and after a time, they wear out. This may contribute to OXIDATIVE STRESS, and other destructive conditions may occur, in theory causing cells to become damaged or die. The NEURODEGENERATIVE disease process of Parkinson's magnifies the consequences of inadequate rest. The body's attempts to compensate result in uncontrollable urges to fall asleep at inappropriate times. Anti-Parkinson's medications, because they alter the biochemical balance of the brain, further contribute to this condition. Inadequate rest stresses the already dysfunctional neuromuscular processes that characterize Parkinson's, worsening symptoms.

Sleep Pattern Changes with Age

Changes in sleep patterns are normal as people grow older. They likely are due to a combination of factors that accompany aging such as slowing of metabolism, decline in hormone levels, reduction of activity, and alterations in brain biochemical processes with APOPTOSIS (programmed, normal cell death) and perhaps other kinds of damage to neurons aside from that of Parkinson's (such as OXIDATION) that affect their functions or cause their death. Researchers are uncertain whether less sleep indicates a diminished need for sleep or difficulty in sleeping that arises from these physiological changes.

Whatever the causative factors, many people find that as they get older they sleep less—they go to bed later or take longer to fall asleep, wake up more frequently throughout the night, and wake earlier in the morning. Most nonetheless feel rested, suggesting that their bodies either adjust to the shortened hours of sleep or do not need them. This is not the case for people with Parkinson's, however, who typically find that the disease magnifies these patterns and creates disturbances that leave them unrested. People who have EARLY-ONSET PARKINSON'S who are generally not yet old enough to be experiencing sleep changes related to aging experience Parkinson-related sleep disturbances as well, although they seem better able to cope with them until later in the disease process.

Insomnia and Nighttime Waking

Insomnia is the inability to fall asleep. Often the person is tired, even so tired that he or she finds it impossible to stay awake, but nonetheless just lies in bed unable to fall asleep. This pattern generates further distress and anxiety. By the middle stages of the disease, many people with Parkinson's have shifted their anti-Parkinson's medication regimens to provide maximal relief of neuromuscular symptoms during waking hours, so the reduced medication coverage during the night allows MUSCLES SPASMS and dystonic events to emerge.

Nighttime waking is another dimension of insomnia in which, after finally falling asleep, the person awakens and then cannot fall asleep again. Many of the factors that originally prevented sleep—motor symptoms, anxiety, "busy" thoughts—contribute again. NOCTURIA (the urge to urinate) interrupts sleep for many people with Parkinson's. Nocturia is a consequence of Parkinson's disease's disruption of smooth muscle function affecting the bladder. When neuromuscular symptoms make it a struggle to get up and go to the bathroom, and then get back into bed and get comfortable enough to fall back to sleep, nocturia can create disturbances that last an hour or longer. Nocturnal MYOCLONUS—jerking of muscle groups—is another physical disturbance that can awaken a person from sleep.

Sleeping during the day disrupts nighttime sleep patterns as well. Many anti-Parkinson's medications cause drowsiness. The person with Parkinson's may take brief or even extended naps during the day as a result, unable to stay awake because of the drug's effect. This napping contributes to the body's "sleep bank," however, and can reduce the need for nighttime sleep because the body's sleep needs are being met throughout the day. Sometimes altering the dosages and schedules of medications can lessen this effect. The medication MODAFINIL (Provigil) is a nonamphetamine stimulant that increases wakefulness and alertness when medication adjustments are ineffective for reducing episodes of sleepiness. Restoring the body's normal cycle of daytime wakefulness improves the ability to sleep at night.

Dreams and Nightmares

Shakespeare's wistful "To sleep, perchance to dream" is not a wish but a dread of many people who have Parkinson's. For them, vivid dreams and nightmares frequently disturb restful sleep. Researchers are unsure why this is, although most believe it is a combination of continued cell death, which alters brain perceptions and activity, and continually fluctuating neurotransmitter levels in the brain. The brain is designed to "expect" certain cycles of physiological events—a predictable rise and fall of biochemical activity. This pattern becomes chaotic in Parkinson's, creating widespread disturbances in brain functions beyond the disruptions of motor function that are the core of the disease. Researchers speculate that this effect contributes to both HALLUCINATIONS and enhanced dream experiences.

Anti-Parkinson's medications, particularly dopaminergics such as LEVODOPA and DOPAMINE AGONISTS (PERGOLIDE, PRAMIPEXOLE) that incidentally activate dopamine receptors in areas of the brain other than the BASAL GANGLIA, trigger brain activity that otherwise would not occur during rest. This effect is manifested through vivid and sometimes frightening or disturbing dreams and nightmares. At times the person with Parkinson's may have a problem distinguishing between dreaming and being awake. The reality of being immobilized by the symptoms of Parkinson's further compounds the sensation of being "frozen" in a dream state. This perception can create considerable anxiety until the person becomes oriented and fully awake. After such experiences, of course, returning to sleep is difficult.

REM Sleep Behavior Disorder (RBD)

Normal sleep occurs in identifiable stages. The stage in which dreams primarily take place is called rapid eye movement (REM). In people with normal brain function, the brain suppresses muscle activity during REM sleep. This mechanism prevents the body from acting out the events of dreams. In people with Parkinson's, this mechanism becomes dysfunctional and the body acts out dreams, sometimes with great physical energy expressed through kicking, thrashing, swinging of the arms, and other actions that can actually be harmful to the person or to a partner who is sharing the bed. Medications that relax the muscles can help to reduce RBD. RBD sometimes emerges or intensifies when the anti-Parkinson's medication regimen is adjusted to mediate increased daytime symptoms, thereby reducing medication coverage at night.

Improving the Potential for Restful Sleep

Finding the optimal blend of conditions to support restful sleep is highly individualized and often requires flexibility to accommodate day-to-day changes in symptoms and activity levels. It generally is helpful to

- Stay awake during the day
- Go to bed and get up at the same times each day, regardless of sleep quality
- Establish a routine of diminishing activity and concentration in the evenings to prepare the body and mind for rest and sleep
- Reduce outside distractions, such as light and noise, as much as possible
- Limit fluid intake after the evening meal to reduce problems with nocturia
- Consider medication for DEPRESSION, if symptoms of depression are present
- Consider sleep medication, if disturbed sleep persists longer than two weeks

Because pharmacotherapy is the primary therapeutic approach for Parkinson's disease at present, the person with Parkinson's typically takes a number of medications. As there generally are choices among the drugs within a particular classification, finding medications that can accomplish more than one mission makes sense. There are, for example, more than a dozen drugs that act as muscle relaxants. These produce varying degrees of sedation. For the person who has trouble sleeping at night because of nocturnal myoclonus and restless muscle activity, choosing a nighttime muscle relaxant with a high sedative effect is helpful. Conversely, it is important to look at the sedative effects of drugs taken during the day, to try to schedule them, or activities, to minimize drowsiness. A person who knows that the morning dose of levodopa causes sleepiness may consider taking a brisk walk at the time drowsiness is most likely to occur, helping to keep the body busy and the mind occupied until the drowsiness passes.

See also BEDROOM COMFORT; DAY–NIGHT REVERSAL; DAYTIME SLEEPINESS; RESTLESS LEG SYNDROME; SLEEP MEDICATIONS.

sleep medications Medications taken to fall asleep and stay asleep. Most sleep medications are sedatives; they reduce neuron communication in the brain, slowing physical and cognitive functions. Often antidepressant sedatives such as trazadone (Desyrel) are utilized to help combat both insomnia and early morning awakening, sometimes even if other symptoms of depression are not evident. Sleep medications such as the mid- to long-acting benzodiazepines FLURAZAPAM (Dalmane), lorazepam (Ativan), diazepam (Valium), and TEMAZEPAM (Restoril) are often used for short-term or occasional relief of insomnia and have less addiction potential than short-acting benzodiazepines such as triazolam (Halcion). Zolpidem (Ambien) is also a less addictive alternative for insomnia, although it can be habit forming and is usually used only for short term or occasionally. Doctors sometimes recommend the over-the-counter antihistamine medication DIPHENHYDRAMINE (Benadryl) as a sleep aid; its antihistamine qualities inherently cause drowsiness, and it has a mild anticholinergic effect that helps to reduce neuromuscular symptoms such as TREMORS. These drugs also act as muscle relaxants, which can help to relieve sleep disturbances such as RESTLESS LEG SYNDROME (RLS) and nocturnal MYOCLONUS.

Sleep medications do alter balance, perception, and muscle control, creating an increased risk for falls if the person has to get up at night. A person who is taking sleep medications should have someone accompany him or her if getting up at night becomes necessary. Sleep medications may also interact with other medications the person is using, particularly muscle relaxants, as many sleep medications belong to this classification of drugs, as well as ANTIDEPRESSANT MEDICATIONS and PAIN RELIEF MEDICATIONS.

See also ADJUNCT THERAPIES; ANTI-PARKINSON'S MEDICATIONS; MEDICATION MANAGEMENT; MEDICATION SIDE EFFECTS; TREATMENT ALGORITHM.

social interaction The process of, and human need for, association with other people. Social interaction helps people to feel connected with one another and with events and circumstances in their communities. Isolation becomes a concern for many people with Parkinson's disease, either because their symptoms limit their ability to seek social interaction independently or embarrass them to the extent that they do not want others to see them. Being with others becomes difficult, too, because the lack of facial expression that Parkinson's can cause (HYPOMIMIA, or masked face) sometimes leads others to perceive incorrectly that the person with Parkinson's is ignoring them or is not interested in what is happening.

Family members, friends, and caregivers provide an important circle of social interaction for the person with Parkinson's. As much as possible, the person also should get out among other people, if only by taking walks in public places or going out to shop. This kind of interaction, even though brief and superficial, provides an important sense of connectedness and a pleasant distraction from routine. This helps to sustain SELF-ESTEEM and to take the person's mind off the Parkinson's for a while. People who enjoyed being around other people before the diagnosis of Parkinson's will still enjoy this interaction after their diagnosis, even though it becomes more difficult.

See also ADJUSTING TO LIVING WITH PARKINSON'S; COMPASSION; EMBARRASSMENT; EMPATHY; FRIENDSHIPS; SHOPPING; TRAVEL.

Social Security A retirement program for employed Americans that the U.S. federal government funds through worker contributions known as Federal Insurance Contributions Act (FICA) taxes, paid through payroll deduction. The Social Security Act of 1935 created the program to assure that working Americans would have a source of income when they retired. Amendments to the act in 1954 added disability benefits. And in the 1960s, the U.S. Congress created MEDICARE to provide medical insurance for people who qualified for Social Security. Today Medicare functions as a separate program and government entity, although eligibility for Medicare coverage remains linked to Social Security eligibility. Social Security exists as two basic components, retirement and disability, that include various kinds of benefits.

Social Security Retirement Insurance

Social Security retirement insurance pays benefits to everyone who contributes as required by law (people who participate in certain private pension programs are exempt from paying into, and cannot collect payments from, Social Security) and who meets the minimal length of employment and age at retirement requirements.

- Length of employment is converted to a system of credits. Each full-time year of employment counts as four credits. A person must accumulate a minimum of 40 credits over a lifetime to qualify for Social Security retirement payments.

- People born before 1938 are eligible for Social Security retirement payments when they reach age 65. The retirement age rises in established increments, presently peaking at age 67 for people born after 1960. It is possible to take early retirement at age 62 and receive reduced benefits.

Social Security retirement payments are based on rates established by Congress and are not affected by disability. Many people who receive regular Social Security retirement benefits also qualify for Social Security Disability Insurance (SSDI).

Social Security Disability Insurance (SSDI)

A person who has Parkinson's disease that prevent him or her from working may be considered disabled under Social Security guidelines and eligible for Social Security Disability Insurance (SSDI) regardless of age. Criteria are related to the person's age and number of credits earned at the time of disability. The medical condition also must be one that the Social Security Administration identifies as capable of causing disability according to its definition. Parkinson's disease (Parkinsonian syndrome) is such a condition. Parkinson's disease alone does not automatically qualify a person for SSDI, however; the person must prove that the disease prevents him or her from working.

The key dimension of disability from the perspective of SSDI is the extent to which the condition interferes with or prevents the person from working and whether the condition is expected to last 12 months or longer or lead to death. Most people with Parkinson's disease, with appropriate treatment, are able to lead a relatively normal life, including working, for years after diagnosis. By the time Parkinson's interferes with daily living to the extent that symptoms preclude working, most people are beyond retirement age. However, people with EARLY-ONSET PARKINSON'S who have severe symptoms may qualify for SSDI.

Filing for SSDI requires statements from physicians and copies of supporting medical records that substantiate that the person's disability prevents him or her from working. It is important that these records be complete in presenting the person's medical circumstances and that they specify the ways in which the impairments of the Parkinson's disease contribute to the person's ability or lack of ability to perform work tasks. FUNCTIONAL CAPACITY assessments and other measures of functional impairment can help to quantify this relationship.

Supplemental Security Income (SSI)

Supplemental Security Income (SSI) is a program that provides payment to people who are disabled, cannot work, and do not have the income or resources to meet their basic needs. As for MEDICAID, SSI qualification criteria are asset-based and vary among states. The Social Security Administration can provide further information specific to an individual's situation.

Eligibility for Social Security Programs and Payments

Because qualification for Social Security programs and payments depends on individual circumstances, it is necessary to contact the Social Security Administration to obtain specific information. Call the Social Security Administration at 1-800-772-1213 (toll-free) or visit the website at www.ssa.gov.

See also ACTIVITIES OF DAILY LIVING; FINANCIAL PLANNING; INSTRUMENTAL ACTIVITIES OF DAILY LIVING; PLANNING FOR THE FUTURE; RETIREMENT.

spasm An intense, involuntary contraction of a muscle or muscle group that can be quite painful. Muscle spasms can occur without apparent reason or be a consequence of overuse or excessive time spent in one position. The DYSTONIA that develops in later stages of Parkinson's is a severe spasm in which the muscles remain held in a contracted state for an extended time, causing pain and awkward positioning. Adjusting the LEVODOPA dosage

sometimes lessens the occurrence of dystonia. RESTLESS LEG SYNDROME (RLS), in which the legs twitch and tingle, often includes muscle spasms. Sometimes massaging the area helps the muscles to relax. MUSCLE RELAXANT MEDICATIONS often are necessary to interrupt the nerve signals causing the contractions when dystonia and spasms become frequent or disruptive.

See also CHOREIFORM DYSKINESIA.

spasticity A sign on examination of abnormal muscle tone in which the muscles contract reflexively to being stretched. Spasticity increases with the speed and direction of the attempted movement since it is activated by stretching. Spasticity is what occurs after injury to the brain or upper parts of the spinal cord, like a stroke, cerebral palsy, or multiple sclerosis, that involve the pyramidal motor system (motor cortex and its primary motor pathways through the brain and spinal cord). Pyramidal tract lesions also display abnormally elevated reflexes and true weakness.

Extrapyramidal disorders such as Parkinson's disease that involve the BASAL GANGLIA are instead associated with RIGIDITY, an increase in stiffness does not change with the speed of movement. The presence of spasticity, or other signs of pyramidal tract lesions, in a person with PARKINSONISM (signs of extrapyramidal dysfunction) would be a sign of either a second disease, or a diagnosis such as multisystem atrophy (MSA), progressive supranuclear palsy (PSP), or disorders other than Parkinson's disease.

speech A complex integration of physical and cognitive abilities that produces an articulation of language using sounds. On the cognitive end, the frontal and temporal lobes of the CEREBRUM that regulate language recognition and processing translate thought processes into the language concepts. This activity takes place primarily in two regions, called Broca's area and Wernicke's area. These are functionally, rather than physically, defined regions in the brain and usually are located in the dominant side of the cerebrum (the left hemisphere in most people; some left-handed people have these regions in the right hemisphere).

Wernicke's area processes incoming language; Broca's area formulates outgoing language.

Outgoing language becomes speech when the cerebral cortex, in coordination with the activities of Broca's area, sends signals to initiate movement of the structures that make speech possible—the lips, mouth, tongue, throat, and vocal cords—as well as of the structures of the chest involved in breathing. In turn, the signals activate the structures of the BASAL GANGLIA, the clusters of nerves that regulate voluntary movement, which send the neuron communications that direct the specific actions of the muscles involved. Signals from the CEREBELLUM coordinate all of this movement, making it smooth and sequential. Interruptions along any part of this pathway disrupt speech.

In Parkinson's disease such interruptions most commonly take place in the basal ganglia, where insufficiency of the level of dopamine causes nerve signals to become jumbled. Muscles on the receiving end of these incomplete or chaotic neuron communications may be slowed (BRADYKINESIA) or fail to respond (AKINESIA). The lips and tongue incompletely shape the appropriate formations for making the sounds of words; the vocal cords do not adjust for the quality of sound the words require; breathing may be inadequate to produce the volume of air necessary to produce adequate sound through the vocal cords. These dysfunctions result in the speech difficulties characteristic of Parkinson's disease such as soft, monotone voice; slowed hesitant, speech; or rapid stuttering speech. When COGNITIVE IMPAIRMENT is a feature of the Parkinson's as well, the cerebrum's language centers also are affected, as manifested by DYSPHASIA (difficulty in finding the right word). Clinicians refer to these difficulties as dysfunctions in phonation, resonation, and articulation.

Speech difficulties generally occur in the later stages of Parkinson's, although in some people a soft, almost whispery voice is one of the earliest signs of the disease (usually recognized in retrospect). SWALLOWING problems often coexist with speech difficulties, as swallowing and speech share common structures and physiological processes. Speech therapy often can help people handle both developments by teaching methods of compensating for diminished functions. Voice volume is a fac-

tor of generating enough breath and sometimes the person with Parkinson's is not able to do so. BRADYKINESIA (slowed muscle response and movement) also can affect the muscles of the chest, the abdomen, and particularly the diaphragm. Although the person's pace and depth of breathing may increase with physical activity as the body demands more oxygen, he or she may have difficulty intentionally taking deep breaths to improve speech. BREATHING EXERCISES, including YOGA breathing, help to maintain maximal BREATH CONTROL.

HYPOMIMIA, or the "masked face" of Parkinson's, tends to contribute to communication problems for people who have speech difficulties, as it eliminates the facial expressions that help to give context to spoken communication. This condition affects the response of others more than the speech of the person with Parkinson's but contributes to the overall challenge of verbal communication. Loved ones can help by being patient when the person with Parkinson's is attempting to articulate the right word. Some people appreciate prompting or filling in elusive words; others find this reaction intrusive and frustrating. It often is worthwhile to ask the person with Parkinson's what he or she prefers. Often speech improves when ANTI-PARKINSON'S MEDICATIONS are at their peak in relieving other motor symptoms and deteriorates during OFF-STATES.

See also DYSARTHRIA; EMBARRASSMENT; EMPATHY; PATIENCE.

speech-language pathology A specialty of health care that focuses on improving the processes of SPEECH and language in a person who has impairments due to disease or injury. People with Parkinson's disease commonly have problems with speech as a consequence of NEURODEGENERATIVE damage that affects control of the muscles necessary for speech and sometimes as a result of COGNITIVE IMPAIRMENT. Early intervention with exercises and methods to maintain optimal speech functions can minimize resulting communication challenges. MEDICARE, most medical insurance plans, and MEDICAID pay for at least some of the costs of speech-language pathology services (sometimes called speech therapy). These interventions also help to improve breathing and swallowing.

A speech-language pathologist (SLP) is a master's-level health care professional who specializes in disorders of speech and language; he or she is sometimes called a speech-language therapist (SLT) or a speech therapist, these are outdated designations and individuals in the profession prefer the title *speech-language pathologist*. Most SLPs have an undergraduate degree in communication disorders and a graduate degree from a program accredited by the American Speech–Language–Hearing Association (ASHA). Most states have licensure and continuing education requirements for SLPs; SLPs should further be certified by the ASHA. Providing support for SLPs are SLP assistants, who typically have associate degrees and carry out defined functions under the direction and supervision of an SLP, and SLP aides, who have vocational or job-based training and perform limited tasks, also under the SLP's direction and supervision.

See also BREATH CONTROL; DYSARTHRIA; DYSPHAGIA; OCCUPATIONAL THERAPY; PHYSICAL THERAPY; SPEECH; SUPPORT THERAPIES; SWALLOWING.

spinal cord   See NERVOUS SYSTEM.

staging of Parkinson's disease   A structure of assessment that denotes the severity of the symptoms of Parkinson's disease and the extent to which they interfere with everyday living. There is no clear correlation between the stage of Parkinson's and any perception of prognosis or life expectancy, unlike in staging scales for other medical conditions such as cancer. Staging systems for Parkinson's disease primarily give perspective as to the disease's relative progression and the range of variation between medicated and nonmedicated states.

The most widely used staging scale is the five-stage Hoehn and Yahr classification system, which the physicians Margaret Hoehn and Melvin Yahr developed in 1967 to assess MOBILITY and MOTOR FUNCTION with and without LEVODOPA, which was at that time a new treatment for Parkinson's disease. The HOEHN AND YAHR STAGE SCALE subsequently has become the standard for assessing the motor symptoms of Parkinson's disease. When a neurologist identifies a person as having "stage II

Parkinson's disease" the reference is to the Hoehn and Yahr staging scale.

There are numerous other approaches to assessing the effect of Parkinson's disease on a person's everyday living experiences, from ACTIVITIES OF DAILY LIVING (ADLs), INSTRUMENTAL ACTIVITIES OF LIVING (IADLs), and the Schwab and England scale of capacity for daily living to various QUALITY OF LIFE assessments such as the PARKINSON'S IMPACT SCALE (PIMS) and the PARKINSON'S DISEASE QUESTIONNAIRE (PDQ-39). Staging scales and assessment systems provide a means of determining whether treatment regimens relieve symptoms. This information is sometimes useful for making decisions about a person's ability to continue employment. Staging scales also can help the person with Parkinson's to understand where he or she is along the continuum of the disease's progression.

See also DIAGNOSING PARKINSON'S.

staring   See HYPOMIMIA.

start hesitation   See GAIT DISTURBANCES.

stem cell   An unspecialized cell that has the ability to reproduce itself over an extended period. Unlike other cells in the body, stem cells have no defined functions or structures. They seem to exist for the purpose of becoming whatever kinds of cells the body needs them to become, a process called differentiation. The therapeutic potential of harnessing this capability is that stem cells could be "grown" into cell types and tissues to replace those damaged or destroyed by disease. At present there remain many unanswered questions about stem cells and their possible use to treat diseases such as Parkinson's. Scientists only partially understand stem cells' origin and function and are just beginning to learn to manipulate their development and differentiation in the laboratory. There are two kinds of stem cells, embryonic and adult.

Embryonic Stem Cells

Embryonic stem cells are the most primal cell structures of the human body. They exist in the earliest stages of human development, when the embryo (called a blastocyst) is no more than a cluster of about 30 cells during the first three to five days after fertilization and before cell differentiation begins. Embryonic stem cells are totipotent—they have the ability to become any kind of cell found in the human body. Genetic encoding determines what kinds of cells they become. In the embryo, differentiation takes place as the genetic blueprint unfolds. In the laboratory, researchers can manipulate embryonic stem cells to differentiate into virtually any kind of cell by introducing the genetic material of the desired type of cell.

The same colony of embryonic stem cells continues to replicate undifferentiated in the laboratory for a year or longer, when sustained in an appropriate culture medium. By taking cells from an established colony and placing them into a separate culture medium, scientists can grow millions of embryonic stem cells from each 30-cell blastocyst. When scientists implant embryonic stem cells into other tissues, the stem cells adopt the genetic code of the adjacent cells and differentiate into cells of that type as they replicate. Embryonic stem cells implanted into the PUTAMEN or the SUBSTANTIA NIGRA, for example, differentiate into dopaminergic neurons.

Such implantation, called embryonic STEM CELL IMPLANT, is investigational as well as a bioethical concern. Embryonic stem cells are obtained from aborted embryos or from embryos created through in vitro fertilization (combining of an ovum, or egg, and a sperm in the laboratory), a treatment for infertility, that are not needed. The moral and legal implications of using human embryos to cultivate embryonic stem cells, and in particular of the potential for researchers to create human embryos for the express purpose of providing such cells, have generated significant controversy within the medical community as well as among the public at large. In 2001, President George W. Bush signed federal legislation restricting embryonic stem cell research to embryonic stem cell cultivations (called stem cell lines) already in existence at about 20 research facilities in the United States. Many other countries also have, or are considering, strict limitations on the sources of embryonic stem cells used in research as well. Conversely, the state of California, as well as some nations like Australia, have passed legislation that control, but specifically permit the use of, embryonic stem cells from in vitro fertilization surpluses and other sources.

Adult Stem Cells

Adult stem cells exist as undifferentiated cells among the differentiated cells that make up numerous body tissues. Scientists have located adult stem cells in the bone marrow, BRAIN, liver, blood vessels, and skin. It is possible that all tissue systems contain stem cells; researchers do not yet know how adult stem cells develop, where they reside, or what activates them to differentiate. They seem to exist in very small numbers and to become activated to differentiate when there is a need to replace tissue, such as when there is an injury. In such circumstances, adult stem cells differentiate at replication, creating new cells of the same type and function as their "host" tissue. But scientists do not understand what mechanisms control this process, or why it does not occur automatically, for example, when a heart attack damages areas of heart tissue. Some adult stem cells are pluripotent: That is, they can differentiate into cells of several kinds of tissues. Scientists are searching for ways to manipulate adult stem cells to differentiate for specific types of cells, in which case they could become treatment options for autoimmune diseases such as diabetes and NEURODEGENERATIVE diseases such as ALZHEIMER'S DISEASE and Parkinson's disease.

Colonies of adult stem cells cultivated in the laboratory have a much shorter life span than cultivated embryonic stem cells, generally living for no longer than six months. Researchers are not sure why this occurs; nor are they sure of the life span of an adult stem cell within the human body. Although one culture can be the foundation for numerous colonies, it is necessary to develop new colonies continually. Also, it is difficult to locate and extract adult stem cells from their native tissues, as there are not many of them and their distribution is diffuse. However, there is little controversy about research and therapy using adult stem cells. Could scientists perfect adult stem cell cultivation and selective differentiation, it would be possible to develop individualized "tissue banks" a person could use as the need arose. The prospect of harnessing the body's own therapeutic potential as a renewable resource has great appeal.

See also ADRENAL MEDULLARY TRANSPLANT; ALLO-GRAFT; BRAIN TISSUE TRANSPLANT; FETAL DOPAMINER-GIC CELL TRANSPLANT; FETAL PORCINE BRAIN CELL TRANSPLANT; GENE MAPPING; GENE MUTATIONS; GENE THERAPY; HOPE FOR A PARKINSON'S CURE; XENOGRAFT.

stem cell implant   Investigational treatment for Parkinson's disease in which neurosurgeons implant embryonic or adult STEM CELLS into the PALLIDUS or PUTAMEN. The procedure also is called stem cell transplant or stem cell therapy. The pallidus and putamen are structures of the BASAL GAN-GLIA that are instrumental to voluntary movement. The stem cells implanted into these areas have already been manipulated to differentiate as dopaminergic neurons and "take root" in the recipient brain. Once well established they produce dopamine just as do native dopaminergic neurons, boosting the brain's supply of endogenous dopamine. This process seems to offset, but does not entirely compensate for, the loss of DOPAMINER-GIC NEURONS from the SUBSTANTIA NIGRA. It is this loss, and the resulting depletion of dopamine, that cause the symptoms of Parkinson's.

Although it would seem reasonable to implant dopaminergic stem cells into the substantia nigra, where they could directly replace dying neurons, researchers have chosen the putamen and pallidus as the recipient sites for stem cell implantation instead, in part because these structures are in close proximity to other structures of the basal ganglia and BRAIN that are involved with movement and have abnormal activity in Parkinson's. Neurons originating in the SUBSTANTIA NIGRA have long dendrite structures that allow them to extend to other structures; implanted cells here would have to be directed to grow these long dendrites as well, which is a difficult proposition. As well, because scientists do not know what causes the substantia nigra's native dopaminergic neurons to die, reseeding the area with new dopaminergic neurons would make little sense.

Results and Effectiveness

The results of investigational stem cell implants for Parkinson's are mixed. Some people who volunteered to participate in stem cell implant studies experienced immediate and dramatic relief of symptoms such as TREMORS and BRADYKINESIA after implant and were able to reduce significantly the amount of LEVODOPA and other ANTI-PARKINSON'S MEDICATIONS they were using, although they could not stop taking them entirely. The rate of positive responders has been much higher in open-label trials than in randomized-controlled trials, suggesting a significant placebo effect. Functional imaging studies in some of the open label trials have confirmed this placebo effect: Many of the patients with an apparent benefit did not have surviving grafts; the implanted cells died and did not form functional connections. In a randomized-controlled trial, only the youngest patients (those under 60) seemed to have had much of a chance of benefit. Other people noticed no appreciable difference in the severity of their symptoms. And still others found that their symptoms worsened, or they developed additional DYSKINESIAS and dystonia because the implanted cells produced too much dopamine; 15 percent of those in the randomized-controlled trial had uncontrollable dyskinesias, even off of all medications. Based upon these results, much of the enthusiasm to conduct human clinical trials with current implantation techniques has waned, with scientists wanting to wait until better techniques, offering a better success rate and less risk of uncontrollable dyskinesias, have been developed.

Because stem cell implant is a relatively new therapeutic approach, scientists do not know how long the effects last or what long-term complications may occur. They do know that the degeneration of dopaminergic neurons continues in the substantia nigra, and the Parkinson's continues to progress. However, the implanted dopaminergic neurons appear capable of sustaining a steady pace of dopamine production in a few people who have received stem cell implants.

Risks and Challenges

There are a number of risks inherent in stem cell implant. One is the transfer of disease to the recipient. Stem cells are taken from other humans, and therefore have the potential to pose a wide range of risks from genetic mutations to infections. Indeed, the risk of infection is itself a potential problem, as stem cell implant requires entering the inner portions of the brain. There is a risk of infection, as well as bleeding, in any kind of surgery. Another risk is the potential for the stem cells to differentiate into cells other than those intended, causing abnormal tissue growth or tumors, even cancerous lesions. Although research centers screen for as many potential problems as possible, this is a very new technology and there just is not enough information about what those possibilities may encompass. Once a stem cell implant takes place, however, its results, good and bad, are permanent. Implanted stem cells cannot be withdrawn or inactivated.

Other challenges confronting this technology are ethical and practical. Embryonic stem cell implants have polarized the research community, people with Parkinson's, and the general public because these cells are harvested from human embryos whose development is arrested to provide them or from embryos that have been aborted. Because even one embryo can provide a virtually endless supply of stem cells, this is a highly controversial topic that has engendered intense debate and resulted in strict federal limitations on embryonic stem cell supplies and research.

Adult stem cell implant is not so controversial, as scientists can harvest adult stem cells without taking or risking the life of the donor. However, adult stem cells exist in limited quantities, are difficult to identify and harvest, and are difficult to cultivate and maintain in the laboratory. As well, most adult stem cells are unipotent: They have the ability to differentiate into cells of the tissue type from which they originate. Adult stem cells found in the brain so far have not demonstrated an ability to differentiate into dopaminergic neurons; research in this area continues.

On either front, stem cell implant is an expensive, high-risk procedure that, at present, offers unpredictable long-term benefits for people with Parkinson's. There are many questions for researchers to answer before this becomes a viable treatment alternative.

See also ADRENAL MEDULLARY TRANSPLANT; ALLOGRAFT; BIOETHICS; BRAIN TISSUE TRANSPLANT; FETAL DOPAMINERGIC CELL TRANSPLANT; FETAL PORCINE BRAIN CELL TRANSPLANT; HOPE FOR A PARKINSON'S CURE; MICHAEL J. FOX FOUNDATION FOR PARKINSON'S RESEARCH; XENOGRAFT.

stereotaxis A method for immobilizing the head and allowing neurosurgeons to guide instruments into the inner portions of the brain precisely during NEUROSURGERY. It also is called stereotaxic surgery or stereotactic surgery. The term means "solid arrangement." A device called a stereotaxic halo is fitted over the person's head and held in place by four screws inserted into the skull. This is done with local anesthesia to numb the areas where the screws are placed; most people experience very little discomfort after the halo is attached. The halo is a lightweight but rigid frame that supports the instruments during surgery, permitting the neurosurgeon to align their insertion into the brain with imagery obtained from MAGNETIC RESONANCE IMAGING (MRI). During surgery the neurosurgeon attaches additional components that hold and guide instruments during surgery. This system allows complete coordination with computer-generated images for surgery that proceeds literally cell by cell. This is especially important in neurosurgery because the brain's structures are less consistent among individuals than are the structures of other organ systems, and mistakes can have permanent and disastrous consequences. MICROELECTRODE RECORDING is often used with stereotaxis as a complementary technique to ensure that the anatomic target neurons exhibit the correct physiology; different neuronal groups have different electrical firing patterns.

See also ABLATION; DEEP BRAIN STIMULATION; MACROELECTRODE; MICROELECTRODE; PALLIDOTOMY; SURGERY; THALAMOTOMY.

stop hesitation See GAIT DISTURBANCE.

stress Circumstances and events that challenge the body's physical and emotional systems. The source of stress can be external, such as the pressures of everyday life. Stress also can be internal, such as the effects of disease. Stress worsens the symptoms of Parkinson's disease.

Physiology of Stress

The body's stress response mechanisms are primitive, designed to give the body the resources it needs to fight or flee—a life-or-death kind of response. When the body perceives stress, a number of physiological events immediately take place: Blood pressure rises, blood peripheral vessels constrict to move blood to vital organs and to the large skeletal muscles, heart rate and breathing increase. The autonomic NERVOUS SYSTEM initiates these actions, stimulating the release of various hormones. Key among them is EPINEPHRINE, which functions as a NEUROTRANSMITTER in the brain and both a neurotransmitter and a HORMONE in the rest of the body. Its increased peripheral circulation heightens muscle activity.

Changes take place at the cell level, preparing tissues to draw more or to conserve energy, depending on their roles. The stomach, for example, slows its activities and the heart boosts its functions. In the normal scheme of things, stress boosts body readiness, the body responds to remove the body from the circumstance causing the stress, and the body returns to normal functions. When the stress is frequent or continual, the body does not have a chance to return to normal and instead remains in a state of heightened readiness. Eventually this state alters body mechanisms.

Physical Stress

Many factors create physical stress to the body. Exposure to toxins and chemicals causes changes in cell functions, sometimes damaging cells and tissues over time. Scientists believe that such long-term stress contributes to Parkinson's disease. Beyond a certain point cells are not able to protect themselves or to recover from damage to their structures or functions, and they die. Genetic defects also can cause physical stress to cells, causing changes in them that result in illness. Researchers believe the TAU deposits characteristic of ALZHEIMER'S DISEASE and the synuclein deposits (LEWY BODIES) characteristic of Parkinson's disease develop as a result of genetic instructions gone awry. These deposits "clog" cells, preventing them from carrying out their normal functions.

Emotional Stress

Continued stress affects emotional stability and well-being. The body's stress reactions further alter the balance of neurotransmitters in the brain, contributing to conditions such as ANXIETY and DEPRES-

SION. When these conditions already are present in the person with Parkinson's, stressful situations often aggravate and exacerbate them. Emotional stress may take the form of anger, frustration, sadness, or worry and often disrupts everyday life. For the person with Parkinson's emotional stress intensifies symptoms. Emotional stress can be more wearing than physical stress, as its causes often are harder to identify and isolate.

Parkinson's Disease and Stress

People with Parkinson's deal with both physical and emotional stress. The disease takes an enormous toll on the body's structures and functions, as neuromuscular degeneration and the resulting symptoms change nearly every aspect of the entire body. Eventually the effect is cascading. Recent research suggests that the dopamine depletion also begins to affect peripheral body systems such as the heart and blood vessels, altering the numbers of epinephrine receptors in the cells of their tissues and changing the way these organs respond to the body's biochemical needs. At present the most effective means of delaying these changes is effective control of symptoms through ANTI-PARKINSON'S MEDICATIONS.

Caregivers and Stress

Just as the person with Parkinson's may feel there is no escape from the disease's physical symptoms, the caregiver often feels confined by the circumstances of the loved one's needs. It is important that caregivers recognize the extent to which stress affects them and take measures to relieve stress. This process includes using STRESS REDUCTION TECHNIQUES and trying to establish ways to be relieved of the demands of caregiving, even for a short time, on a regular basis.

See also COMPASSION; COPING WITH ONGOING CARE OF PARKINSON'S; EMOTIONS; EMPATHY; OXIDATIVE STRESS.

stress reduction techniques Methods to cope with the effects of stress. People find relief in many ways; the "best" are the ones that work for each individual and that the person can and will use. Stress reduction techniques include

• Breathing exercises: Calm, deep, slow breaths help to slow the body's pace and ease anxiety. Drawing a series of deep breaths at frequent intervals throughout the day can restore a sense of control and groundedness.

- Meditation: Quiet reflection and focus still the mind and relax the body. There are many forms of meditation, from the structured methods of Transcendental Meditation to the informal practice of taking a few minutes to concentrate on the breathing.

- Exercise: Activities that put the body in motion help to dissipate energy the body has readied for fight or flight, returning body functions to normal. Walking is one of the easiest and most effective and has the added advantage of diverting the attention of the mind.

- Yoga: This ancient Eastern practice integrates physical postures with breath control and meditation. Most people benefit from taking a class to learn how to perform the postures safely and correctly. Then yoga can be used anywhere, any time. Most people find yoga as relaxing and restorative, physically and emotionally.

- Tai chi: An ancient form of martial arts, tai chi employs slow, flowing movements that calm the body and the mind. Generally done in groups or classes, tai chi is also probably useful for improving balance and posture.

- Aromatherapy: Certain fragrances are soothing and relaxing.

It is important to recognize anxiety and depression, and to treat them appropriately with medications if indicated. Many people find support groups helpful outlets for expressing concerns and worries, relieving emotional stress. Psychotherapy can help people to understand the sources or causes of stress and take actions to alleviate or mediate them to the extent possible. Psychotherapy also can teach specific coping mechanisms.

See also ALTERNATIVE THERAPIES; BIOFEEDBACK; SUPPORTIVE THERAPIES.

striatonigral degeneration See MULTIPLE SYSTEM ATROPHY.

striatum A part of the BASAL GANGLIA, the cluster of neurons deep within the BRAIN that regulates voluntary movement. The striatum consists of the PUTAMEN and the CAUDATE, two components of the basal ganglia, and controls the smoothness and coordination of movement. The name means "striped," a reference to the striatum's cordlike appearance. The striatum is primarily a bidirectional conduit linking the basal ganglia and other structures of the brain that participate in movement. Striatal neurons in the putamen are the main targets in the basal ganglia for DOPAMINE from the substantia nigra, the key NEUROTRANSMITTER affected by Parkinson's disease. It provides inhibitory (mainly GABA) outputs to the globus pallidus, THALAMUS, and brainstem.

The substantia nigra produces most of the dopamine that these structures require. The pigmented dopamine-producing neurons of the substantia nigra have long projections, called the NIGROSTRIATAL FIBERS, that carry dopamine to the putamen. These fibers are lost as Parkinson's progresses. The STRIATONIGRAL FIBERS conduct signals from the striatum and the thalamus to the substantia nigra; this pathway seems to remain intact as Parkinson's progresses, although the diminished supply of dopamine alters neuron function just as it does elsewhere in the basal ganglia.

The striatum also produces and circulates small amounts of ACETYLCHOLINE, a neurotransmitter that facilitates communication between neurons and muscle cells. Although acetylcholine levels do not change in Parkinson's disease, researchers believe the imbalance between dopamine and acetylcholine that results when dopamine becomes depleted allows acetylcholine to become hyperactive, overstimulating neurons to the extent that nerve signals overwhelm muscle cells. Such changes in the striatum may cause the TREMORS characteristic of Parkinson's disease. Surgical treatment that targets the globus pallidus or especially the thalamus, structures that receive and send nerve signals through the striatum, is sometimes successful in controlling tremors for an extended time.

See also MULTIPLE SYSTEM ATROPHY; PALLIDOTOMY; PARKINSON'S PLUS SYNDROMES; THALAMOTOMY.

structured treatment interruption (STI) See DRUG HOLIDAY.

substantia nigra   A structure within the BASAL GANGLIA (a collection of nerve clusters that regulate voluntary movement) that produces nearly all of the DOPAMINE that the BRAIN requires for communication of NEURONS related to movement. The name is Latin for "black substance," a reference to the dark pigmentation of some of the cells of this structure. A protein called neuromelanin accounts for the pigmentation; it accumulates as a result of dopamine metabolism. Although biochemically neuromelanin is very similar to the melanin that pigments skin, there is no correlation between skin pigmentation and the amount of neuromelanin in the substantia nigra.

The substantia nigra is integral to voluntary movement. It has two distinct parts, the substantia nigra pars compacta (SNc), which means "dense part," and the substantia nigra pars reticulata (SNr), which means "networked part." The names are references to the appearances of the different tissues. Although both the SNc and the SNr communicate with other structures of the basal ganglia, the SNc does so through dopamine and the SNr through another neurotransmitter, GAMMA-AMINOBUTYRIC ACID (GABA).

The SNc transmits nerve signals to and from the CAUDATE and PUTAMEN (known collectively as the STRIATUM) that affect motor function throughout the body. The SNr receives nerve signals from the striatum that are largely specific for movements of the head and eyes, which it then conveys to the THALAMUS and cerebral cortex. The SNc and the SNr do not have much interaction with each other. In the context of Parkinson's disease, references to the substantia nigra generally indicate the SNc.

It is the SNc that deteriorates in Parkinson's, cutting brain dopamine production. Dopamine is the key NEUROTRANSMITTER essential for modulating the basal ganglia outputs that regulate voluntary movement, and its depletion causes the motor disruptions that characterize Parkinson's. This is the foundation of Parkinson's disease, although scientists do not know what causes this sequence of events to begin or continue. The symptoms of Parkinson's disease become apparent when fewer than 20 percent of the SNc's dopaminergic neurons remain.

It is sometimes possible to detect and monitor the loss of dopaminergic neurons by using sophis-ticated FUNCTIONAL IMAGING STUDIES such as SINGLE PHOTON EMISSION COMPUTED TOMOGRAPHY (SPECT) or POSITRON EMISSION TOMOGRAPHY (PET). However, there is little clinical value in such studies unless the neurologist is looking for evidence of effectiveness of a regimen of ANTI-PARKINSON'S MEDICATIONS.

See ACCELERATED AGING; AGING; APOPTOSIS; PARKINSON'S DISEASE, CAUSES OF; PALLIDUM; STRIATUM; THALAMUS.

subthalamic nucleus   (STN)   See SUBTHALAMUS.

subthalamus   An area that includes the subthalamic nucleus (STN), a structure of the BASAL GANGLIA, specialized nerve clusters in the BRAIN that direct voluntary movement. It is located between the THALAMUS, the substantia nigra, and the HYPOTHALAMUS, and as are other structures in the brain it is a paired, or bilateral, structure. The subthalamus has a number of distinctive cell clusters that have different but integrated roles in voluntary movement. The functions of some of these areas and their roles in motor function are poorly understood.

Subthalamic Nucleus (STN)

The area of significance in Parkinson's disease is the subthalamic nucleus (STN), a dense cluster of NEURONS in the center of the subthalamus. The STN receives nerve signals from the globus PALLIDUS externus (external pallidus, or GPe) and sends nerve signals to the globus pallidus internus (internal pallidus, or GPi). These signals integrate with neuron communication from other structures of the basal ganglia. The GPi then sends on the mix of nerve signals to the THALAMUS, which in turn filters and organizes them before passing them through to the cerebral cortex (the part of the cerebrum that initiates the "call to action" setting into motion the sequence of events necessary for voluntary movement).

The dopamine depletion characteristic of Parkinson's disease allows the STN to become overactive in generating nerve signals to inhibit muscle activity. These signals flood the thalamus, which in turn decreases excitation of the cerebral cortex. Scientists believe this action is what causes motor symptoms such as bradykinesia and rigidity.

Subthalamotomy

Creating LESIONS in the STN, in surgical techniques similar to PALLIDOTOMY and THALAMOTOMY, is an INVESTIGATIONAL TREATMENT used to provide long-term relief of these symptoms by interrupting or blocking some of the STN's cells from functioning. Neurosurgeons have performed this surgery, called subthalamotomy, on about two dozen people who had late stage Parkinson's disease in OPEN-LABEL STUDIES. The majority experienced significant improvements in their Parkinson's symptoms and were able to reduce the levels of ANTI-PARKINSON'S MEDICATIONS they had been taking before the experimental surgery. However, as with almost all other surgical procedures for Parkinson's, the damage of Parkinson's continues to progress.

The STN is a much smaller structure within the brain than either the thalamus or the pallidus. Targeting it requires great precision, and the margin of error is very narrow. As with other ablative procedures, deep brain stimulation (DBS) offers many safety advantages over subthalamotomy. It remains unclear whether subthalamotomy offers any advantages over the more established ablative procedures of pallidotomy and thalamotomy, which also entail significant risk but target larger and better understood structures of the brain's movement system and therefore have a somewhat more comfortable margin of error.

See also SURGERY.

suicide   The act of taking one's own life. Suicide is a significant risk of DEPRESSION. Depression is among the symptoms of Parkinson's, affecting close to half of people who have the disease. It is difficult to know how prevalent thoughts about suicide are among people with Parkinson's. Statistics show that fewer of them commit suicide when compared to the general public even though depression is four to six times more common among people with Parkinson's. It is also sometimes hard to know when a person's comments and actions cross the line between what he or she experiences and expresses as the normal spectrum of emotions that accompany having a chronic, neurodegenerative disease and the point of concern. Sudden changes in behavior, such as giving away possessions or "getting things ready," are potential warning signs.

Thoughts of suicide may occur when a person feels hopeless and helpless and does not want to continue his or her current experience of life. Although the situation may not appear so bleak to those on the outside, the narrow focus of the person's perspective limits his or her ability to see beyond what appears to be an insurmountable problem or situation. The cause may be current physical symptoms that now preclude favorite activities or constrain independence or a projection of such restrictions into the future. Some people worry about the strain their debilitation, present or prospective, places on family members and in their despondent state believe it would be better to spare them this anguish. To the loved one this is frightening and extreme, but the person with depression cannot see other options.

It is important that the person with Parkinson's have someone to talk to, whether or not he or she is depressed, who will just listen without being judgmental or dismissive and without putting forth solutions or giving advice. Sometimes just sitting quietly with the person, letting the person know he or she is not alone, is enough for the moment. Most people who are feeling suicidal or who have thoughts of suicide try to talk about their feelings. Because of the difficulty of hearing or understanding such expressions, loved ones naturally responded by attempting to comfort the person or fix the perceived problems. A family member or caregiver who is concerned that a loved one with Parkinson's may be suicidal should contact a local suicide hotline (look in the telephone book's entry for "suicide") or the person's physician for advice about what to do and how best to help. Sometimes a person who is feeling suicidal finds it easier to speak with a counselor or therapist.

It is most important to treat depression when it does exist; doctors should regularly check for depression using objective clinical assessments. Many specialists in Parkinson's disease believe that depression is underrecognized and underdiagnosed and consequently undertreated. In Parkinson's disease the imbalances among neurotransmitters in the brain fluctuate, often widely, in correlation with medication dosages. There really is no stable or steady state, biochemically, and that affects all brain functions to some extent including those related to mood and emotion. Researchers believe this is why depression is common among people with Parkinson's and why depression typically responds well to treatment with ANTIDEPRESSANT MEDICATIONS such as the SELECTIVE SEROTONIN REUPTAKE INHIBITORS (SSRIs), which act to rebalance the brain's biochemicals.

See also ANXIETY; BECK DEPRESSION INVENTORY; COPING WITH DIAGNOSIS OF PARKINSON'S; EMOTIONS; HAMILTON DEPRESSION RATING SCALE; PSYCHOTHERAPY; QUALITY OF LIFE; SUPPORT GROUPS.

sundowning Episodes of DELUSIONS, HALLUCINA-TIONS, AGITATION, and increased DEMENTIA that intensify in the evening. Clinicians do not fully understand the timing of sundowning episodes. Theories include correlations with hormonal cycles in the body, fluctuations in brain neurotransmitter levels that result from medication peaks and troughs, a "crash" letdown+ from the activities of the day, and the somewhat surrealistic images that can occur as a combination of artificial lighting and shadows as evening begins. As are other dimensions of neurodegenerative diseases, it is likely a combination of all of these factors. Sundowning is a particularly common manifestation in ALZHEIMER'S DISEASE; its appearance in a person with Parkinson's disease suggests that dementia is present.

Sundowning is stressful for caregivers because they know it is coming and they know it is unpredictable. Agitation reaches a peak when family members are also tired and ready to relax, and the resources they need to be innovative and supportive are often wearing thin by this time of the day. Sometimes the loved one responds to efforts to keep activities and the surroundings calm and quiet. Other times, it seems that nothing family members try makes any difference. Sometimes changes in the ANTI-PARKINSON'S MEDICATION regimen improve the situation. Although in the person with Alzheimer's disease ANTIPSYCHOTIC MEDICATIONS are sometimes helpful, these drugs are a more limited option for the person with Parkinson's because the risk of motor side effects or intensified symptoms of Parkinson's is significant. Quetiapine, clozapine, and perhaps aripiprazole are thought to be the best antipsychotics for people with Parkinson's.

Establishing a predictable routine seems to be the most consistently helpful approach for manag-

ing sundowning. The routine should start while there is still plenty of daylight and should take place every day regardless of the day's activities. This schedule can be confining for family members and the person's response will continue to vary from day to day, but the sense of structure is useful to caregivers as well. Other recommendations include making sure to turn on lights in the house before darkness sets in and having someone stay with the person during the transitional time between daylight and darkness. Most people who experience sundowning become calm again as night falls.

See also COPING WITH ONGOING CARE OF PARKINSON'S; PSYCHOSIS; SUPPORT GROUPS.

support groups Organized gatherings of people who have common interests and concerns. There are support groups for people with Parkinson's and for caregivers and family members of people with Parkinson's. Many support groups are open to anyone who wishes to attend meetings; others are more restrictive. Various organizations sponsor support groups. Many are affiliated with Parkinson's organizations such as the NATIONAL PARKINSON FOUNDATION and the AMERICAN PARKINSON DISEASE ASSOCIATION. Hospitals, medical centers, neurology practices, senior centers, and churches also sponsor Parkinson's support groups. Appendix I lists resources for support groups.

Support groups provide a safe forum for sharing experiences, concerns, fears, and frustrations. Those who attend often find this process of exchange both informational and helpful for relieving STRESS, a chance to vent their feelings and EMOTIONS. Sometimes people with Parkinson's are reluctant to join support groups because their situation is stable and they do not want to hear about the symptoms that other people are experiencing, fearing the prospect of facing the potential of such symptoms themselves. But the course of Parkinson's is widely variable, and most people do not experience the full range of possible symptoms. Other people appreciate the opportunity to talk freely, because they sometimes cannot with family members and friends, and draw encouragement and reassurance from their involvement with a support group. Talking with others who live with

Parkinson's helps to give a broader perspective of the disease and the many ways in which it is possible to adjust and adapt to have a fairly normal experience of life. In support groups, too, people share their experiences and information about various treatment approaches, CLINICAL RESEARCH STUDIES, and INVESTIGATIONAL TREATMENTS.

See also DENIAL AND ACCEPTANCE; FRIENDSHIPS; PSYCHOSOCIAL FACTORS.

supportive therapies Treatment approaches, sometimes called ancillary services, that address the wide range of symptoms and difficulties associated with Parkinson's disease. While ANTI-PARKINSON'S MEDICATIONS and other treatment options such as SURGERY target the direct symptoms of Parkinson's, supportive therapies focus on improving or maintaining functions that those symptoms affect.

See also ADJUNCT THERAPIES; ALTERNATIVE THERAPIES; CARE MANAGEMENT AND PLANNING; MONOTHERAPY; TREATMENT ALGORITHM.

surgery Invasive intervention to alter the functions of brain structures involved in movement that become dysfunctional in Parkinson's disease. Surgeries may involve the creation of lesions, or scars, through a technique called ABLATION (burning a very small segment of tissue, often just selective neurons) to interrupt the flow of nerve signals, the installation of deep brain stimulation electrodes to remodulate pathologic patterns of neuronal output, the implantation of tubes for the infusion of neurotrophic factors, the implantation of dopamine producing cells, or other possible interventions to improve Parkinson's symptoms such as TREMORS, BRADYKINESIA, AKINESIA, and other DYSKINESIAS. Because the risks associated with any surgery of the brain are relatively high, surgery to treat Parkinson's typically becomes an option only when ANTI-PARKINSON'S MEDICATIONS no longer suppress motor symptoms. The most common surgical procedures are:

- DEEP BRAIN STIMULATION (DBS), which is temporary and modifiable

COMMON SUPPORTIVE THERAPIES

Supportive Therapy	Helps with	Covered by Insurance or Medicare
Physical therapy	Joint range of motion; muscle strength and tone; flexibility and movement; gait; freezing; balance	Yes, with limits
Occupational therapy	Use of adaptive equipment and assist devices; new ways to perform functions and tasks; home environment changes to improve safety and mobility; systems to compensate for memory problems (such as medication sets); functional nutrition counseling	Yes, with limits
Speech-language pathology (speech therapy)	Speech clarity; chewing and swallowing; breath control	Yes, with limits
Massage therapy	Muscle spasms and cramps caused by dyskinesias; dystonia	Sometimes
Meditation	Pain relief; relaxation; stress relief	No
Home health care	Feeding tube; dressing changes and wound care; injury care; IV or parenteral lines	Yes, with limits
Psychotherapy	Depression; anxiety; emotional distress; coping; stress relief	Yes, with limits
Acupuncture	Pain relief; stress relief	Sometimes
Biofeedback	Pain relief; stress relief	Sometimes
Chiropractic	Joint range of motion; muscle tone; flexibility	Yes, with limits
Tai chi	Movement; balance; breath control; stress relief	No
Yoga	Flexibility; balance; breath control; stress relief	No

- PALLIDOTOMY, which creates a lesion in the PAL-LIDUS to relieve bradykinesia, akinesia, and other dyskinesias

- THALAMOTOMY, which creates a lesion in the THALAMUS to relieve tremors

Researchers are exploring other surgical treatments that are still investigational, too, such as subthalamotomy, STEM CELL IMPLANT, FETAL DOPAMINERGIC CELL TRANSPLANT, and FETAL PORCINE BRAIN CELL TRANSPLANT.

Neurosurgeons use stereotactic frames, structures that attach to the skull, to assure precise placement of electrodes for these surgeries. This procedure allows computer-guided probe advancement, minimizing the risk of damage to adjacent tissues and to cells along the path of the probe. MAGNETIC RESONANCE IMAGING (MRI) helps neurosurgeons to locate and reach the sites within the brain where they wish to place the MACROELECTRODES to create the ablations or to implant macroelectrodes for deep brain stimulation. Microelectrodes are often inserted prior to the macroelectrode so that the electrical activity of target cells can be determined to see if they match the expected activity of the target (for example, cells firing in synchrony with the tremor in the thalamus, or cells that fire with passive movement of the involved limb in the globus pallidus) in a technique known as microelectrode recording. The person is mildly sedated for relaxation during the surgery but awake so the electrophysiology remains optimal for microelectrode recording and he or she can respond to questions and instructions from the neurosurgeons. The person's responses help the surgeon ensure proper placement of the microelectrodes and test the effectiveness of the ablation or stimulation by using a brief test stimulation to ensure both efficacy and lack of side effects. Many results from ablative procedures are immediately apparent, although during the recovery period of eight to 10 weeks most people notice fluctuations in their symptoms as the tissue surrounding the ablated lesion first swells and then recedes, as a normal aspect of the healing process.

Benefits of Surgery

Surgical procedures can provide long-term relief from the most troublesome symptoms of Parkin-son's. As with medical treatments for Parkinson's, it is difficult to predict exactly how a person's symptoms will respond, partly because the physiology of the brain is unique from individual to individual and partly because the surgery disrupts only the consequences of Parkinson's and cannot stop its progression. Eventually the disease progresses and symptoms will likely return and worsen. Most people continue to take anti-Parkinson's medications after surgery although some surgeries are associated with significant expected reductions in the amount of medication required, which improves dopaminergic side effects.

Risks of Surgery

The risks of surgery for Parkinson's disease are substantial, as they are for any procedure that enters the brain. Even with impeccable sterile technique it is impossible to rid the surface of the skin of bacteria completely; surgical instruments can carry bacteria into the brain, where they can cause infection. As well, bleeding can occur within the brain and cause damage to neurons. The consequences of such side effects can be minimal or catastrophic, depending on the areas of the brain that they affect and whether neurosurgeons can intervene to treat them.

A key risk of the surgeries for Parkinson's is damage to adjacent tissues and structures during the placement of the microelectrodes and the macroelectrodes; these structures are not clearly delineated or consistent in terms of their physical location and structure. The pallidus and thalamus are very close to the optic tract, the path of nerve structures that manage vision. The neurosurgeon repeatedly asks the person whether he or she sees flashes of light or any other visual representations, which are a clear sign that the probe is very near the optic tract. Damage to the optic tract can result in permanent vision problems. It also is possible for the probe used to guide electrode placement to cause damage along the path of its progression into the thalamus or globus pallidus, with potential to cause temporary or permanent movement dysfunctions other than those of the Parkinson's, including localized, regional, or extensive paralysis. Although many complications are obvious immediately, others do not appear until weeks or even months after the surgery.

Determining Whether and When
Surgery Is Appropriate

Perhaps only 20 percent of people with Parkinson's are likely to benefit from current surgery options. Those who experience the greatest level of success

- Are younger than age 70. People who are older have a more difficult recovery from the stress of surgery and seem to experience less substantial effects from surgical interventions.

- Have been taking anti-Parkinson's medications and have reached the point at which they have significant fluctuations with good ON-STATES and either severe on-dyskinesias or significant OFF-STATE symptoms.

- For subthalamic or pallidal targets, have primarily bradykinesia and akinesia.

- For thalamic targets have only tremors.

People who generally do not benefit significantly from surgery for Parkinson's

- Derive reasonable control of symptoms through anti-Parkinson's medications, with minimal off-state episodes.

- Have a PARKINSON'S PLUS SYNDROME or rapidly advancing, severe Parkinson's symptoms that do not respond well to anti-Parkinson's medications.

- Have other significant health problems such as hypertension (high blood pressure), heart disease, or diabetes.

- Have dementia or significant cognitive impairment.

It is important that the person to have appropriate expectations and a full understanding of the potential benefits and risks. Surgery cannot cure Parkinson's disease; nor can it eliminate the need for, at a minimum, LEVODOPA. It is not possible to know how an individual will respond, or how long the effects will last. Each person must consider his or her unique circumstances.

See also CLINICAL RESEARCH STUDIES; GENE THERAPY; HOPE FOR A PARKINSON'S CURE; INVESTIGATIONAL TREATMENT; MACROELECTRODE; NEUROTROPHIC FACTORS; STEREOTAXIS.

surgery, ablative   See ABLATION.

surgery, stimulative   See DEEP BRAIN STIMULATION.

swallowing   A sequence of actions that moves food and liquids from the mouth to the stomach. Movement of the muscles of the mouth, including the tongue, is voluntary. Parkinson's disease often affects the function of these muscles, causing the same kinds of symptoms that affect the muscles of mobility such as BRADYKINESIA (slowed muscle response) and lack of coordination. Putting a bite of food into the mouth activates the swallowing sequence—normally the lips close, the jaw muscles move the jaw up and down and side to side to allow the teeth to break the food into pieces small enough to swallow, and the tongue mixes the pieces with saliva to make them soft enough to swallow. The tongue then presses against the roof of the mouth to move the food to the back of the mouth and into the throat.

At this juncture a series of involuntary movements take over, propelling the food down the esophagus and into the stomach. The epiglottis, a small flap of tissue, closes over the opening to the trachea to keep the food out of the lungs, and a series of powerful, wavelike contractions (peristalsis) carry the food down the esophagus. The sphincter muscle at the opening to the stomach relaxes, and the food drops into the stomach. The force of this involuntary sequence is so powerful that it can move food from the throat to the stomach even when a person is upside-down.

A slowed response at any part of the voluntary sequence affects the rest of the movements. Uncoordinated jaw movements result in inadequate pressure and motion to chew the food. If the tongue does not move properly, the food remains dry, making it harder to swallow. Parkinson's can cause problems with the involuntary sequence of swallowing as well, especially if the person is taking ANTICHOLINERGIC MEDICATIONS to treat TREMORS, which have the effect of slowing the actions of involuntary muscles such as those in the esophagus and the rest of the digestive tract.

Swallowing problems, called DYSPHAGIA, affect the person's ability to eat. The manifestations of dysphagia can be fairly minor, such as DROOLING or leaking of food from the mouth during the voluntary phase of swallowing. Although these conditions seldom have health consequences, they often are embarrassing to the person with Parkinson's. Aspirating food or liquid into the lungs is a significant health risk that can cause choking (a piece of food blocks the airways) and aspiration pneumonia (food particles settle into the lungs and cause infection). Both of these conditions can be life-threatening; everyone living in the household should know how to perform the HEIMLICH MANEUVER, a method for dislodging food that becomes stuck in the airways.

Some people with Parkinson's have less saliva than they need to chew safely and effectively, usually as a side effect of medications such as anticholinergics, which dry out mucous membranes such as the lining of the mouth. Sometimes doctors prescribe anticholinergics specifically for this purpose, when saliva accumulates in the mouth and drooling becomes a problem. Most people with Parkinson's have adequate saliva but lack the muscle control to swallow it. It is important to make a conscious effort to swallow saliva regularly, to prevent it from pooling in the mouth. However, saliva can present as significant a choking or aspiration risk as food.

SPEECH-LANGUAGE PATHOLOGY can help a person improve control of the muscles involved in swallowing and learn new methods for coping with symptoms such as bradykinesia. Swallowing and speech use many of the same physical structures, including muscle sequences. Techniques to improve one invariably improve the other. If choking and aspirating become more frequent than not as a result of worsening Parkinson's symptoms, using a FEEDING TUBE to bypass the swallowing process may be necessary. Although many people resist use of a feeding tube, perceiving it as a capitulation to the disease process or a means of artificially sustaining life, it can relieve discomfort with minimal intrusion. Sometimes the symptoms of Parkinson's more significantly affect the structures of the mouth and throat, leaving other voluntary muscle functions less affected or even intact. In such situations the person with Parkinson's is not at the end of life but cannot get enough nutrition to meet the body's needs. A feeding tube can alleviate these problems.

Dehydration and malnutrition are risks for people who have swallowing difficulties, who may consciously choose not to eat or drink or not eat or drink because of their difficulty. It is important for the person with Parkinson's to drink adequate fluids and eat foods that are nutritious. For a person who has swallowing problems, soft or pureed foods often are easier to manage.

See also EATING; NUTRITION AND DIET; PARENTERAL NUTRITION.

sweating Excessive and even drenching episodes of sweating are common in Parkinson's, particularly in mid to late stages of the disease, when OFF-STATES begin to occur. Excessive sweating can be a consequence of damage to the autonomic NERVOUS SYSTEM as Parkinson's progresses or a side effect of ANTI-PARKINSON'S MEDICATIONS.

The autonomic nervous system regulates the body's autonomic, or automatic, functions such as heartbeat, blood pressure, and temperature control. The DOPAMINE depletion that characterizes Parkinson's affects the functions of autonomic nervous system structures including parts of the BASAL GANGLIA that participate in directing smooth (involuntary) muscle activity. The SUBTHALAMIC NUCLEUS (STN) and the THALAMUS, a structure in the midbrain that modulates nerve signals to and from the CEREBELLUM, play roles in transmitting nerve signals that control smooth muscle tissue such as in the walls of the blood vessels. Dilation of the blood vessels is part of the body's process for cooling itself, moving larger volumes of blood closer to the skin's surface. This process releases heat from within the body. Sweating is an element of this process and typically occurs in coordination with blood vessel dilatation.

People who have Parkinson's often experience sweating when LEVODOPA and other dopaminergic drugs reach peak levels in the body and during off-states. Such sweating can be intense, drenching the person within minutes. Adjusting medication dosages sometimes relieves or at least moderates this response; a dance to find dosages high enough to relieve Parkinson's symptoms without causing such responses ensues. ANTICHOLINERGIC MEDICATIONS such as BENZTROPINE (Cogentin) and BIPERIDEN (Akineton) provide relief by suppressing the actions of ACETYLCHOLINE on smooth muscle. ALPHA-ADRENERGIC BLOCKER (ANTAGONIST) medications such as Prazozin (Minipress) and CLONIDINE (Catapres) suppress the actions of EPINEPHRINE to similar effect.

Temperature regulation is a complex process that involves a number of body systems including the endocrine system, a network of hormone-producing structures and their hormones. Thyroid imbalance, which becomes increasingly common with advancing age, also can be a culprit in dysfunctions of temperature regulation. Usually a few simple blood tests can determine whether the thyroid gland is properly functioning, and thyroid replacement hormone can correct imbalances. Episodes of excessive sweating often are embarrassing as well as uncomfortable for the person with Parkinson's. Changing into dry clothing when the sweating episode ends restores comfort and prevents the further discomfort of chilling. Some people with Parkinson's find that warm temperatures trigger excessive sweating or experience chronic excessive sweating involving the face and head. This condition can exacerbate skin problems such as DANDRUFF and sebaceous dermatitis.

See also DERMATITIS, SEBACEOUS; DROOLING; HYGIENE.

Symmetrel See AMANTADINE.

symptoms of Parkinson's disease See PARKINSON'S DISEASE.

synapse See NEURON.

tacrine An ACETYLCHOLINESTERASE INHIBITOR medication taken to improve COGNITIVE FUNCTION. Tacrine (Cognex) is U.S. Food and Drug Administration–(FDA)-approved in the United States for treatment of COGNITIVE IMPAIRMENT and DEMENTIA of people with ALZHEIMER'S DISEASE. Its use in people with Parkinson's is open-label. Because there is a significant overlap in disease processes between Alzheimer's and Parkinson's, some neurologists prescribe acetylcholinesterase inhibitors for people with Parkinson's who have dementia, MEMORY LOSS, HALLUCINATIONS, and cognitive impairment even when Alzheimer's is not present. Though there are reports of its effectiveness in Lewy body dementia and the dementia of Parkinson's disease, its effectiveness is inconsistent; some people notice measurable improvement, and others experience no difference. There does not appear to be a way to assess who is likely to respond and who is not; when significant cognitive impairment is a factor in Parkinson's, many people consider it worth the effort to try tacrine to see whether it produces improvement. However, tacrine can cause worsened motor function in people with Parkinson's.

Tacrine and other acetylcholinesterase inhibitors work by preventing the ENZYME ACETYLCHOLINESTERASE from metabolizing ACETYLCHOLINE, a brain NEUROTRANSMITTER important to cognitive function that becomes depleted in Alzheimer's disease. Acetylcholine also affects muscle activity and in excess causes TREMORS, DYSTONIA, and other DYSKINESIAS. By extending acetylcholine's availability in the brain, tacrine can significantly worsen the neuromuscular symptoms of Parkinson's or cause such symptoms to emerge in people with Alzheimer's. Each acetylcholinesterase inhibitor has somewhat different actions in the brain, so if tacrine is ineffective or causes undesired side effects, one of the other medications in this classification may be more effective. RIVASTIGMINE has the most evidence of both its usefulness and safety in people with Parkinson's, hence it is currently the first choice of Parkinson's experts for treating dementia.

See also DONEPEZIL; DYSKINESIA; GALANTAMINE; OFF-LABEL DRUG; RIVASTIGMINE.

tai chi A form of martial art that emphasizes slow, smooth, flowing movements. Tai chi, which originated in China in the 16th century, integrates physical postures with MEDITATION. The premise of tai chi is that it encourages the free flow of life energy, called *chi* in Eastern medicine. From the Western perspective the gentle nature of this structured exercise belies its ability to stretch and tone muscles, improving overall fitness, joint flexibility, and balance. The meditation aspect provides relaxation and stress relief. As in all martial arts, BREATH CONTROL and breathing exercises are essential components of tai chi.

Many health clubs, community centers, and senior centers offer classes in tai chi. Although the movements are easy to learn and perform, many people enjoy the social environment of doing them in groups. There are many different movements that combine into sequences called forms; in a class or group there is a leader who presents an organization of forms for a 20- or 30-minute session. The group leader can help individuals adapt tai chi movements and forms to accommodate specific limitations or needs. Groups often meet outdoors, weather permitting, in parks and other areas where the movements can interact with the natural environment. Doing tai chi regularly (several times a week to daily) provides the most benefit.

The National Institutes of Health (NIH) and others have conducted controlled studies of tai chi's health benefits, concluding that it is a generally safe and effective way, especially for seniors to improve and maintain mobility, reducing risks related to poor motor skills such as falls. It is believed that tai chi probably provides the same mobility and balance benefits in those with Parkinson's.

See also STRESS; STRESS REDUCTION TECHNIQUES; YOGA.

tardive dyskinesia (TD) Involuntary, repetitive, and often contorted movements that develop as side effects of ANTIPSYCHOTIC MEDICATIONS and other neuroleptic drugs such as the antinausea medications prochlorperazine (Compazine) and promethazine (Phenergan). Other drugs that alter the brain's biochemical balance can sometimes cause TD as well; those taken to control PSYCHOSIS, DEMENTIA, and other disturbances of behavior related to brain function carry the highest risk. *Tardive* means "late" or "delayed;" TD develops after these medications have been used over an extended period and reflects permanent damage to the brain's neurochemical structures and networks. The dyskinesias can involve any muscle or muscle group and often affect the face and mouth, appearing as repetitive grimacing or movements of the lips and tongue.

The newer antipsychotics, called atypical because they affect the brain differently than conventional antipsychotic drugs do, such as clozapine (Clozaril) quetiapine (Seroquel), clanzapine (Zyprexa), risperidone (Risperdal), and ariprazole (Abilify) are less likely to cause tardive dyskinesia and should be the first drugs tried. Older antipsychotics such as CHLORPROMAZINE (Thorazine), HALOPERIDOL (Haldol), thioridazine (Mellaril), and thiothixene (Navane) carry a high risk of motor side effects including TD. Doctors have traditionally prescribed these medications for people with Alzheimer's disease who have moderate to severe dementia, some of whom also have Parkinson's disease.

See also MEDICATION MANAGEMENT; MEDICATION SIDE EFFECTS.

task simplification A process of dividing tasks and activities into small steps to make accomplishing them easier. This eases the anxiety people with Parkinson's often feel about being unable to complete activities and helps to accommodate the motor limitations that develop as the disease progresses. Daily activities such as bathing, dressing, toileting, preparing meals, and even walking can be overwhelming to the person who struggles with DEXTERITY, COORDINATION, and BALANCE, particularly in the middle to late stages of the disease. Although people tend to view everyday functions as single events, they actually are sequences of steps. COGNITIVE IMPAIRMENT, even mild, and the disruptions to thought processes (drowsiness and difficulty concentrating or paying attention) that ANTI-PARKINSON'S MEDICATIONS often cause can affect a person's ability to connect the steps into actions that once were commonplace. Family members and caregivers can make daily functions more efficient and less traumatic by helping to organize them into their component steps.

- Establish routines that break tasks into the smallest possible steps. Rather than looking at morning hygiene as a process of toileting, showering, brushing teeth, shaving, and combing hair, approach the process step by step. Toileting, for example, entails several actions: step into bathroom, turn on light, lift toilet lid, turn around, pull down pants, sit down.

- Allow enough time to carry out each step and maintain a consistent routine for this time allocation. Although some mornings the person with Parkinson's may complete the steps of showering in 30 minutes, other mornings those steps may require an hour. It always is better to take each step without rushing and to finish ahead of schedule.

- Lay out items of personal hygiene, clothing, kitchen utensils—whatever items the person needs to complete the task. Lay them out in the sequence in which they are used.

- When GAIT DISTURBANCES such as start hesitation and difficulty in changing direction become problems, encourage the person to think of each component of mobility separately. Sometimes it is overwhelming for the person with Parkinson's to consider entering a room to sit down and watch television. Breaking down the actions into small units makes them less intimidating and gives the person a specific focus. This may involve establishing markers within the room, such as taking three steps to the coffee table.

The person's needs will change over time as the Parkinson's progresses. It is important to remain observant; if the person seems to struggle with what appear to be simple steps, look for ways to make the actions even more basic. Ask the person what would make them easier. Often solutions are possible but not obvious.

See also ACTIVITIES OF DAILY LIVING; ADAPTIVE EQUIPMENT AND ASSIST DEVICES; ADJUSTING TO LIVING WITH PARKINSON'S; BATHING AND BATHROOM ORGANIZATION; BEDROOM COMFORT; COPING WITH ONGOING CARE OF PARKINSON'S; KITCHEN EFFICIENCY.

Tasmar See TOLCAPONE.

tau A protein that accumulates in the BRAIN NEURONS of people with Alzheimer's disease, creating entanglements and disrupting neuron activity. Tau is important to nerve cell functions and to maintenance the neuron's cellular structure and integrity. The tau gene controls tau metabolism; it appears that a defect in this gene allows either excessive tau production or incomplete tau metabolism, leading to accumulations of tau deposits within neurons. Doctors can detect deposits only at autopsy after death. Some people with Parkinson's disease also have tau deposits. Researchers are not certain whether the deposits indicates that such people also had the beginnings of, or undetected, Alzheimer's disease at the time of death or that there are connections between dysfunctions with tau metabolism and that of the synuclein (a different brain protein) that composes the LEWY BODY deposits in brain neurons that are characteristic of Parkinson's disease. Scientists do suspect a connection as there appear to be overlaps in the disease processes of Alzheimer's and Parkinson's.

See also GENE MUTATIONS; GENE THERAPY; LEWY BODIES; ALPHA-SYNUCLEIN GENE.

telecommuting Working from home or a distant location and communicating with the workplace through the Internet via computer and other electronic connections. As many jobs become more dependent on electronic processes, the physical location in which they take place has less relevance. A computer, modem, and telephone line can allow the work to take place in virtually any location. Telecommuting often is a viable alternative for people with Parkinson's who have mobility restrictions that create difficulty in commuting or moving around in an office yet are otherwise capable of performing the tasks of their job. Sometimes telecommuting is the preferred workplace accommodation for an employer and a person who has Parkinson's disease.

See also ADAPTIVE EQUIPMENT AND ASSIST DEVICES; AMERICANS WITH DISABILITIES ACT; INSTRUMENTAL ACTIVITIES OF DAILY LIVING; WORKPLACE ACCOMMODATIONS FOR PARKINSON'S; WORKPLACE RELATIONSHIPS.

temazepam A SLEEP MEDICATION in the BENZODIAZEPINE family of drugs. Temazepam (Restoril) is fast-acting, generally producing significant drowsiness within 30 minutes. Its effect lasts about six hours, helping to prevent waking in the middle of the night. Most people do not feel any lingering effects the next morning. Its intended action is to produce drowsiness, which alters judgment and balance. A person who gets up during the night, for instance, to use the bathroom, may be disoriented and confused and experience difficulty with coordination. This condition increases the risk of problems such as FALLS.

As with other benzodiazepines, resistance and dependence can develop when temazepam is used for more than a few weeks; this risk is highest with short-acting agents such as alprazolam (Xanax), triazdam (Halcion), and oxazepam (Serax). Other medications, particularly other benzodiazepines taken as MUSCLE RELAXANTS or as ANTIANXIETY MEDICATIONS, that cause drowsiness can result with pronounced sleepiness. Benzodiazepines doctors often prescribe for people with Parkinson's include LORAZEPAM (Ativan) and CLONAZEPAM (Klonopin). Some anti-Parkinson's medications also cause drowsiness, including dopaminergics such as LEVODOPA and DOPAMINE AGONIST MEDICATIONS such as BROMOCRIPTINE (Parlodel).

See also RESTLESS LEG SYNDROME (RLS); SLEEP DISTURBANCES.

thalamotomy   A surgical procedure that creates a LESION (scar) in the THALAMUS to disrupt the nerve signals between the BRAIN and the muscles. The thalamus regulates neuron communication between the cerebral CORTEX, which initiates voluntary movement, and the structures of the brain that participate in controlling and coordinating voluntary movement (primarily the BASAL GANGLIA, brainstem, and cerebellum). Thalamotomy is effective for reducing TREMORS in some people with Parkinson's disease but does not usually have a significant effect on other symptoms such as BRADYKINESIA and AKINESIA; PALLIDOTOMY, a similar lesioning procedure that targets the pallidus rather than the thalamus, is more effective for reducing these symptoms.

Neurosurgeons first used thalamotomy in the 1950s, before the computer and imaging technology used today to assure precision in placement of the lesion was available. In its early years, thalamotomy had a high rate of complications that often included other neuromuscular disturbances such as DYSKINESIAS (involuntary, abnormal movements) and even paralysis. When LEVODOPA debuted in 1967 as a viable DOPAMINE replacement therapy for Parkinson's disease, it supplanted the riskier surgical treatments as the treatment of first choice.

As computer technology has made great precision in placing lesions now possible, however, thalamotomy has again become a treatment option for a select few people with Parkinson's; the greatest success in long-term symptom relief occurs in those who have TREMOR-DOMINANT PARKINSON'S affecting only one side of the body. Thalamotomy also is an effective treatment alternative for ESSENTIAL TREMOR, another neuromuscular disorder that produces tremors. The thalamus is a paired structure, with one on either side of the brain. Bilateral procedures are avoided since they have a high risk of causing problems with swallowing (dysphagia), speaking (dysarthria), or thinking. Unilateral procedures are safer, but they carry some risk of causing numbness, gait problems, dysarthria, balance problems, or thinking changes. Neurosurgeons typically target a small area of the thalamus called the ventral intermediate nucleus (VIM), the cells of which become overly active in Parkinson's disease targeting the thalamus that is opposite the side of the body experiencing the more severe tremors. This is done because nerve structures cross when they leave the brainstem, controlling activity on the opposite side of the body.

Thalamotomy is generally a treatment that becomes a reasonable option only when medications do not control symptoms. As in all neurosurgery, thalamotomy carries risks of infection, bleeding, and damage to other parts of the brain. It is not an effective alternative for people who have PARKINSON'S PLUS SYNDROMES or for those who are doing well with ANTI-PARKINSON'S MEDICATIONS. People who have bilateral tremors (tremors equally affecting both sides of the body) may not receive adequate relief as tremors continue on the nonlesioned side.

Thalamotomy generally is performed as inpatient surgery; the person spends the nights before and after the procedure in the hospital. The day before the surgery, the neurosurgeon affixes the stereotaxic halo, a device attached to the skull that allows the precision of computer-assisted placement of the microelectrodes that deliver the ablative lesion. MAGNETIC RESONANCE IMAGING (MRI) determines the location for placing the lesion, and the halo allows the computer to guide electrode induction and placement. Although the ABLATION can be performed by radiosurgery, which requires no sedation, most procedures are open procedures that use thermocoagulation to destroy the tissue. During surgery the person receives mild sedation to relieve anxiety but remains awake to respond to directions from the neurosurgeon, to allow for normal neuronal activity so that microelectrode recording patterns may be used to confirm the location of tremor synchronous firing thalamic neurons, and to assess the effect of the lesion, which is immediate. The person's participation helps to ensure that the lesion is in the correct place and to minimize inadvertent damage to adjacent brain structures.

The healing process takes about eight weeks, during which the lesion first swells and then recedes into a permanent scar. During the swelling phase the person sometimes experiences dyskinesias and even DYSTONIA (extreme rigidity that often causes unnatural and uncomfortable positions). As healing progresses, these problems usually abate. Tremors often, but not always, completely disappear when healing of the lesion is complete. Rigidity usually improves as well, as both symptoms result from excessive stimulation of muscle tissues. The person still needs anti-Parkinson's medications to relieve other neuromuscular symptoms such as bradykinesia, although often dosages can be reduced significantly. Although the effects of thalamotomy are permanent, tremors generally return within 18 months to three years as the surgery cannot stop the progression of the Parkinson's.

See also ABLATION; CARE MANAGEMENT AND PLANNING; MACROELECTRODE STIMULATION; MEDICAL MANAGEMENT; MICROELECTRODE RECORDING; SURGERY; TREATMENT ALGORITHM.

thalamus A structure in the BRAIN that filters and organizes nerve signals passing between the cerebral CORTEX and other brain structures that control movement, primarily the BASAL GANGLIA, brainstem, and cerebellum. It is a paired structure made of GRAY MATTER (dense neuron bodies) that straddles the upper portion of the brainstem; each side is about the size and shape of a walnut. The thalamus also processes sensory signals and is the site within the brain where pain recognition begins.

A small area within the center of the thalamus, called the ventral intermediate nucleus (VIM), becomes overactive in Parkinson's disease and many other tremor disorders. It is theorized that the imbalance of neurotransmitters in the brain that results from the dopamine depletion that characterizes Parkinson's creates chaotic neuron communications that barrage the thalamus, overwhelming its ability to inhibit them. This

causes Dysfunctional movements that manifest as TREMORS and RIGIDITY (muscles in continual contraction).

Dopaminergic ANTI-PARKINSON'S MEDICATIONS that replace or extend the presence of dopamine, such as LEVODOPA and the DOPAMINE AGONISTS, help to restore the brain's neurotransmitter balance, putting neuron communication under control and reducing the numbers and chaos of nerve signals to the thalamus. This effect calms the signals that travel to the muscles in the body, relieving the tremors and rigidity for the duration of the medication's effectiveness. As Parkinson's disease progresses, these medications are less effective and symptoms persist or worsen. Some people with Parkinson's have what doctors call TREMOR-PREDOMINANT PARKINSON'S, in which their primary symptoms are tremors; these can be severe enough to be debilitating. THALAMOTOMY (surgery to interrupt the flow of nerve signals from the thalamus) often can relieve symptoms in these cases, although not all those with Parkinson's who reach such a stage are good candidates for surgery. Other health problems such as heart disease or diabetes, and other symptoms of Parkinson's disease such as BRADYKINESIA and AKINESIA, which do not improve after thalamotomy can tip the balance on surgery's overall effectiveness in providing relief.

See also COPING WITH ONGOING CARE NEEDS OF PARKINSON'S; MEDICAL MANAGEMENT; MEDICATION MANAGEMENT; THERAPEUTIC WINDOW; TREATMENT ALGORITHM.

therapeutic window An opportunity of timing during which certain treatments for Parkinson's disease have the highest likelihood of success. Traditionally neurologists have viewed the time immediately after diagnosis as the optimal window of opportunity for treatment with LEVODOPA to restore depleted DOPAMINE levels to ensure optimal quality of life during the course of Parkinson's. Levodopa is used because at the disease's start there are still functioning dopamine-producing neurons and levodopa can be fairly low and yet produce significant beneficial effects. As the Parkinson's progresses, dopamine producing neurons continue to die leaving the surviving dopamine producing neurons overwhelmed and unable to convert all of the increasing amounts of levodopa into the needed dopamine. Levodopa sometimes begins to lose its efficacy as a treatment after just five to seven years, when motor fluctuations commonly begin to appear. There is research that suggests that methods to provide more continuous dopaminergic activity (either via adding on COMT inhibitors or dopamine agonists) may prolong levodopa's therapeutic window.

New DOPAMINE AGONIST MEDICATIONS such as ropinirole (Requip), pramexipole (Mirapex), and pergolide (Permax) that have entered the market in the past few years, coupled with advances in understanding the pathological processes of Parkinson's disease have become the drugs of choice among most neurologists in the initial therapy of most Parkinson's patients. These medications appear able to postpone the need to begin levodopa therapy for up to three years and to have equal effectiveness in relieving symptoms in Parkinson's disease's early stages. Starting levodopa later not only extends its coverage to later in the disease, lengthening the time for which medications can manage symptoms but combining it with an agonist also may increase the therapeutic window.

There are more clearly defined, and narrow, therapeutic windows for other ANTI-PARKINSON'S MEDICATIONS. AMANTADINE, for example, is effective in relieving symptoms when taken as MONOTHERAPY in DE NOVO PARKINSON'S (previously untreated disease). Once there has been treatment with other medications (especially with levodopa), however, amantadine is no longer effective alone. It is not clear whether this effect is related to the drug's actions in the brain, the progression of Parkinson's that takes it beyond the range for which amantadine can be effective, the effects of nonendogenous dopamine on brain neurons, or—most likely—a combination of all of these factors. Amantadine often is a component of ADJUNCT THERAPIES later in the course of the disease, however, being particularly useful in diminishing levodopa-induced dyskinesias. As well, these medications are most effective in the early stages of Parkinson's. When the disease progresses beyond a certain point, these medications, may

not add anything to symptom relief may create more troubling symptoms of their own in the form of undesired side effects.

See also CARE MANAGEMENT AND PLANNING; MEDICATION MANAGEMENT; MEDICATION SIDE EFFECTS; TREATMENT ALGORITHM.

3,4-dihydroxyphenylalanine (DOPA) An AMINO ACID structure formed from the hydroxylation (metabolic conversion) of TYROSINE in the brain. The enzyme DOPA DECARBOXYLASE (DDC) then converts DOPA to DOPAMINE, the NEUROTRANSMITTER essential for facilitating nerve signals in the structures of the BASAL GANGLIA that direct COORDINATION and smooth movement.

3,4-dihydroxyphenylacetic acid (DOPAC) One of the key substances, or metabolites, of DOPAMINE produced through the action of MONOAMINE OXIDASE (MAO). DOPAC is in turn converted to 3-methoxy-4-hydroxyphenylacetic acid (HVA) by COMT, hence COMT-INHIBITOR MEDICATIONS taken to treat Parkinson's disease cause DOPAC to accumulate, shifting the equilibrium of the DOPA-DOPAC reaction so that DOPA preferentially enters the pathway of conversion into dopamine.

3-methoxy-4-hydroxyphenylacetic acid (HVA) One of the key substances, or metabolites, produced through the action of both CATECHOL-O-METHYLTRANSFERASE (COMT) and monoamine oxidase (MAO) in series on dopamine. This substance is also called homovanillic acid, commonly known as HVA. High levels of HVA are correlated to low levels of DOPAMINE. COMT-INHIBITOR drugs taken to treat Parkinson's disease slow or suppress HVA production to extend the period that dopamine remains active in the brain.

3-methoxytyramine (3-MT) One of the key substances, or metabolites, that result from the metabolism of DOPAMINE. The enzyme CATECHOL-O-METHYLTRANSFERASE (COMT) converts dopamine into 3-MT, hence into other substances high levels of 3-MT are correlated to low levels of dopamine. COMT-INHIBITOR drugs taken to treat Parkinson's disease slow or suppress 3-MT production. This effect extends the period that dopamine remains active in the brain.

See also LEVODOPA; WEARING-OFF STATE.

3-O-methyldopa (3-OMD) One of the key substances, or metabolites, that result from the metabolism of LEVODOPA by CATECHOL-O-METHYLTRANSFERASE (COMT). 3-OMD cannot cross the BLOOD-BRAIN BARRIER, so preventing its formation increases the amount of levodopa that can enter the brain to be converted to DOPAMINE in dopaminergic neurons. COMT-INHIBITOR drugs used to treat Parkinson's disease can block 3-OMD production, making more levodopa available for conversion to dopamine.

See also WEARING-OFF STATE.

tocopherol See ALPHA-TOCOPHEROL.

tolcapone A powerful CATECHOL-O-METHYLTRANSFERASE (COMT) INHIBITOR medication that delays the action of the ENZYME CATECHOL-O-METHYLTRANSFERASE (COMT) to metabolize LEVODOPA into 3-O-METHYLDOPA (3-OMD) in the bloodstream, extending the amount of levodopa that crosses the BLOOD-BRAIN BARRIER to be metabolized into dopamine in the BRAIN. COMT is also present in the brain to convert dopamine to 3-methoxytyramine (3-MT), so COMT inhibition probably also extends the life of dopamine inside the brain. Tolcapone (Tasmar) was the first COMT inhibitor marketed, after its U.S. Food and Drug Administration (FDA) approval in the United States in 1993. It marked a major advance in medication treatment for Parkinson's disease, allowing people with Parkinson's to take lower and less frequent dosages of levodopa and derive greater benefit from them.

Tolcapone is effective as one of the ADJUNCT THERAPIES used in middle to late stages of the disease when increasingly higher dosages of levodopa are required to relieve symptoms. Side effects include DIARRHEA and DYSKINESIAS. Rarely tolcapone can cause serious and sometimes fatal liver dysfunction, which has caused it to be removed from the market in Canada and many European countries, although it remains available in the United States. Because of this potential risk, tol-

capone should be the second choice of COMT inhibitors, and ENTACAPONE (Comtan) generally the first choice, even though tolcapone is a more potent inhibitor of COMT than entacapone.

See also ANTI-PARKINSON'S MEDICATIONS; DOPA DECARBOXYLASE (DDC); DOPA DECARBOXYLASE INHIBITOR (DDCI) MEDICATIONS; MEDICATION MANAGEMENT; MEDICATION SIDE EFFECTS.

touch therapy See ALTERNATIVE THERAPIES.

traditional Chinese medicine (TCM) See ALTERNATIVE THERAPIES.

tramadol A moderately strong nonnarcotic PAIN RELIEF MEDICATION taken to relieve RESTLESS LEG SYNDROME (RLS), supported by the results of an open-label trial, and other causes of nocturnal (nighttime) and chronic pain. Though tramadol (Ultram) is not a narcotic, it can cause dependence with long-term use. It usually does not cause CONSTIPATION, however, unlike narcotic pain medications. Common side effects include drowsiness, euphoria, confusion, and disorientation. Tramadol also seems to have a mild antidepressant effect.

See also DEPRESSION; EXERCISE AND ACTIVITY; PAIN; PAIN MANAGEMENT; SLEEP DISTURBANCES.

tranquilizer See ANTIANXIETY MEDICATION.

trauma, role of in causing Parkinson's See PARKINSON'S DISEASE, CAUSES OF.

trazodone An atypical ANTIDEPRESSANT MEDICATION that derives some of its effect from blocking the reuptake of SEROTONIN, a brain neurotransmitter important to mood and emotion, and has other mechanisms that are not completely understood. It causes DROWSINESS, therefore it is usually given at night and is particularly effective in people with insomnia or other disturbances of sleep (used even as a chronic sleep aid in people without depression). Trazodone (Desyrel) also can cause HEADACHE, ORTHOSTATIC HYPOTENSION (a drop in blood pressure with a change in position), heart arrhythmias, and sexual dysfunctions including priapism (extended erection), ejaculation dysfunction, erectile dysfunction, and inability to reach orgasm. Because these side effects are fairly common, this is a medication to consider when other antidepressant medications are inappropriate. Trazodone generally does not have interactions with ANTI-PARKINSON'S MEDICATIONS, however.

See MEDICATION MANAGEMENT; MEDICATION SIDE EFFECTS; MONOAMINE OXIDASE INHIBITOR MEDICATIONS; SELECTIVE SEROTONIN REUPTAKE INHIBITOR MEDICATIONS; TRICYCLIC ANTIDEPRESSANTS.

treatment algorithm   A clinical "decision tree" used for determining which treatments are appropriate for specific symptoms and the course of disease. Symptoms vary so widely among people with Parkinson's that establishing a standard treatment protocol is impossible. Neurologists follow general guidelines that consider symptom clusters, the disease's stage, the risks of side effects, and a THERAPEUTIC WINDOWS of opportunity for optimal relief. Much of the process is continual adjustment to keep pace with the changing pathological processes of Parkinson's as it progresses, variable response to treatments, treatment resistance, and the person's ability to tolerate specific ANTI-PARKINSON'S MEDICATIONS. The most effective approach to treatment decisions is based on collaboration between the physician and the person with Parkinson's.

Although LEVODOPA is the cornerstone of medical treatment of Parkinson's, people respond to it in different ways at different points in the disease process. It becomes important to present a balance of approaches that provide optimal relief from the range of primary and secondary symptoms. Other medications, and for some people, surgical interventions such as THALAMOTOMY, PALLIDOTOMY, or DEEP BRAIN STIMULATION (DBS), offer unique benefits and risks for each individual.

See also ADJUNCT THERAPIES; CARE MANAGEMENT AND PLANNING; MEDICATION MANAGEMENT; MEDICATION SIDE EFFECTS; MONOTHERAPY; SURGERY; THERAPEUTIC WINDOW.

trembling   Rhythmic, involuntary movements that are often the earliest indication of Parkinson's disease. Sometimes described as shaking and clini-

cally called TREMORS, these movements commonly affect a hand or the head. In Parkinson's disease the trembling usually begins on just one side of the body; in other neuromuscular disorders in which tremors are symptoms, the movements often occur on both sides.

See also CARDINAL SYMPTOMS; CONDITIONS SIMILAR TO PARKINSON'S; DIAGNOSING PARKINSON'S.

tremors   One of the four CARDINAL SYMPTOMS of Parkinson's disease and often the first symptom to cause a person to seek medical attention. The tremor of Parkinson's is slow and steady, about four hertz; and generally is more prevalent at rest than with activity. Tremor indicates malfunction of neuronal circuits involving the THALAMUS, which filters nerve signals that enter and leave the cerebral CORTEX, the midbrain, the basal ganglia, or the CEREBELLUM. In Parkinson's, the imbalance of NEUROTRANSMITTERS in the basal ganglia permits erratic and chaotic communication among NEURONS. This effect overwhelms the thalamus, which passes on many of these signals to the cerebral cortex, where they become messages of action to the muscles.

Tremors generally improve with ANTI-PARKINSON'S MEDICATIONS such as ANTICHOLINERGIC MEDICATIONS, which suppress ACETYLCHOLINE, the neurotransmitter that conveys nerve signals to the muscles, and with DOPAMINERGIC MEDICATIONS, which supplement or restore brain dopamine levels and restore the brain's neurotransmitter balance. LEVODOPA, the standard dopaminergic therapy, creates a nonendogenous source the brain can use to synthesize additional dopamine; the DOPAMINE AGONISTS act like artificial dopamine in the brain, directly stimulating dopamine receptors.

Tremors are not painful and often the person who has them does not notice them, in the early stages of Parkinson's, unless he or she happens to notice a hand that is trembling. Often using the limb that has tremors ends them, at least for the duration of the activity. However, tremors can become so severe that they cause nearly complete debilitation, interfering with COORDINATION and DEXTERITY to the extent that the person cannot hold objects or manage simple daily living tasks such as dressing. Tremors that affect the feet and legs can make walking difficult or impossible. When tremors do not respond to medication, sometimes surgery can relieve them.

See also ABLATION; ARCHIMEDES SPIRALS; DEEP BRAIN STIMULATION; DIAGNOSING PARKINSON'S; DYSKINESIA; MICROGRAPHIA; PALLIDOTOMY; PARKINSON'S DISEASE; THALAMOTOMY.

tremor-predominant Parkinson's A presentation of Parkinson's disease in which the primary and obvious symptom is TREMOR. In about half of people with Parkinson's the disease starts this way; as it runs its course, other symptoms such as BRADYKINESIA and rigidity become more evident. Tremor-predominant Parkinson's sometimes is difficult to differentiate from ESSENTIAL TREMOR, a common and chronic but not progressive disorder, though the tremors of the two disorders are usually fairly distinct to a trained observer. The key clinical factor is responsiveness to dopaminergic medications, particularly LEVODOPA. In tremor-predominant Parkinson's, the tremors almost always improve with such medications, whereas essential tremor usually does not change. As well, the tremors of Parkinson's are most apparent at rest and are asymmetrical (one-sided); the tremors of essential tremor are most apparent during activity and tend to be symmetrical (bilateral, or affecting both sides of the body equally).

See also CARDINAL SYMPTOMS; CONDITIONS SIMILAR TO PARKINSON'S.

tricyclic antidepressant medications A classification of medications taken to relieve the symptoms of DEPRESSION, though they are also useful for treating chronic (particularly neuropathic) pain. They work primarily by extending the availability of certain NEUROTRANSMITTERS in the brain. Each tricyclic drug does this in a somewhat different way; most have the strongest influence on suppressing the reuptake of SEROTONIN and NOREPINEPHRINE and do not affect MONOAMINE OXIDASE (MAO) or DOPAMINE directly. The tricyclic antidepressants have been on the market since the 1950s. Once therapy with tricyclics begins, it can require

up to eight weeks, and sometimes longer, for the full antidepressant effect to become established. Stopping a tricyclic antidepressant should be done gradually over about two weeks.

Depression is four to six times as common in people with Parkinson's as in the general public, affecting 40 percent or more of those with Parkinson's at some stage of the disease. Depression is often one of the earliest symptoms of Parkinson's; however, the disease is not recognized until other symptoms begin to appear. The dopamine depletion that characterizes Parkinson's upsets the balance of neurotransmitters in the brain, altering the functions of them all. Antidepressant medications help to restore balance to the neurotransmitters that are most involved with mood and emotion.

Tricyclic antidepressants interact with numerous other medications including many ANTI-PARKINSON'S MEDICATIONS. In particular, tricyclic antidepressants can decrease the amount of LEVODOPA that enters the bloodstream from the intestines.

Commonly prescribed tricyclic antidepressants include

- AMITRIPTYLINE (Elavil, Endep)
- Desipramine (Norpramine)
- Imipramine (Tofranil)
- Nortriptyline (Pamelor)

Tricyclic antidepressants have a variety of side effects that vary somewhat by drug. Common among them are drowsiness, constipation, dry mouth, and cardiac arrhythmias (a key factor in their lethality even if just several days' worth of medication is taken as an intentional overdose). Tricyclics also rarely can worsen the symptoms of Parkinson's or cause other extrapyramidal symptoms such as DYSTONIA and choreic dyskinesias. They cannot be used at the same time as MONOAMINE OXIDASE INHIBITOR (MAOI) MEDICATIONS (including SELEGILINE) or SELECTIVE SEROTONIN REUPTAKE INHIBITOR (SSRI) MEDICATIONS. The SSRIs have become the antidepressants of choice for people with Parkinson's disease, as they have the fewest drug interactions and side effects.

See also ANXIETY; MEDICATION MANAGEMENT; MEDICATION SIDE EFFECTS.

trigger event A circumstance that spurs the development of Parkinson's disease. This may be repeated head trauma, as in the case of the former heavyweight boxing champion MUHAMMAD ALI, or exposure to CHEMICAL TOXINS such as pesticides. As Parkinson's disease appears to develop as an intersection of various genetic and environmental (internal and external) factors, there are likely numerous possible trigger events. Most people probably do not know what caused the disease's development. Limiting exposure to known risk factors for Parkinson's disease makes sense, although the extent to which these are trigger events remains uncertain.

See also PARKINSON'S DISEASE, CAUSES OF; DIAGNOSING PARKINSON'S DISEASE.

trihexyphenidyl A medication with antispasmodic and anticholinergic properties taken to relieve symptoms of Parkinson's such as tremors and rigidity as well as drug-induced neuromuscular side effects of other medications (particularly ANTIPSYCHOTIC MEDICATIONS). Trihexyphenidyl (Artane) works by blocking the actions of ACETYLCHOLINE, a NEUROTRANSMITTER that conveys nerve signals to muscle tissues. It can be given alone in tremor-predominant Parkinson's disease or given adjunctively with other anti-Parkinson's medications. Trihexyphenidyl also slows the response of smooth muscle tissue and can cause CONSTIPATION and URINARY RETENTION. Other common side effects include drowsiness and dry mouth. Trihexyphenidyl should not be taken at the same time as tricyclic ANTIDEPRESSANT MEDICATIONS, AMANTADINE, or other ANTICHOLINERGIC MEDICATIONS.

See also ADJUNCT THERAPIES; ANTI-PARKINSON'S MEDICATIONS; MEDICATION MANAGEMENT; MEDICATION SIDE EFFECTS.

tryptophan An essential AMINO ACID (one the body must obtain from outside sources) that is a serotonin precursor (a substance the BRAIN requires to produce the NEUROTRANSMITTER SEROTONIN). Serotonin is important for NEURON communication related to mood and emotion; below-normal levels of serotonin cause DEPRESSION and ANXIETY and contribute to PSYCHOSIS. The body obtains tryptophan from dietary proteins such as meats, dairy products, whole grains and whole grain products, soy-based foods, and legumes. There are also dietary supplement products that deliver this amino acid in the form of L-tryptophan.

People who have Parkinson's disease, particularly middle and late stage, often do not obtain enough tryptophan from their diet because of PROTEIN RESTRICTIONS. Dietary protein competes with levodopa, also a protein, for absorption from the intestines into the bloodstream. When it becomes necessary to take higher dosages of levodopa to mitigate the symptoms of Parkinson's, this competition becomes a problem. The solution is to eat meals high in carbohydrates during the day, to aid in levodopa's absorption, and to consume the daily protein requirement with the evening meal when the levodopa dosage is smaller. For many people, however, this is hard to do, and as a result they do not receive adequate protein. Compounding the situation are the symptoms of Parkinson's that affect the ability to chew and swallow, which make eating meat, the most common source of protein in the U.S. diet, difficult. People with advanced Parkinson's disease and weight loss or other signs of low protein intake should probably consider nutritional supplements that include L-tryptophan to attempt to meet the body's needs for this essential amino acid. It is important to avoid taking such supplements at the same time as levodopa dosages and to consult the doctor before beginning such supplements as they may contain other ingredients that can interact with ANTI-PARKINSON'S MEDICATIONS or therapeutic reasons for not taking them. A nutritionist's consultation may also be helpful in making this decision.

See also ANTIDEPRESSANT MEDICATIONS; METABOLIC NEEDS; NUTRITION AND DIET.

turning, problems with See GAIT DISTURBANCE.

2 beta-carboxymetholoxy-3 beta (4-iodophenyl) tropane (beta-CIT) (DOPASCAN) An injectable radioactive chemical that concentrates in cells in the SUBSTANTIA NIGRA, making them detectable by SINGLE PHOTON EMISSION COMPUTED TOMOGRAPHY (SPECT). This technique makes it possible to assess the levels of dopamine in the brain by measuring

the density of DOPAMINE-PRODUCING CELLS. Developed, marketed, and licensed for worldwide distribution by Guilford Pharmaceuticals Inc., DOPASCAN is in phase III clinical trials in the United States and other countries. Researchers hope this and other BIOMARKERS currently in development will make it possible to diagnose Parkinson's disease conclusively as well as to measure the effectiveness of treatment objectively. The base radioisotope for DOPASCAN is iodine-123.

See also CLINICAL PHARMACOLOGY TRIALS; DIAGNOSING PARKINSON'S.

tyrosine   An AMINO ACID that the BRAIN uses to synthesize (manufacture) DOPAMINE through the actions of the ENZYME tyrosine hydroxylase, which converts the tyrosine to endogenous (naturally occurring) LEVODOPA in the brain. The enzyme DOPA DECARBOXYLASE then metabolizes levodopa, whether endogenous or therapeutic, into dopamine. The body's supply of tyrosine comes from dietary proteins. Some CLINICAL RESEARCH STUDIES have investigated the therapeutic value of tyrosine supplements, but have not found that they increase brain dopamine levels significantly enough to affect the symptoms of Parkinson's disease.

See also NUTRITION AND DIET; PROTEIN RESTRICTIONS, DIETARY.

ubiquinone   See COENZYME Q-10.

ubiquitin   A PROTEIN family important in the sequence of events, called the ubiquitin proteasome system, through which cells eliminate the waste by-products of their functions. The Latin word *ubique* means "everywhere," an apt foundation for this protein's name. Nearly all cells in the human body contain ubiquitin, and ubiquitin is the most prevalent protein in the brain. Malfunctions of the ubiquitin proteasome system allow protein molecules to accumulate within cells, where they can disrupt normal cell functions and damage and even kill the cell. Genes regulate ubiquitin synthesis (production) and function. Scientists have discovered a number of mutations in the genes that regulate ubiquitin in people with neurodegenerative diseases such as ALZHEIMER'S DISEASE and PARKINSON'S DISEASE, suggesting that there are connections between malfunctioning ubiquitin processes and the accumulations of proteins such as TAU (in Alzheimer's, cortical-basal ganglionic degeneration, and progressive supranuclear palsy) and ALPHA-SYNUCLEIN (in Parkinson's, multiple system atrophy, and Lewy body dementia) that characterize these diseases.

The Ubiquitin Proteasome System

The ubiquitin proteasome system is an intricate, and not yet completely understood, process through which cells identify and "tag" molecules they no longer need. These molecules may be the waste by-products of the cell's metabolic function, or molecules that have aged beyond their ability to be functional. It appears that there is a sequence of tagging, or ubiquitin encoding, that takes place. When the right encoding tags a molecule, an enzyme structure called a proteasome ("protein body") interacts with the molecule and degrades it (takes it apart). The ubiquitin molecules attached to the molecule seem also to participate in this degradation, although scientists are not certain of their roles. The cell then recycles the component particles to feed its adenosine triphosphate (ATP) energy production needs and to perform other cell functions.

Researchers do not know how much of the ubiquitin proteasome system is genetic and how much is environmental (influenced by cell activity). They do know that when the system malfunctions, damaged and ineffective protein molecules remain within the cell. This molecular clutter eventually interferes with the cell's ability to function, damaging the entire cell or leading to its death. Ubiquitin also has roles in repair of cell deoxyribonucleic acid (DNA), in mitochondrial metabolism, and in the process of APOPTOSIS (programmed cell death), although the precise nature of this involvement also is among the aspects of ubiquitin's function that scientists do not fully understand.

Ubiquitin, Alpha-Synuclein, and Parkin

Although Parkinson's LEWY BODIES predominantly contain ALPHA-SYNUCLEIN, they also contain PARKIN and ubiquitin. The ubiquitin genes, which regulate the body's production and use of ubiquitin, exist in close proximity to genes that regulate various protein functions linked to Parkinson's (parkin and alpha-synuclein) and Alzheimer's (TAU). Some scientists suspect that mutations of these genes are interrelated and affect the functioning of all of these proteins. Others believe that ubiquitin gene mutations affect only the ways in which ubiquitin functions to tag and degrade other proteins, including alpha-synuclein and tau; that it is a malfunction of ubiquitin tagging that allows these proteins to accumulate as the deposits found in the tau entanglements of Alzheimer's disease and the LEWY BODIES of Parkinson's disease; and that other factors (genetic and environmental) determine the disease process that results.

See also MITOCHONDRIAL DYSFUNCTION; MITOCHONDRIAL ELECTRON TRANSPORT CHAIN; OXIDATION.

Udall, Morris K. A U.S. congressional representative of the state of Arizona from 1961 to 1991. Udall's diagnosis with Parkinson's in 1979 called the disease to public attention. Udall resigned from Congress in 1991 because of his health and died in 1998 as a consequence of Parkinson's. During his congressional career, Udall was noted for his support of environmental and Native American issues; today the Morris K. Udall Foundation is a federal agency that extends his legacy through scholarships for these fields of study.

In Udall's honor, the U.S. Congress passed the MORRIS K. UDALL PARKINSON'S RESEARCH ACT OF 1997, which generated the first significant federal funding of Parkinson's disease research. The act established awards for Excellence in Parkinson's Disease Research to develop Morris K. Udall Centers at leading medical centers throughout the United States. In 2003, there were 11 such centers.

See also ALI, MUHAMMAD; FOX, MICHAEL J.; MICHAEL J. FOX FOUNDATION FOR PARKINSON'S RESEARCH; MUHAMMAD ALI PARKINSON RESEARCH CENTER.

undergarments, protective Products worn under regular clothing to contain leakage of urine or stool due to INCONTINENCE. There are many designs and styles, most of which either men or women can use and some specifically styled for men or for women. These products are disposable; most are made of materials that are highly absorbent but low-bulk.

- Pads and liners are lightweight and narrow, accommodate minor urine leaks, and attach with a peel-and-stick adhesive to the inside of regular underpants.

- Guards are thicker and wider than pads or liners and offer more protection for urine leaks. They are designed primarily for women and attach to the inside of regular underpants.

- Shields are wider and longer than pads or liners, attach to regular underpants, and accommodate minor urine and stool leaks.

- Disposable underpants (such as the brand name product Depends) have absorbent padding and a leakproof exterior. Some designs pull on and off as regular underpants do, some are like oversized pads and are held in place with a special belt, and others have open sides that are sealed with tape closures. These offer maximal protection for urine and stool incontinence.

- Condom catheters are for men only. Known technically as external collection devices, catheters have a latex sheath that fits over the penis as a condom does, with a tube at the end that drains urine into a sealed collection bag usually attached to the thigh. The catheter must be changed every 24 hours to prevent skin damage.

Women sometimes use products designed for menstruation to accommodate urinary leaks. However, these products are designed for the thicker consistency of blood and do not collect or wick fluid in the same way as do products designed for urinary incontinence. Although a menstrual pad or sanitary napkin is a handy choice in a pinch as most women's public restrooms sell them in dispensers, products designed specifically to absorb urine provide better protection and less irritation to tissues.

Product selection depends on personal preference, level of need, and level of activity. Thick pads and disposable underpants are more bulky and can interfere with movement. As well, their bulk makes them apparent under most clothing and can cause embarrassment. Some designs feature high-density absorbent materials that have less bulk, but generally less bulk means more frequent changes. Many people who use protective undergarments wear lighter products during the day and use more extensive protection at night.

See also URINARY FREQUENCY AND URGENCY; URINARY RETENTION.

Segment	Area	Rates
Part I	Mentation, behavior, and mood	Intellectual impairment, thought disorder, depression, motivation, and initiative
Part II	Activities of daily living (ADLs)	Key areas of daily function including speech, swallowing, handwriting, dressing, food handling and eating, personal hygiene, and basic mobility
Part III	Motor examination	Speech, facial expressions, tremors (resting and active), rigidity, repetitive movements, posture, changing positions, gait, stability
Part IV	Complications of therapy	Dyskinesias, dystonia, on–off fluctuations, sleep disturbances, orthostatic hypotension
Part V	Modified Hoehn and Yahr staging	Assigns staging of motor function on graduated scale, no signs to bedridden, with 1.5 and 2.5 increments added
Part VI	Schwab and England activities of daily living scale	Scaled assessment of overall function from completely independent to vegetative, 100% to 0% in increments of 10%

Unified Parkinson's Disease Rating Scale (UPDRS)

An extensive assessment of the progression, symptoms, and functional limitations of an individual's experience with Parkinson's disease. Introduced in 1987, the UPDRS has six components, two of which incorporate other rating systems, to give a comprehensive presentation of the disease for ON-STATE and OFF-STATE.

Doctors and researchers use the UPDRS to monitor changes in response to medication as well as disease progression.

See also ACTIVITIES OF DAILY LIVING; PARKINSON'S DISEASE QUALITY OF LIFE QUESTIONNAIRE; PARKINSON'S DISEASE QUESTIONNAIRE; PARKINSON'S IMPACT SCALE; QUALITY OF LIFE; SHORT FORM 36; SICKNESS IMPACT PROFILE.

unilateral symptoms   See ASYMMETRICAL SYMPTOMS.

urinary frequency and urgency   Sensation of a need to empty the bladder often or intensely, even when the bladder is not full. These are common and related problems in Parkinson's disease, as well as in aging, and sometimes are called overactive bladder. Either can result in urinary INCONTINENCE, an involuntary leaking of urine that occurs with or without stress (such as coughing or sneezing). Urinary frequency and urgency account for most NOCTURIA, the need to get up at night to go to the bathroom. As with many SECONDARY SYMPTOMS, it is important to make sure there are no underlying causes of these problems.

Urinary tract infections cause both frequency and urgency, as well as burning, and are far more common in women than in men. Generally when there is an infection, the urine has a foul smell and may be cloudy or discolored; however, CATECHOL-O-METHYLTRANSFERASE INHIBITOR (COMT) medications such as ENTACAPONE (Comtan) also turn urine dark orange. Another condition that causes similar symptoms is interstitial cystitis, also significantly more common in women. In men the prostate gland enlarges with age and can interfere with the flow of urine. Sometimes a consultation with a urologist (physician who specializes in disorders of the urinary tract) is necessary to determine whether these conditions exist.

The disease process of Parkinson's is itself largely responsible for these symptoms, as it affects the function of smooth muscle tissue such as composes the bladder and other structures of the urinary tract. ANTI-PARKINSON'S MEDICATIONS, especially ANTICHOLINERGIC MEDICATIONS, further contribute by blocking the action of ACETYLCHOLINE, to reduce smooth muscle motility. Sometimes adjusting the choice or dosage of medication can eliminate or reduce frequency and urgency.

Following a FREQUENT VOIDING SCHEDULE, in which the person urinates at planned intervals of two to four hours whether or not there is a need to empty the bladder, sometimes helps relieve the sensations of urgency. It also can relieve the anxiety that many people have about finding a bathroom when the urge strikes. Some people attempt to stave off the sensations of urgency and frequency by limiting the amount of water and other liquids that they drink during the day. This is generally not a good idea, as dehydration can result. As well, adequate hydration helps to fend off another common problem in Parkinson's disease, constipation.

Various medications also can relieve symptoms. Among those commonly prescribed are oxybutynin (Ditropan), tolterodine (Detrol), propantheline (Pro-Banthine), dicyclomine (Bentyl), and flavoxate (Urispas), which are anticholinergics. For men with prostate enlargement doctors sometimes prescribe prazosin (Minipress), a medication also used to treat high blood pressure and that has a clear risk of potentiating orthostatic hypotension in people with Parkinson's. All of these medications can cause drowsiness and have various other side effects, although they generally do not interact with ANTI-PARKINSON'S MEDICATIONS.

See also UNDERGARMENTS, PROTECTIVE; URINARY RETENTION.

urinary incontinence   See INCONTINENCE.

urinary retention   Incomplete emptying of the bladder with urination. There are many reasons this can occur, from poor muscle tone of the bladder to inability to sense whether the bladder is empty. Urinary retention becomes more common with aging and is also common in later stages of Parkinson's as the smooth muscles that control bladder function become impaired. It can lead to INCONTINENCE and urinary tract infections and can cause sensations of URINARY FREQUENCY AND URGENCY. Treatment for urinary retention depends on the underlying cause. Medications that relieve urinary frequency and urgency sometimes help to restore normal bladder function. ANTI-PARKINSON'S MEDICATIONS, especially ANTICHOLINERGIC MEDICATIONS, which slow smooth muscle contractions, often affect bladder function. Altering the medication regimen can sometimes improve bladder emptying. It is important to evaluate urinary retention as an independent medical condition rather than assuming that it is a SECONDARY SYMPTOM of Parkinson's, as its cause may be unrelated to Parkinson's disease, especially in men for whom prostatic enlargement that obstructs urinary outflow from the bladder is a very common cause.

Valium   See DIAZEPAM.

ventral intermediate nucleus   See THALAMUS.

Viagra   See SILDENAFIL.

vision problems   Many people with Parkinson's have problems with vision that arise from the neurodegeneration taking place in the brain and its effects on the muscles that move the eye and eyelid. Difficulty in moving the eyes creates problems with focus and with tracking (following a line of vision). While some difficulties with eye movements are fairly common as Parkinson's progresses, early presenting or severe eye movement difficulties would be suggestive of an alternative diagnosis such as MULTIPLE SYSTEM ATROPHY (MSA) or, particularly, progressive supranuclear palsy (PSP) as abnormal vertical eye movements are a cardinal feature of PSP. BLEPHAROSPASMS (DYSTONIA of the eyelids) and eyelid opening APRAXIA sometimes force the eyes closed. DYSAUTONOMIA can also be a factor if it affects the ability of the pupils to contract, causing blurry vision, or if perfusion of the retinas, the part of the eye that receives and translates into images the light signals that enter the eye, is compromised.

Parkinson's slows (BRADYKINESIA) and reduces (AKINESIA, HYPOMIMIA) many normal movements, including a reduction in blinking. The healthy eye blinks every five to 10 seconds, or six to 12 times a minute. A person who has Parkinson's may blink once or twice a minute or may not blink for several minutes. The effect is lessening of the frequency with which tears rinse the eyes, which causes debris to remain and become irritating to the eye. It also allows the delicate tissues of the eye to dry out, further increasing irritation. At the same time excessive tearing, the eye's natural response to irritation, often occurs. Unless the eyelid blinks to move the tears across the eye, however, the tears pool and eventually spill over the lower lids, giving the impression that the person is crying.

Disturbances of color vision also are common in Parkinson's. The retina is one of the two locations in the body other than the brain that have cells that produce DOPAMINE (the other is the adrenal medulla). As scientists study the effects of Parkinson's on these other dopaminergic cells, they are finding that the cells' activity diminishes as Parkinson's progresses. It is not yet clear whether the retina's dopaminergic cells die, as do the dopaminergic cells in the SUBSTANTIA NIGRA and other structures of the BASAL GANGLIA in the BRAIN, or whether they simply slow their production of dopamine. Whatever the cause, retinal dopamine levels decline in Parkinson's disease, and researchers believe this decline affects the quality of visual images transmitted to the brain, decreasing the resolution, or sharpness, of black and white signals and dulling the perception of colors. This effect degrades the quality of the visual images that travel to the brain, which interprets them as blurry and lackluster.

It does not appear that Parkinson's disease affects vision itself, other than in the dopamine changes in the retina. The structures that participate in vision—optic nerves, cranial nerves, optic tract, and occipital lobes in the CEREBRUM—remain intact and fully functional. Other circumstances can cause vision problems. Cataracts, cloudy discolorations of the lens, commonly develop with increasing age and cause blurring and loss of visual acuity. It is also possible for the eyes to become infected; infection usually causes symptoms that include extreme sensitivity to light, itching, burning, and the desire to keep the eyes closed. An ophthalmologist (physician who specializes in care and diseases of the eyes) should evaluate all vision and eye difficulties, even when they appear to be related to the Parkinson's.

See also ADRENAL GLANDS; ADRENAL MEDULLARY TRANSPLANT; BLINK RATE; BLURRY VISION; COLOR PERCEPTION; NERVOUS SYSTEM; READING.

vitamins   Naturally occurring chemicals that are necessary for the processes and functions of the human body. Food supplies nearly all of vitamins that people ingest, although the skin produces vitamin D in response to sunlight. Different vitamins are essential for specific functions in the body. When the diet cannot meet the body's nutritional needs (for vitamins as well as minerals and other nutrients), doctors and nutritionists recommend vitamin supplements. The B vitamins (thiamin, riboflavin, pyridoxine, cyanocobalamin, niacin, pantothenic acid, biotin, and folic acid) and vitamin C are water-soluble; they dissolve in water and in the bloodstream. These are vitamins the body

Vitamin	Recommended Dietary Allowance (RDA)		Common Food Sources	Uses in Body
	Men	Women		
WATER-SOLUBLE VITAMINS				
Thiamin (B$_1$)	1.2 mg	1.1 mg	Fortified breads and cereals; ham; pork; fish	Mitochondrial electron transport chain (energy production)
Riboflavin (B$_2$)	1.3 mg	1.1 mg	Fortified breads and cereals; dairy products; green leafy vegetables	Mitochondrial electron transport chain (energy production)
Niacin	1.6 mg	1.4 mg	Fortified breads and cereals; beef; pork; poultry; legumes; beans	Mitochondrial electron transport chain (energy production)
Pyridoxine (B$_6$)	1.6 mg	1.4 mg	Fortified breads and cereals; bananas; potatoes; pork; fish; poultry; legumes; beans	Mitochondrial electron transport chain (energy production); red blood cell manufacture
Pantothenic acid	5 mg	5 mg	Fortified breads and cereals; fish; eggs; vegetables	Mitochondrial electron transport chain (energy production)
Biotin	30 mg	30 mg	Fortified breads and cereals; bananas; grapefruit; watermelon; mushrooms; cruciferous vegetables	Mitochondrial electron transport chain (energy production); amino acid metabolism
Folic acid	0.4 mg	0.4 mg	Fortified breads and cereals; green leafy vegetables; peas; mushrooms; eggs	Mitochondrial electron transport chain (energy production); DNA synthesis
Cyanocobalamin (B$_{12}$)	2.4 mg	2.4 mg	Beef; pork; fish; poultry; dairy products	Neuron maintenance; new cell production
C	90 mg	70 mg	Oranges; tomatoes; green leafy vegetables; strawberries	Tissue growth, repair, and healing
FAT-SOLUBLE VITAMINS				
A (beta-carotene)	0.9 mg	0.7 mg	Dairy products; carrots; apricots; fish oil	Maintenance of structures and functions of vision; immune system
D	0.5 mg–1.5 mg	0.5 mg–1.5 mg	Dairy products; salmon; tuna; eggs	Strengthening of bones and teeth
E (alpha-tocopherol)	15 mg	15 mg	Vegetable oil; beef; pork; poultry; green leafy vegetables; eggs	Antioxidant
K	120 mg	90 mg	Green leafy vegetables; cheese; pork	Blood clotting

cannot store, so it needs a steady and regular intake to meet its needs. Vitamins A, D, E, and K are fat-soluble; they dissolve only in fatty acids (lipids). The body can and does store these vitamins, so it needs smaller amounts of them in the diet.

The B vitamins are particularly important because they supply the COENZYMES necessary for MITOCHONDRIAL ELECTRON TRANSPORT CHAIN activity, the process through which cells generate energy. This property makes them essential for nearly every bodily function; chronic insufficiency results in numerous and widespread health problems. People who are chronically malnourished, such as those who cannot eat an adequate diet, sometimes require cyanocobalamin (vitamin B$_{12}$) injections to meet the body's need for this important B vitamin. Laboratory tests to measure blood levels can determine whether there is a deficiency of vitamin B$_{12}$.

Vitamin Therapy

Many people take vitamin supplements as a means of bolstering the body's natural immune and repair systems. As long as dosages are within the recommended dietary allowance (RDAs), there is no harm in this practice. Whether there is benefit remains a matter of debate. For people with poor nutrition that cannot be remedied through changes in the diet, as when the abilities to chew and swallow become compromised as in the later stages of Parkinson's, vitamin supplements often are necessary to meet the body's needs. Health care providers typically recommend a general multivitamin that also contains minerals, as minerals and vitamins work together in the body.

Megadose Vitamins

Excessive dosages of vitamins seldom have any therapeutic value and can be harmful. The body excretes excess amounts of water-soluble vitamins, but toxicity is still possible particularly in people with compromised kidney function. Excessive dosages of fat-soluble vitamins can be toxic, causing serious health problems and, rarely, death. Although it is generally difficult to overdose on any particular vitamin via food, routine supplementation of any particular vitamin or mineral that greatly exceeds the recommended allowance should be avoided unless thorough research supports no expected ill effects. There is no research-supported evidence that higher than recommended dosages of any vitamins relieve Parkinson's symptoms or slow the course of the disease. For a time there was hope that the antioxidant functions of vitamin E (ALPHA-TOCOPHEROL) could slow Parkinson's, but controlled clinical research studies have not borne this out.

See also ANTIOXIDANT; ANTIOXIDANT THERAPY; COMPLEX I; NUTRITION AND DIET; METABOLIC NEEDS.

walking   An activity that has several dimensions for the person with Parkinson's. The neuromuscular symptoms of Parkinson's such as BRADYKINESIA (slowed muscle response and movement) and AKINESIA (freezing) prominently interfere with walking, restricting MOBILITY and limiting INDEPENDENCE. It is among the first functions to show the signs of Parkinson's, through characteristic changes in GAIT and BALANCE. Walking also is one of the best activities for maintaining as much function as possible. It exercises all of the body's major muscle groups and reinforces balance and coordination. MOBILITY AIDS such as walking sticks, canes, and walkers can provide additional support and stability when walking becomes challenging. Walking provides a means of diversion and relaxation, and of interaction with other people.

See also AMBULATION; EXERCISE AND ACTIVITY; GAIT DISTURBANCE; POSTURAL INSTABILITY.

walking aids   See MOBILITY AIDS.

wearing-off state   A period during which dosage of one of the ANTI-PARKINSON'S MEDICATIONS should still be effective but is not. Wearing-off is an indication that LEVODOPA is losing its ability to meet the brain's DOPAMINE needs. Some people benefit from switching to a controlled release formula of SINEMET, the most common form of levodopa therapy used to provide a longer steady-state level of medication, and then supplement as needed with dosages of the regular release formulation. ADJUNCT THERAPIES such as DOPAMINE AGONIST MEDICATIONS and CATECHOL-*O*-METHYLTRANSFERASE (COMT) INHIBITOR MEDICATIONS also can extend ON-STATES.

During a wearing-off state, the person with Parkinson's experiences some but not complete or predictable relief from symptoms. Wearing-off is frustrating for the person with Parkinson's because there can be no predictability to it and it can be demoralizing as it is a sign of disease progression. Maintaining a sense of HUMOR about unexpected situations and remaining calm when the body refuses to respond are helpful responses. Wearing-off is not quite as disruptive as the OFF-STATES that occur later in Parkinson's, in which the disease's progression exceeds the ability of medications to control symptoms, which become both extensive and dominant.

See also CONTROLLED RELEASE MEDICATION; COPING WITH ONGOING CARE OF PARKINSON'S; FLUCTUATING RESPONSE; ON-STATE.

weight management   The ability to achieve and maintain a body weight that is healthy and desirable. Many people with Parkinson's disease experience carbohydrate cravings that prompt them to eat sweets. Doctors are not sure why this happens, although carbohydrates do aid in LEVODOPA absorption and some researchers speculate that craving sweets may be one of the body's ways to attempt to improve its condition. When eating of sweets not counterbalanced with regular exercise and physical activity, particularly in the early stages of Parkinson's, when appetite and nutrition are normal, the consequence is weight gain. As well, a person who was accustomed to a high level of physical activity before Parkinson's is likely to maintain the same eating habits even when his or her activity level drops off and experience weight gain. Control of TREMOR and DYSKINESIAS can also contribute to weight gain due to the decreased burning of calories, which might partially explain the weight gain that happens after PARKINSON'S

SURGERY, particularly after DEEP BRAIN STIMULATION of the SUBTHALAMIC NUCLEUS.

Excess body weight can contribute to numerous other health problems and increases challenges with BALANCE, COORDINATION, and MOBILITY as the symptoms of Parkinson's progress. Health care providers generally advise the person who is more than 20 percent overweight to lose weight through increased activity and more nutritious eating habits.

In the later stages of Parkinson's, low body weight often becomes a problem. Chewing and swallowing difficulties change eating habits, and people tend to eat less food because the process of eating takes considerable effort. Appetite and tastes change, too, and PROTEIN RESTRICTIONS related to levodopa dosages affect food choices. Low body weight, particularly when it reaches 10 to 20 percent below what is considered a healthy weight for the person's height, disrupts the body's hormonal and immune systems. It also indicates that the person is not receiving adequate nutrition; when food intake is inadequate to maintain weight, usually nutrient intake is also insufficient. Lack of nourishment can further weaken muscles and lower stamina. When body weight drops to such a level, health care providers generally recommend nutritional supplements, often liquid for ease of swallowing, that are high in calories and nutrients.

Most people with Parkinson's commonly benefit from consultation with a NUTRITIONIST or a dietitian who can help them assess their nutritional needs and plan meals that meet them.

See also DAILY LIVING CHALLENGES; DIETITIAN, REGISTERED; FOOD PREPARATION; FOODS TO AVOID; FOODS TO EAT; KITCHEN EFFICIENCY; NUTRITION AND DIET.

weight shifting   See GAIT.

white matter   See BRAIN.

White, Maurice   A founding member and lead singer of the rhythm and blues group Earth, Wind, and Fire who was diagnosed with Parkinson's disease in early 1990 after he noticed TREMOR in his hands. White was 50 years old at the time of his diagnosis, and, as do many public figures, initially kept his Parkinson's diagnosis under wraps. He

announced his diagnosis in 2000 in an interview for *Rolling Stone* magazine when Earth, Wind, and Fire was inducted into the Rock and Roll Hall of Fame. White toured with the band for five years after his diagnosis, controlling his symptoms with ANTI-PARKINSON'S MEDICATIONS, before retiring in 1994 to devote his efforts to producing rather than performing.

See also ALI, MUHAMMAD; FOX, MICHAEL J.; MORRIS K. UDALL PARKINSON'S RESEARCH ACT; RENO, JANET; UDALL, MORRIS K.

wills   See ESTATE PLANNING.

Wilson's disease   A rare disorder of copper metabolism that results from liver dysfunction in which copper accumulates in the liver and in the BRAIN. Copper deposits in the brain cause neurological symptoms that may appear similar to the symptoms of Parkinson's disease such as TREMORS, BRADYKINESIA, AKINESIA, STOOPED POSTURE, and GAIT DISTURBANCES. Commonly other signs of neurologic (such as cerebellar ataxia), psychiatric, or liver disease are also present.

A gene mutation on chromosome 13 causes Wilson's disease. Most commonly, the faulty gene is inherited from both parents who are unaffected carriers (autosomal recessive inheritance) although many cases are thought to result from new (*de novo*) mutations, hence there is usually no history of the disorder in the family. Copper accumulations begin at birth and reach a point of causing damage usually when a person is in the 20s and 30s, although symptoms can appear earlier or later. Typically there is significant liver damage long before there are any signs of brain damage, so most people with Wilson's disease are diagnosed long before they exhibit symptoms similar to those of Parkinson's. However, a doctor may suspect Parkinson's disease when a person in his or her 40s has primarily neurological symptoms. Results of laboratory tests to measure the levels of copper in the urine, or the amount of the copper transporting protein ceruloplasm in the blood, are very helpful in making the diagnosis but a biopsy to confirm excess copper deposition in the liver produce a conclusive diagnosis. Treatment to lower copper levels can avert further damage, although it cannot repair damage that has already occurred. Untreated Wilson's disease is fatal.

See also ACERULOPLASMINEMIA; CHELATION; CONDITIONS SIMILAR TO PARKINSON'S; DIAGNOSING PARKINSON'S; HALLERVORDEN–SPATZ SYNDROME.

workplace adaptations to accommodate Parkinson's
Many people who are still employed when they receive the diagnosis of Parkinson's disease wish to, and are able to, continue working. The AMERICANS WITH DISABILITIES ACT of 1990 established requirements that employers make "reasonable accommodations" to permit people with disabilities to remain at their job. What this means depends on the employer, the person's abilities, and the requirements of the job. ANTI-PARKINSON'S MEDICATIONS keep most symptoms at bay usually for at least the first five to 10 years of the disease in most people, often making the Parkinson's unnoticeable to coworkers and others. In such situations, workplace adaptations often are unnecessary. It is important to notice whether anti-Parkinson's medications cause drowsiness, and whether they do so predictably. It may be necessary to adjust job responsibilities or even the work schedule to accommodate drowsiness. The diagnosis of Parkinson's is a good opportunity to evaluate job tasks and to make appropriate changes to improve the efficiency of performing them:

- Clear workspaces and offices of clutter and unnecessary furnishings, to reduce the risk for falls and make navigation of the area easier.

- Organize work accoutrements—tools, supplies, equipment—so items are within easy reach and in the order in which they are likely to be used. This arrangement reduces the amount of movement necessary to complete job tasks, minimizing strain on muscle groups.

- Activate appropriate disability features on COMPUTER software to accommodate personal needs, such as for large print or high-contrast display. Voice transcription software also is helpful to minimize writing or the use of a computer keyboard.

- A large-button telephone makes dialing telephone numbers easier; there are overlays for certain designs of phones to adapt an existing keypad. A headset eliminates the need to pick up and hold the receiver to make or receive calls, and one with adjustable microphone volume can amplify a soft voice.

- In jobs that require standing, make arrangements to sit for five minutes of every half-hour to rest and relax the muscles. In jobs that require sitting, stand up for five minutes of every half-hour to stretch and move around. Changing positions frequently helps prevent muscles from becoming stiff and achy.

- Allow time for rest breaks. Parkinson's disease puts physical stress on the body, causing people to tire easily. Regular rest breaks, stepping away from the work station if possible, give the body a chance to recharge. Taking a short nap during the lunch break is very helpful for avoiding afternoon fatigue and sleepiness.

When the symptoms of Parkinson's interfere with the ability to perform the tasks of the job, it is necessary to discuss options with the employer. Tremors often are embarrassing to people, as anti-Parkinson's medications may relieve all but a mild tremor. As Parkinson's tremor usually improves when the limb is active, it is rarely disabling until the mid or late stages of the disease. Slowness of movement (BRADYKINESIA), RIGIDITY, GAIT DISTURBANCES, IMBALANCE, WEARING OFF, DYSKINESIAS, and COGNITIVE IMPAIRMENT can affect the ability to perform work tasks. Early in Parkinson's, changing the medication regimen often resolves the problem. As the disease progresses, this may not be effective and it may be necessary to make decisions about the work. This is a very individualized process. Sometimes job modifications are easy to make. Other job tasks are essential.

See also ACTIVITIES OF DAILY LIVING; ADAPTIVE EQUIPMENT AND ASSIST DEVICES; FUNCTIONAL CAPACITY; GOING PUBLIC; HYPOPHONIA; INSTRUMENTAL ACTIVITIES OF DAILY LIVING; LIFESTYLE FACTORS; RETIREMENT; WORKPLACE RELATIONSHIPS.

workplace relationships Coworkers often are unsure of how to respond to learning that a person has Parkinson's disease. Some may have suspected something was wrong because of symptoms such as TREMORS; to others the diagnosis may come as a surprise. Most people have a limited understanding of what Parkinson's is and how it affects a person. Those who have had relatives or friends with the disease may have ideas that are outdated, as treatment options today differ from those just five years ago. The person with Parkinson's finds that some people in the workplace ask far too many questions, and others ask nothing because of respect for the person's privacy. Many people with Parkinson's do not make their diagnosis public, telling only the few people at work who may need to know such as supervisors and coworkers with whom they work closely. There is no single right approach.

Although the AMERICANS WITH DISABILITIES ACT and changing attitudes are reshaping the workplace into an environment of increasing tolerance, people with Parkinson's do sometimes encounter biases among coworkers. Direct and honest responses to questions and challenges generally are most effective in helping others to understand what it means to have Parkinson's. Coworkers who are friends are understandably concerned about the person's well-being. Those who are work acquaintances may only be curious. Others in the workplace may worry that they will have to pick up additional job responsibilities or that the person with Parkinson's will make mistakes that will jeopardize the entire work team. In time, of course, they will see that such mistakes are likely after a diagnosis of Parkinson's than before.

See also FRIENDSHIPS; GOING PUBLIC; WORKPLACE ADJUSTMENTS TO ACCOMMODATE PARKINSON'S.

xenograft Tissue transplanted or implanted into a human recipient from a donor of another species, also called a xenotransplant. FETAL PORCINE BRAIN CELL TRANSPLANT, in which dopaminergic neurons from fetal pigs are transplanted into the BRAIN of a person with Parkinson's, is a xenograft procedure being explored as an INVESTIGATIONAL TREATMENT for Parkinson's disease. Xenograft tissues are generally more available than ALLOGRAFT tissues, are taken from human donors. As well, they present fewer risks of infection, as most pathogens (disease-causing substances) are species-specific. Conversely, it is much more difficult for the body to not reject tissue that is from another species.

See also AUTOGRAFT; BIOETHICS; CLINICAL RESEARCH STUDIES; NEURAL GRAFT; STEM CELL.

yoga A centuries-old method of exercise that blends the body and mind through physical postures and MEDITATION. Yoga may be very beneficial for people with Parkinson's because it gently improves flexibility, BALANCE, MUSCLE STRENGTH, and MUSCLE TONE. Postures range from simple to challenging and can be modified to accommodate individual physical limitations. Although many people practice yoga alone, it is best to learn yoga through classes in which experienced yogis, or yoga teachers, can demonstrate the proper ways to perform the postures and provide guidance for making any necessary modifications. Breath control and breathing exercises are at the core of yoga and are very effective for relaxation and relieving stress.

Yoga's mountain pose is one that most people with Parkinson's (and caregivers) can do and can experience benefits from doing. It also is easy to modify.

- Stand with the feet as close together as balance tolerates. In the full mountain pose the feet touch and toes point straight ahead. People with Parkinson's who have balance problems may feel comfortable starting with the feet at shoulder width.
- Hold the back, neck, and head straight and tall. The chin should be level, eyes looking straight ahead.
- Let the arms hang at the sides, fingers together and pointing down.
- Breathe in through the nose, slowly and smoothly, to a count of 10. Pull the breath deep into the belly, letting it push the belly out. Keep the eyes open and looking straight ahead.
- Hold the breath for a count of 10. Feel the energy it gives to the body; feel the energy enter each cell to give it strength and vitality.
- Slowly let out the breath over a count of 10. Feel the belly tighten as it pushes the air back out of the body.
- Repeat this sequence three to five times, and do the sequences as often during the day as desired.

If Parkinson's makes standing difficult, modify the mountain pose by sitting in a chair. Sit as upright as possible, with spine, neck, and head straight. Follow the preceding steps. The body and the mind may feel refreshed and recharged after a yoga session.

See also EXERCISE AND ACTIVITY; MINDFULNESS; STRESS REDUCTION TECHNIQUES; TAI CHI.

zolpidem A mild SLEEP MEDICATION. Zolpidem (Ambien) is fast-acting and usually clears the body quickly, so most people who take it do not experience any "hangover" effect the next morning. Taking zolpidem regularly for longer than a few weeks carries a risk of dependency, and of increased sleeping difficulty when it is no longer taken. Its intended effect is to cause drowsiness, and it can cause DISORIENTATION and CONFUSION when a person gets out of bed at night, which can rarely "hangover" into the morning. Side effects can include headache, DIZZINESS, and unusual or vivid dreams. Although zolpidem is not a benzodiazepine, it has many of the same actions and should not be taken with BENZODIAZEPINE MEDICATIONS such as ALPRAZOLAM (Xanax) or DIAZEPAM (Valium) that may be prescribed as muscle relaxants or to treat anxiety.

See also ANTIANXIETY MEDICATIONS; SLEEP DISTURBANCES.

APPENDIXES

APPENDIX I
ORGANIZATIONS AND RESOURCES

Listings in **bold** have entries in the book that provide information about the organization or resource.

I. INFORMATION, RESOURCES, SUPPORT, AND REFERRALS

American Parkinson Disease Association, Inc.
1250 Hylan Boulevard
Suite 4B
Staten Island, NY 10305-4399
(718) 981-8001 or (800) 223-2732
http://www.adaparkinsons.org

Bachmann-Strauss Dystonia & Parkinson Foundation, Inc.
One Gustave L. Levy Place
P.O. Box 1490
New York, NY 10029
(212) 241-5614
http://www.dystonia-parkinsons.org

National Parkinson Foundation, Inc.
Bob Hope Parkinson Research Center
1501 NW 9th Avenue
Bob Hope Road
Miami, FL 33136-1494
(800) 327-4545 or (305) 547-6666
http://www.parkinson.org

Parkinson Alliance
211 College Road East
3rd Floor
Princeton, NJ 08540
(800) 579-8440 or (609) 688-0870
http://www.parkinsonalliance.net

Parkinson Foundation of Canada
710-390 Bay Street
Toronto, Ontario M5H 2Y2

Canada
(800) 565-3000 or (416) 366-0099
http://www.parkinson.ca

Parkinson's Action Network (PAN)
300 N. Lee Street
Suite 500
Alexandria, VA 22314
(800) 850-4726 or (703) 518-8877
http://www.parkinsonaction.org

Parkinson's Support Group of America
11376 Cherry Hill Road, #204
Beltsville, MD 20705
(301) 937-1545

Parkinson's Disease Foundation
William Black Medical Building
Columbia-Presbyterian Medical Center
710 West 168th Street
New York, NY 10032-9982
(800) 457-6676 or (212) 923-4700
http://www.pdf.org

Parkinson's Disease Society
215 Vauxhall Bridge Road
London SW1V 1EJ
020 7931 8080
http://www.parkinsons.org.uk

Parkinson's Resource Organization
74-090 El Paseo
Suite 102
Palm Desert, CA 92260-4135
(760) 773-5628 or (877) 775-4111
http://www.parkinsonresource.org

United Parkinson Foundation
833 West Washington Boulevard
Chicago, IL 60607
(312) 733-1893

World Parkinson Disease Association
Via Zuretti, 35
20125 Milano, Italy
(39) 02 66713111
http://www.wpda.org

Worldwide Education & Awareness for Movement Disorders (WE MOVE)
204 West 84th Street
New York, NY 10024
(800) 437-MOV2 (6682) or (212) 875-8312
http://www.wemove.org

Young Onset Parkinson's Association
P.O. Box 50936
Albuquerque, NM 87181
(505) 293-5612
http://www.yopa.org

II. PARKINSON'S DISEASE RESEARCH

The Michael J. Fox Foundation for Parkinson's Research
Grand Central Station
P.O. Box 4777
New York, NY 10163
http://www.michaeljfox.org

Muhammad Ali Parkinson Research Center
Barrow Neurological Institute
500 W. Thomas Road
Suite 720
Phoenix, AZ 85013
(602) 406-4931 or (800) 273-8182
http://www.thebni.com
http://www.aliproject.org

National Human Genome Research Institute
National Institutes of Health
Building 31, Room 4B09
31 Center Drive, MSC 2152
9000 Rockville Pike
Bethesda, MD 20892-2152
(301) 402-0911
http://www.genome.gov

National Institute of Neurological Disorders and Stroke (NINDS)
P.O. Box 5801
Bethesda, MD 20824
(800) 352-9424 or (301) 496-5751
(301) 468-5981 (TTY)
http://www.ninds.nih.gov

National Institutes of Health
Building 1
1 Center Drive
Bethesda, MD 20892
(301) 496-4000
http://www.nih.gov

Morris K. Udall Centers for Excellence in Parkinson's Disease Research
Brigham and Women's Hospital Center for Neurological Diseases
Harvard Medical School
75 Francis Street, Boston, MA 02115
(617) 732-5500
http://www.brighamandwomens.org

Duke University Medical Center
Udall PDRCE
P.O. Box 2903
Durham, NC 27710
(919) 681-5696
www.chg.mc.duke.edu/udall/

Johns Hopkins School of Medicine
Morris K. Udall Parkinson's Disease Research Center of Excellence (PDRC)
600 North Wolfe Street
Baltimore, MD 21287
(410) 614-3359
http://www.hopkinsmedicine.org/parkinsons

Mailman Research Center at McLean Hospital, Harvard Medical School
McLean Hospital, MRC I
115 Mill Street
Belmont, MA 02478
(617) 855-3283
http://www.neuroregeneration.org

Udall Center at the Mayo Clinic
Birdsall Research 234
4500 San Pablo Road
Jacksonville, FL 32224
(904) 953-2855
http:/www.mayo.edu/fpd

UCLA Udall Center
University of California Los Angeles
UCLA School of Medicine Brain Research Institute
Los Angeles, CA 90095
http://www.bri.ucla.edu

University of Kentucky Chandler Medical Center
The Morris K. Udall Parkinson's Disease Research
 Center of Excellence
Rose Street
Lexington, KY 40536
(859) 323-5000
http://www.mc.uky.edu/parkinsons

University of Virginia
Neurosciences Service Center
Parkinson's Disease Treatment
#800566 UVA Health System
Charlottesville, VA 22908
(434) 924-5888
http://www.hsc.virginia.edu/neurology-care/
 parkinsons.html

III. PHYSICIAN GROUPS FOR RESEARCH AND PARKINSON'S PATIENT CARE

Parkinson Study Group
PSG Central Office
University of Rochester
1351 Mt. Hope Avenue
Suite 220
Rochester, NY 14620
http://www.parkinson-study-group.org

The Parkinson's Institute
1170 Morse Avenue
Sunnyvale, CA 94089-1605
(800) 786-2958 or (408) 734-2800
http://www.parkinsonsinstitute.org

IV. WEBSITE-BASED INTERNET RESOURCES

Healthfinder
http://www.healthfinder.gov/

MEDLINE Plus Health Information
http://www.nlm.nih.gov/medlineplus/

National Institutes of Health Clinical Trials Database
http://www.clinicaltrials.gov/

P-I-E-N-O Parkinson, international email and website about Parkinson's
http://www.parkinsons-information-exchange-
 network-online.com

Somerset Pharmaceuticals, Inc.
http://www.parkinsonsinfo.com

V. WORKPLACE ACCOMMODATIONS

Alliance for Technology Access
2175 E Francisco Boulevard
Suite L
San Rafael, CA 94901
(415) 455-4575 (Voice)
(415) 455-0491 (TTY)
http://www.ataccess.org

Job Accommodation Network (JAN)
West Virginia University
P.O. Box 6080
Morgantown, WV 26506-6080
(800) 526-7234 (Voice or TTY)
http://www.jan.wvu.edu

U.S. Department of Justice
950 Pennsylvania Avenue NW
Americans with Disabilities Act
Civil Rights Division
Disability Rights Section—NYAVE
Washington, DC 20530
(800) 514-0301 (Voice)
(800) 514-0383 (TTY)
http://www.ada.gov

U.S. Department of Health and Human Services
DHHS Working Group for ADA/Olmstead
c/o Center for Medicaid and State Operations
CMS, Room S2-14-26, DEHPG
7500 Security Boulevard
Baltimore, MD 21244-1850
http://www.cms.hhs.gov/olmstead/

U.S. Department of Labor
Office of Disability Employment Policy
200 Constitution Avenue NW, Room S-1303
Washington, DC 20210
(202) 693-7880 (Voice)
(202) 693-7881 (TTY)
http://www.dol.gov/odep/

U.S. Administration on Aging
Administration on Aging
Washington, DC 20201
(202) 619-0724
http://www.aoa.gov

AoA Region I—CT, MA, ME, NH, RI, VT
John F. Kennedy Bldg.
Rm. 2075
Boston, MA 02203
(617) 565-1158

AoA Regions II, III—NY, NJ, PR, VI, DC, DE, MD, PA, VA, WV
26 Federal Plaza
Rm. 38-102
New York, NY 10278
(212) 264-2976

AoA Region IV—AL, FL, GA, KY, MS, NC, SC, TN
61 Forsyth St., SW, #5M69
Atlanta, GA 30303
(404) 562-7600

AoA Region V—IL, IN, MI, MN, OH, WI
233 N. Michigan Avenue
Suite 790
Chicago, IL 60601-5519
(312) 353-3141

AoA Region VI—AR, LA, OK, NM, TX
1301 Young St.
Rm. 736
Dallas, TX 75201
(214) 767-2971

AoA Region VII—IA, KS, MO, NE
601 East 12th St.
Rm. 1731
Kansas City, MO 64106
(816) 426-3511

AoA Region VIII—CO, MT, ND, SD, UT, WY
1961 Stout St.
Rm 1022
Federal Office Bldg.
Denver, CO 80294-3538
(303) 844-2951

AoA Region IX—AS, AZ, CA, CNMI, GU, HI, NV
50 United Nations Plaza
Rm. 455
San Francisco, CA 94102
(415) 437-8780

AoA Region X—AK, ID, OR, WA
Blanchard Plaza, MS-RX-33
2201 Sixth Avenue
Rm. 1202
Seattle, WA 98121-1828
(206) 615-2298

APPENDIX II
DIRECTORY OF STATE MEDICAID OFFICES

Alabama
Alabama Medicaid Agency
501 Dexter Avenue
P.O. Box 5624
Montgomery, AL 36103-5624
(334) 242-5600
http://www.medicaid.state.al.us

Alaska
Division of Medical Assistance
Department of Health and Social Services
P.O. Box 110660
Juneau, AK 99811
(907) 465-3355
http://www.hss.state.ak.us/dma/

American Samoa
Medicaid Program Director
LBJ Tropical Medical Center
Pago Pago, AS 96799
(011 684) 633-4590

Arizona
Arizona Health Care Cost
Containment System (AHCCCS)
801 East Jefferson
Phoenix, AZ 85034
(800) 654-8713 (In-state)
(800) 523-0231 (Out-of-state)
http://www.ahcccs.state.az.us/

Arkansas
Division of Medical Services
Department of Human Services
P.O. Box 1437, Slot 1100
103 E. 7th Street
Little Rock, AR 72203
(501) 682-8292
(501) 682-6789 (TDD)
http://www.medicaid.state.ar.us/

California
Medical Care Services
Department of Health Services
714 P Street
Room 1253
Sacramento, CA 95814
(916) 654-0391
http://www.dhs.ca.gov/mcs/

Colorado
Office of Medical Assistance
Department of Health Care Policy & Financing
1575 Sherman Street
Denver, CO 80203-1714
(303) 866-2868
(303) 866-3883 (TDD)
http://www.chcpf.state.co.us/

Connecticut
Medical Care Administration
Department of Social Services
25 Sigourney Street
Hartford, CT 06106
(800) 842-1508
(800) 842-4524 (TDD)
http://www.dss.state.ct.us/

Delaware
Medical Services
Department of Health and Social Services
P.O. Box 906, Lewis Building
New Castle, DE 19720
(888) 295-5156 (In-state)
(302) 744-5617 (Out-of-state)
http://www.state.de.us/dhss/dph/

Washington, D.C.
Medical Assistance Administration
Department of Health
825 North Capitol Street NE
Washington, DC 20002

(202) 442-5999
http://www.dchealth.dc.gov/

Florida
Agency for Health Care Administration
2727 Mahan Drive, Building 3
Tallahassee, FL 32308
(850) 488-3560
http://www.fdhc.state.fl.us/Medicaid/

Georgia
Department of Medical Assistance
2 Peachtree Street NW
Atlanta, GA 30303
(404) 656-4507
http://www.communityhealth.state.ga.us/

Guam
Bureau of Health Care Financing
Department of Public Health and Social Services
P.O. Box 2816
Agana, GU 96910
(671) 735-7269

Hawaii
Department of Human Services
601 Kamokila Boulevard
Room 518
Kapolei, HI 96707
(808) 692-8050
http://www.state.hi.us/dhs/

Idaho
Department of Health and Welfare
Division of Medicaid
3380 Americana Terrace
Suite 230
Boise, ID 83706
(208) 334-5747
http://www.state.id.us/dhw/medicaid/

Illinois
Medical Programs
Illinois Department of Public Aid
201 S. Grand Avenue, East
Springfield, IL 62763-0001
(214) 782-2570
http://www.state.il.us/dpa/

Indiana
Medicaid Policy & Planning
Family & Social Services Administration
402 W. Washington Street
Room W382

Indianapolis, IN 46204-2739
(800) 457-4584
http://www.state.in.us/fssa/servicedisabl/medicaid/

Iowa
Division of Medical Services
Department of Human Services
1305 East Walnut Street
Des Moines, IA 50319
(515) 281-8433
http://www.dhs.state.ia.us/MedicalServices/

Kansas
Director of Medical Policy
Department of Social and Rehabilitation Services
915 SW Harrison Street
Topeka, KS 66612
(785) 296-3959
http://www.srskansas.org/

Kentucky
Department for Medicaid Services
275 East Main Street
Frankfort, KY 40621
(800) 635-2570
http://www.chs.state.ky.us/dms/

Louisiana
Bureau of Health Services Financing
1201 Capitol Access Road
P.O. Box 91030
Baton Rouge, LA 70821-9030
(225) 342-5774
http://www.dhh.state.la.us/medicaid/

Maine
Bureau of Medical Services
Department of Human Services
442 Civic Center Drive
11 Statehouse Station
Augusta, ME 04333
(207) 624-7539
(800) 321-5557 (In-state)
http://www.state.me.us/bms/

Maryland
Department of Health and Mental Hygiene
201 West Preston Street
Baltimore, MD 21201
(410) 767-6860
(877) 463-3464 (In-state)
http://www.dhmh.state.md.us/

Massachusetts
MassHealth
Division of Medical Assistance
600 Washington Street
Boston, MA 02111
(800) 841-2900 (In-state)
(800) 497-4648 (In-state) (TTY)
http://www.state.ma.us/dma/

Michigan
Department of Community Health
320 S. Walnut, 6th Floor
Lansing, MI 48913
(517) 373-3500
(517) 373-3573 (TDD)
http://www.mdch.state.mi.us/msa/mdch_msa/

Minnesota
Department of Human Services
MinnesotaCare
444 Lafayette Road
St. Paul, MN 55155-3852
(651) 297-3862
(800) 657-3672 (In-state)
(800) 627-3529 (In-state) (TDD)
http://www.dhs.state.mn.us/healthcare/

Mississippi
Office of the Governor
Division of Medicaid
239 North Lamar Street
Jackson, MS 39201-1399
(601) 359-6050
http://www.dom.state.ms.us/

Missouri
Division of Medical Services
615 Howerton Court
P.O. Box 6500
Jefferson City, MO 65102
(573) 751-3425
(800) 735-2966 (In-state) (TDD)
http://www.dss.state.mo.us/dms/

Montana
Department of Public Health & Human Services
1400 Broadway
Helena, MT 59601
(406) 444-4540
http://www.dphhs.state.mt.us/hpsd/

Nebraska
Medical Services Division
Department of Health & Human Services
P.O. Box 95026
301 Centennial Mall South, 5th Floor
Lincoln, NE 68509
(402) 471-2306
http://www.hhs.state.ne.us/med/

Nevada
Division of Health Care Financing and Policy
1100 E. Williams Street
Suite 101
Carson City, NV 89710
(775) 684-3676
http://dhcfp.state.nv.us/

New Hampshire
Health Policy & Medicaid
Department of Health and Human Services
Office of the Commissioner
129 Pleasant Street
Concord, NH 03301-6521
(603) 271-3676
http://www.state.nh.us/

New Jersey
Division of Medical Assistance & Health Services
Department of Human Services
P.O. Box 712
Trenton, NJ 08625-0712
(609) 588-2600
http://www.state.nj.us/humanservices/dmahs/

New Mexico
Medical Assistance Division
Department of Human Services
P.O. Box 2348
Sante Fe, NM 87504-2348
(505) 827-3100
(888) 997-2583 (In-state)
http://www.state.nm.us/hsd/mad/

New York
Office of Medicaid Management
Department of Health
Empire State Plaza
Room 1466
Corning Tower Building
Albany, NY 12237
(718) 557-1399
http://www.health.state.ny.us/nysdoh/medicaid/

North Carolina
Division of Medical Assistance
Department of Health & Human Services
1985 Umstead Drive

Raleigh, NC 27699-2517
(919) 733-4261
(919) 733-4851 (TDD)
http://www.dhhs.state.nc.us/dma/

North Dakota
Medical Services Division
North Dakota Department of Human Services
600 E. Boulevard Avenue, Dept. 325
Bismarck, ND 58505-0261
(701) 328-2321
(800) 755-2604 (In-state)
http://www.lnotes.state.nd.us/dhs/dhsweb.nsf/
    ServicePages/MedicalServices

Ohio
Ohio Department of Job and Family Services
Ohio Health Plans
30 East Broad Street, 31st Floor
Columbus, OH 43215-3414
(614) 644-0140
http://www.state.oh.us/odjfs/ohp/

Oklahoma
Oklahoma Health Care Authority
4545 N. Lincoln Boulevard
Suite 124
Oklahoma City, OK 73105
(405) 522-7300
http://www.ohca.state.ok.us/

Oregon
Department of Human Resources
Office of Medical Assistance Programs
500 Summer Street
Salem, OR 97310-1014
(503) 945-5772
(800) 527-5772 (In-state)
(800) 375-2863 (In-state) (TDD)
http://www.omap.hr.state.or.us/

Pennsylvania
Department of Public Welfare
Office of Medical Assistance Programs
    (OMAP)
Health and Welfare Building
Room 515
Harrisburg, PA 17105-2675
(717) 787-1870
http://www.dpw.state.pa.us/omap/

Puerto Rico
Office of Economic Assistance to the Medically Indigent
Department of Health

Call Box 70184
San Juan, PR 00936
(787) 250-7429

Rhode Island
Division of Health Care Quality
Department of Human Services
Louis Pasteur Building
600 New London Avenue
Cranston, RI 02920
(401) 462-3113
http://www.dhs.state.ri.us/dhs/

South Carolina
Department of Health & Human Services
P.O. Box 8206
1801 Main Street
Columbia, SC 29202-8206
(803) 898-2500
http://www.dhhs.state.sc.us/

South Dakota
Medical Services
Department of Social Services
Kneip Building
700 Governors Drive
Pierre, SD 57501
(605) 773-3495
http://www.state.sd.us/social/medical/

Tennessee
Department of Finance & Administration
TennCare
729 Church Street
Nashville, TN 37247-6501
(615) 741-0213
http://www.state.tn.us/tenncare/

Texas
Texas Department of Human Services
701 W 51st Street
P.O. Box 149030
Austin, TX 78711
(888) 834-7406
(888) 425-6889 (TDD)
http://www.dhs.state.tx.us/programs/Elderly/

Utah
Department of Health
Division of Health Care Financing
Martha S. Hughes Cannon Building
P.O. Box 143106
288 North 1460 West
Salt Lake City, UT 84114-3106

(800) 662-9651 (In-state)
(801) 538-6155 (Out-of-state)
http://hlunix.hl.state.ut.us/medicaid/

Vermont
Office of Vermont Health Access
Department of Social Welfare
Agency of Human Services
103 South Main Street
Waterbury, VT 05671-1201
(800) 250-8427 (In-state)
http://www.dsw.state.vt.us/districts/ovha/

Virginia
Department of Medical Assistance Services
600 East Broad Street
Richmond, VA 23219
(804) 786-4231
http://www.dmas.state.va.us/

Virgin Islands
Bureau of Health Insurance and Medical
   Assistance
210-3A Altona
Suite 302
Frostco Center
St. Thomas, US Virgin Islands 00802
(340) 774-4624
http://www.gov.vi/

Washington
Medical Assistance Administration
Department of Social & Health Services

P.O. Box 45080
Olympia, WA 98504-5080
(800) 562-3022 (In-state)
(360) 902-7807
http://www.maa.dshs.wa.gov/

West Virginia
Bureau for Medical Services
Department of Health & Human Resources
350 Capitol Street
Room 251
Charleston, WV 25301-3706
(304) 558-1700
http://www.wvdhhr.org/bms/

Wisconsin
Division of Health Care Financing
Dept. of Health and Family Services
1 West Wilson Street
Room 350
P.O. Box 309
Madison, WI 53701-0309
(608) 266-8922

Wyoming
Office of Medicaid
Health Care Access & Resource Division
154 Hathaway Building
2300 Capitol Avenue
Cheyenne, WY 82002
(307) 777-7848
http://www.wdh.state.wy.us/

SELECTED BIBLIOGRAPHY AND FURTHER READING

BOOKS: CLINICAL AND SCIENTIFIC

Gordin, Ariel, ed. *Parkinson's Disease: Advances in Neurology,* vol. 91. New York: Lippincott, Williams & Wilkins, 2002.

Jankovic, Joseph and Eduardo Tolosa, M.D., eds. *Parkinson's Disease and Movement Disorders.* 4th ed. New York: Lippincott, Williams & Wilkins, 2002.

Playfer, Jeremy and John V. Hindle, eds. *Parkinson's Disease in the Older Patient.* Oxford: Oxford University Press, 2002.

Schapira, Anthony, ed. *Mitochondrial Function and Dysfunction,* vol. 53. New York: Elsevier Science, 2003.

Starkstein, Sergio and Marcello Merello. *Psychiatric and Cognitive Disorders in Parkinson's Disease.* Cambridge: Cambridge University Press, 2002.

Tarsy, Daniel, ed. *Surgical Treatments of Parkinson's Disease and Other Movement Disorders.* Totawa, N.J.: Humana Press, 2003.

Turkington, Carol. *Encyclopedia of the Brain and Brain Disorders.* New York: Facts On File, 2002.

Waters, Cheryl H. *Diagnosis and Management of Parkinson's Disease,* 3d ed. Caddo, Okla.: Professional Communications, 2002.

Webster, Roy, ed. *Neurotransmitters, Drugs, and Brain Function.* New York: John Wiley & Sons, 2001.

BOOKS: ABOUT PARKINSON'S FOR PEOPLE WITH PARKINSON'S AND FOR CAREGIVERS

Argue, John. *Parkinson's Disease and the Art of Moving.* Oakland, Calif.: New Harbinger Publications, 2000.

Cram, David L. *Answers to Frequently Asked Questions in Parkinson's Disease: A Resource Book for Patients and Families.* San Francisco: Acorn Books, 2002.

———. *Understanding Parkinson's Disease: A Self-Help Guide.* Omaha, Nebr.: Addicus Books, 2001.

Houser, Robert and Theresa Zesiewicz. *Parkinson's Disease Questions and Answers,* 3d ed. West Palm Beach, Fla.: Merit Publishing International, 2000.

Lierberman, Abraham. *Shaking up Parkinson's Disease: Fighting Like a Tiger, Thinking Like a Fox.* Boston: Jones & Bartlett Publishers, 2001.

———. *100 Questions and Answers about Parkinson's Disease.* Boston: Jones & Bartlett Publishers, 2003.

Rosenstein, Ann A. *Water Exercises for Parkinson's: Maintaining Balance, Strength, Endurance, and Flexibility.* Ravensdale, Wash.: Idyll Arbor, 2002.

Weiner, William J., Lisa M. Schulman, and Anthony E. Lang. *Parkinson's Disease: A Complete Guide for Patients and Families.* Baltimore: Johns Hopkins University Press, 2001.

BOOKS: PERSONAL EXPERIENCES AND LIVING WITH PARKINSON'S

Blake-Krebs, Barbara and Linda Herman, eds. *When Parkinson's Strikes Early: Voices, Choices, Resources, and Treatment.* Alameda, Calif.: Hunter House Publishers, 2001.

Chearney, Lee Ann. *Visits Caring for an Aging Parent: Reflections and Advice.* New York: Three Rivers Press, 1998.

Fox, Michael J. *Lucky Man: A Memoir.* New York: Hyperion Press, 2002.

Havemann, Joel. *A Life Shaken: My Encounter with Parkinson's Disease.* Baltimore: Johns Hopkins University Press, 2002.

Kondracke, Morton. *Saving Milly: Love, Politics, and Parkinson's Disease.* New York: Public Affairs Books, 2001.

McGoon, Dwight C. *The Parkinson's Handbook.* New York: W. W. Norton & Company, 1990.

ARTICLES

Albin, R. L. "Sham Surgery Controls: Intracerebral Grafting of Fetal Tissue for Parkinson's Disease and Proposed Criteria for use of Sham Surgery Controls." *Journal of Medical Ethics 28* (2002): 322–325.

Apaydin, H. et al. "Parkinson Disease Neuropathology: Later-Developing Dementia and Loss of the Levodopa Response." *Archives of Neurology 59* (2002): 102–112.

Bronte-Stewart, H. M. et al. "Postural Instability in Idiopathic Parkinson's Disease: The Role of Medication and Unilateral Pallidotomy." *Brain: A Journal of Neurology* 125 (2002): 2100–2114.

Dawson, T. M., and V. L. Dawson. "Rare Genetic Mutations Shed Light on the Pathogenesis of Parkinson Disease." *Journal of Clinical Investigation* 111 (2003): 145–151.

Fine, J. et al. "Long-Term Follow-up of Unilateral Pallidotomy in Advanced Parkinson's Disease." *New England Journal of Medicine* 342 (2000): 1708–1714.

Foltynie, T. et al. "The Genetic Basis of Parkinson's Disease." *Journal of Neurology, Neurosurgery and Psychiatry* 73 (2002): 363–370.

Freed, C. R. et al. "Transplantation of Embryonic Dopamine Neurons for Severe Parkinson's Disease." *New England Journal of Medicine* 344 (2001): 710–719.

Growdon, J. H. et al. "Levodopa Improves Motor Function without Impairing Cognition in Mild Non-Demented Parkinson's Disease Patients." *Journal of Neurology* 50 (1998): 1327–1331.

Hauser, R. A. et al. "Bilateral Human Fetal Striatal Transplantation in Huntington's Disease." *Neurology* 58 (2002): 687–695.

Henderson, J. M. et al. "Loss of Thalamic Intralaminar Nuclei in Progressive Supranuclear Palsy and Parkinson's Disease: Clinical and Therapeutic Implications." *Brain: A Journal of Neurology* 123 (2000): 1410–1421.

Jankovic, J. et al. "Evolution of Diagnosis in Early Parkinson's Disease." *Archives of Neurology* 57 (2000): 369–372.

Limousin, P. et al. "Electrical Stimulation of the Subthalamic Nucleus in Advanced Parkinson's Disease." *New England Journal of Medicine* 339 (1998): 1105–1111.

Lücking, C. et al. "Association between Early-Onset Parkinson's Disease and Mutations in the *Parkin* Gene." *New England Journal of Medicine* 342 (2000): 1560–1567.

Lyons, K. E. et al. "Gender Differences in Parkinson's Disease." *Clinical Neuropharmacology* 21 (1998): 118–121.

Marder, K. et al. "Postmenopausal Estrogen Use and Parkinson's Disease with and without Dementia." *Neurology* 50 (1998): 1141–1143.

McDermott, M. P. et al. "Factors Predictive of the Need for Levodopa Therapy in Early, Untreated Parkinson's Disease." *Archives of Neurology* 52 (1995): 565–570.

Morris, H. R. et al. "Pathological, Clinical and Genetic Heterogeneity in Progressive Supranuclear Palsy." *Brain: A Journal of Neurology* 125 (2002): 969–975.

Mouradian, M. M. "Recent Advances in the Genetics and Pathogenesis of Parkinson Disease." *Neurology* 58 (2002): 179–185.

Obeso, J. A. et al. "Deep-Brain Stimulation of the Subthalamic Nucleus or the Pars Interna of the Globus Pallidus in Parkinson's Disease." *New England Journal of Medicine* 345 (2001): 956–963.

Olanow, C. W., R. L. Watts, and W. C. Koller. "An Algorithm (Decision Tree) for the Management of Parkinson's Disease." *Neurology* 56 (2001): S1–S88.

Parkinson Study Group. "DATATOP: A Multi-Center Controlled Clinical Trial in Early Parkinson's Disease." *Archives of Neurology* 46 (1989): 1052–1060.

———. "Impact of Deprenyl and Tocopherol Treatment on Parkinson's Disease in DATATOP Subjects Not Requiring Levodopa." *Annals of Neurology* 39 (1996): 29–36.

Parkinson Study Group and J. Friedman. "Low Dose Clozapine for the Treatment of Drug-Induced Psychosis in Parkinson's Disease." *New England Journal of Medicine* 340 (1999): 757–763.

Parkinson Study Group and R. Holloway. "A Randomized Controlled Trial Comparing Pramipexole with Levodopa in Early Parkinson's Disease: Design and Methods of the CALM-PD Study." *Clinical Neuropharmacology* 23 (2000):34–44.

Parkinson Study Group and K. Marek. "A Multicenter Assessment of Dopamine Transporter Imaging with DOPASCAN/SPECT in Parkinsonism." *Neurology* 55 (2000): 1540–1547.

Parkinson Study Group and N. Shetty. "The Placebo Response in Parkinson's Disease." *Clinical Neuropharmacology* 22 (1999): 207–212.

Rascol, O. et al. "A Five-Year Study of the Incidence of Dyskinesia in Patients with Early Parkinson's Disease Who Were Treated with Ropinirole or Levodopa." *New England Journal of Medicine* 342 (2000): 1484–1491.

Roberts-Warrior, D. et al. "Postural Control in Parkinson's Disease after Unilateral Posteroventral Pallidotomy." *Brain: A Journal of Neurology* 123 (2000): 2141–2149.

Rosenberg, R. N. "Mitochondrial Therapy for Parkinson Disease." *Archives of Neurology* 59 (2002): 1523.

Schlossmacher, M. G. et al. "Parkin Localizes to the Lewy Bodies of Parkinson Disease and Dementia with Lewy Bodies." *American Journal of Pathology* 160 (2002): 1655–1667.

Schuurman, P. R. "A Comparison of Continuous Thalamic Stimulation and Thalamotomy for Suppression of Severe Tremor." *New England Journal of Medicine* 342 (2000): 461–468.

Waters, C. H. "Advances in Managing Parkinson's Disease." *Hospital Practice* (15 June 2001).

West, A. B. et al. "Functional Association of the *Parkin* Gene Promoter with Idiopathic Parkinson's Disease." *Human Molecular Genetics* 22 (2002): 2787–2792.

INDEX

electroencephalogram in 111
for essential tremor 118
fMRI in study of 192
for gait disturbance 144
macroelectrode in 191
microelectrode recording in 206
for multiple system atrophy 220
muscle tone and 221
of pallidum 31
in planning 272
for rigidity 296
of subthalamic nucleus 31
vs. subthalamotomy 324
weight management and 349–350
degenerative condition 49, 50, **81**. *See also* neurodegenerative; *specific conditions*
dehydration, risk of 110, 238, 329
delirium **81–82,** 83
delusion **82–83**
from cognitive impairment 263
from dementia 83
vs. hallucinations 153
from Lewy body disease 184
olanzapine for 243
in paranoia 253
in psychosis 282
in schizophrenia 299
in sundowning 325
dementia **83–85**
acetylcholine and 3
acetylcholinesterase and 3
acetylcholinesterase inhibitor for 4
in Alzheimer's disease 17
antipsychotic medications for 300, 332
donepezil for 97
in Guam ALS-PDC 151
haloperidol for 154
rivastigmine for 297
tacrine for 331
antipsychotic medications for 154, 332
apathy in 22
benztropine and 34
burnout and 46

cabergoline and 47
choline acetyltransferase and 58
from cognitive impairment 263
confusion from 72
with delirium 82
with delusions 83
in diffuse Lewy body disease 94
disorientation in 94–95
emotional behavior with 33
estate planning and 118
estrogen for 120
galantamine for 144–145
in Hallervorden-Spatz syndrome 152
hallucinations from 153
Lewy bodies and 183
from Lewy body disease 184
in mental status 204
neuropsychiatry for 233–234
in off-state 243
olanzapine for 243
paranoia in 253
in Parkinson's diagnosis 50
pons and 44
in progressive supranuclear palsy 278
vs. psychosis 282
residential care and 292
in sundowning 325
surgery and 328
tacrine for 331
treatment for, drug-induced Parkinson's from 103
dendrite **85**
axon and 27
in neuron structure 232, 235
of Purkinje's cells 43
denial and acceptance **85–87**
in adjustment to Parkinson's 8
in coping with diagnosis 74
mindfulness for 207
second opinion and 300
de novo Parkinson's disease **87**
amantadine for 242, 336
cabergoline for 47
carbidopa for 50
monotherapy for 215
selegiline for 214, 302

dental care and hygiene **87,** 195
dental insurance records 289
deoxyribonucleic acid (DNA), of mitochondria 208
Deprenyl. *See* selegiline
Deprenyl and Tocopherol Antioxidative Therapy for Parkinson's Disease (DATATOP) 214, 246, 302
depression **87–90.** *See also* antidepressant medication
in adjustment to Parkinson's 8
anxiety in 22
apathy in 22
body image and 39
burnout and 46
from Creutzfeldt-Jakob disease 76
daily living challenges and 78
delusions from 83
diagnosis of 32
dopamine in 301
electroconvulsive therapy for 111
embarrassment and 113
emotional stress and 321
from frustration 137
in mental status 204
mindfulness for 207
monoamine oxidase in 212–213
neurotransmitters and 211
in pain management 249
in Parkinson's disease 212, 259, 339
in Parkinson's Impact Scale 263
in Parkinson's personality 263
psychotherapy for 282
quality of life and 285
as risk factor 89–90
scale for 154–155
serotonin in 301, 340
sleep disturbances from 313
suicide and 324
symptoms of 92
dermatitis, sebaceous 38, 79, **90**
desipramine **90,** 339
Desyrel. *See* trazodone
dexterity, mental **90–91,** 102

cisapride and 61
COMT inhibitors and 55–56
cooking and 73
coping with 74
with dizziness 95
from dopaminergic
medications 101
driving and 102
in early-onset Parkinson's 107
eating and 109
from entacapone 115
from fetal dopaminergic brain
cell transplant 130
from fluctuating phenomenon
132
gamma aminobutyric acid in
145
from haloperidol 154
from lesions 231
in levodopa treatment 181,
182
MAOIs for 24
metabolic rate affected by 205
in multiple system atrophy
219
neurons in 232
nortriptyline and 239
in off-state 243
in olivopontocerebellar
atrophy 219
in on-state 244
pallidotomy for 251
pallidum and 252
proprioception and 280
reading and 288
from rescue drugs 290
reserpine for 291
in secondary parkinsonism
257
sexual dysfunction and 304
from stem cell transplant 319
surgery for 234, 326
from thalamotomy 334, 335
weight management and 349
workplace and 351
dyskinesia, levodopa-induced. See
levodopa
dysphagia 105. See also
swallowing
cisapride for 61
gastric motility and 145
parenteral nutrition and 254

dysphasia 105, 316
dystonia 105
from antipsychotic
medications 185
baclofen for 29
botulinum toxin therapy for
40
chiropractic for 57
vs. choreiform dyskinesia 60
clonazepam for 63–64
from corticobasal degeneration
75
diazepam for 94
in early-onset Parkinson's
129–130
electroconvulsive therapy for
111
exotoxin for 122
from fluctuating phenomenon
132
gamma aminobutyric acid in
145
in Hallervorden-Spatz
syndrome 152
from haloperidol 154
in Huntington's disease 165
insomnia from 311–312
from levodopa 132
lorazepam for 189
from midbrain tumors 44
in multiple system atrophy
219
in off-state 182, 243
in olivopontocerebellar
atrophy 219
in on-state 244
pain from 248
pallidotomy for 251
pallidum and 252
from rescue drugs 290
from selegiline 303
spasms of 315
from SSRIs 302
from thalamotomy 335
from tricyclic antidepressants
339

E

early menopause. See menopause
early morning off-medication
dyskinesia. See off-state

early-onset Parkinson's 106–109,
258
age-related Parkinson's and
12
cabergoline for 47
diagnosis of 92
dystonia in 129–130
embarrassment and 113
end of life care planning and
115
family history and 125–126
financial planning for 131
of Fox, Michael J. 135
gait analysis and 141
gait disturbance in 144
genes related to 60, 255, 296
going public with 149
increase in diagnosis of 168
pregnancy in 276
retirement and 294
second opinion on 300
sleep disturbances in 311
SSDI for 315
early retirement 294
early symptoms. See Parkinson's
disease
eating 109–110. See also nutrition
and diet
choking during 157
depression and 88
feeding tube for 129
fluctuating phenomenon and
133
food preparation and 134
loss of interest in 49
metabolic needs and 205
patience with 267
slowed peristalsis and 269
swallowing in 328
ECT (electroconvulsive therapy)
89, 111
edema 110, 130
EDS (excessive daytime
sleepiness). See daytime
sleepiness
EEG. See electroencephalogram
efficacy 110
Elavil. See amitriptyline
Eldepryl. See selegiline
Eldercare Locator 110–111
electrical cords 124, 159–160
electrical outlets 159–160